CANCER TREATMENT - CONVENTIONAL AND INNOVATIVE APPROACHES

Edited by **Letícia Rangel**

Cancer Treatment - Conventional and Innovative Approaches
http://dx.doi.org/10.5772/45937
Edited by Letícia Rangel

Contributors

Letícia Rangel, Renata Dalto?, Alice Herlinger, Taciane Ladislau, Klesia Pirola Madeira, Isabella Guimarães, Sarah Teixeira, Paulo Lyra-Junior, Iuri Valadão, Gustavo Amorim, Diandra Santos, Karina Rangel Demuth, Yi Luo, Eric Askeland, Mark Newton, Michael O'Donnell, Jonathan Henning, Maurizio Amichetti, Dante Amelio, Marco Cianchetti, Sabina Vennarini, Barbara Rombi, Giuseppe Minniti, Francesco Dionisi, Georgios Tsoulfas, Polyxeni Agorastou, Júlio César Nepomuceno, Bassam Abdul Rasool Hassan, Khanh Luong, Gianfranco Baronzio, Jose Antonio March Villalba, Raoul Saggini, Varisa Pongrakhananon, Diana Averill-Bates, Ahmed Bettaieb, Paulina K. Wrzal, Sergio Huerta, Brent Herron, Alex Herron, Kathryn Howell, Luann Roads, Daniel Chin, Anne Dagnault, Julie Goudreault, Hiroyuki Abe, Pan, Shouji Shimoyama, Mônica Oliveira, Sávia Lopes, Cristiane Dos Santos Giuberti, Talita Rocha, Diego Ferreira, Elaine Leite, Rodriguez-Macias Wallberg, Marina Shaduri, Roberta Di Pietro, Francesca D'Auria, Takanori Moriyama

Published by InTech
Janeza Trdine 9, 51000 Rijeka, Croatia

Publishing Process Manager Danijela Duric
Technical Editor InTech DTP team
Cover InTech Design team

Additional hard copies can be obtained from orders@intechopen.com

Cancer Treatment - Conventional and Innovative Approaches , Edited by Letícia Rangel
p. cm.
ISBN 978-953-51-1098-9

For EU product safety concerns:
IN TECH d.o.o., Prolaz Marije Krucifikse Kozulić 3, 51000 Rijeka, Croatia,
info@intechopen.com or visit our website at intechopen.com.

Meet the editor

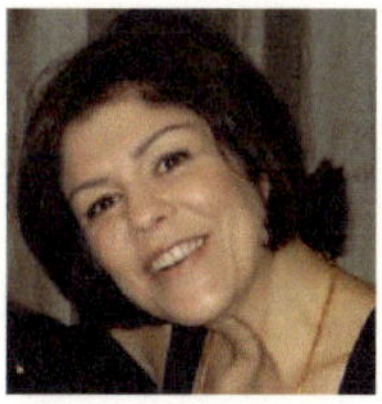

Letícia B. A. Rangel, Pharm.D., Ph.D., is an Associate Professor of the Department of Pharmaceutical Sciences and a member of the Biotechnology Program at the Federal University of Espirito Santo (UFES). As the head of the Laboratory of Cellular and Molecular Biology of Human Cancer, coordinates projects on ovarian cancer, breast, lung and kidney, with emphasis on the cellular and molecular mechanisms of these diseases, the development of biotechnology products and processes, and the discovery of new anticancer molecules. Her scientific network includes the Department of Chemistry (UFES), the Institute of Biophysics Carlos Chagas Filho (Federal University of Rio de Janeiro), the Division of Clinical Research of the Brazilian National Cancer Institute, The Department. of Molecular Medicine, University of Texas at San Antonio (USA), and the Department of Pathology at the Johns Hopkins University (USA), as well as the private sector. Aside from papers published on international journals, and ongoing patents negotiations, she has been awarded by the Brazilian government in recognition to her contribution in cancer research.

Contents

Preface XI

Section 1 Cancer Treatment: Conventional and Innovative Pharmacological Approaches 1

Chapter 1 **Conventional Cancer Treatment 3**
Isabella dos Santos Guimarães*, Renata Dalmaschio Daltoé*, Alice Laschuk Herlinger, Klesia Pirola Madeira, Taciane Ladislau, Iuri Cordeiro Valadão, Paulo Cilas Morais Lyra Junior, Sarah Fernandes Teixeira, Gustavo Modesto Amorim, Diandra Zipinotti dos Santos, Karina Rangel Demuth and Leticia Batista Azevedo Rangel

Chapter 2 **Target Cancer Therapy 37**
Taciane Ladislau, Klesia P Madeira, Renata D Daltoé, Isabella S Guimarães, Sarah F Teixeira, Paulo CM Lyra-Júnior, Iuri C Valadão, Leticia BA Rangel and Alice L Herlinger

Chapter 3 **Anticancer Properties of Cardiac Glycosides 65**
Varisa Pongrakhananon

Chapter 4 **Liposomes as Carriers of Anticancer Drugs 85**
Sávia Caldeira de Araújo Lopes, Cristiane dos Santos Giuberti, Talita Guieiro Ribeiro Rocha, Diêgo dos Santos Ferreira, Elaine Amaral Leite and Mônica Cristina Oliveira

Section 2 Combinatorial Strategies to Fight Cancer: Surgery, Radiotherpay, Backytherapy, Chemotherapy, and Hyperthermia 125

Chapter 5 **The Role of Surgery in the Treatment of Hepatocellular Carcinoma 127**
Georgios Tsoulfas and Polyxeni Agorastou

Chapter 6 **Laparoscopic Surgery in Genitourinary Cancer Treatment 147**
March Villalba José Antonio

Chapter 7 **Current Strategies in the Management of Adenocarcinoma of the Rectum 163**
Sergio Huerta and Sean P. Dineen

Chapter 8 **Mesothelioma: An Evidence-Based Review 177**
Julie Goudreault and Anne Dagnault

Chapter 9 **Definitive Chemo-Radiotherapy for Resectable Esophageal Cancer — Unresolved Problems Remain 201**
Shouji Shimoyama

Chapter 10 **A Review of Radiation Therapy's Role in Early-Stage Breast Cancer and an Introduction to Electronic Brachytherapy 223**
Brent Herron, Alex Herron, Kathryn Howell, Daniel Chin and Luann Roads

Chapter 11 **Radiosurgery and Hypofractionated Stereotactic Irradiation with Photons or Protons for Tumours of the Skull Base 239**
Dante Amelio, Marco Cianchetti, Barbara Rombi, Sabina Vennarini, Francesco Dionisi, Maurizio Amichetti and Giuseppe Minniti

Chapter 12 **Hyperthermia: Cancer Treatment and Beyond 257**
Ahmed Bettaieb, Paulina K. Wrzal and Diana A. Averill-Bates

Chapter 13 **Glioblastomas, Astrocytomas: Survival Amelioration Adding Hyperthermia to Conformal Radiotherapy and Temozolomide — Use of Pegylated Doxorubicin and Hyperthermia in the Treatment of a Recurrent Case 285**
Gianfranco Baronzio, Gurdev Parmar, Michela De Santis and Alberto Gramaglia

Section 3 The Immunotherapy of Cancer 297

Chapter 14 **Targeted Cancer Therapy by Dendritic Cell Vaccine 299**
Hiroyuki Abe, Touko Shimamoto, Shinichiro Akiyama and Minako Abe

Chapter 15 **Immunotherapy of Urinary Bladder Carcinoma: BCG and Beyond 319**
Yi Luo, Eric J. Askeland, Mark R. Newton, Jonathan R. Henning and Michael A. O'Donnell

Chapter 16 **Anti-Angiogenic Active Immunotherapy for Cancers: Dawn of a New Era? 363**
Jianping Pan and Lihuang Zhang

Section 4 Multidisciplinarity in Cancer Therapy: Nutrition and Beyond 389

Chapter 17 **Nutrigenomics and Cancer Prevention 391**
Júlio César Nepomuceno

Chapter 18 **The Impact of Vitamin D in Cancer 417**
Khanh vinh quoc Luong and Lan Thi Hoang Nguyen

Chapter 19 **The Treatment of Cancer: A Comprehensive Therapeutic Model Entailing a Complex of Interaction Modalities 455**
R. Saggini and M. Calvani

Section 5 Supportive Care for Cancer Patients 485

Chapter 20 **Supportive and Palliative Care in Solid Cancer Patients 487**
Bassam Abdul Rasool Hassan, Zuraidah Binti Mohd Yusoff, Mohamed Azmi Hassali and Saad Bin Othman

Chapter 21 **Impact of Cancer Treatment on Reproductive Health and Options for Fertility Preservation 519**
Kenny A. Rodriguez-Wallberg

Section 6 Perspectives in Cancer Biology and Modeling 539

Chapter 22 **Sialyl Salivary–Type Amylase Associated with Ovarian Cancer 541**
Takanori Moriyama

Chapter 23 **Role of CREB Protein Family Members in Human Haematological Malignancies 555**
Francesca D'Auria and Roberta Di Pietro

Chapter 24 **Life-Cycling of Cancer: New Concept** **583**
Marina Shaduri and Marc Bouchoucha

Preface

Notwithstanding the advances in the cancer research field, the related epidemiology data remain dramatic and clearly point to an urge to optimize and innovate the therapeutic approaches to fight cancer. Indeed, the elucidation of important aspects of cancer biology and human tumorigenesis has progressively enabled oncologists to provide more accurate cancer diagnosis; thus, guiding more efficiently the treatment of multiple cancer types and subtypes. Nonetheless, cancer treatment still challenges researchers and clinicians, as proven by the still impressive and increasing number of worldwide cancer-related deaths, caused either by the disease late diagnosis, surgical limitations or radio/chemoresistance. Adding complexity to the inter-individual variables, cancer comprises multiple diseases harboring diverse genetic and epigenetic signatures, which types and subtypes respond differentially to treatment, and are associated to distinct clinical outcomes.

Cancer Treatment: Conventional and Innovative Approaches is an attempt to integrate into a book volume the various aspects of cancer treatment, compiling comprehensive reviews written by an international team of experts in the field. The volume is presented in six sections: i) Section 1: Cancer treatment: Conventional and innovative pharmacological approaches; ii) Section 2: Combinatorial strategies to fight cancer: Surgery, radiotherapy, backytherapy, chemotherapy, and hyperthermia; iii) Section 3: The immunotherapy of cancer; iv) Section 4: Multidisciplinarity in cancer therapy: nutrition and beyond; v) Section 5: Supportive care for cancer patients; vi) Section 6: Perspectives in cancer biology and modeling. Ultimately, we hope this book can enlighten important issues involved in the management of cancer, summarizing the state-of-the-art knowledge regarding the disease control and treatment; thus, providing means to improve the overall care of patients that daily battle against this potentially lethal condition.

Prof. Letícia Rangel
Federal University of Espírito Santo, Brazil

Section 1

Cancer Treatment: Conventional and Innovative Pharmacological Approaches

Chapter 1

Conventional Cancer Treatment

Isabella dos Santos Guimarães*,
Renata Dalmaschio Daltoé*,
Alice Laschuk Herlinger, Klesia Pirola Madeira,
Taciane Ladislau, Iuri Cordeiro Valadão,
Paulo Cilas Morais Lyra Junior,
Sarah Fernandes Teixeira,
Gustavo Modesto Amorim,
Diandra Zipinotti dos Santos,
Karina Rangel Demuth and
Leticia Batista Azevedo Rangel

Additional information is available at the end of the chapter

http://dx.doi.org/10.5772/55282

1. Introduction

The era of cancer chemotherapy began in the 1940s with the first use of nitrogen mustards and antifolate drugs. The practice of cancer medicine has changed dramatically allowing treatments for many previously fatal cancers. Furthermore, the adjuvant chemotherapy and hormonal therapy can extend life and prevent disease recurrence following surgical resection of diferent types of malignancies.

Concurrently with the new discoveries of chemotherapeutic agents, the remarkable scientific and technological development allowed understanding of cell biology of human cancer cells and thereby the emergence of targeted therapy. Although the targeted therapy drugs have had outstanding successes in selected types of cancer, new therapies are not likely to replace cytotoxic agents in the foreseeable future. Rather, clinical trials have demonstrated potent synergy between targeted molecules and traditional cytotoxic agents.

The compounds used in cancer therapy are quite varied in structure and mechanism of action, including: alkylating agents, antimetabolite analogs, natural products, hormones and hormone antagonists and a variety of agents directed at specific molecular targets.

In this chapter we will discuss the history, applications and toxicity, among other aspects, of these agents that, in spite of systemic toxicity and severe side effects, became a mainstay of cancer treatment. As molecularly targeted agents have been used on a quite widespread way among different cancers, it can already be considered a conventional cancer therapy. Even more, as a full chapter of this book will be dedicated to these agents this subject will not be discussed in the present chapter.

2. Alkylating agents

Alkylating agents are genotoxic drugs which affect the nucleic acids and their function by direct binding to the DNA, interfering with replication and transcription resulting in mutations. In this way, the goal of using these agents is to induce DNA damage in cancer cells, severe enough to provoke them to enter into apoptosis. Alkylating agents act by replacing a hydrogen atom into another molecule by an alkyl radical through the electrolytic attack by the alkylating agent; however, this compound can also react with molecules containing an atom in a lower valence state that will undergo electrolytic attack instead of hydrogen.

Alkylating agents can be divided in several subgroups which include nitrogen mustards, various alkylating agents and platinum coordination complexes. Each one of these groups will be discussed below.

2.1. Nitrogen mustards

Nitrogen mustards were the first clinically useful anticancer agents [1] and its derivatives, such as cyclophosphamide, are still among the most widely used antitumor drugs [2].

Cyclophosphamide is a derivative of nitrogen mustards with a modified chemical structure that confers it a greater specificity for cancer cells [3]. The rational on developing cyclophosphamide was that cancer cells express higher levels of phosphamidase, which is able to cleave the phosphorus-nitrogen (P-N) bond, releasing the nitrogen mustard within the cancer cell [4]; this premise was later proven inaccurate [5]. The first clinical trials with cyclophosphamide occurred in 1958, when this drug was found to be the most effective anticancer compound against 33 cancer types on a 1,000 compounds screening trial [6]. In 1959, cyclophosphamide was approved by the Food and Drug Administration (FDA) as a cytotoxic anticancer compound, and up until now, over 50 years of its approval, it is still one of the most successful anticancer drugs [5]. Cyclophosphamide is used for the treatment of lymphoma, leukemias, breast and ovary cancers [7-10].

Cyclophosphamide is administered as a prodrug which is highly stable and requires hepatic mixed function oxidase system to be metabolically activated. Hepatic cytochrome P-450 systems are responsible for generating 4-hydroxycyclophosphamide by the hydroxylation of the oxazaphosphorine ring on cyclophosphamide. Several metabolites are generated but 4-hydroxycyclophosphamide is considered the most significant as it distributes throughout the body, including reaching the tumor where it is preferentially converted into the active nitrogen mustard as described above [11].

Afterwards, the active nitrogen mustard will form adducts in the DNA in a sequential alkylation process in which each drug molecule will react with two different nucleotides: firstly it forms a monofunctional adduct followed by a second adduct on the opposite strand of the DNA, forming an interstrand cross-link. This cross-link will prevent strands from separating during replication, inhibiting DNA synthesis [12].

Iphosphamide is chemically related to cyclophosphamide by transposition of a chloroethyl group from the exocyclic to endocyclic nitrogen. Clinical investigations have highlighted the lower toxicity of iphosphamide in comparison to that observed for cyclophosphamide [13]. Doxorubicin and iphosphamide remain the backbone of chemotherapy in patients with locally advanced or metastatic soft tissue sarcoma [14]. In the mid 1980s, iphosphamide was found to be effective in patients with refractory germ cell tumors [15].

2.2. Diverse alkylating agents

2.2.1. Nitrosoureas

Nitrosoureas were synthesized at the National Cancer Institute (NCI) following rational design based on structure-activity relation [16]. Nitrosoureas can react through alkylation with both nucleic acids and proteins or specifically through carbamylation with the latter. In order to acquire its alkylating and carbamylating properties these compounds undergo a nonenzymatic decomposition to form a 2-chloroethyl carbonium ion, which is highly electrophile and capable of alkylating guanine, cytidine, and adenine. Some compounds of this drug category are: (i) 2-chloroethylnitrosoureas (*CENUs*); (ii) 1-(2-chloroethyl)-3-cyclohexyl)-1-nitrosourea (*CCNU*, lomustine); (iii) bis(chloroethyl) nitrosourea (*BCNU*, carmustine); (iv) 1-(2-chloroethyl)-3-(4-methylcyclohexyl)-1-nitrosourea (*methyl-CCNU*, semustine); (v) chlorozotocin. The most used nitrosoureas in chemotherapy are the lipid soluble agents CCNU and BCNU. Actually, hydrophobicity is an important feature of this drug category since it allows them trespassing blood-brain barrier promoting their wide usage for brain tumor's treatment as well as non-Hodgkin's lymphoma.

2.2.2. Triazenes

Triazene compounds of clinical interest, dacarbazine and temozolomide, are a group of alkylating agents with similar chemical, physical, antitumor and mutagenic properties. Their mechanism of action is mainly related to methylation of *O*6-guanine, mediated by methyldiazonium ion, a highly reactive derivative of the two compounds. The cytotoxic/mutagenic effects of these drugs are based on the presence of DNA *O*6- methylguanine adducts that generate base/base mismatches with cytosine and with thymine. These adducts lead to cell death, or if the cell survives, provoke somatic point mutations represented by C:G→T:A transition in DNA helix. Triazene compounds have excellent pharmacokinetic properties and limited toxicity [17].

Temozolomide is an oral alkylating agent with established antitumor activity in patients with melanoma and primary brain tumors, due to its excellent bioavailability in the central nervous system [18]. Dacarbazine is employed to treat Hodgkin disease and malignant melanoma [19,20].

2.3. Platinum complexes

Rosenberg and colleagues reported, in 1965 the discovery that platinum complexes present in nutrient medium in low concentrations can inhibit cell division of *Escherichia coli* and cause the development of long filaments [21]. In the seventies the efficacy in human cancer patients was established [22].

Since then, over 3,000 platinum derivatives have been synthesized and tested against cancer cells [23]. Because of renal, oto and neurotoxicities of cisplatin, there were intensive efforts to devise analogs with fewer of these serious side effects. Moreover, analogs of cisplatin have been developed in an attempt not only to lessen the toxicity of the parent compound, but also to try to overcome the problem of platinum resistance, which may be present either in the outset of the disease, or emerging during its course or yet be acquired as a result of the treatment [24]. This effort led to the development of carboplatin, which produces primarily hematopoietic toxicity and has antitumor effects similar to those of cisplatin. Other platinum compounds have been developed and evaluated, as described later, although they haven't showed any significant advantages over cisplatin and carboplatin [25].

Today, six platinum compounds are used clinically: cisplatin (available since 1978); carboplatin and oxaliplatin (world-wide 2nd generation analogs); nedaplatin (also a 2nd generation analog); and lobaplatin and heptaplatin (3rd generation analogs). Some platinum complexes are still under clinical investigation, including those developed for oral administration.

Cytotoxicity of platinum compounds is believed to result from the formation of platinum-DNA adducts [26]. In fact, these platinum drugs can be considered as prodrugs, yielding after aquation the active diaquo-platinum compound. The main differences between these prodrugs can be related to the different kinetics of activation. Hydrolysis of cisplatin is extremely rapid, whereas it is slower for carboplatin and nedaplatin. The diaquo-platinum species react with the amine groups of proteins, RNA and DNA. The latter reaction yields platinum-DNA adducts, which appears to be associated with antitumor activity. Aquated platinum reacts preferentially with the N-7 position of guanine and adenine and produces cross-links between bases in the same strand (intrastrand) or opposite strands (interstrand). The efficacy of platinum agents against cancer cells may be mediated with the inhibition of DNA synthesis or saturation of the cellular capacity to repair platinum adducts on DNA [22].

Cisplatin is used alone and in combination with a wide range of other drugs. In combination with bleomycin, etoposide, iphosphamide, or vinblastine, cures 90% of patients with testicular cancer. Cisplatin or carboplatin used with paclitaxel induces complete response in the majority of patients with ovary carcinoma. Cisplatin produces responses in bladder, head and neck, cervix, and endometrium cancers; all forms of lung carcinoma; anal and rectal carcinomas; and neoplasms of childhood [27,25].

Resistance and the spectrum of clinical activity of carboplatin are similar to those of cisplatin. Carboplatin is relatively well tolerated clinically, causing less nausea, neurotoxicity, ototoxicity, and nephrotoxicity than cisplatin. Instead, the dose-limiting toxicity is myelosuppression, primarily thrombocytopenia [27].

Oxaliplatin exhibits a variety of antitumor activity such as against colorectal and gastric cancers which differs from other platinum agents [27]. A great number of phase II and III trials in solid tumors administering oxaliplatin in combination with other drugs have suggested increased activity as compared to oxaliplatin alone. Further, in comparison to cisplatin, oxaliplatin has not demonstrated nephrotoxic effects, which is due to the absence of platinum accumulation in plasma [28].

3. Antimetabolites

Antimetabolites are cytotoxic agents developed for more than 65 years and considered a mainstay in cancer chemotherapy. The antimetabolites can be divided according with their structure and function as folic acid analogs, purine analogs, pyrimidine analogs and cytidine analogs.

These agents are structurally similar to natural metabolites, which are essential for normal biochemical reactions in cells. The mechanism of action of antimetabolites include: competition for binding sites of enzymes that participate in essential biosynthetic processes and incorporation into nucleic acids, which inhibits their normal function triggering the apoptosis process.

3.1. Folic acids analogs

In 1948, aminopterin, an antifolate drug, was the first drug to induce temporary remissions in children with acute lymphoblastic leukemia (ALL) [29]. This success stimulated research into new antimetabolites less toxic than aminopterin. A few years later another antifolate drug, methotrexate (MTX) showed anticancer property. Currently, this drug category plays an important role in cancer treatment acting in several ways. Mostly they compete with folates for uptake into cells and prevent the formation of folates coenzymes primarily by inhibiting dihydrofolate reductase (DHFR) or thymidylate synthase (TS).

Mammalian cells lack the ability to synthesize their own reduced folate derivatives and therefore must obtain them from exogenous sources (i.e. food and dietary supplements). In normal and cancer cells, folic acid is reduced to dihydrofolate (FH_2) and then to active tetrahydrofolate (FH_4) by the enzyme DHFR. FH_4 is a cofactor that provides methyl groups for the synthesis of precursors of DNA (thymidylate and purines) and RNA (purines). TS catalyses transfer of the carbon from the FH_4 to the target molecules by oxidizing the folate ring of the FH_4, reverting it back into a FH_2 [30].

3.1.1. Methotrexate

Although several antifolate drugs have been developed, MTX is the antifolate with the widest spectrum of use. MTX is extensively used in lymphoma, ALL and osteosarcoma. Moreover, MTX is part of chemotherapeutic schemes for choriocarcinoma, breast, bladder and head and neck cancer [27].

MTX enters the cells via reduced folate carrier (RFC) or via the membrane folate binding protein (FBP) and is polyglutamated by folylpolyglutamate synthetase (FPGS) in MTX-polyglutamate, which is retained in cells for longer periods compared with MTX [31,32]. The main target of MTX and MTX-polyglutamate is the inhibition of DHFR enzyme, leading to partial depletion of the FH_4 cofactors required for the synthesis of new thymidylate and purines nucleotides. Consequently, there will be a decrease of DNA and RNA synthesis. In addition, MTX-polyglutamates are also inhibitors of other folate-requiring enzymes such as: TS and two enzymes related with de novo purine synthesis - glycinamide ribonucleotide transformylase (GART) and aminoimidazole carboxamide ribonucleotide transformylase (AICART) [31].

In normal cells a decreased polyglutamation is observed when compared to malignant cells, which partially explains the selectivity of MTX for malignant tissue [33]. Despite this predilection for malignant cells, MTX can kill rapidly dividing normal cells such as those of the intestinal epithelium and bone marrow [34]. Common side effects are cytopenia, serious infections, liver damage, mucocutaneous problems, alopecia and allergic interstitial pneumonitis [35].

3.1.2. Pemetrexed

Pemetrexed is a multitargeted antifolate chemotherapy agent approved by FDA in 2004 for the treatment of malignant pleural mesothelioma (MPM) and advanced or metastatic non-small cell lung cancer (NSCLC). Ongoing clinical trials are evaluating pemetrexed efficacy in other malignancies such as breast, colorectal, bladder, cervical, gastric and pancreatic cancer [36].

Likewise MTX, pemetrexed inhibits DHFR and as a polyglutamate, it inhibits even more potently GART and TS [37]. The inhibition of TS and GART predominates because pemetrexed's usage produces little changes in the pool of reduced folates.

Currently, this agent is employed as a monotherapy or in combination with cisplatin. It is generally a well-tolerated drug and the most common adverse reactions with its usage as single-agent are fatigue, nausea, and anorexia. Myelosuppression is the most common and dose-limiting toxicity, predominantly developed as neutropenia [38].

3.2. Purine analogs

Purine nucleoside analogues (PNA) were identified for the first time by Hitchings and Elion in 1942 with antileukemic and immunosuppressant properties [39]. The 6-mercaptopurine (6-MP) is the oldest PNA approved for clinical use, employed in the treatment of acute leukemias. The next generation of PNAs has been available worldwide since the 1990s, comprising primarily the cladribine, pentostatin, and fludarabine. PNAs have an important role as chemotherapeutic agents in hematological malignancies [40].

3.2.1. 6-Mercaptopurine

The 6-mercaptopurine (6-MP) was one of the first chemotherapeutic agents to be used in acute leukemia, remaining up today as one of the most useful drugs in acute leukemia's treatment [41,42]. In 1953 FDA approved the usage of 6-MP after a short 2 years mean time period of its synthesis. At this time there were only MTX and steroids as established treatment options for ALL, the commonest childhood cancer [43].

This chemotherapeutic agent is a prodrug, analogue of hypoxanthine, a naturally occurring purine derivative. 6-MP requires intracellular conversion into 6-thioinosine-5'-monophosphate (TIMP) by the hypoxanthine guanine phosphoribosyl transferase (HGPRT). TIMP is a substrate of thiopurine S-methyltransferase (TPMT) producing methylated TIMP which is an effective inhibitor of de novo purine biosynthesis. The TIMP that is not involved in catabolism is further metabolized by inosine monophosphate dehydrogenase (IMPDH) and later metabolized by a series of kinases and reductases to produce deoxy-6-thioguanosine5′triphosphate (thio-dGTP). Incorporation of thio-dGTP has been shown to trigger cell-cycle arrest and apoptosis involving the DNA mismatch repair [44].

3.2.2. Fludarabine

Fludarabine phosphate (FAMP) has activity in various indolent B cell malignancies and it was approved in 1991 for clinical usage in the treatment of chronic lymphocytic leukemia (CLL). FAMP is a prodrug that requires metabolic conversion to exert cytotoxic activity. It is rapidly dephosphorylated to 9-β-D-arabinosyl-2-fluoroadenine (F-ara-A), transported into cells and then phosphorylated by deoxycytidine kinase to the active form 2-fluoro-ara-ATP (F-ara-ATP) [45,46]. The F-ara-ATP is the only metabolite of FAMP that have cytotoxic activity, acting through different mechanisms that affect DNA synthesis.

F-ara-ATP inhibits ribonucleotide reductase (RNR), responsible for the conversion of ribonucleotides into deoxyribonucleotides which in turn are one of the key components at the construction of DNA strands. Furthermore F-ara-ATP incorporates into DNA, at the 3′-terminus, resulting in repression of DNA polymerization as well as inhibition of DNA ligase, an enzyme involved in DNA replication [47] and DNA primase, an accessory protein that synthesizes an RNA primer required for initiation of synthesis by DNA polymerase [48].

The most frequent adverse events associated with FAMP regimens are myelosuppression lymphocytopenia and infection, typically on respiratory tract. Despite the minor occurrence, severe neurotoxicity is one of the complications associated with FAMP [49].

3.2.3. Cladribine

Likewise FAMP, cladribine (2-CdA; 2-chloro-2'-deoxyadenosine) is phosphorylated and accumulated as 2-chlorodeoxyadenosine triphosphate (2-CdA-TP) in cells [50]. This metabolite disrupts cell metabolism by incorporating into the DNA then inhibits DNA synthesis and repair, leading to accumulation of DNA strand breaks [50]. In addiction 2-CdA-TP is a potent inhibitor of RNR.

2-CdA was shown to have potent and long-term effects in the treatment of low-grade B-cell neoplasms, approved by FDA for clinical use in hairy cell leukemia (HCL). It shares the same adverse effects of FAMP, being the bone marrow suppression its major toxic effect, associated with severe infections.

3.2.4. Pentostatin

Pentostatin (deoxycoformycin; DCF) is a natural product first isolated from the culture of *Streptomyces antibioticus* [51] in 1974. This antimetabolite was the first effective agent against HCL, but nowadays its usage has largely been superseded by cladribine.

The primary site of action is the inhibition of adenosine deaminase (ADA), an enzyme that participates in purine salvage metabolic pathways. Inhibition of ADA leads to accumulation of adenosine and deoxyadenosine nucleotides in cells, which can block DNA synthesis by inhibiting RNR. Another important action of pentostatin is the inactivation of S-adenosyl homocysteine hydrolase by deoxyadenosine, resulting in accumulation of S-adenosyl homocysteine, an intermediate in the synthesis of cysteine and adenosine particularly toxic to lymphocytes. Pentostatin also has adverse effects related with the bone marrow suppression.

3.3. Pyrimidine analogs

Pyrimidine analogs sparked the interest of scientists from the observation that rat malignant tissue used pyrimidine uracil more rapidly than normal tissues [52]. In the late 1950s Charles Heidelberger and colleagues synthesized the fluoropyrimidine 5-fluorouracil (5-FU) [53], which demonstrated specific uracil antagonism within antitumor capabilities. Others pyrimidine analogs were developed later (e.g. capecitabine, cytosine arabinoside and gemcitabine) and this class is currently extensively used in cancer therapy.

3.3.1. Fluouracil

5-FU is the mainstay of treatment for many common malignant diseases, particularly for colorectal cancer. It's also used in breast, pancreatic and head and neck cancers [52]. This antimetabolite exerts its antitumor effects through several mechanisms including inhibition of the enzyme TS, related to thymidine synthesis from uridine, and incorporation of its metabolites into RNA and DNA. 5-FU enters into cells rapidly and is converted intracellularly by metabolic enzymes into its active metabolite 5-fluoro-2'-deoxyuridine-5'-monophosphate (FdUMP). FdUMP inhibits TS leading to nucleotide pool imbalance, decreasing thymine concentration which leads to uracil incorporation into DNA causing DNA strand breaks [52]. Another 5-FU metabolite, fluorouridine triphosphate (FUTP) is extensively incorporated into RNA, disrupting normal RNA processing and function.

Usual side effects of 5-FU are gastrointestinal, including nausea, vomiting, diarrhea, and stomatitis. Hematologic effects are also common, like myelosuppression and thrombocytopenia. Although considered unusual, cardiotoxicity has been reported as well as adverse neurological effects [54,55].

3.3.2. *Capecitabine*

Capecitabine (N^4-pentyloxycarbonyl-5′-deoxy-5-fuorocytidine) is an oral prodrug of 5-FU developed with the objective of improving tolerability and intratumor drug concentrations through tumor-specific conversion to the active drug. This selectivity is due the presence at higher levels of thymidine phosphorylase (TP), the final enzyme responsible for conversion to the active drug, in cancer cells [56].

In 1998, capecitabine was approved by FDA for the treatment of women with taxane- and anthracycline-refractory advanced breast cancer. Afterwards, this antimetabolite received the approval for metastatic colorectal carcinoma.

The most common toxicities related to treatment with capecitabine are gastrointestinal effects (diarrhea, nausea and vomiting) and hand-foot syndrome [57]. Other adverse effects were also observed such as alopecia, myelosuppression and cardiotoxicity [57,55].

3.3.3. *Gemcitabine*

The deoxycytidine analogue gemcitabine (difluorodeoxycytidine, dFdC) received its first approval by FDA in 1996 for the treatment of patients with pancreatic cancer and NSCLC. Furthermore, gemcitabine was approved for the first-line treatment of patients with metastatic breast cancer and advanced ovarian cancer, in 2004 and 2006, respectively.

Gemcitabine is phosphorylated by deoxycytidine kinase (DCK) to its 5′-monophosphate form (dFdCMP) and additionally metabolized by several other enzymes to its 5′-diphosphate (dFdCDP) and 5′-triphosphate derivatives (dFdCTP). Then, this last metabolite dFdCTP is incorporated into DNA, inhibiting DNA replication and inducing apoptosis [58].

The major dose-limiting toxicity of gemcitabine is myelosuppression, but other adverse effects are related with the therapy such as flu-like symptoms, nausea, vomiting and rash [59].

3.3.4. *Cytarabine*

Cytarabine (1-β-D-arabinofuranosylcytosine; ara-C) had its first approval by FDA in 1969 as a chemotherapeutic agent to be used with other drugs for the treatment of adult and pediatric acute myelogenous leukemia (AML). According to the NCI, cytarabine is also approved to treat ALL, chronic myelogenous leukemia (CML) and as a single agent to prevent and treat meningeal leukemia.

Since its approval by FDA in 1969, the clinical effectiveness of this drug has increased with knowledge of its pharmacologic and biologic properties. Ara-C is a prodrug and needs to be converted to its active form, ara-C 5′-triphosphate (Ara-CTP), by a series of intracellular enzyme-dependent phosphorylation steps [60].

Its mechanism of action is similar to that of the deoxycytidine analogue Gemcitabine: Ara-C is transported into the cell and once it is inside, it is phosphorylated into ara-C monophosphate (ara-CMP) by DCK and eventually to ara-C triphosphate (ara-CTP) which then competes with deoxycytidine triphosphate (dCTP) for incorporation into DNA and subsequently blocking DNA synthesis causing cell death [60].

Treatment with ara-C is associated with several adverse side effects, including myelosuppression (mostly leukopenia, thrombocytopenia and severe anemia), infections, mucositis, neurotoxicity, and acute pulmonary syndrome [61,27]

4. Microtubule-target agents

Microtubules are dynamic structures composed of α–β-tubulin heterodimers and microtubule-associated proteins representing one of the major components of the cytoskeleton. Microtubules are involved in many cellular processes including maintenance of cell structure, protein transportation and mitosis. Because of the central role of microtubules in mitosis, drugs that affect microtubule are useful in cancer chemotherapy. In this context, Microtubule-Targeted Agents (MTAs) constitute a class of anticancer drugs largely used in the clinics to treat solid tumors and hematological malignancies, either alone or as part of different combination regimens. MTA are potent mitotic poisons that are broadly classified into microtubule-stabilizing (e.g. taxanes and epothilones) and microtubule-destabilizing (e.g. vinca alkaloids) drugs.

4.1. Vinca alkaloids

The first natural anticancer agents approved to clinical use were the vinca alkaloids vincristine and vinblastine, introduced in the late 1960s. Vinca alkaloids were originally isolated from the Madagascar periwinkle *Catharanthus roseus* and over thirty alkaloids have been obtained of which a few are known definitely to be active [62]. Actually, there are three major vinca alkaloids in clinical use: vinblastine, vincristine and vinorelbine.

Vincas are classified as destabilizing agents due to their ability to cause microtubule depolymerization, suppress treadmilling and dynamic instability, blocking mitotic progression, and ultimately result in cell death by apoptosis. Vinca akaloids bind in one of three sites on tubulin, called the "vinca" domain, located near the exchangeable GTP binding site [63-65].

Vinca alkaloids differ in their chemotherapeutic effectiveness being part of therapeutic schemes in different types of malignancies. Vincristine is used in combination chemotherapy for treating pediatric leukemias, Hodgkin and non-Hodgkin lymphoma, as well as solid tumors such as Wilms tumor and neuroblastoma [66-68]. Vincristine can occasionally be used in the treatment of small cell lung cancer (SCLC). Currently, vinblastine is a standard component of regimens for treating lymphomas including Hodgkin's disease. It´s also used for the treatment of bladder cancer, testicular carcinomas, germ cell malignancies and breast cancer [66,69]. Moreover the semisynthetic derivate of vinblastine, vinorelbine, has activity against NSCLC and breast cancer [70,71].

Furthermore these compounds diverge in their toxicities. While severe neurotoxicity is observed less frequently with vinorelbine and vinblastine, this side effect is frequently noticed with vincristine [72,73]. Myelosuppression, in turn, predominates with vinblastine and vinorelbine [74] and is the main dose-limiting toxicity of those drugs.

Vinca alkaloids and the others MTAs can present resistance in cancer cells due to: (i) cellular efflux of the anticancer agents, especially by the overexpression of drug efflux pumps, such as P-glycoprotein and multidrug resistance-associated protein 1 (MRP1) [75]; (ii) mutations in tubulin at the drug binding sites [76,77]; (iii) changes in the tubulin isotype composition of microtubules [78] and; (iv) changes in micro-tubule-regulatory proteins [79].

4.2. Taxanes

Taxanes are natural cytotoxic diterpenes classified as microtubule-stabilizing anticancer agents. Paclitaxel and the semisynthetic analog docetaxel are considered to be among the most important anticancer drugs in cancer chemotherapy.

Paclitaxel was identified in 1971 as part of a NCI program that screened medicinal plants for potential anticancer activity, whereof the researchers found cytotoxic effects on solid tumors and leukemic cells [80]. Paclitaxel was initially derived from the bark of the Pacific yew (*Taxus brevifolia*) in a process that a centenary tree provides only a gram of the compound. This lead to a semi-synthetic method that use the 10-deacetylbaccatin-III, which is extracted from more abundant yew species such as the European yew *Taxus baccata* [81].

Docetaxel, in turn, is an esterified derivative of 10-deacetylbaccatin-III, produced by Potier and his colleagues in 1986 [82]. The structures of paclitaxel and docetaxel differ on the ester side chain attached at C-13 and in substitutions at the C-10 taxane ring position, which confers docetaxel slightly more water solubility than paclitaxel [83,25]

These drugs interact with β-tubulin promoting tubulin polymerization and formation of stable microtubules, even in the absence of GTP- and microtubule-associated proteins, which are usually essential for these processes. This inhibition of microtubule depolymerization results in mitotic arrest leading to apoptosis of the cancer cells [84]. Furthermore, taxanes have been demonstrated to induce many other cellular effects that may or may not relate to their disruptive effects on microtubule dynamics, including the directly phosphorylation, hence inactivation, of proteins that blocks apoptosis in cancer cells (such as bcl-2) [85].

Paclitaxel was approved by the FDA in 1992 for the treatment of refractory breast cancer and refractory ovarian cancer. Currently this agent has a central role in the treatment of breast, ovarian, NSCLC and AIDS-related Kaposi's sarcoma. In turn, docetaxel received the approval in 1995 for the treatment of metastatic breast cancer. Furthermore was approved for use in hormone refractory prostate cancer (HRPC), advanced squamous cell carcinoma of the head and neck, breast cancer, gastric adenocarcinoma and NSCLC.

Treatment with these drugs often results in a number of undesirable side effects, as well as resistance in cancer cells, as mentioned previously. In order to overcome those problems, novel taxanes are in development as well as novel formulations. In 2005 Abraxane® (paclitaxel albumin-bound nanoparticles, solvent-free) was approved for advanced breast cancer. Abraxane® prevent the hypersensitivity reactions typically associated with paclitaxel, which are generally related to the solvent suspension of polyoxyethylated castor oil (Cremophor EL) [86-88].

Taxanes exerts its primary toxic effects on the bone marrow, mainly neutropenia, and may cause neuropathy [89]. Docetaxel causes greater degrees of neutropenia than paclitaxel. Furthermore, docetaxel can cause fluid retention leading to peripheral edema and pulmonary edema, in extreme cases. Despite the high incidence of major hypersensitivity reactions due to the Cremophor EL vehicle, these reactions are no longer a serious problem due to the advent of effective premedication regimens [90] and new formulations [88].

4.3. Epothilones

Epothilones are a new class of natural cytotoxic antineoplastic microtubule-stabilizing agents. Ixabepilone, a semisynthetic analog of the natural product epothilone B, is the only epothilone approved for cancer therapy, indicated for metastatic breast cancer.

The epothilones competitively inhibit the binding of paclitaxel to polymerized tubulin, indicating that the two compounds share a common binding site despite significant structural differences [90,91]. It has been reported that ixabepilone is less susceptible to drug-resistance mechanisms that limit the efficacy of taxanes, like P-glycoprotein mediated efflux and the overexpression of class III β-tubulin, due to its reduction in polymerization rate of microtubules [91,92].

Likewise taxanes, ixabepilone is also formulated in Cremophor EL yielding hypersensitivity reactions. Other side effects related to its use are neuropathy, neutropenia, severe diarrhea and fatigue [93,94].

5. Camptothecin analogs

Likewise paclitaxel, camptothecin was discovered as part of a NCI program in 1966 by Wall and Wani [95]. Camptothecin is a pentacyclic quinoline alkaloid present in wood, bark, and fruit of the Asian tree *Camptotheca acuminate,* that specifically target the topoisomerase I (Top-I), a nuclear enzyme that plays a critical role in DNA replication and transcription [96].

Top-I promote relaxation of the supercoiled DNA, prior to transcription, through the formation of a single strand break and religation. The camptothecins bind the covalent Top-I-DNA complex, known as the "cleavable complex", stabilizing it and inhibiting reannealing of the parent DNA. Consequently, camptothecins lead to reversible accumulation of double-stranded DNA breaks and tumor cell death [97-99].

Several derivatives of camptothecin have been synthesized, but only irinotecan and topotecan have been approved for clinical use. Irinotecan and topotecan, which are more soluble and less toxic analogs, are currently used in a wide spectrum of cancers. Topotecan is part of regimens to treat ovarian, lung and cervical cancer. Irinotecan is a prodrug, currently used for metastatic colorectal cancer.

Irinotecan and topotecan produces dose-limiting side effects restricting safety administration and then their anti-tumor efficacy. Diarrhea is the principal side effect related to irinotecan. Moreover the use of this drug can cause nausea, vomiting, anorexia, fatigue, abdominal pain, alopecia and neutropenia. The principal toxicity of topotecan when administered at standard doses is neutropenia, while the nonhematological toxicities are usually mild [100,101].

6. Epipodophyllotoxins

Podophyllotoxin was first isolated in 1880, but its structure was determined later by Hartwell and Schrecker [102]. Despite the antineoplastic activity, podophyllotoxin was not used in clinical practice due to its toxicity. Several less toxic analogs of podophyllotoxin were produced and two analogs were approved for clinical use (etoposide and teniposide).

While etoposide is most widely used to treat lung cancer and testicular cancer, it is also effective for Hodgkin and non-Hodgkin lymphomas, acute nonlymphocytic leukemia, gastric cancer, and soft-tissue sarcomas. Teniposide has significant activity in SCLC and in the treatment of childhood lymphomas and leukemias [103-105].

The cellular target for etoposide and teniposide is topoisomerase II (Top-II) [106,107]. Top-II enzymes regulate essential cellular processes, including DNA replication and chromosome segregation, by altering the topology of chromosomal DNA. These enzymes induce transient double-stranded breaks in the DNA allowing DNA strands to pass through each other and unwind or unknot tangled DNA. Etoposide and teniposide inhibit Top-II to religate cleaved DNA molecules [108]. This phenomenon leads to accumulation of covalent complexes Top-II-DNA resulting in permanent DNA strand breaks, which trigger mutagenic and cell death pathways [109].

In addition to causing cell death, these agents may, under certain circumstances, lead to neoplastic transformation. Epipodophyllotoxin therapy can cause AML characterized by chromosomal translocations, especially in chromosome 11q23 [110,111]. Other common side effects related to antineoplastic drugs might arise, such as bone marrow suppression, nausea, vomiting and alopecia.

7. Antibiotics

7.1. Anthracyclines and anthracenediones

The anthracyclines, which include doxorubicin, daunorubicin, epirubicin and idarubicin, are a class of antibiotic chemotherapeutic agents routinely used in the treatment of several cancers. While daunorubicin and idarubicin are more effective in acute leukemias, doxorubicin and epirubicin display broader activity against human solid tumors. Doxorubicin has a central role in the therapy of breast, lung, gastric, ovarian, thyroid, non-Hodgkin's and Hodgkin's lymphoma, sarcoma and pediatric cancers. Epirubicin is an epimer of doxorubicin indicated as component of therapy for breast cancer [112,113].

These chemotherapeutic agents attack cancer cells by multiple mechanisms (i) intercalation with DNA and disruption of Top-II, directly affecting DNA replication and repair, (ii) generation of quinone-type free radicals and their damage to cellular membranes, DNA and proteins and (iii) triggering of apoptotic cell death through complex signaling pathways [27,113].

Despite the large use, the most serious toxicity associated with anthracyclins is cardiotoxicity which can be cumulative and irreversible [114]. However, liposomal formulation of doxorubicin was shown to be less cardiotoxic than traditional doxorubicin without compromising efficacy in adults with solid tumors [115].

Another important antibiotic chemotherapeutic agent is the anthracenediones, which also inhibit Top-II. Mitoxantrone is the most active compound in the anthracenediones class and has been approved for use in AML and prostate cancer [116,117]. It is relevant to point that mitoxantrone has limited ability to produce quinone-type free radicals and causes less cardiac toxicity than does doxorubicin.

7.2. Bleomycin

Bleomycins are a group of glycopeptides antibiotics, isolated in the early 1960s from *Streptomyces verticillis* [118]. Its cytotoxic properties result from generation of free radicals leading to single- and double-stranded breaks in DNA.

Bleomycins are attractive components of chemotherapy regimens due to minimal myelotoxicity and immunosuppression whilst the pulmonary toxicity related to its use limits the applicability of this drug [119]. Currently bleomycins have antitumor activity against certain types of lymphoma, testicular tumors, head and neck cancers, Kaposi sarcoma, cervical cancer and germ-cell tumors.

8. Enzymes

8.1. L-Asparaginase (L-ASNase)

L-Asparaginases (L-ASNase) are effective antineoplastic agents used in first-line treatment of a variety of lymphoproliferative disorders, especially in ALL. It has been used in combination with other agents, including methotrexate, doxorubicin, vincristine, and prednisone [120]. Currently, there are three preparations of L-ASNase available for clinical use: native enzyme from *Escherichia coli* (Elspar®); a pegylated *E. coli* L-ASNase (Oncospar®), and native erwinia enzyme from *Erwinia chrysanthemi* (Erwinase®).

The mechanism of action of L-ASNase is based on the assumption that tumor cells, especially leukemic cells, require a huge amount of amino acid asparagine (Asn) to maintain their rapid malignant growth. Those cells lack adequate amounts of asparagine synthetase and are dependent on an exogenous source of Asn for survival. L-ASNase catalyzes the hydrolysis of L-ASN to L-aspartic acid and ammonia, significantly depleting the circulating asparagines from plasma [27,121].

The most common side effect is related to inhibition of protein synthesis and allergic reactions. Hypersensitivity reactions can be solved by use of modified versions of L-ASNase such as polyethylene glycol (PEG)-conjugated asparaginase (pegasparaginase). Pegasparaginase reduce immunogenic reactions and posses a considerably longer half-life, reducing the number of injections for the patient. In recent years, clinical trials have established the importance of pegasparaginase in frontline pediatric and adult ALL therapy [120,122]

Resistance arises through induction of asparagine synthetase in tumor cells [123] and administrations of ASNase may induce the development of antibodies that neutralize the enzyme [120, 121,124].

9. Diverse agents

9.1. Hydroxyurea

The synthesis of Hydroxyurea (HU) occurred for the first time in 1869 by Dresler and Stein [125], meanwhile its biological activities as a myelossupressive drug were only demonstrated 60 years later [126]. Further studies regarding its mechanism of action were able to demonstrate its activity at impairing DNA synthesis through blocking its deoxyribonucleotides subunits formation by acting at the ribonucleotide reductase (RNR) enzyme [127]. The RNR enzyme inhibited by HU is responsible for the conversion of ribonucleotides into deoxyribonucleotides which in turn are one of the key components at the construction of DNA strands. Once HU is mainly effective at the S phase of the cell cycle, when its target, e.g. the catalytic subunit of RNR, is highly activated in cells, it also provides synergistic effect with radiotherapy [128]. Additionally, regardless of the origin of the HU-induced release of nitric oxide [129,130], its contribution to the antineoplastic effect of HU remains relatively unexplored.

HU is currently used in combination therapies along with other chemotherapeutic agents and radiation regimens to treat resistant chronic myelocytic leukemia (CML), cervical carcinomas, malignant melanomas, head and neck cancers and brain tumors (e.g., glioma, meningioma) [127,128].

HU is well-known by its dose-limiting myelosuppressive effect which appears within a few days after the beginning of its use and is mostly reversed through the discontinuation of the drug. Skin and nail hyperpigmentation, malleolar ulcerations and solar hypersensitivity are some of the most observed cutaneous side effects in long-term exposed patients [131,132]. Multiple skin tumors as well as its precursor lesions may also develop after sun exposure [133,134].

9.2. Thalidomide

In the late 1950s thalidomide was introduced by Chemie Grunenthal company into the market as a sedative drug and within a few years later the disseminated teratogenic consequences of its use during pregnancy practically banned its worldwide commercialization [135]. Further studies demonstrated the antiangiogenic activity of thalidomide *in vivo* through inhibition of bFGF/VEGF as well as its immunomodularory effects by suppression of the pro-inflamatory TNF-alfa synthesis and T-cell co-stimulatory activity [136]. Those properties encouraged further studies regarding its advantages of usage in a series of cancers, such as multiple myeloma (MM), renal cell carcinoma, prostate cancer, among others [135]. Thalidomide has currently been used in combination with dexamethasone in the treatment of MM [137]. Thalidomide has at least a partial benefit in response to cancer-related cachexia, mitigating the total weight and lean body mass reduction [138,139].

The most common adverse effects associated with thalidomide's employment include constipation and sedation. Meanwhile cardiovascular effects like hypotension and bradycardia, somnolence, thromboembolism and peripheral neuropathy are the most severe toxic events related to this drug and may require the withdrawal of it, which is generally sufficient to achieve clinical improvement [140,141].

9.3. Estramustine

Estramustine is a nitrogen mustard derivative formed by the union of normustine (nitrogen mustard) and estradiol-17beta-phosphate with antineoplastic effects that rely on its properties as an anti-mitotic drug through disruption of the microtubule organization in HRPC cells as well as by pro-apoptotic events [142]. Recently concluded trials also assigned an additional benefit in treating prostate cancer with the addition of other chemotherapeutics, e.g. docetaxel, in comparison to the administration of estramustine alone [143].

The most common side effects observable within the use of estramustine are vomiting and nausea, affecting nearly 50% of the patients. Meanwhile the pro-estrogenic consequences (gynecomastia, impotence) and thromboembolic events are some of the most severe adverse effects. The latter, specifically is also due to the contribution of the disease itself [143].

9.4. Bortezomib

Bortezomib was the first proteasome inhibitor approved by the FDA in 2003 as an alternative treatment for refractory MM. Its approval was extended in 2008 for the treatment of newly diagnosed MM. Bortezomib's usage as an anticancer agent was also approved by the FDA in 2006 for the treatment of relapsed or refractory mantle cell lymphoma (MCL) [144].

This drug acts through inhibition of the 26S proteasome by blocking its 20S core subunit's chymotrypsin-like activity, which affects several intracellular signaling pathways, as the NF-kB anti-apoptotic pathway. The NF-kB molecule is found directly attached to its inhibitor (IkB) which in turn becomes ubiquitinated and degraded at the proteasome in response to specific stressful situations, releasing NF-kB to enter the nucleus and exert its pro-survival effects. By this means, targeting the proteasome structure would lead to inhibition of NF-kB activation. Additionally, bortezomib may also promotes cancer cells to sensitization towards cytotoxic drugs [145].

The commonest toxic effects related to the use of bortezomib are fatigue, gastrointestinal disturbances, thrombocytopenia, paresthesia and peripheral neuropathy. Besides the adverse events aforementioned, intrinsic/acquired resistance and unsatisfactory response toward solid tumors represent some of the disadvantages associated with the utilization of bortezomib [145].

9.5. Zoledronic acid

Zoledronic acid is a heterocyclic nitrogen-containing bisphosphonate [146]. Bisphosphonates, such as zoledronic acid, are anti-resorptive agents approved for treatment of skeletal complication associated with metastatic breast cancer and prostate cancer. These agents act on osteoclasts, key cells in the bone microenvironment, inhibiting bone resorption [147, 148].

Moreover, zoledronic acid is used extensively in diseases with high bone turnover such as MM. Nephrotoxicity can be observed with use of this drug, and is related to dose, infusion time and plasma concentration. Furthemore, zoledronic acid has a long renal half-life, contributing to renal damage. Osteonecrosis of the jaw is also associated with zoledronic acid [149,150].

10. Hormones and related agents

10.1. Glucocorticoids

Glucocorticoids are primary stress hormones that function to maintain homeostasis regulating many biological processes, including immune function, skeletal growth, reproduction, cognition, behavior, and cell proliferation and survival [151]. Glucocorticoids act through their binding to a specific physiological receptor that translocates to the nucleus and induces antiproliferative and apoptotic responses in sensitive cells [27]. These actions are important in their usage as therapeutic agents in cancer treatment.

Glucocorticoids, dexamethasone and prednisone, are widely used for the treatment of leukemias and lymphomas because of their effects on cell cycle progression and apoptosis. They are also adopted as a co-medication in the therapy of solid tumors, either because of their effectiveness in treating the malignancy or for decreasing edema, pain, electrolyte imbalance, nausea and emesis or yet to reduce cytotoxic reactions caused by other treatment regimens [152].

10.2. Progestins

Progesterone is an essential regulator of normal human female reproductive function in the uterus, ovary, mammary gland and brain, and also plays an important role in non-reproductive tissues such as the cardiovascular system, bone and the central nervous system. This highlights the widespread role of this hormone in normal physiology. The effects of progesterone are mediated through the nuclear progesterone receptor (PR), which interacts with transcriptional coregulators, moves into nuclear aggregates and regulates gene expression [153].

Progestational agents, such as the agonists of the PR megestrol and megestrol acetate, have been used as second-line hormonal therapy for metastatic hormone-dependent breast cancer and in the management of endometrial carcinoma previously treated by surgery and radiotherapy [27].

10.3. Antiestrogens and antiandrogens

Antiestrogens and antiandrogens inhibit the binding of the natural endogenous ligands with the estrogen and androgen receptors (ER; AR) respectively. Thus they act preventing exacerbation of these receptors signaling pathways frequently observable in cancer cells. This fact lead to inhibition of cancer cells division [154, 155].

Fulvestrant is an antiestrogen approved by the FDA in 2002 for the treatment of hormone receptor positive metastatic breast cancer in post-menopausal women refractory to previous tamoxifen regimen [156]. Fulvestrant is a complete antagonist of the ER-alfa/ER-beta and inhibits estrogen signaling by promoting mainly the degradation of ER-alfa and PRs after binding to the ER [157]. The most observable side effects due to the usage of fulvestrant include hot flashes, thrombosis, joint disorders, pain and gastrointestinal events [158].

Flutamide, Bicalutamide and Nilutamide are non-steroidal antiandrogens introduced in the 1970s in order to preclude the unwanted effects caused by the nonselective profile of steroidal agents. These non-steroidal agents are only used in combination with other drugs, mostly with GnRH agonists, for the treatment of prostate cancer in order to counterbalance the effect of the released testosterone following GnRH administration. Bicalutamide has been recently approved in the European Union for the treatment of locally advanced prostate cancer and present the best schedule and adverse effects profiles. Toxic effects include hot flashes, hepatotoxicity, diarrhea, decreased libido and gynecomastia. Patients in treatment with nilulatamide may experience ocular alterations [155].

10.4. Selective Estrogen Receptor Modulators (SERMs)

Selective estrogen receptor modulators (SERMs) are tissue-selective compounds and depending on the site of action, exhibit agonistic (bone, liver, brain, cardiovascular system), antagonistic (brain, breast) and mixed agonist/antagonist (uterus) effects. This phenomenon occurs due to different ER subtypes expression throughout the body among other factors [159,160].

The currently SERMs approved by the FDA are tamoxifen, toremifene and raloxifen. Raloxifen is used in osteoporosis's treatment and prevention for postmenopausal women and reduction of invasive breast cancer's risk for women with osteoporosis or at increased risk of invasive breast cancer.

Tamoxifen is used in the treatment of metastatic breast cancer as well as in the adjuvant treatment of node-positive breast cancer. Additionally, tamoxifen demonstrates preventive effects in women at high-risk of developing breast cancer [161]. Toremifene is used in the treatment of metastatic breast cancer in postmenopausal women with ER+ or tumors with unknown ER status [162].

Due to its agonistic properties, tamoxifen significantly increases the risk of endometrial cancer, pulmonary embolism and stroke, rendering the treatment based on aromatase inhibitors an interesting alternative, which demonstrate reduced frequency of the aforementioned adverse effects, though not without a high risk of loss in bone mineral density (BMD) and, consequently, fractures [160]. Raloxifen and toremifene demonstrates similar effectiveness in comparison to tamoxifene regarding reduction of risks in developing advanced and invasive breast cancer respectively. They also show evidence of lower incidence of venous thromboembolic events and endometrial cancer [163,164].

10.5. Aromatase inhibitors

The aromatase enzyme is responsible for the conversion of androgens to estrogens and represent the primary source of estrogens in post-menopausal women. Accordingly, the aromatase inhibitors (AI) provide reduction of estrogen concentration within ER+ breast cancer cells. There are three generations of AI, which may also be classified as belonging to the type 1 (steroidal) and type 2 (non-steroidal) [27]. Aminoglutethimide is a 1st generation nonsteroidal AI which was utilized in association to glucocorticoid in the treatment of breast cancer and is currently replaced by the following generations of AI. Formestane, a 2nd generation steroidal AI, administrated via intramuscular-injection, led to localized reactions. It also presents clinical benefits within the group of patients that experienced progressive disease after treatment with tamoxifen and nonsteroidal AI [25,165]. Exemestane is an irreversible 3rd generation orally administrated steroidal AI, which exhibits higher estrogen deprivation effect in comparison to formestane in the treatment of ER+ breast cancer progressive cases previously treated with tamoxifen. Anastrozole and letrozole are 3rd generation nonsteroidal AI which have demonstrated improved results with respect to disease free survival, recurrence rate and time to recurrence when compared to tamoxifen. This observation regards early, advanced and metastatic ER+ breast cancer treatment, irrespective of functioning as a first line adjuvant or post-tamoxifen drug. Despite the aforementioned improved clinical outcome provided by 3rd generation AIs, further long-term studies should be conducted in order to assess whether its safety profiles are superior when compared to that of tamoxifen [164,166-170).

11. Conclusion

Despite the increased number of therapeutic options, the cancer therapy remains a challenge for physicians and researchers, especially with regards to the tumor resistance. In this scenario, a better understanding about the molecular basis of cancer will enable the improvement and development of therapeutic strategies that allow an effective combat against this malignancy and better quality of life for patients.

Author details

Isabella dos Santos Guimarães*, Renata Dalmaschio Daltoé*, Alice Laschuk Herlinger, Klesia Pirola Madeira, Taciane Ladislau, Iuri Cordeiro Valadão, Paulo Cilas Morais Lyra Junior, Sarah Fernandes Teixeira, Gustavo Modesto Amorim, Diandra Zipinotti dos Santos, Karina Rangel Demuth and Leticia Batista Azevedo Rangel

Laboratory of Cellular and Molecular Biology of Human Cancer, Federal University of Espirito Santo, Brazil

*These authors equally contributed to the elaboration of this chapter

References

[1] Gilman A & Phillips FS. The Biological Actions and Therapeutic Applications of the B-Chloroethyl Amines and Sulfides. Science 1946;103(2675): 409-436.

[2] Haskell C M. Cancer Treatment. Philadelphia: Saunders; 1990.

[3] Arnold H, Bourseaux F, Brock N. Chemotherapeutic action of a cyclic nitrogen mustard phosphamide ester (B 518-ASTA) in experimental tumours of the rat. Nature 1958;181(4613): 931.

[4] Friedman OM, Seligman AM. Preparation of N-phosphorylated derivatives of bis-P-chloroethylamine. Journal of the American Chemical Society 1954;76: 655-658.

[5] Emadi A, Jones RJ, Brodsky RA. Cyclophosphamide and cancer: golden anniversary. Nature Reviews Clinical Oncology 2009;6: 638-647.

[6] Brock N, Wilmanns H. Effect of a cyclic nitrogen mustard-phosphamidester on experimentally induced tumors in rats; chemotherapeutic effect and pharmacological properties of B518 ASTA. Deutsche Medizinische Wochenschrift 1958;83: 453-458.

[7] Mey U, Hitz F, Lohri A, Pederiva S, Taverna C, Tzankov A, Meier O, Yeow K, Renner C. Diagnosis and treatment of diffuse large B-cell lymphoma. Swiss Medical Weekly 2012; 142:0.

[8] Hillmen P. Using the biology of chronic lymphocytic leukemia to choose treatment. American Society of Hematology Education Program 2011;2011: 104-109.

[9] López-Tarruella S, Martín M. Recent advances in systemic therapy: advances in adjuvant systemic chemotherapy of early breast cancer. Breast Cancer Research 2009;11: 204.

[10] Clowse ME, Behera MA, Anders CK, Copland S, Coffman CJ, Leppert PC, Bastian LA. Ovarian preservation by GnRH agonists during chemotherapy: a meta-analysis. Journal of Womens Health (Larchmt) 2009;18: 311-319.

[11] Siddik ZH. Mechanism of action of cancer chemotherapeutic agents: DNA-interactive alkylating agents and antitumour platinum-based drugs. In The cancer handbook. Edited by Alison M R. New Jersey: John Wiley & Sons 2002.

[12] Colvin ME, Sasaki JC, Tran NL. Chemical factors in the action of phosphoramidic mustard alkylating anticancer drugs: roles for computational chemistry. Current Pharmaceutical Design 1999;5: 645-663.

[13] Corsi A, Calabresi F, Greco C. Comparative effects of cyclophosphamide and isophosphamide on Lewis lung carcinoma. British Journal of Cancer 1978;38: 631-633.

[14] Penel N, Van Glabbeke M, Marreaud S, Ouali M, Blay JY, Hohenberger P. Testing new regimens in patients with advanced soft tissue sarcoma: analysis of publications from the last 10 years. Annals of Oncology 2011;22: 1266-1272.

[15] Voss MH, Feldman DR, Bosl GJ, Motzer RJ. A review of second-line chemotherapy and prognostic models for disseminated germ cell tumors. Hematology/Oncology Clinics of North America 2011;25: 557-576.

[16] Wasserman TH, Slavik M, Carter SK. Clinical comparison of the nitrosoureas. Cancer 1975;36: 1258-1268.

[17] Marchesi F, Turriziani M, Tortorelli G, Avvisati G, Torino F, De Vecchis L. Triazene compounds: mechanism of action and related DNA repair systems. Pharmacological Research 2007;56: 275-287.

[18] Neyns B, Tosoni A, Hwu WJ, Reardon DA. Dose-dense temozolomide regimens: antitumor activity, toxicity, and immunomodulatory effects. Cancer 2010;116(12): 2868-2877.

[19] Advani R. Optimal therapy of advanced Hodgkin lymphoma. American Society of Hematology Education Program 2011;2011: 310-316.

[20] Flaherty KT. Chemotherapy and targeted therapy combinations in advanced melanoma. Clinical Cancer Research 2006;12: 2366-2370.

[21] Rosenberg B, Vancamp L, Krigas T. Inhibition of cell division in Escherichia coli by electrolysis products from a platinum electrode. Nature 1965;205: 698-699.

[22] Desoize B. Metals and metal compounds in cancer treatment. Anticancer Research 2004;24(3a): 1529-1544.

[23] Boulikas T, Pantos A, Bellis E, Christofis P. Designing platinum compounds in cancer: structures and mechanisms. Cancer Therapy 2007;5: 537-583.

[24] Gore ME, Fryatt I, Wiltshaw E, Dawson T, Robinson BA & Calvert AH. Cisplatin/carboplatin cross-resistance in ovarian cancer. British Journal of Cancer 1989;60: 767-769.

[25] Hong WK, Bast Jr RC, Hait WN, Kufe DW, Pollock RE, Weichselbaum RR, Holland JF & Frei III E. Cancer Medicine 8. American Association for Cancer Research 2010.

[26] Saris CP, van de Vaart PJ, Rietbroek RC, Blommaert FA. In vitro formation of DNA adducts by cisplatin, lobaplatin and oxaliplatin in calf thymus DNA in solution and in cultured human cells. Carcinogenesis 1996;17(12): 2763-2769.

[27] Brunton LL, Chabner BA & Knollmann BC. Goodman & Gilman's. The Pharmacological Basis of Terapeutics. New York: McGraw-Hill Companies 2011.

[28] Pasetto LM, D'Andrea MR, Brandes AA, Rossi E & Monfardini S. The development of platinum compounds and their possible combination. Critical Reviews in Oncology Hematology 2006;60: 59-75.

[29] Farber S, Diamond LK. Temporary remissions in acute leukemia in children produced by folic acid antagonist, 4-aminopteroyl-glutamic acid. New England Journal of Medicine. 1948; 238(23):787-793.

[30] Zhao R & Goldman ID. Resistance to antifolates. Oncogene 2003;22(47): 7431-7457.

[31] Chabner BA, Allegra CJ, Curt GA, Clendeninn NJ, Baram J, Koizumi S, Drake JC, Jolivet J. Polyglutamation of methotrexate. Is methotrexate a prodrug? The Journal of Clinical Investigation 1985;76(3): 907-912.

[32] Cho RC, Cole PD, Sohn KJ, Gaisano G, Croxford R, Kamen BA, Kim YI. Effects of folate and folylpolyglutamyl synthase modulation on chemosensitivity of breast cancer cells. Molecular Cancer Therapy 2007;6(11): 2909-2920.

[33] Fabre I, Fabre G, Goldman ID. Polyglutamylation, an important element in methotrexate cytotoxicity and selectivity in tumor versus murine granulocytic progenitor cells in vitro. Cancer Research. 1984;44(8): 3190-3195.

[34] Holmboe L, Andersen AM, Mørkrid L, Slørdal L, Hall KS. High dose methotrexate chemotherapy: pharmacokinetics, folate and toxicity in osteosarcoma patients. British Journal of Clinical Pharmacology 2012;73(1): 106-114.

[35] Salliot C & Van der Heijde D. Long-term safety of methotrexate monotherapy in patients with rheumatoid arthritis: a systematic literature research. Annals of the Rheumatic Diseases 2009;68(7): 1100-1104.

[36] Buqué A, Muhialdin JS, Muñoz A, Calvo B, Carrera S, Aresti U, Sancho A, Rubio I, López-Vivanco G. Molecular mechanism implicated in Pemetrexed induced apoptosis in human melanoma cells. Molecular Cancer 2012;11(1): 25.

[37] Scagliotti GV, Parikh P, von Pawel J, Biesma B, Vansteenkiste J, Manegold C, Serwatowski P, Gatzemeier U, Digumarti R, Zukin M, Lee JS, Mellemgaard A, Park K, Patil

S, Rolski J, Goksel T, de Marinis F, Simms L, Sugarman KP, Gandara D. Phase III study comparing cisplatin plus gemcitabine with cisplatin plus pemetrexed in chemotherapy-naive patients with advanced-stage non-small-cell lung cancer. Journal of Clinical Oncology 2008;26(21): 3543-3551.

[38] Adjei AA. Pharmacology and mechanism of action of pemetrexed. Clinical Lung Cancer 2004;5Suppl2: S51-55.

[39] Hitchings GH Jr. Nobel lecture in physiology or medicine - 1988. Selective inhibitors of dihydrofolate reductase. In Vitro Cellular Developmental Biology 1989;25(4): 303-310.

[40] Galmarini CM, Mackey JR, Dumontet C. Nucleoside analogues and nucleobases in cancer treatment. The Lancet Oncology 2002;3(7): 415-424.

[41] Stanczyk M, Sliwinski T, Trelinska J, Cuchra M, Markiewicz L, Dziki L, Bieniek A, Bielecka-Kowalska A, Kowalski M, Pastorczak A, Szemraj J, Mlynarski W, Majsterek I. Role of base-excision repair in the treatment of childhood acute lymphoblastic leukaemia with 6-mercaptopurine and high doses of methotrexate. Mutation Research 2012;741(1-2): 13-21.

[42] Dervieux T, Blanco JG, Krynetski EY, Vanin EF, Roussel MF, Relling MV. Differing contribution of thiopurine methyltransferase to mercaptopurine versus thioguanine effects in human leukemic cells. Cancer Research 2001;61(15): 5810-5816

[43] Elion GB. Nobel lecture in physiology or medicine - 1988. The purine path to chemotherapy. In Vitro Cell Development Biology 1989;25(4): 321-330.

[44] Karran P & Attard N. Thiopurines in current medical practice: molecular mechanisms and contributions to therapy-related cancer. Nature Review Cancer 2008;8(1): 24-36.

[45] Plunkett W, Huang P, Gandhi V. Metabolism and action of fludarabine phosphate. Seminars Oncology 1990;17(5): 3-17.

[46] Chun HG, Leyland-Jones B, Cheson BD. Fludarabine phosphate: a synthetic purine antimetabolite with significant activity against lymphoid malignancies. Journal of Clinical Oncology 1991;9(1): 175-188.

[47] Yang SW, Huang P, Plunkett W, Becker FF, Chan JY. Dual mode of inhibition of purified DNA ligase I from human cells by 9-beta-D-arabinofuranosyl-2-fluoroadenine triphosphate. The Journal of Biological Chemistry 1992;267(4): 2345-2349.

[48] Catapano CV, Perrino FW, Fernandes DJ. Primer RNA chain termination induced by 9-beta-D-arabinofuranosyl-2-fluoroadenine 5'-triphosphate. A mechanism of DNA synthesis inhibition. Journal of Biological Chemistry 1993;268(10): 7179-7185.

[49] Cheson BD, Vena DA, Foss FM, Sorensen JM. Neurotoxicity of purine analogs: a review. Journal of Clinical Oncology 1994;12(10): 2216-2228.

[50] Beutler E. Cladribine (2-chlorodeoxyadenosine). Lancet 1992;340(8825): 952-956.

[51] Klohs WD & Kraker AJ. Pentostatin: future directions. Pharmacological Reviews 1992;44(4): 459-477.

[52] Longley DB, Harkin DP, Johnston PG. 5-Fluorouracil: Mechanisms of action and clinical strategies. Nature 2003;3: 330-338.

[53] Lamont EB & Schilsky RL. The Oral Fluoropyrimidines in Cancer Chemotherapy. Clinical Cancer Research 1999;5: 2289-2296.

[54] Han R, Yang YM, Dietrich J, Luebke A, Mayer-Pröschel M, Noble M. Systemic 5-fluorouracil treatment causes a syndrome of delayed myelin destruction in the central nervous system. Journal of Biology 2008;7(4): 12.

[55] Stewart T, Pavlakis N, Ward M. Cardiotoxicity with 5-fluorouracil and capecitabine: more than just vasospastic angina. Internal Medicine Journal 2010;40(4): 303-307.

[56] Miwa M, Ura M, Nishida M, Sawada N, Ishikawa T, Mori K, Shimma N, Umeda I, Ishitsuka H. Design of a novel oral fluoropyrimidine carbamate, capecitabine, which generates 5-fluorouracil selectively in tumours by enzymes concentrated in human liver and cancer tissue. European Journal of Cancer 1998;34(8): 1274–1281.

[57] Johnston PG & Kaye S. Capecitabine: a novel agent for the treatment of solid tumors. Anticancer Drugs 2001;12(8): 639-646.

[58] Qiu MT, Ding XX, Hu JW, Tian HY, Yin R, Xu L. Fixed-dose rate infusion and standard rate infusion of gemcitabine in patients with advanced non-small-cell lung cancer: a meta-analysis of six trials. Cancer Chemotherapy and Pharmacology 2012; DOI: 10.1007/s00280-012-1974-z.

[59] Hui YF & Reitz J. Gemcitabine: A cytidine analogue active against solid tumors. American Journal of Health-System Pharmacy 1997;54: 162-170.

[60] Kim KI, Huh IS, Kim IW, Park T, Ahn KS, Yoon SS, Yoon JH, Oh JM. Combined interaction of multi-locus genetic polymorphisms in cytarabine arabinoside metabolic pathway on clinical outcomes in adult acute myeloid leukaemia (AML) patients. European Journal of Cancer 2012;DOI: 10.1016/j.ejca.2012.07.022.

[61] Hartford CM, Duan S, Delaney SM, Mi S, Kistner EO, Lamba JK, Huang RS, Dolan ME. Population-specific genetic variants important in susceptibility to cytarabine arabinoside cytotoxicity. Blood 2009;113(10): 2145–2153.

[62] Johnson IS, Wright HF, Svoboda GH, Vlantis J. Antitumor principles derived from Vinca rosea Linn. I. Vincaleukoblastine and leurosine. Cancer Research 1960;20: 1016-1022.

[63] Jordan MA, Thrower D, Wilson L. Mechanism of inhibition of cell proliferation by vinca alkaloids. Cancer Research 1991;51(8): 2212-2222.

[64] Jordan MA & Wilson L. Microtubules as a target for anticancer drugs. Nature Reviews Cancer 2004;4: 253-265.

[65] Dumontet C & Jordan MA. Microtubule-binding agents: a dynamic field of cancer therapeutics. Nature Reviews Drug Discovery 2010;9(10): 790-803.

[66] Kingston DG. Tubulin-interactive natural products as anticancer agents. Journal Natural Products 2009;72: 507-515.

[67] Lucas DM, Still PC, Pérez LB, Grever MR & Kinghorn AD. Potential of Plant-Derived Natural Products in the Treatment of Leukemia and Lymphoma. Current Drug Targets 2010;11: 812–822.

[68] Groninger E, Meeuwsen-de Boar T, Koopmans P, Uges D, Sluiter W, Veerman A, Kamps W, de Graaf S. Pharmacokinetics of vincristine monotherapy in childhood acute lymphoblastic leukemia. Pediatric Research 2002;52(1): 113-118.

[69] Rowinsky EK & Donehower RC. The clinical pharmacology and use of antimicrotubule agents in cancer chemotherapeutics. Pharmacology & Therapeutics 1991;52: 35-84.

[70] Mano M. Vinorelbine in the management of breast cancer: New perspectives, revived role in the era of targeted therapy. Cancer Treatment Reviews 2006;32: 106-118

[71] Gralla RJ, Gatzemeier U, Gebbia V, Huber R, O'Brien M, & Puozzo C.Oral vinorelbine in the treatment of non-small cell lung cancer: rationale and implications for patient management. Drugs 2007;67: 1403-1410.

[72] Quasthoff S & Hartung HP. Chemotherapy-induced peripheral neuropathy. Journal of Neurology 2002;249(1): 9-17.

[73] Canta A, Chiorazzi A, Cavaletti G. Tubulin: a target for antineoplastic drugs into the cancer cells but also in the peripheral nervous system. Current Medicinal Chemistry 2009;16(11): 1315-1324.

[74] Goa KL & Faulds D. Vinorelbine. A review of its pharmacological properties and clinical use in cancer chemotherapy. Drugs Aging 1994;5(3): 200-234.

[75] Gottesman MM, Fojo T, Bates SE. Multidrug resistance in cancer: role of ATP-dependent transporters. Nature Reviews Cancer 2002;2(1): 48-58.

[76] Natarajan K, Senapati S. Understanding the basis of drug resistance of the mutants of αβ-tubulin dimer via molecular dynamics simulations. PLoS One 2012;7(8):e42351 1-13.

[77] Gonzalez-Garay ML, Chang L, Blade K, Menick DR, Cabral F.A beta-tubulin leucine cluster involved in microtubule assembly and paclitaxel resistance. The Journal of Biological Chemistry 1999;274(34): 23875-23882.

[78] Burkhart CA, Kavallaris M, Band Horwitz S. The role of beta-tubulin isotypes in resistance to antimitotic drugs. Biochimica et Biophysica Acta (BBA) – Proteins and Proteomics 2001;1471(2): O1-9.

[79] Zhang CC, Yang JM, White E, Murphy M, Levine A, Hait WN. The role of MAP4 expression in the sensitivity to paclitaxel and resistance to vinca alkaloids in p53 mutant cells. Oncogene 1998;16(12): 1617-1624.

[80] Wani MC, Taylor HL, Wall ME, Coggon P, McPhail AT. Plant antitumor agents VI. The isolation and structure of taxol, a novel antileukemic and antitumor agent from Taxus brevifolia. Journal of the American Chemical Society 1971;93(9): 2325-2327.

[81] Wall ME, Wani MC. Camptothecin and taxol: discovery to clinic--thirteenth Bruce F. Cain Memorial Award Lecture. Cancer Research 1995;55(4): 753-760.

[82] Guenard D, Gueritte-Voegelein F, Potier P. Taxol and taxotere: discovery, chemistry, and structure-activity relationships. Accounts of Chemical Research 1993;26(4): 160–167.

[83] Rowinsky EK. The development and clinical utility of the taxane class of antimicrotubule chemotherapy agents. Annual Reviews Medicine 1997;48: 353-374.

[84] Horwitz SB, Cohen D, Rao S, et al. Taxol: mechanisms of action and resistance. Journal of the National Cancer Institute 1994;15: 63–67.

[85] Haldar S, Chintapalli J, Croce CM. Taxol induces bcl-2 phosphorylation and death of prostate cancer cells. Cancer Research 1996; 56: 1253–1255.

[86] Weiss RB, Donehower RC, Wiernik PH, Ohnuma T, Gralla RJ, Trump DL, Baker JR Jr, Van Echo DA, Von Hoff DD, Leyland-Jones B. Hypersensitivity reactions from taxol. Journal of Clinical Oncology 1990;8(7): 1263-1268.

[87] Rowinsky EK, Donehower RC (1995) Paclitaxel (taxol). New England Journal of Medicine 1995;332: 1004–1014

[88] Miele E, Spinelli GP, Miele E, Tomao F, Tomao S. Albumin-bound formulation of paclitaxel (Abraxane ABI-007) in the treatment of breast cancer. International Journal of Nanomedicine 2009;4: 99-105.

[89] Rowinsky EK, Eisenhauer EA, Chaudhry V, Arbuck SG, Donehower RC. Clinical toxicities encountered with paclitaxel (Taxol). Seminars in Oncology 1993;20(Suppl 3): 1-15.

[90] Cortes J & Baselga J. Targeting the microtubules in breast cancer beyond taxanes: the epothilones. Oncologist 2007;12: 271-280.

[91] Nettles JH, Li H, Cornett B, Krahn JM, Snyder JP, Downing KH. The binding mode of epothilone A on α,β-tubulin by electron crystallography. Science 2004;305: 866–869

[92] Bode CJ, Gupta ML Jr, Reiff EA, Suprenant KA, Georg GI & Himes RH. Epothilone and paclitaxel: unexpected differences in promoting the assembly and stabilization of yeast microtubules. Biochemistry 2002;41: 3870–3874.

[93] de Jonge M & Verweij J. The epothilone dilemma. Journal of Clinical Oncology 2005;23(36): 9048-9050.

[94] Goodin S, Kane MP, Rubin EH. Epothilones: mechanism of action and biologic activity. Journal of Clinical Oncology 2004;22(10): 2015-2025.

[95] Wall ME, Wani MC, Cook CE, Palmer KH. Plant antitumor agents, I: the isolation and structure of camptothecin, a novel alkaloidal leukemia and tumor inhibitor from Camptotheca acuminate. Journal of the American Chemical Society 1966;88: 3888–3890

[96] Pommier Y. Topoisomerase I inhibitors: camptothecins and beyond. Nature Reviews Cancer 2006;6(10): 789-802.

[97] Hsiang YH, Hertzberg R, Hecht S, Liu LF. Camptothecin induces protein-linked DNA breaks via mammalian DNA topoisomerase I. The Journal of Biological Chemistry 1985;260(27): 14873–14878.

[98] Eng WK, Faucette L, Johnson RK, Sternglanz R. Evidence that DNA topoisomerase I is necessary for the cytotoxic effects of camptothecin. Molecular Pharmacology 1988;34(6): 755–760.

[99] Jaxel C, Kohn KW, Wani MC, Wall ME, Pommier Y. Structure-activity study of the actions of camptothecin derivatives on mammalian topoisomerase I: evidence for a specific receptor site and a relation to antitumor activity. Cancer Research 1989;49(6): 1465–1469.

[100] Grochow LB, Rowinsky EK, Johnson R, Ludeman S, Kaufmann SH, McCabe FL, Smith BR, Hurowitz L, DeLisa A, Donehower RC, et al. Pharmacokinetics and pharmacodynamics of topotecan in patients with advanced cancer. Drug Metabolism and Disposition 1992;20(5): 706-713.

[101] Ormrod D, Spencer CM. Topotecan: a review of its efficacy in small cell lung cancer. Drugs. 1999;58(3): 533-551.

[102] Hartwell JL & Schrecker AW. Components of Podophyllin. V. The Constitution of Podophyllotoxin. Journal of the American Chemical Society 1951;73(6): 2909–2916.

[103] Lucas DM, Still PC, Pérez LB, Grever MR, Kinghorn AD. Potential of plant-derived natural products in the treatment of leukemia and lymphoma. Current Drug Targets 2010;11(7): 812-822.

[104] Hande KR. Topoisomerase II inhibitors. Update on Cancer Therapeutics 2006;1: 3-15.

[105] Hande KR. Etoposide: four decades of development of a topoisomerase II inhibitor. European Journal of Cancer 1998;34: 1514-1521.

[106] Long BH, Casazza AM. Structure-activity relationships of VP-16 analogues. Cancer Chemotherapy Pharmacology 1994;34: 26-31.

[107] Ross W, Rowe T, Glisson B, Yalowich J, Liu L. Role of topoisomerase II in mediating epipodophyllotoxin-induced DNA cleavage. Cancer Research 1984;44: 5857–5860.

[108] Osheroff N. Effect of antineoplastic agents on the DNA cleavage/religation reaction of eukaryotic topoisomerase II: inhibition of DNA religation by etoposide. Biochemistry 1989;28: 6157–6160.

[109] Fan JR, Peng AL, Chen HC, Lo SC, Huang TH, Li TK. Cellular processing pathways contribute to the activation of etoposide-induced DNA damage responses. DNA Repair 2008;7(3): 452-463.

[110] Blanco JG, Dervieux T, Edick MJ, Mehta PK, Rubnitz JE, Shurtleff S, Raimondi SC, Behm FG, Pui CH, Relling MV. Molecular emergence of acute myeloid leukemia during treatment for acute lymphoblastic leukemia. Proceedings of National Acadamy of Sciences of the United States of America 2001;98(18): 10338-10343.

[111] Ratain MJ, Rowley JD. Therapy-related acute myeloid leukemia secondary to inhibitors of topoisomerase II: from the bedside to the target genes. Annals of Oncology 1992;3(2): 107-111.

[112] Cortés-Funes H & Coronado C. Role of anthracyclines in the era of targeted therapy. Cardiovascular Toxicology 2007;7: 56-60.

[113] Thorn CF, Oshiro C, Marsh S, Hernandez-Boussard T, McLeod H, Klein TE & Altman RB. Doxorubicin pathways: pharmacodynamics and adverse effects. Pharmacogenetics and Genomics 2011;21: 440-446.

[114] Pai VB, Nahata MC. Cardiotoxicity of chemotherapeutic agents: incidence, treatment and prevention. Drug Safety 2000;22(4): 263-302.

[115] Batist G, Ramakrishnan G, Rao CS, Chandrasekharan A, Gutheil J, Guthrie T, Shah P, Khojasteh A, Nair MK, Hoelzer K, Tkaczuk K, Park YC, Lee LW. Reduced cardiotoxicity and preserved antitumour efficacy of liposome-encapsulated doxorubicin and cyclophosphamide compared with conventional doxorubicin and cyclophosphamide in a randomized, multicenter trial of metastatic breast cancer. Journal of Clinical Oncology 2001;19: 1444–1454.

[116] Trifilio SM, Rademaker AW, Newman D, Coyle K, Carlson-Leuer K, Mehta J, Altman J, Frankfurt O, Tallman MS. Mitoxantrone and etoposide with or without intermediate dose cytarabine for the treatment of primary induction failure or relapsed acute myeloid leukemia. Leukemia Research 2012;36: 394-396.

[117] Doggrell SA. Which drug combination for hormone-refractory prostate cancer?. Expert Opinion on Pharmacotherapy 2005;6: 667-670.

[118] Umezawa H. Natural and artificial bleomycins: chemistry and antitumor activities. Pure and Applied Chemistry 1971;28: 665–680.

[119] Chen J & Stubbe J. Bleomycins: towards better therapeutics. Nature Reviews Cancer 2005;5: 102-112.

[120] Masetti R & Pession A. First-line treatment of acute lymphoblastic leukemia with pegasparaginase. Biologics 2009;3: 359-368.

[121] Avramis VI. Asparaginases: A Successful Class of Drugs Against Leukemias and Lymphomas. Journal of Pediatric Hematology/Oncology 2011;33: 573-579

[122] Dinndorf PA, Gootenberg J, Cohen MH, Keegan P, Pazdur R. FDA drug approval summary: pegaspargase (oncaspar) for the first-line treatment of children with acute lymphoblastic leukemia (ALL). The Oncologist 2007;12(8): 991-998.

[123] Hutson RG, Kitoh T, Moraga Amador DA, Cosic S, Schuster SM, Kilberg MS.Amino acid control of asparagine synthetase: relation to asparaginase resistance in human leukemia cells. The American Journal of Physiology 1997;272(5): 1691-1699.

[124] Albertsen BK, Schroder H, Jakobsen P, et al. Antibody formation during intravenous and intramuscular therapy with Erwinia asparaginase. Medical and Pediatric Oncology 2002;38: 310–316

[125] Dresler WFC, Stein R. Uber den Hydroxylharnstoff. Justus Liebigs Annalen der Chemie 1869;150(2): 242-252.

[126] Rosenthal F, Wislicki L, Koller L. Uber die Bziehungen von schwertsen Blutgiften zu Abauprodukten des Einweisses: ein Beitrag zum Enstehungmechanismus der pernizosen Anemie. Klin Wochenschr 1928;7: 972-977.

[127] Saban N, Bujak M. Hydroxyurea and hydroxamic acid derivatives as antitumor drugs. Cancer Chemotherapy and Pharmacology 2009;64(2): 213-221.

[128] Madaan K, Kaushik D, Verma T. Hydroxyurea: a key player in cancer chemotherapy. Expert Review of Anticancer Therapy 2012;12(1): 19-29.

[129] Cokic VP, Smith RD, Beleslin-Cokic BB, Njoroge JM, Miller JL, Gladwin MT, Schechter AN. Hydroxyurea induces fetal hemoglobin by the nitric oxide-dependent activation of soluble guanylyl cyclase. Journal of Clinical Investigation 2003;111(2): 231-239.

[130] Huang J, Kim-Shapiro DB, King SB. Catalase-mediated nitric oxide formation from hydroxyurea. Journal of Medicinal Chemistry 2004;47(14): 3495-3501.

[131] Kennedy BJ, Smith LR, Goltz RW. Skin changes secondary to hydroxyurea therapy. Archives of Dermatology 1975;111(2): 183-187.

[132] Friedrich S, Raff K, Landthaler M, Karrer S. Cutaneous ulcerations on hands and heels secondary to long-term hydroxyurea treatment. European Journal of Dermatology 2004;14(5): 343-346.

[133] Best PJ, Petitt RM. Multiple skin cancers associated with hydroxyurea therapy. Mayo Clinic Proceedings: Mayo Clinic 1998;73(10): 961-963.

[134] Sanchez-Palacios C, Guitart J. Hydroxyurea-associated squamous dysplasia. Journal of the American Academy of Dermatology 2004;51(2): 293-300.

[135] Matthews SJ, McCoy C. Thalidomide: a review of approved and investigational uses. Clinical Therapeutics 2003;25(2): 342-395.

[136] Bartlett JB, Dredge K, Dalgleish AG. The evolution of thalidomide and its IMiD derivatives as anticancer agents. Nature Reviews Cancer 2004;4(4): 314-322.

[137] FDA - U.S. Food and Drug Administration. FDA: Thalidomide (marketed as Thalomid) Information. www.fda.gov/Drugs/DrugSafety/PostmarketDrugSafetyInformationforPatientsandProviders/ucm107296.htm (accessed 01 August 2012)

[138] Bruera E, Neumann CM, Pituskin E, Calder K, Ball G, Hanson J. Thalidomide in patients with cachexia due to terminal cancer: preliminary report. Annals of Oncology 1999;10(7): 857-859.

[139] [139]. Gordon JN, Trebble TM, Ellis RD, Duncan HD, Johns T, Goggin PM. Thalidomide in the treatment of cancer cachexia: a randomised placebo controlled trial. Gut 2005; 54(4): 540-545.

[140] [140]. Grover JK, Uppal G, Raina V. The adverse effects of thalidomide in relapsed and refractory patients of multiple myeloma. Annals of Oncology 2002;13(10): 1636-1640.

[141] Dimopoulos MA, Eleutherakis-Papaiakovou V. Adverse effects of thalidomide administration in patients with neoplastic diseases. American Journal of Medicine 2004;117(7): 508-515.

[142] Mohan R, Panda D. Kinetic stabilization of microtubule dynamics by estramustine is associated with tubulin acetylation, spindle abnormalities, and mitotic arrest. Cancer Research 2008;68(15): 6181-6189.

[143] Ravery V, Fizazi K, Oudard S, Drouet L, Eymard JC, Culine S, Gravis G, Hennequin C, Zerbib M. The use of estramustine phosphate in the modern management of advanced prostate cancer. BJU International 2011;108(11): 1782-1786.

[144] U.S. Food and Drug administration. FDA: FDA approves bortezomib (Velcade) for the treatment of patients with mantle cell lymphoma who have received at least one prior therapy. www.fda.gov/AboutFDA/CentersOffices/OfficeofMedicalProductsandTobacco/CDER/ucm094929.htm (accessed 01 August 2012)

[145] Chen D, Frezza M, Schmitt S, Kanwar J, Dou QP. Bortezomib as the first proteasome inhibitor anticancer drug: current status and future perspectives. Current Cancer Drug Targets 2011;11(3): 239-253.

[146] Major P. The use of zoledronic acid, a novel, highly potent bisphosphonate, for the treatment of hypercalcemia of malignancy. The Oncologist 2002;7: 481-491.

[147] Green JR. Antitumor effects of bisphosphonates. Cancer 2003;97(3 Suppl): 840-847.

[148] Rogers TL & Holen I. Tumour macrophages as potential targets of bisphosphonates. Journal of Translational Medicine 2011;179: 177.

[149] Pozzi S & Raje N. The role of bisphosphonates in multiple myeloma: mechanisms, side effects, and the future. The Oncologist 2011;16: 651-662.

[150] Richardson PG, Laubach JP, Schlossman RL, Ghobrial IM, Mitsiades CS, Rosenblatt J, Mahindra A, Raje N, Munshi N & Anderson KC.The Medical Research Council Myeloma IX trial: the impact on treatment paradigms. European Journal of Haematology. 2012;88: 1-7.

[151] Oakley RH & Cidlowski JA. Cellular processing of the glucocorticoid receptor gene and protein: new mechanisms for generating tissue-specific actions of glucocorticoids. The Journal of Biological Chemistry 2011;286: 3177-3184.

[152] Schlossmacher G, Stevens A & White A. Glucocorticoid receptor-mediated apoptosis: mechanisms of resistance in cancer cells. Journal of Endocrinology 2011;211: 17-25.

[153] Scarpin KM, Graham JD, Mote PA & Clarke CL. Progesterone action in human tissues: regulation by progesterone receptor (PR) isoform expression, nuclear positioning and coregulator expression. Nuclear Receptor Signaling 2009;7: e009. www.nursa.org/article.cfm?doi=10.1621/nrs.07009 (accessed 20 October 2012).

[154] Heldring N, Pike A, Andersson S, Matthews J, Cheng G, Hartman J, Tujague M, Ström A, Treuter E, Warner M, Gustafsson JA. Estrogen receptors: how do they signal and what are their targets. Physiological Reviews 2007;87(3): 905-931.

[155] Chen Y, Clegg NJ, Scher HI. Anti-androgens and androgen-depleting therapies in prostate cancer: new agents for an established target. Lancet Oncology 2009;10(10): 981-991.

[156] U.S. Food and Drug administration. FDA: Drug Databases: Drugs@FDA: Fulvestrant Label and Approval History: Labeling Revision (11/09/2012). www.accessdata.fda.gov/drugsatfda_docs/label/2012/021344s019s020lbl.pdf. (accessed 20 November 2012)

[157] Robertson JF. Fulvestrant (Faslodex) -- how to make a good drug better. Oncologist 2007;12(7): 774-784.

[158] Valachis A, Mauri D, Polyzos NP, Mavroudis D, Georgoulias V, Casazza G. Fulvestrant in the treatment of advanced breast cancer: a systematic review and meta-analysis of randomized controlled trials. Critical Reviews in Oncology/Hematolology 2010;73(3): 220-227.

[159] Lewis JS, Jordan VC. Selective estrogen receptor modulators (SERMs): mechanisms of anticarcinogenesis and drug resistance. Mutation Research 2005;591(1-2): 247-263.

[160] Pickar JH, MacNeil T, Ohleth K. SERMs: progress and future perspectives. Maturitas 2010;67(2): 129-138.

[161] U.S. Food and Drug administration. FDA: Drug Databases: Drugs@FDA: Nolvadex Label and Approval History: Labeling Revision (03/17/2005). www.accessdata.fda.gov/drugsatfda_docs/label/2005/17970s053lbl.pdf. (accessed 20 November 2012)

[162] U.S. Food and Drug administration. FDA: Drug Databases: Drugs@FDA: Fareston Label and Approval History: Labeling Revision (03/21/2011). www.accessdata.fda.gov/drugsatfda_docs/label/2011/020497s006lbl.pdf. (accessed 20 November 2012)

[163] Vogel VG, Costantino JP, Wickerham DL, Cronin WM, Cecchini RS, Atkins JN, Bevers TB, Fehrenbacher L, Pajon ER Jr, Wade JL 3rd, Robidoux A, Margolese RG, James J, Lippman SM, Runowicz CD, Ganz PA, Reis SE, McCaskill-Stevens W, Ford LG, Jordan VC, Wolmark N; National Surgical Adjuvant Breast and Bowel Project (NSABP). Effects of tamoxifen vs raloxifene on the risk of developing invasive breast cancer and other disease outcomes: the NSABP Study of Tamoxifen and Raloxifene (STAR) P-2 trial. JAMA 2006;295(23): 2727-2741.

[164] Cuzick J, Sestak I, Baum M, Buzdar A, Howell A, Dowsett M, Forbes JF; ATAC/LATTE investigators. Effect of anastrozole and tamoxifen as adjuvant treatment for early-stage breast cancer: 10-year analysis of the ATAC trial. Lancet Oncology 2010;11(12): 1135-1341

[165] Johnston SR, Dowsett M. Aromatase inhibitors for breast cancer: lessons from the laboratory. Nature Reviews Cancer 2003;3(11): 821-831.

[166] Dowsett M, Cuzick J, Ingle J, Coates A, Forbes J, Bliss J, Buyse M, Baum M, Buzdar A, Colleoni M, Coombes C, Snowdon C, Gnant M, Jakesz R, Kaufmann M, Boccardo F, Godwin J, Davies C, Peto R. Meta-analysis of breast cancer outcomes in adjuvant trials of aromatase inhibitors versus tamoxifen. Journal of Clinical Oncology 2010;28(3): 509-518

[167] Huiart L, Dell'Aniello S, Suissa S. Use of tamoxifen and aromatase inhibitors in a large population-based cohort of women with breast cancer. British Journal of Cancer 2011;104(10): 1558-1563.

[168] Jakesz R, Jonat W, Gnant M, Mittlboeck M, Greil R, Tausch C, Hilfrich J, Kwasny W, Menzel C, Samonigg H, Seifert M, Gademann G, Kaufmann M, Wolfgang J; ABCSG and the GABG. Switching of postmenopausal women with endocrine-responsive early breast cancer to anastrozole after 2 years' adjuvant tamoxifen: combined results of ABCSG trial 8 and ARNO 95 trial. Lancet 2005;366(9484): 455-462.

[169] Regan MM, Neven P, Giobbie-Hurder A, Goldhirsch A, Ejlertsen B, Mauriac L, Forbes JF, Smith I, Láng I, Wardley A, Rabaglio M, Price KN, Gelber RD, Coates AS, Thürlimann B; BIG 1-98 Collaborative Group; International Breast Cancer Study Group (IBCSG). Assessment of letrozole and tamoxifen alone and in sequence for postmenopausal women with steroid hormone receptor-positive breast cancer: the BIG 1-98 randomised clinical trial at 8-1 years median follow-up. Lancet Oncology 2011;12(12): 1101-1108.

Chapter 2

Target Cancer Therapy

Taciane Ladislau, Klesia P Madeira, Renata D Daltoé,
Isabella S Guimarães, Sarah F Teixeira,
Paulo CM Lyra-Júnior, Iuri C Valadão,
Leticia BA Rangel and Alice L Herlinger

Additional information is available at the end of the chapter

http://dx.doi.org/10.5772/55284

1. Introduction

Over the past decade, cancer therapy has changed drastically by the introduction of the target therapies, which focus on unique molecules present in tumors or protein whose expression or function is enriched within the neoplastic tissue; the so called molecular targets. In this context, target therapies may include monoclonal antibodies, drugs or small inhibitors capable of inhibiting specific molecules, such as kinases. The major targets in cancer therapy are pathways directing cell growth, proliferation and survival, as well as, those interfering on tumors microenvironmental aspects, such as angiogenesis. On the other hand, an emerging field on target therapy is the use of epigenetic drugs, which aim the restoration of the normal epigenetic landscape in cancer cells by targeting the epigenetic machinery of cells. Despite some major side effects associated to some target drugs, these therapies are well tolerated by patients. Moreover, it bears the possibility of developing personal therapies to each individual patient, which is considered the optimum choice in oncology.

2. Kinases and their hole on tumor progression

Kinases are by definition proteins capable of catalyzing the transfer of the terminal phosphate of ATP to substrates that contain, in most cases, a serine, threonine or tyrosine residue. The importance of targeting kinases to fight cancer relies on the central role that these molecules play on tumorigenesis, as uncontrolled tissue growth, and the capacity of cells to invade and metastasize [1]. Considering that, kinases involved in cell growth, division, migration and differentiation, as well as, angiogenesis and metastasis have been exploited and targeted in therapeutic oncology [2].

RAF/MEK/ERK and PI3K/AKT/mTOR are particularly important, as aberrant activation of these pathways is frequently observed in many types of cancers. Of interest, they are involved in chemoresistance to conventional chemotherapy, hormonal therapies and radiaotherapy. In addition, upstream elements of these signaling pathways, such as growth factors and growth factor receptors, as well as kinases exclusively found on cancer cells, as the kimeric kinases derived from Philadelphia chromosome (Ph), can also be target for cancer therapy. Thus, inhibitors targeting any of these molecules can potentially suppress tumorigenesis and bypass resistance to conventional treatments to cancer [3, 4, 5].

3. Small molecule kinase inhibitors in cancer therapy

Kinase inhibitors (KI) are divided into several classes based on the site they bind to at the enzyme. Types 1 and 2 bind to the ATP site of kinases, acting as ATP competitors. The difference between these two types is that whereas type I inhibitors target the active conformation of the kinase, type 2 bind to the inactive one. On the other hand, type 3 KI bind outside the ATP site, inhibiting kinases on an allosteric manner. This class of KI is usually more selective, since they bind to unique sequences from specific kinases. The forth class of KI are the covalent inhibitors, which irreversibly bind to the kinase active site, usually by reacting with a nucleophilic cystein residue [6]. KI already approved by the US Food and Drug Administration (FDA) will be discussed next, followed by KI currently under trial.

3.1. Kinase inhibitors approved by FDA for cancer treatment

3.1.1. EGFR and HER2 kinase activity inhibitor

Gefitinib was approved under FDA's accelerated approval regulation in 2003. It acts by inhibiting the phosphorylation of a series of intracellular kinases associated with epidermal growth factor receptor (EGFR), among others. At its initial approval it was recommended for the treatment of patients with locally advanced or metastatic non-small cell lung carcinoma (NSCLC) after the failure of both platinum-based and docetaxel chemotherapies. However, in 2005, FDA published a labeling revision due to the failure demonstrated by gefitinib in increasing NSCLC patients' survival. Since this revision, gefitinib has only been prescribed for patients who are benefiting or have benefited from gefitinib.

In 2004, FDA approved **erlotinib**, which also inhibits the phosphorylation of EGFR-associated TKs, for the treatment of locally advanced or metastatic NSCLC after failure of at least one prior chemotherapy regimen. On the next year, the indication for the use of erlotinib in combination with gemcitabine for the first-line treatment of patients with locally advanced, unresectable or metastatic pancreatic cancer (PC).

Different from the above mentioned KIs, **lapatinib**, approved by FDA in 2007, is a direct inhibitor of the intracellular kinase domain of both EGFR and human growth epidermal growth factor 2 (HER2/neu), inhibiting the tumor driven cell growth. Its initial indication was for the treatment of patients with advanced or metastatic breast cancer (BC) whose tumors overexpress HER2 and who have received prior therapy including an anthracycline, a taxane, and trastuzumab. In 2012, the indications for lapatinib include the combined use of this drug with: capecitabine, for the treatment of patients with advanced or metastatic BC in the same conditions as mentioned above; letrozole for the treatment of postmenopausal women with hormone receptor positive metastatic BC that overexpress the HER2 receptor for whom hormonal therapy is indicated.

3.1.2. Raf inhibitors

A variety of agents have been discovered to interfere with RAF kinases, each of which acting on different ways in order to block Raf protein expression, c-Ras/Raf interaction, Raf kinase activity, Raf's ATP-binding site, or the kinase activity of the Raf target protein MAPKK.

Among these, **sorafenib tyosilate**, a c-Raf inhibitors, has been approved by FDA in 2005. This bi-aryl urea was initially identified as an adenosine triphosphate competitive inhibitor of the c-Raf kinase. Sorafenib targets two kinase classes known to be involved in both tumor proliferation and angiogenesis [7]. The drug blocks the enzyme c-Raf kinase it self, a critical component of the Ras/Raf/MEK/ERK signaling pathway, which is responsible for controlling cell division and proliferation. In addition, sorafenib inhibits the vascular endothelial growth factor receptor (VEGFR)-2/platelet-derived growth factor receptor (PDGFR)-beta signaling cascade, thereby blocking tumor growth and angiogenesis. Sorafenib has been evaluated as a single therapy agent and in combination with various chemotherapy drugs in a number of clinical trials [8-10]. At its first approval sorafenib tosylate was indicated for the treatment of adenois cyst carcinoma (ACC) patients; latter on, at the latest review, in 2012, the indication for the treatment of unresectable hepatocellular carcinoma (HCC) patients was included.

Later on, in 2011, vemurafenib, which targets the mutated form of BRAF protein BRAFv600, was approved by FDA [11]. It has been approved for the treatment of patients with metastatic melanoma (MM) whose tumors presented the mutation, as detected by a FDA approved test. However, it is not recommended for the treatment of MM patients who harbors the wild-type BRAF gene. It has been no review on vermurafenib label so far.

Raf inhibitors that are currently under clinical evaluation have shown promising signs of anti-cancer efficacy with a very tolerable safety profile [12], and will be further discussed on this chapter.

3.1.3. MEK inhibitors

Although MEK mutations are rare in human cancer, MEK inhibitors have been developed as a therapeutic strategy to combat B-RAF inhibitor resistance by targeting downstream effectors. To date, these MEK inhibitors have shown poor efficacy and activity in the clinic. However, with the emergence of resistance to B-RAF therapy, and a higher than previously thought frequency of somatic MEK mutations, these inhibitors are finding renewed clinical use [13].

Several MEK inhibitors have been identified: PD184352 (CI-1040), Selumetinib (AZD6244, ARRY-142886), PD0325901, XL518, GSK1120212 (JTP-74057), ARRY-438162. Worth noticing, most of the known MEK inhibitors are noncompetitive (ie, they do not bind to the ATP–binding site of the kinase) [14]. Despite ATP-biding pockets are highly conserved among human kinases [15], structural analysis of demonstrates tha it harbors a unique site adjacent to the ATP binding site [16]. Thus, biding of inhibitos to this unique MEK site explain the high degree of specificity of the MEK inhibitors compared to other kinase inhibitors with competitive activity.

PD184352 is an orally active highly selective and potent chemical inhibitor of MEK1/2 and was the first MEK inhibitor to enter clinical trials. Selumetinib is the second MEK inhibitor to go into clinical trial after the first MEK inhibitor, CI-1040, demonstrated poor clinical efficacy. Selumetinib is a benzimidazole derivative with reported nanomolar activity against the purified MEK1 enzyme. Through a series of studies using preclinical cell cultures and animal models, it was shown that Selumetinib suppresses the growth of melanoma cells through the induction of cytostasis, but Selumetinib has a limited ability to induce apoptosis or block angiogenesis [17,18].

3.1.4. mTOR inhibitors

Rapamycin, the canonical mTOR inhibitor, was identified in 1975 as a potent antifungal isolated from *Streptomyces hygroscopicus*, nowadays it is recognized for its immunosuppressive and antitumor activities. However, rapamycin has limited bioavailability duo to its poor aqueous solubility. In an effort to improve its pharmacokinetic characteristics, several rapamycin analogues, named **rapalogs**, have been developed, such the first generation mTOR inhibitors **temsirolimus, everolimus**, and **ridaforolimus** [19-21].

In mammalian cells, members of this pharmacological class associate with the intracellular receptor FK506 binding protein 12 (FKBP12). Then, this complex interacts with FKBP12-rapamycin binding (FRB) domain, performing an allosteric mechanism of inhibition of mammalian target of rapamycin (mTOR) kinase activity. Traditionally the rapalogs inhibit only mTOR complex (mTORC) 1, probably because FRB domain is occluded in mTORC2. However, some studies have shown that these compounds are able to disrupt mTORC2 in a dose-, time- and cell type-dependent manner [20, 22]. A possible mechanism by which rapamycin and rapalogs could inhibit mTORC2 would be that rapamycin- or rapalogs-FKBP12 complexes would interact with newly synthesized mTOR molecules. In turn, this interaction would prevent mTOR interaction with RICTOR, inhibiting mTORC2. Indeed, it has been shown that prolonged treatment of cancer cells with rapamycin can promote its binding to mTOR before mTORC2 assembly, and subsequently inhibit Akt signaling [23]. In addition, treatment with temsirolimus or everolimus in acute myeloid leukemia (AML) cell lines blocked mTORC1 as well mTORC2 assembly [24]. In this way, rapalogs inhibit the signal transduction through the mTORCs downstream effectors, as 4E-BP1 and S6K1, resulting in reduction of protein synthesis and cell proliferation, also inhibit cell-cycle progression and angiogenesis, and promote apoptosis. Despite this positive action against cancer cells, these compounds, when inhibiting only mTORC1, lead to relieve negative feedback loop from S6K1 to IRS-1 resulting in PI3K/AKT pathway activation, and, consequently, could promote cell survival and chemoresistance [21, 25].

Temsirolimus and everolimus have been approved by FDA for the treatment of renal cell carcinoma (RCC). Everolimus has been approved for pancreatic neuroendocrine tumors, and recently for HER2-negative BC in combination with exemestane, after letrozole or anastrozole treatment fails. These antineoplastic agents have been investigated in clinical trials for malignancies from many tissues, including breast, gynecologic, gastrointestinal, lung and melanoma, alone or in association with hormonal therapies, EGFR inhibitors, and cytotoxic drugs [3, 19, 26, 27].

The efficacy of rapalogs is partially limited by compensatory mechanism of mTOR activation driven by the loss of negative feedback and because mTOR can be regulated by other signaling pathways such as Ras/Raf/MEK/ERK. Thereby, the inhibition of this pathway alone provides a transient benefit that may result in treatment resistance. It has already been shown the benefits of using mTOR inhibitors in combination with anti-insulin-like growth factor 1 receptor (IGF-1R) monoclonal antibodies. Thus, in order to overcome possible mechanisms of resistance, it would be interesting to establish therapeutic schemes that use combinations of different drugs [4, 27]. Inhibitors of mTOR (TORKinhibs) are still under development/trial, as well as the dual mTOR/PI3K inhibitors and will be discussed further on this chapter.

3.1.5. Ph chromosome-related kinase inhibitors.

In 2003, FDA approved **imatinib mesylate**, a Bcr-Abl fusion tyrosine kinase, leading to impaired proliferation and apoptosis induction of cancer cells. Its indications were for newly diagnosed adult patients with Ph chromosome positive chronic myelogeneous leukemia (CML) in chronic phase, as well as for patients with CML in blast crisis, accelerated phase, or in chronic phase after failure of interferon (IFN)-alfa therapy. Apart from that, imatinib mesylate was also indicated for the treatment of patients with c-Kit positive unresected and/or metastatic malignant gastrointestinal stroma tumors (GIST). The most recent FDA revision on this drug label, from 2012, indicates imatinib mesylate for the treatment of all diseases mentioned above, as well as for: adult patients with relapsed or refractory Ph chromosome positive acute lymphoblastic leukemia (ALL); adult patients with myelodysplastic/myeloproliferative diseases (MDS/MP) associated with PDGFR gene re-arrangements; adult patients with aggressive systemic mastocytosis (ASM) without the D816V c-Kit mutation or with c-Kit mutational status unknown; adult patients with hypereosinophilic syndrome (HES) and/or chronic eosinophilic leukemia (CEL) who have the FIP1L1PDGFRα fusion kinase (mutational analysis or FISH demonstration of CHIC2 allele deletion) and for patients with HES and/or CEL who are FIP1L1-PDGFRα fusion kinase negative or unknown status; adult patients with unresectable, recurrent and/or metastatic dermatofibrosarcoma protuberans (DFSP); and, adjuvant treatment of adult patients following complete gross resection of c-Kit positive GIST.

Dasatinib is a KI of Bcr-Abl, SRC family, c-Kit, ephrin type-A receptor 2 (EPHA2) and PDGFRβ developed to overcome the imatinib-resistance observed in relapsed patients with accelerated phase or blast crisis phase CML [28]. It was approved by FDA in 2006 and is predicted, based on modeling studies, to bind to multiple conformations of ABL kinase. It was initially approved for the treatment of patients with chronic, accelerated, myeloid or lymphoid blast phase CML with resistance or intolerance to prior therapy including imatinib mesylate, as well as for the treatment of adults with Ph chromosome-positive ALL resistant or intolerant to prior therapy. The 2012 label review for this drug also includes its indication for the treatment of newly diagnosed adults with Ph chromosome-positive CML in chronic phase.

Nilotinib hydrochloride monohydrate was approved by FDA in 2007 for the treatment of chronic and accelerated phase Ph chromosome-positive CML adult patients which have developed resistance or intolerance to prior therapy that included imatinib. In 2012, apart from these previous indications, nilotinib hydrochloride monohydrate has also been indicated for the treatment of newly diagnosed adult patients with Ph chromosome-positive CML in chronic phase.

3.1.6. Multi-kinase inhibitors

In 2006 FDA approved **sunitinib malate**, a multi-kinase inhibitor targeting several receptor tyrosine kinases (RTK), such as PDGFR-α and -β, VEGFR-1,-2 and -3, c-Kit, Fms-like tyrosine kinase-3 (FLT3), colony stimulating factor receptor Type 1 (CSF-1R) and the glial cell-line derived neurotrophic factor receptor (RET). At its first approval, sunitinib malate was indicated for the treatment of GIST after disease progression or intolerance to imatinib mesylate; and, for the treatment of advanced RCC, this based on the partial response rates and duration of responses observed for this drug. On the latest FDA review on sunitinib malate indications, in 2012, it was included the indication for the treatment of progressive, well-differentiated pancreatic neuroendocrine tumors (NET) in patients with unresectable locally advanced or metastatic disease.

In 2009, FDA approved the multi-kinase inhibitor **pazopanib hydrochloride** targeting VEGFR-1,-2 and -3, PDGFR-α and –β, fibroblast growth factor receptor (FGFR)-1 and -3, c-Kit, interleukin -2 receptor inducible T-cell kinase (Itk), leukocyte-specific protein kinase (Lck), and transmembrane glycoprotein receptor tyrosine kinase (c-Fms). At its first approval, pazopanib hydrochloride was indicated for the treatment of RCC patients, and at its latest label review, in 2012, it was also indicated for the treatment of patients with advanced soft tissue sarcoma (STS) who have received prior chemotherapy, except for patients with adipocytic STS or GIST, for which pazopanib hydrochloride's efficacy has not been proved.

During the year of 2011, two KIs with different targets and indications have been approved by FDA. Firstly, **vandetanib** a KI with multiple targets, including VEGFR and EGFR, has been approved for the treatment of symptomatic or progressive medullary thyroid cancer (MTC) in patients with unresectable locally advanced or metastatic disease. Also, **crizotinib** was approved for the treatment of patients with anaplasic lymphoma kinase (ALK) -positive locally advanced or metastatic NSCLC. There was no indication review for this drug so far.

In early 2012, the VEGFR-1, -2 and -3 inhibitor **axitinib** was approved by FDA. This KI was capable of decreasing VEGF-mediated endothelial cell proliferation and growth both in vitro and in animal models. It is indicated for the treatment of advanced RCC patients after failure of previous systemic therapy.

3.2. Kinase inhibitor currently under development or in clinical trial

3.2.1. The PKC inhibitor PKC412/Midostaurin

One of the most promising KI under trial is PKC412/midostaurin. It is a N-Benzoil derivative capable of inhibiting classical protein kinase C (PKC) α, β, γ and the calcium-dependent PKCs δ, ε, η, as well as TK pathways [29]. In 2001, Propper and colleagues published a phase I and pharmacokinetics study on this compound [30]. This study engaged 32 subjects with different types of tumor, which were either refractory to conventional therapy or unresponsive to standard treatment, exposed to seven doses of PKC412/midostaurin (12.5 mg/day – 300 mg/day). From this study it was concluded the PKC412/midostaurin has had as main toxicity nausea/vomiting and fatigue, with significant side effects as diarrhea, anorexia, and headache. A dose-related suppression on circulating lymphocyte and monocyte number was observed after 28 days of treatment. The overall conclusion of this work was that PKC412/midostaurin at 150mg/day would be well tolerated chronically. Currently, 7 active clinical trials using PKC412/midostaurin as single drug or in combination with others can be assessed at the Clinical Trial Search engine from National Cancer Institute [31], as well as, at the U.S. National Institute of Health clinical trial database [32].

Among studies using PKC412/midostaurin in combination with other drugs, two trials from Novartis (CPKC412A2114 and CPCK412AUS06T) evaluate the combined therapy of PKC412/midostaurin with the epigenetic drugs 5-azacytidine and decitabine, respectively. The first trial has been carried out with refractory or relapsed ALL and MDS patients' under 18 years old; the second has been carried out with newly diagnosed or relapsed AML patients over 60 years old. Also from Novartis, a trial (NCT01477606) evaluates PKC412/ midostaurin in several combinations with the epigenetic drug cytarabine and the anthracycline daunorubicin, or as single agent, for the treatment of AML patients which express the RTK FLT3-ITD. From the Washington University of Medicine, a study (NCT01161550) evaluated the combination of PKC412/midostaurin with either epigenetic drug cladribine or cytarabine in AML patients. Furthermore, PKC412/midostaurin has been evaluated on a collaborative trial (NCT01174888) from Novartis and Millennium Pharmaceuticals, Inc. in combination with bortezomib (a proteasome inhibitor), mitoxantrone hydrochloride (an anthracenedione), etoposide (a topoisomerase inhibitor) or cytarabine (an epigenetic drug) for the treatment of patients with relapsed or refractory AML. Finally, PKC412/midostaurin has been tested in combination with radiation therapy and 5-fluorouracil for the treatment of patients with advanced rectal cancer in a study (NCT01282502) sponsored by the Massachusetts General Hospital. As a single agent, PKC412/midostaurin has been tested by Novartis (NCT00866281) for the treatment of relapsed or refractory pediatric patients with AML and

ALL. Of interest, by the time this chapter was written, all the above mentioned trials were recruiting participants.

3.2.2. The EGFR inhibitor icotinib

Icotinib has been approved by the State Food and Drug Administration from China, in 2011, under the trade name of Conmana (Beta Pharma Inc.), but it was not yet approved by FDA. It is a reversible EGFR KI capable of inhibiting growth of tumor cell overexpressing EGFR, which underwent two phase I studies reported in 2011 [33, 34]. Both studies demonstrated that icotinib is safe and well tolerated by NSCLC patients and shows positive clinical anti-tumor activities.

3.2.3. PI3 kinase inhibitors

PI3K inhibitors target the p110 catalytic subunit of PI3K, and may be divided into two groups, isoform-specific inhibitors or pan-PI3K inhibitors; the latter can inhibit all class IA PI3Ks. In this way, they block the signal transduction through the PI3K/AKT/mTOR pathway exerting antiproliferative effects. The first-generation of PI3K inhibitors included wortmannin, an irreversible PI3K inhibitor isolated from *Penicillium wortimannin*, and LY294002, a synthetic and reversible PI3K inhibitor. However there are limiting features for their clinical use, which involve low selectivity for PI3K isoforms, poor solubility and toxicity in animals [35, 36].

Several other PI3K inhibitors have been developed in an attempt to overcome these initial limitations. Firstly, CAL-101 has 14 trials on phase I, II or III registered [37]. From these 11 are active, and evaluate either safety or efficacy of the drug alone or in combination with others, for the treatment of indolent non-Hodgkin lymphoma (NHL), chronic lymphocytic leukemia (CLL), mantle cell lymphoma (MCL), follicular lymphoma, small lymphocytic lymphoma (SLL), Hodgkin lymphoma, AML, among others. On the other hand, AMG 319 has only one phase I trial registered on the same data base. This trial is currently recruiting patients with hematologic malignancies. Moreover, XL147 has been on nine clinical trials which evaluate its safety and efficacy, alone or in combination, for the treatment of lymphoma, as well as, several solid tumors such as BC, NSCLC and ovarian cancer (OVCA), among others. Furthermore, GDC-0941 has been on 12 clinical trial, nine of which active. From these, a phase I trials evaluate its effect on solid tumors such as BC and NSCLC, as well as in NHL. Two phase II trial are also active, one with NSCLC patients and the other with BC patients. Other PI3K inhibitor, BYL719, has been on five active phase I and II trials with patients with several solid tumors. Additionally, PX-866 has been on seven pahse I and II trials, five of which active, also for the treatment of solid tumors. Lastly, BKM-120 has been on 43 trials, 42 active, evaluating its effects mostly on solid tumors, such as BC, NSCLC, endometrial carcinoma and glioblastoma, among others [32, 38, 39]. Compounds specifics for a given isoform can be used at lower doses avoiding side effects. Moreover, these isoform-specific compounds have achieved good results in certain cancers. For instance, a specific p110β inhibitor was shown to be more effective in PTEN-deficient cancer [40], whilst it was suggested that PI3K inhibitor specific for p110α might block angiogenesis [41]. However, it is believed that inhibition of one single isoform can lead to activation of another as a compensatory mechanism [42].

3.2.4. *Raf inhibitors*

As previously mentioned, Raf inhibitors have shown good results on clinical trials. Among these, dabrafenib has been tested as sigle agent or in combination for the treatment of cancer patients, mainly with melanoma. Also, a phase III randomized trial has recently been completed, however the early results have not been relieased by the time this chapter was concluded [43]. Moreover, RAF-265 is currently under phase I and II clinical trials with malignant melanoma patients. This compound is a potent inhibitor of Raf with a highly selective profile and inhibits all 3 isoforms of RAF, as well as mutant BRAF, with high potency [44]. Additionaly, XL281, a specific inhibitor of RAF kinases, including the mutant form of BRAF, and has finished Phase I testing [45].

3.2.5. *MEK inhibitors*

Although MEK mutations are rare in human cancer, MEK inhibitors have been developed as a therapeutic strategy to combat B-RAF inhibitor resistance by targeting downstream effectors. To date, these MEK inhibitors have shown poor efficacy and activity in the clinic. However, with the emergence of resistance to B-RAF therapy, and a higher than previously thought frequency of somatic MEK mutations, these inhibitors are finding renewed clinical use [13].

Several MEK inhibitors have been identified and are ubdergoing clinical trials: i.e. PD184352 (CI-1040), selumetinib (AZD6244, ARRY-142886), PD0325901, GDC-0973/XL518, trametinib (GSK1120212), MEK162 (ARRY-438162). Worth noticing, most of the known MEK inhibitors are noncompetitive (ie, they do not bind to the ATP–binding site of the kinase) [14]. Despite ATP-biding pockets are highly conserved among human kinases [15], structural analysis of demonstrates tha it harbors a unique site adjacent to the ATP binding site [16]. Thus, biding of inhibitos to this unique MEK site explain the high degree of specificity of the MEK inhibitors compared to other kinase inhibitors with competitive activity.

PD184352 is an orally active highly selective and potent chemical inhibitor of MEK1/2 and was the first MEK inhibitor to enter clinical trials. Selumetinib is the second MEK inhibitor to go into clinical trial after the first MEK inhibitor, CI-1040, demonstrated poor clinical efficacy. Selumetinib is a benzimidazole derivative with reported nanomolar activity against the purified MEK1 enzyme. Through a series of studies using preclinical cell cultures and animal models, it was shown that Selumetinib suppresses the growth of melanoma cells through the induction of cytostasis, but Selumetinib has a limited ability to induce apoptosis or block angiogenesis [17, 18].

3.2.6. *AKT inhibitors*

Akt inhibition promotes decreasing cancer cell survival and proliferation by preventing signal transduction through its downstream effectors as mTOR. Target Akt is an interesting pharmacological approach due to the Akt activation in consequence of the feedback loop release when mTOR is inhibited. Within this group, we can mention allosteric Akt inhibitors (mK2206), Akt catalytic sites inhibitors (PX316, GSK690693, AT-13148, A-443654) and lipid-based phosphatidylinositol (perifosine, triciribine) [32, 36, 39].

The allosteric Akt inhibitors act preventing the translocation of Akt to the plasma membrane, a crucial step for the activation of this molecule, and are more specific for one Akt isoform than the Akt catalytic sites inhibitors which can target all AKT isoforms [42]. Perifosine, the best-characterized Akt inhibitor, is a lipid-based antitumor agent that inhibits Akt Pleckstrin homology (PH) domain preventing the Akt recruitment to the cell membrane and its activation. Perifosine has shown great efficacy in vitro and in vivo against several human cancers such as breast, ovarian, multiple myeloma and glioma and has been tested in clinical trials [30, 32].

3.2.7. mTOR inhibitors

The ATP-competitive inhibitors of mTOR (TORKinhibs) directly inhibit the mTOR kinase activity affecting both mTORC1 and mTORC2. Thus, resulting in antiproliferative effects by decreasing protein synthesis, inducing cell cycle arrest, and inhibiting angiogenesis in several cancer cell lines [22]. Many TORKinhibs have been developed, including Torin1, Torin2, PP242, PP30, KU0063794, WAY-600, WYE-687, WYE-354, XL-388, INK-128, AZD-2014, AZD8055 and OSI-027. Some of them are currently being tested in human subjects with hematological malignancies, glioma and advanced solid tumors in phase I trials [3, 21, 32].

TORKinhibs have achieved better results than rapamycin and rapalogs. This is due to the additional inhibition of mTORC2, which prevents Akt phosphorylation at S473, and also can inhibit mTORC1 with a higher potency. It has been postulated that complete inhibition of mTORC1 is responsible for this enhanced response to treatment, overcoming the limitations of rapamycin. However, it has been found that loss of feedback on PI3K results in activation of downstream effectors other than Akt. Furthermore, these drugs induce phosphorylation of Akt at residue T308, mediated by PDK-1, configuring a resistance mechanism that requires a different therapeutic approach [18, 22, 46].

3.2.8. PI3K and mTOR dual inhibitors

A strategy to overcome the limitations of rapalogs and TORKinhibs is to target two molecules in the PI3K/Akt/mTOR pathway, PI3K and mTOR. The dual PI3K/mTOR inhibitors include NVP-BEZ235, BGT226, XL765, SF1126, GDC-0980, PI-103, PF-04691502, PKI-587, and SK2126458. These drugs inhibit the catalytic activity of mTOR, targeting both mTORC1 and mTORC2 like the TORKinhibs, beyond that they also inhibit PI3K catalytic subunit. Thus, they act on two fronts in the PI3K/AKT/mTOR signaling pathway decreasing cell proliferation, angiogenesis, apoptosis, and inducing cell cycle arrest [21, 47].

The dual PI3K/mTOR inhibitors have demonstrated a greater antitumor efficacy than rapamycin but also have increased toxicity. Nevertheless, some of them are in phase I/II clinical trials for the treatment of lymphoma, glioma, advanced and refractory solid tumors and presented overall good tolerability [8]. Their potent antitumor effect can be explained by the inhibition of AKT phosphorylation at two sites, S473 and T308, blocking downstream signaling more efficiently than rapamycin/rapalogs and TORinhibs alone, as demonstrated in preclinical studies of NVPBEZ-235 and PI-103 [3, 22, 47].

4. Epigenetic drugs

4.1. Histona deacetylace inhibitors

Due to its ability to regulate gene transcription, histone acetylation has been increasely studied. Histone deacetylases (HDACs) are a group of enzymes that, in conjunction with histone acetyltransferases (HATs), regulate the acetylation status of histone tails. HATs acetylate lysine residues on histone tails resulting in neutralization of their charge and decreased affinity for DNA [48].

There are 18 HDACs, which are classified according to functional and phylogenetic criteria [49]. They are divided into Zn2+-dependent (class I, II and IV), Zn2+-independent and NAD-dependent (classIII) enzymes. Most inhibitors currently under development as anti-cancer agents target class I, II and IV enzymes [50].

There are numerous studies demonstrating that HDACs and HATs also regulate acetylation of nonhistone proteins, including transcription factors, chaperone proteins, and signaling molecules involved in cancer development and progression, such as the tumor suppressor p53 [51]. Furthermore, these enzymes are often overexpressed in various types of cancers, compared with the corresponding normal tissues, and their overexpression is correlated with a poor prognosis [52], because they can drive the silencing of tumor suppressor genes or activation of oncogenes [53].

Over recent years, it has been found that the epigenetic silencing of tumor suppressor genes induced by overexpression of HDACs plays an important role in carcinogenesis, above all in hematological cancers [54]. Thus, HDAC inhibitors (HDACi) have emerged as promising accessory therapeutic agents for multiple human malignancies, as, through their action, tumor suppressor gene expression can be restore, cell differentiation can be induce, and both intrinsic and extrinsic apoptotic pathways can be activated [55]. Also, by targeting HDAC6, for example, these inhibitors can stimulate cell cycle arrest, autophagy, and anti-angiogenic effects, can induce oxidative injury, and interfere with tubulin assembly, and cause disruption of the aggregosome pathways [50].

Several HDACi derived both from natural or synthetic sources have been identified. These compounds share a common pharmacophore containing a cap, a connecting unit, a linker and a zinc binding group that chelates the cation in the catalytic domain of the target HDAC [56]. Thus, this class of inhibitors can be separated into several structurally distinct classes according to their chemical structure [53, 57], and each agent varies in its ability to inhibit individual HDACs.

Regarding short chain fatty acids class, **valproate** (valproic acid, VPA) has been used as an anticonvulsant for three decades, and has only recently been recognized as an HDAC inhibitor. It specifically targets 2 of the 4 classes of HDACs: class I, subclasses Ia and Ib, and class II, subclass IIa. Within subclass IIa, HDAC9 is an exception to this modulation, being activated by VPA, which is also true for HDAC11 [58]. **Butyrate**, also a short chain fatty acid, naturally produced by bacterial fermentation in the colon, has been designated as the most potent fatty acid in arresting cell proliferation [59].

Another class of these inhibitors includes hydroxamic acids. In this group, **vorinostat** (SAHA) and **panobinostat** (LBH 589) are the most extensively studied drugs. The latter is currently under phase II/III clinical trials, and the former has been approved by FDA for the treatment of relapsed and refractory cutaneous T-cell lymphoma [60]. Vorinostat represents the second generation of the polar-planar compounds and is a relatively selective inhibitor for class I HDACs; that is, by inhibiting HDAC-1, −2, −3 and −8, but also with mild activity against class II HDAC-6, −10 and −11 [61]. However, vorinostat lacks activity against class II HDAC-4, −5, −7 and −8. **Belinostat**, other compound of this group, has shown efficacy as monotherapy, and has been the basis for the first pivotal phase I trial of this agent to treat relapsed or refractory peripheral T-cell lymphoma [62]. Belinostat's anticancer effect is thought to be mediated through multiple mechanisms of action, including the inhibition of cell proliferation, induction of apoptosis, inhibition of angiogenesis, and induction of differentiation [63]. Moreover, it has been demonstrated that **resminostat** inhibits proliferation and induces apoptosis in multiple myeloma cells [64]. HDACi **PCI-24781** has been shown to enhance chemotherapy-induced apoptosis in multidrug- resistant sarcoma cell lines [65]. **Givinostat** is currently being tested on three trials, but none of these on neoplasias [32], and **JNJ-26481585** shows results in blood malignancies in phase I trial as monotherapy and in combination with proteasome inhibitor (bortezomib).

On benzamides, **entinostat** (MS-275) is an isotype-selective synthetic benzamide derivative HDACi with predominant class I inhibition. Entinostat has been investigated in patients with advanced refractory acute leukemias, mainly acute myeloid leukemia [66]. Whereas, **mocetinostat** is well-tolerated and exhibits favorable pharmacokinetic and pharmacodynamic profiles indicating target inhibition and clinical responses. It induces cell death and autophagy, synergizes with proteasomal inhibitors and affects non-histone targets, such as microtubules [67]. Yet, mocetinostat shows selectivity for HDAC I/II. It has been used in clinical trials mostly for hematological malignancies, such as AML, CML, NHL and refractory Hodgkin disease, where it has shown very encouraging results [68].

Regarding cyclic tetrapeptides, **romidepsin** (ISTODAX®) shows potential as a new agent, having revealed remarkable activity in the treatment of T-cell lymphomas in preclinical studies and early-phase clinical trials. In 2006, it was approved by FDA for the treatment of CTCL in patients who have received at least one prior systemic therapy [69].

Preclinical studies in cell lines and animal models, HDACi have been proven to be very successful as single-modality agents for the treatment of a variety of cancers. Thus, several structurally different HDACi have been used in numerous clinical trials to test their toxicity and effectiveness [32]. The most common adverse effects associated with HDAC inhibitors include thrombocytopenia, neutropenia, diarrhea, nausea, vomiting and fatigue. Extensive studies have been performed to determine whether HDAC inhibitors are associated with cardiac toxicities. Until now, there is little conclusive evidence to determine whether some or all HDAC inhibitors cause electrocardiac changes [70].

Mechanisms of resistance to HDACi are not well elucidated; however it's believed that it may reflect drug efflux, epigenetic alterations, stress response mechanisms and anti-apoptotic, and pro-survival mechanisms [71]. In this context, it is known that DNA hyper-methylation may cause resistance to HDACi, inducing compact nucleosomes, blocking the access to acetylases, which leads to tumor suppression genes silencing [49].

4.2. Rational combination of HDAC inhibitors with current cancer therapy

HDACi have revealed promise in the clinic but there is clearly space for improvement of therapeutic index. One way to achieve greater clinical efficacy is to use HDACi in combination with other chemotherapeutic agents [53, 72]. There have been numerous preclinical and clinical studies examining rational combinations of HDACi with many current therapies for the treatment of hematological and solid malignancies [60]. Indeed, it has been described that HDACi have synergistic or additive effect with different anticancer agents, including radiation therapy, chemotherapy, hormonal therapies and new targeted agents.

Regarding HDACi in combination with radiotherapy, these inhibitors, including vorinostat, TSA, valproic acid and PCI-24781, enhance the radiosensitivity of cancer cells [73]. Chemotherapeutic agents with additive or synergistic effects with HDACi therapy includes: antitubulin agent (docetaxel) [74]; topoisomerase II inhibitors (doxorubicin, etoposide, and ellipticine) [75, 76]; and DNA cross-linking reagent (i.e. cisplatin) [77].

HDACi combinations with hormonal therapy are also possible. In this context, clinical trials are in progress for BC and prostate cancer (PC). As a monotherapy, the HDACi vorinostat has not shown effectiveness in metastatic BC and PC [78]. On the other hand, preclinical studies have demonstrated that HDACi potentiates the antitumor activity of tamoxifen in a variety of ER-positive BC cell lines [79]; whereas in PC the addition of an HDACi to the anti-androgen bicalutamide have resulted in a synergistic increase in cytotoxicity on hormone-sensitive and resistant preclinical models [80].

Recent studies showed that the combination of some of the specific RTK-targeted therapies with HDCAi can represent a novel way for suppressing tumor growth. Combined therapies with transtuzumab [81], erlotinib and gefitinib [82], sorafenib [83], everolimus [84], imatinib [85], heat shock protein-90 inhibitor 17-N-allylamino-17-demethoxygeldanamycin [86] and bortezomide, a proteasome inhibitor [87], have been studied. The obtained data indicate that, although preclinical studies demonstrated a benefit, it is too early to know whether this combination will prove more beneficial than treatment with RTK pathway inhibitors alone.

Hematological malignancies appear to be particularly sensitive to HDACi therapy. There are well over 100 clinical trials ongoing with HDACi as monotherapy or in combination therapy for several carcinomas. The available results for these clinical trials have recently been reviewed [50]. As mentioned, vorinostat and romidepsin have been approved by FDA for the treatment advanced and refractory cutaneous T-cell lymphoma (CTCL). The clinical value of HDACi in other malignancies remains to be determined.

5. PARPs inhibitors

Poly ADP ribose polymerases (PARPs) are a family of 17 proteins pooled together based on their structural similarity, specifically, they are composed by two ribose moieties and two phosphates per polymer unit [88]. Known since 1963, these enzymes function is to catalyses the polymerization and formation of highly negatively charged poly ADP ribose chains on target proteins, therefore modifying their action [89]. Furthermore, PARPs contain three zinc finger motifs which bind with high affinity to DNA breaks and triggers the enzyme's catalytic module and synthesis of negatively-charged, branched polymers of poly(ADP-ribose) (PAR) from NAD+ [90]. Currently, PARP 1 and PARP 2 are the best understood of these proteins and their key role is to maintain genomic integrity, in particular the repair of single strand DNA lesions and breaks, using the base excision repair (BER) pathway [91]. Moreover, PARPs are also involved in activating apoptosis on both caspase dependent or independent fashion; however this PARP hole is not yet fully understood and will not be discussed in this chapter [92].

5.1. PARPs inhibitors in cancer therapy

Durkacz and colleagues proposed, in 1980, that modulating PARP-1 might augment the effect of alkylating chemotherapy [93]. So far the modulation of its activity by stimulation or inhibition can be applied in therapy or prevention of several pathologies including cardiac infarct [94], septic shock [95], diabetes [96], inflammation [97], neurodegenerative disorders [98], and acute necrotizing pancreatitis [99]. Lately a new potential strategy for therapy has emerged, the PARP inhibitors, using the synthetic lethality and exploiting tumor-specific genetic alterations. Synthetic lethality is defined as the premise, whereby, deletion of one of two genes independently has no effect on cellular viability, whereas, simultaneous loss of both genes is lethal [100]. It has become clear that the genomic instability of some tumor cells allows PARP inhibitors to have selectivity for the tumor cells over normal cells, what explains why this class of drugs shows fewer side effects as a single agent. Taken together, inhibition of these enzymes and, therefore, the BER pathway causes persistence of single strand breaks (SSBs) leading to cell death. Also, PARP inhibitors, when in combination with cytotoxic agents, prevent repair of SSBs caused by these agents in cells with underlying homologous recombination (HR) defects [101].

It has been shown that cancer cells with mutations in the breast and ovarian susceptibility genes BRCA1 and BRCA2 are extremely sensitive to small molecule inhibitors of PARP-1 [102, 103]. Thus, PARP inhibitors have raised as a promise in phase I and phase II clinical trials for the treatment of BRCA1/2-deficient breast, ovarian and prostate tumors [104-106]. However, a recently completed phase III study combining PARP inhibition with chemotherapy did not generate the anticipated survival gains; suggesting that additional, as yet unidentified, molecular factors may influence the *in vivo* anti-tumor effectiveness of this class of drugs [107, 108].

5.2. PARPs inhibitors under clinical development

Some PARP inhibitors, targeting both PARP-1 and PARP-2, were recently under clinical development, which include Pfizer's PF 01367338 (AG014699), AstraZeneca's olaparib (AZD2281, KU-0059436), Sanofi-Aventis' iniparib (BSI 201) and Abbott Laboratories' veliparib (ABT 888) [109].

The first agent analyzed clinically was AG014699 (the phosphate salt of AG14361), in 2003. Publications described preclinical data for 39 OVCA cell lines (without reporting BRCA status of these cell lines) with AG014699 as single-agent or in combination (with carboplatin, doxorubicin, gemcitabine, paclitaxel, or topotecan) using combination index/isobologram analysis for multiple drug effect analysis. The investigators noted a concentration-dependent efficacy across the different cell lines to different degrees. The greatest impact appears to be in combination with carboplatin, topotecan, and doxorubicin. Therefore, an initial phase I was conducted with temozolide (TMZ), both given for 5 days in 28-day cycles, with patients with solid tumors. A subsequent phase II study with melanoma patients has been reported. Overall, there was modest activity with significant myelosuppression. The study started using one-half standard dose (100 mg/m^2) of TMZ and AG014699 was escalated to PARP inhibitory dose (PID) as evaluated from peripheral blood mononuclear cell (PBMCs). The PID, defined as at least 50% of decrease in PARP activity 24 hours after dosing, was determined to be 12 mg/m^2 and at this dose there was 74-97% inhibition of peripheral blood mononuclear cells (PBMCs) PARP. The mean terminal half-life was 7.4-11.7 hours. The PARP in the PBMCs recovered at least 50% function by 72 hours after dosing. The dose limiting toxicity (DLT) for the highest dose level tested of 18 mg/m^2 in combination with standard dose TMZ and lead to myelosuppression [110]. The phase II study evaluated the efficacy of AG014699 at 12 mg/m^2 with TMZ at 200 mg/m^2 in 40 chemotherapy-naive patients with advanced multiple melanoma. Myelosuppression was more significant in the phase II trial than seen in the phase I trial. It was reported several signs of toxicity besides fatigue and nausea: 12% grade four thrombocytopenia, 15% neutropenia, and one death from febrile neutropenia. There were four partial responses (PRs), four prolonged stable diseases, and 10 patients were too early to evaluate at the time of the report [111].

Olaparib is an oral PARP inhibitor (IC_{50} = 4.9 nM for PARP 1) extensively studied for BRCA tumors treatment in combination or as single agent. In a phase I trial, olaparib was given at days 1-4, cisplatin at day 3, and gemcitabine at days 3 and 10, every 21 days. As toxicities effects, five of six patients experienced grade three or four thrombocytopenia. Two PRs were reported in 1 pancreatic cancer and 1 NSCLC patient [112]. Another phase I, this time focusing olaparib as single-agent, enrolled 60 patients with solid tumors, including 22 BRCA mutation patients. This study supported the synthetic lethality concept. Patients were treated at escalating doses and duration. Doses of 10 mg QD 2 out of 3 weeks to 600 mg BID continuously were evaluated. The initial cohort was not restricted to BRCA-deficient patients but was enriched for this population. In the expansion cohort, patients had to have BRCA mutation to enroll and were treated at 200 mg BID continuously. Eight PRs, by response evaluation criteria in solid tumors (RECIST), were observed out of the 15 patients with BRCA mutation-related advanced OVCA group. All the responses in OVCA were seen in BRCA mutated tumors [105].

Iniparib (BSI 201 or 4-iodo-3-nitrobenzamide) is a prodrug which irreversibly inhibits PARP-1 and it is the first PARP inhibitor to show survival advantage in triple-negative breast cancer (TNBC) patients. It has entered in phase III study despite the fact its active metabolite is still unknown. Iniparib is given intravenously twice a week. The phase I study included 23 patients with solid tumors. The concentration that brought about efficacy in preclinical models was 20-30 ng/mL, so achievable levels were well over the preclinical efficacious levels. The 2.8 mg/kg dose caused PARP inhibition in PBMCs by more than 50% with the first dose. Subsequent dosing increased the amount of PARP inhibition to more than 80%. Six of the 23 heavily pretreated patients had stable disease for at least 2 months (up to over 9 months in 1 patient) [113].

Veliparib has been shown to be a potent inhibitor of PARP, as well as, to have a good bioavailability. In pre-clinical studies veliparib potentiated TMZ, platinum agents, cyclophosphamide, and radiation in syngeneic and xenograft tumor models [114]. Combined with topotecan, veliparib has showed significant myelosuppression. The original schedule was topotecan at days 8 and 2-5 at 1.2 mg/m^2, and veliparib 10 mg BID at days 1-7. The schedule was changed to topotecan at days 1-5 when 0.9 mg/m2 of it was not tolerated [115]. Furthermore, PARP inhibitors also augmented the effect of irradiation *in vivo,* as shown in mouse colon cancer xenograft model, where combined therapy increased survival from 23 days with radiation alone to 36 days. One subject also presented complete remission (CR) [108].

Unfortunately, as well as for other therapies, resistance to PARP inhibitors has already been reported. A possible explanation for that would be that a second mutation, a compensatory mutation or a crossover could reestablish the wild-type BCRA protein, reversing the BCRA deficiency [109]. Additionally, upregulation of p-glycoprotein efflux pump, 53BP1 silencing 53BP1 and increased expression of PARP by the tumor have also been shown as a resistance mechanism for PARP inhibitors [116]. Nevertheless, overcoming this resistance could be achieved by: a third mutation on BCRA, which converts the cell back to the mutated form; a mutation that inhibits HR; downregulation of the P-glycoprotein pump; or, upregulation of 53BP1. Recently 6-thioguanine (6-TG) has been shown to be active in cells resistant to PARP inhibitors in BRCA2 deficient tumors [117].

6. Conclusions

Despite the difficulties encountered by physicians and patients in the fight against cancer, we are currently witnessing an ever growing spectrum of new targets and strategies to combat this disease. Considering that an optimal therapy for cancer would be developed based on specific aspect of each patient, target therapies appear as important alternatives to overcome the hurdles presented by currently available strategies. Moreover, as different molecules can be targeted at once, in combination or not with conventional therapies, issues associated to resistance are thought to be milder than with chemotherapy alone. Altogether, we consider that target therapy brings the possibility of increasing patients' overall survival, quality of life, and, maybe, could point to the possibility of vanquishing this disease.

Author details

Taciane Ladislau, Klesia P Madeira, Renata D Daltoé, Isabella S Guimarães, Sarah F Teixeira, Paulo CM Lyra-Júnior, Iuri C Valadão, Leticia BA Rangel and Alice L Herlinger

Laboratory of Cellular and Molecular Biology of Human Cancer, Federal University of Espírito Santo State, Brazil

Authors Taciane Ladislau and Klesia P Madeira equally contributed to the elaboration of this chapter

References

[1] Blume-jensen, P, & Hunter, T. Oncogenic kinase signaling. Nature (2001). , 411, 355-365.

[2] Dancey, J, & Sausville, E. A. Issues and progress with protein kinase inhibitors for cancer treatment. Nature Reviews Drug Discovery (2003). , 2(4), 296-313.

[3] Willems, L, Tamburini, J, Chapuis, N, & Lacombe, C. Mayeux P & Bouscary D. PI3K and mTOR signaling pathways in cancer: new data on targeted therapies. Current Oncology Reports (2012). , 14, 129-138.

[4] Ogita S & LoRuss PTargeting phosphatidylinositol 3 kinase (PI3K)-Akt beyond rapalogs. Targeted Oncology (2011). , 6, 103-117.

[5] Roberts, P. J. Der CJ. Targeting the Raf-MEK-ERK mitogen-activated protein kinase cascade for the treatment of cancer. Oncogene (2007). , 26(22), 3291-310.

[6] Zhang, J, Yang, P. L, & Gray, N. S. Targeting cancer with small molecule kinase inhibitors. Nature Reviews Cancer (2009). , 9(1), 28-39.

[7] Adnane, L, Trail, P. A, Taylor, I, & Wilhelm, S. M. Sorafenib (BAY 43-9006, Nexavar), a dual-action inhibitor that targets RAF/MEK/ERK pathway in tumor cells and tyrosine kinases VEGFR/PDGFR in tumor vasculature. Methods in Ezymology (2006). , 407, 597-612.

[8] Egberts, F, Kahler, K. C, Livingstone, E, & Hauschild, A. Metastaticmelanoma: Scientific rationale for sorafenib treatment and clinical results. Onkologie (2008). , 3, 398-403.

[9] Eisen, T, Ahmad, T, Flaherty, K. T, Gore, M, Kaye, S, Marais, R, Gibbens, I, Hackett, S, James, M, Schuchter, L. M, Nathanson, K. L, Xia, C, Simantov, R, Schwartz, B, Poulin-costello, M, Dwyer, O, & Ratain, P. J. MJ. Sorafenib in advanced melanoma: A phase II randomised discontinuation trial analysis. British Journal of Cancer (2006). , 95(5), 581-586.

[10] Gupta-abramson, V, Troxel, A. B, Nellore, A, Puttaswamy, K, Redlinger, M, Ransone, K, Mandel, S. J, Flaherty, K. T, Loevner, L. A, Dwyer, O, Brose, P. J, & Phase, M. S. II Trial of sorafenib in advanced thyroid cancer. Journal of Clinical Oncology (2008). , 26(29), 4714-4719.

[11] Keating, G. M. Vemurafenib: in unresectable or metastatic melanoma. BioDrugs (2012). , 26(5), 325-324.

[12] Gollob, J. A, Wilhelm, S, Carter, C, & Kelley, S. L. Role of Raf kinase in cancer: therapeutic potential of targeting the Raf/MEK/ERK signal transduction pathway. Seminars in Oncology (2006). , 33(4), 392-406.

[13] Bromberg-white, J. L, Andersen, N. J, & Duesbery, N. S. MEK genomics in development and disease. Briefings in Functional Genomics (2012). , 11(4), 300-310.

[14] Wallace, E. M, Lyssikatos, J. P, Yeh, T, Winkler, J. D, & Koch, K. Progress towards therapeutic small molecule MEK inhibitors for use in cancer therapy. Current Topics in Medicinal Chemistry (2005). , 5(2), 215-229.

[15] Messersmith, W. A, Hidalgo, M, Carducci, M, & Eckhardt, S. G. Novel targets in solid tumors: MEK inhibitors. Clinical Advances in Hematology and Oncology (2006). , 4(11), 831-836.

[16] Ohren, J. F, Chen, H, Pavlovsky, A, Whitehead, C, Zhang, E, Kuffa, P, Yan, C, Mcconnell, P, Spessard, C, Banotai, C, Mueller, W. T, Delaney, A, Omer, C, Sebolt-leopold, J, Dudley, D. T, Leung, I. K, Flamme, C, Warmus, J, Kaufman, M, Barrett, S, Tecle, H, & Hasemann, C. A. Structures of human MAP kinase kinase 1 (MEK1) and MEK2 describe novel noncompetitive kinase inhibition. Nature Structural & Molecular Biology (2004). , 11(12), 1192-1197.

[17] Allen, L. F, Sebolt-leopold, J, & Meyer, M. B. CI-1040 (PD184352), a target signal transduction inhibitor of MEK (MAPKK). Seminars in Oncology (2003). , 30(5), 105-116.

[18] Davies, B. R, Logie, A, Mckay, J. S, Martin, P, Steele, S, Jenkins, R, Cockerill, M, Cartlidge, S, & Smith, P. D. AZD6244 (ARRY-142886), a potent inhibitor of mitogen-activated protein kinase/extracellular signal-regulated kinase kinase 1/2 kinases: mechanism of action in vivo, pharmacokinetic/pharmacodynamic relationship, and

potential for combination in preclinical models. Molecular Cancer Therapeutics (2007)., 6(8), 2209-2219.

[19] Liu, Q, Thoreen, C, & Wang, J. Sabatini D & Gray NS. mTOR mediated anti-cancer drug discovery. Drug Discovery Today: Therapeutic Strategies (2009)., 6, 47-55.

[20] Alvarado, Y, Mita, M. M, & Vemulapalli, S. Mahalingam D & Mita AC. Clinical activity of mammalian target of rapamycin inhibitors in solid tumors. Targeted Oncology (2011)., 6, 69-94.

[21] Zaytseva, Y. Y, & Valentino, J. D. Gulhati P & Evers BM. mTOR inhibitors in cancer therapy. Cancer Letters (2012)., 319, 1-7.

[22] Guertin DA & Sabatini DMThe Pharmacology of mTOR Inhibition. Science Signaling (2009)., 2, 24-30.

[23] Sarbassov, D. D, Ali, S. M, Sengupta, S, Sheen, J. H, Hsu, P. P, Bagley, A. F, Markhard, A. L, & Sabatini, D. M. Prolonged rapamycin treatment inhibits mTORC2 assembly and Akt/PKB. Molecular Cell (2006)., 22, 159-168.

[24] Zeng, Z. Sarbassov dos D, Samudio IJ, Yee KW, Munsell MF, Ellen Jackson C, Giles FJ, Sabatini DM, Andreeff M & Konopleva M. Rapamycin derivatives reduce mTORC2 signaling and inhibit AKT activation in AML. Blood (2007). , 109, 3509-3512.

[25] Guertin DA & Sabatini DMDefining the role of mTOR in cancer. Cancer Cell (2007)., 12, 9-22.

[26] Food, U. S. and Drug Administration. FDA: Drugs. http://www.fda.gov/Drugs/default.htmaccessed 7 August (2012).

[27] Diaz-padilla, I, & Duran, I. Clarke BA & Oza AM. Biologic rationale and clinical activity of mTOR inhibitors in gynecological cancer. Cancer Treatment Reviews (2012)., 38, 767-775.

[28] Weisberg, E, Manley, P, Mestan, J, Cowan-jacob, S, Ray, A, & Griffin, J. D. AMN107 (nilotinib): a novel and selective inhibitor of BCR-ABL. British Journal of Cancer (2006)., 94(12), 1765-1769.

[29] Propper, D. J, Mcdonald, A. C, Man, A, Thavasu, P, Balkwill, F, Braybrooke, J. P, Caponigro, F, Graf, P, Dutreix, C, Blackie, R, Kaye, S. B, Ganesan, T. S, Talbot, D. C, Harris, A. L, Twelves, C, & Phase, I. and pharmacokinetic study of PKC412, an inhibitor of protein kinase C. Journal of Clinical Oncology (2001)., 19(5), 1485-92.

[30] Sun W & Modak SEmerging treatment options for the treatment of neuroblastoma: potential role of perifosine. Journal of Onco Targets and Therapy (2012)., 5, 21-29.

[31] National Cancer InstituteNCI: Search for Clinical Trials. http://www.cancer.gov/clinicaltrials/searchaccessed 6 August (2012).

[32] U.S. National Institute of Health clinicaltrials.gov. http://clinicaltrials.gov/ct2/search (accessed 7 August 2012).

[33] Wang, H. P, Zhang, L, Wang, Y. X, Tan, F. L, Xia, Y, Ren, G. J, Hu, P, Jiang, J, Wang, M. Z, & Xiao, Y. Phase I trial of icotinib, a novel epidermal growth factor receptor tyrosine kinase inhibitor, in Chinese patients with non-small cell lung cancer. Chinese Medical Journal (English Edition) (2011).

[34] Zhao, Q, Shentu, J, Xu, N, Zhou, J, Yang, G, Yao, Y, Tan, F, Liu, D, Wang, Y, & Zhou, J. Phase I study of icotinib hydrochloride (BPI-2009H), an oral EGFR tyrosine kinase inhibitor, in patients with advanced NSCLC and other solid tumors. Lung Cancer (2011)., 73(2), 195-202.

[35] LoPiccolo JBlumenthal GM, Bernstein WB & Dennis PA. Targeting the PI3K/Akt/mTOR pathway: effective combinations and clinical considerations. Drug Resistance Updates (2008)., 11, 32-50.

[36] Liu, P, & Cheng, H. Roberts TM & Zhao JJ. Targeting the phosphoinositide 3-kinase (PI3K) pathway in cancer. Nature Reviews Drug Discovery (2009)., 8, 627-644.

[37] Mccubrey, J. A, Steelman, L. S, Abrams, S. L, Lee, J. T, Chang, F, Bertrand, F. E, Navolanic, P. M, Terrian, D. M, Franklin, R. A, Assoro, D, Salisbury, A. B, Mazzarino, J. L, Stivala, M. C, & Libra, F. M. Roles of the RAF/MEK/ERK and PI3K/ PTEN/AKT pathways in malignant transformation and drug resistance. Advances in Enzyme Regulation (2006)., 46(1), 249-279.

[38] Schatz, J. H. Targeting the PI3K/AKT/mTOR pathway in non-Hodgkin's lymphoma: results, biology, and development strategies. Current Oncology Reports (2011). , 13398-406.

[39] Hernandez-aya, L. F, & Gonzalez-angulo, A. M. Targeting the phosphatidylinositol 3-kinase signaling pathway in breast cancer. The Oncologist (2011)., 16, 404-414.

[40] Jia, S, Liu, Z, Zhang, S, Liu, P, Zhang, L, Lee, S. H, Zhang, J, Signoretti, S, & Loda, M. Roberts TM & Zhao JJ. Essential roles of PI(3)K-in cell growth, metabolism and tumorigenesis. Nature (2008)., 110beta.

[41] Graupera, M, Guillermet-guibert, J, Foukas, L. C, Phng, L. K, Cain, R. J, Salpekar, A, Pearce, W, Meek, S, Millan, J, Cutillas, P. R, Smith, A. J, Ridley, A. J, & Ruhrberg, C. Gerhardt H & Vanhaesebroeck B. Angiogenesis selectively requires the isoform of PI3K to control endothelial cell migration. Nature (2008)., 110alpha.

[42] Engelman, J. A, & Targeting, P. I. K signalling in cancer: opportunities, challenges and limitations. Nature Reviews Cancer (2009)., 9, 550-562.

[43] Anforth, R. M, Blumetti, T. C, Kefford, R. F, Sharma, R, Scolyer, R. A, Kossard, S, Long, G. V, & Fernandez-peñas, P. Cutaneous Manifestations of Dabrafenib (GSK2118436): A Selective Inhibitor of Mutant BRAF in patients with Metastatic Melanoma. British Journal of Dermatology (2012)., 1365-2133.

[44] James, J, Ruggeri, B, Armstrong, R. C, Rowbottom, M. W, Jones-bolin, S, Gunawardane, R. N, Dobrzanski, P, Gardner, M. F, Zhao, H, Cramer, M. D, Hunter, K, Nepomuceno, R. R, Cheng, M, Gitnick, D, Yazdanian, M, Insko, D. E, Ator, M. A, Apuy, J. L, Faraoni, R, Dorsey, B. D, Williams, M, Bhagwat, S. S, & Holladay, M. W. CEP-32496: a novel orally active BRAF(inhibitor with selective cellular and in vivo antitumor activity. Molecular Cancer Therapie (2012). , 600E

[45] Beeram, M, Patnaik, A, & Rowinsky, E. K. Raf: a strategic target for therapeutic development agains cancer. Journal of Clinical Oncology (2005). , 23(27), 6771-6790.

[46] Thoreen, C. C, Kang, S. A, Chang, J. W, Liu, Q, Zhang, J, Gao, Y, Reichling, L. J, Sim, T, Sabatini, D. M, & Gray, N. S. An ATP-competitive mammalian target of rapamycin inhibitor reveals rapamycin-resistant functions of mTORC1. The Journal of Biological Chemistry (2009). , 284, 8023-32.

[47] Manara, M. C, Nicoletti, G, Zambelli, D, Ventura, S, Guerzoni, C, Landuzzi, L, Lollini, P. L, Maira, S. M, García-echeverría, C, & Mercuri, M. Picci P & Scotlandi K. NVP-BEZ235 as a new therapeutic option for sarcomas. Clinical Cancer Research (2010). , 16, 530-40.

[48] Hong, L, Schroth, G. P, Matthews, H. R, Yau, P, & Bradbury, E. M. Studies of the DNA binding properties of histone H4 amino terminus. Thermal denaturation studies reveal that acetylation markedly reduces the binding constant of the H4 "tail" to DNA. Blood (1993). , 268, 305-314.

[49] Marks, P. A, & Xu, W. S. Histone deacetylase inhibitors: Potential in cancer therapy. Journal of Cellular Biochemistry (2009). , 107, 600-608.

[50] Khan, O. La Thangue NB. HDAC inhibitors in cancer biology: emerging mechanisms and clinical applications. Immunology and Cell Biology (2012). , 90, 85-94.

[51] Gu, W, & Roeder, R. G. Activation of sequence-specific DNA binding by acetylation of the p53 C-terminal domain. Cell (1997). , 53.

[52] Weichert, W, Röske, A, Gekeler, V, Beckers, T, Stephan, C, Jung, K, Fritzsche, F. R, Niesporek, S, Denkert, C, Dietel, M, & Kristiansen, G. Histone deacetylases 1, 2 and 3 are highly expressed in prostate cancer and HDAC2 expression is associated with shorter PSA relapse time after radical prostatectomy. British Journal of Cancer (2008). , 98, 604-610.

[53] Miller, C. P, & Singh, M. M. Rivera-Del Valle N, Manton CA, Chandra J. Therapeutic strategies to enhance the anticancer efficacy of histone deacetylase inhibitors. Journal of Biomedicine and Biotechnology (2011). , 2011, 1-17.

[54] Pan, L. N, Lu, J, & Huang, B. HDAC inhibitors: a potential new category of anti-tumor agents. Cellular & Molecular Immunology (2007). , 4, 337-343.

[55] Xu, W, Ngo, L, Perez, G, Dokmanovic, M, & Marks, P. A. Intrinsic apoptotic and thioredoxin pathways in human prostate cancer cell response to histone deacetylase inhibitor. Proceedings of the National Academy of Sciences (2006). , 103, 15540-15545.

[56] Bertrand, P. Inside HDAC with HDAC inhibitors. The European Journal of Medicinal Chemistry (2010). , 45, 2095-2116.

[57] Dickinson, M, Johnstone, R. W, & Prince, H. M. Histone deacetylase inhibitors: potential targets responsible for their anti-cancer effect. Investigational New Drugs (2010). , 28, 3-20.

[58] Bradbury, C. A, Khanim, F. L, Hayden, R, Bunce, C. M, White, D. A, Drayson, M. T, Craddock, C, & Turner, B. M. Histone deacetylases in acute myeloid leukaemia show a distinctive pattern of expression that changes selectively in response to deacetylase inhibitors. Leukemia (2005). , 19, 1751-1759.

[59] Louis, M, Rosato, R. R, Brault, L, Osbild, S, Battaglia, E, Yang, X. H, Grant, S, & Bagrel, D. The histone deacetylase inhibitor sodium butyrate induces breast cancer cell apoptosis through diverse cytotoxic actions including glutathione depletion and oxidative stress. International Journal of Oncology (2004). , 25, 1701-1711.

[60] Thurn, K. T, Thomas, S, Moore, A, & Munster, P. N. Rational therapeutic combinations with histone deacetylase inhibitors for the treatment of cancer. Future Oncology (2011). , 2, 263-283.

[61] Matalon, S, Palmer, B. E, Nold, M. F, Furlan, A, Kassu, A, Fossati, G, Mascagni, P, & Dinarello, C. A. The histone deacetylase inhibitor ITF2357 decreases surface CXCR4 and CCR5 expression on CD4(+) T-cells and monocytes and is superior to valproic acid for latent HIV-1 expression in vitro. Journal of Acquired Immune Deficiency Syndromes (2010). , 54, 1-9.

[62] Zain, J. M, & Connor, O. O. Targeted treatment and new agents in peripheral T-cell lymphoma. International Journal of Hematology (2010). , 92, 33-44.

[63] Kapoor, S. Inhibition of HDAC6-dependent carcinogenesis: emerging, new therapeutic options besides belinostat. International Journal of Cancer (2009). , 124, 509-520.

[64] Mandl-weber, S, Meinel, F. G, Jankowsky, R, Oduncu, F, Schmidmaier, R, & Baumann, P. The novel inhibitor of histone deacetylase resminostat (RAS2410) inhibits proliferation and induces apoptosis in multiple myeloma (MM) cells. British Journal of Haematology (2010). , 149, 218-528.

[65] Yang, C, Choy, E, Hornicek, F. J, Wood, K. B, Schwab, J. H, Liu, X, Mankin, H, & Duan, Z. Histone deacetylase inhibitor PCI-24781 enhances chemotherapy-induced apoptosis in multidrug-resistant sarcoma cell lines. Anticancer Research (2011). , 31, 1115-1123.

[66] Gojo, I, Tidwell, M. L, Greer, J, Takebe, N, Seiter, K, Pochron, M. F, Johnson, B, Sznol, M, Karp, J. E, & Phase, I. and pharmacokinetic study of Triapine, a potent ribonucleo-

tide reductase inhibitor, in adults with advanced hematologic malignancies. Leukemia Research (2007). , 31, 1165-1173.

[67] Boumber, Y, Younes, A, & Garcia-manero, G. Mocetinostat (MGCD0103): a review of an isotype-specific histone deacetylase inhibitor. Expert Opinion on Investigational Drugs (2011). , 20, 823-829.

[68] Tambaro, F. P. Dell'aversana C, Carafa V, Nebbioso A, Radic B, Ferrara F, Altucci L. Histone deacetylase inhibitors: clinical implications for hematological malignancies. Clinical Epigenetics (2010).

[69] Jain, S, & Zain, J. Romidepsin in the treatment of cutaneous T-cell lymphoma. Journal of Blood Medicine (2011). , 2, 37-47.

[70] Münster, P, Marchion, D, Bicaku, E, Schmitt, M, Lee, J. H, Deconti, R, Simon, G, Fishman, M, Minton, S, Garrett, C, Chiappori, A, Lush, R, Sullivan, D, & Daud, A. Phase I trial of histone deacetylase inhibition by valproic acid followed by the topoisomerase II inhibitor epirubicin in advanced solid tumors: a clinical and translational study. Journal of Clinical Oncology (2007). , 15, 1979-1985.

[71] Fantin, V. R, & Richon, V. M. Mechanisms of resistance to histone deacetylase inhibitors and their therapeutic implications. Clinical Cancer Research (2007). , 13, 7237-7242.

[72] Bots, M, & Johnstone, R. W. Rational combinations using HDAC inhibitors. Clinical Cancer Research (2009). , 15, 3970-3977.

[73] Munshi, A, Kurland, J. F, Nishikawa, T, Tanaka, T, Hobbs, M. L, Tucker, S. L, Ismail, S, Stevens, C, & Meyn, R. E. Histone deacetylase inhibitors radiosensitize human melanoma cells by suppressing DNA repair activity. Clinical Cancer Research (2005). , 11, 4912-4922.

[74] Owonikoko, T. K, Ramalingam, S. S, Kanterewicz, B, Balius, T. E, Belani, C. P, & Hershberger, P. A. Vorinostat increases carboplatin and paclitaxel activity in non-small-cell lung cancer cells. Internacional Journal of Cancer (2010). , 126, 743-755.

[75] Lopez, G, Liu, J, Ren, W, Wei, W, Wang, S, Lahat, G, Zhu, Q. S, Bornmann, W. G, Mcconkey, D. J, Pollock, R. E, & Lev, D. C. Combining PCI-24781, a novel histone deacetylase inhibitor, with chemotherapy for the treatment of soft tissue sarcoma. Clinical Cancer Research (2009). , 15, 3472-3483.

[76] Das, C. M, Aguilera, D, Vasquez, H, Prasad, P, Zhang, M, Wolff, J. E, & Gopalakrishnan, V. Valproic acid induces and topoisomerase-II (alpha/beta) expression and synergistically enhances etoposide cytotoxicity in human glioblastoma cell lines. Journal of Neuro-Oncology (2007). , 21.

[77] Noguchi, H, Yamashita, H, Murakami, T, Hirai, K, Noguchi, Y, Maruta, J, Yokoi, T, & Noguchi, S. Successful treatment of anaplastic thyroid carcinoma with a combination

of oral valproic acid, chemotherapy, radiation and surgery. Endocrinology Journal (2009). , 56, 245-249.

[78] Luu, T. H, Morgan, R. J, Leong, L, Lim, D, Mcnamara, M, Portnow, J, Frankel, P, Smith, D. D, & Doroshow, J. H. Wong. A phase II trial of vorinostat (suberoylanilide hydroxamic acid) in metastatic breast cancer: a California Cancer Consortium study. Clinical Cancer Research (2008). , 14, 7138-7142.

[79] Biçaku, E, Marchion, D. C, Schmitt, M. L, & Münster, P. N. Selective inhibition of histone deacetylase 2 silences progesterone receptor-mediated signaling. Cancer Research (2008). , 68, 1513-1519.

[80] Pfeiffer, M. J, Mulders, P. F, & Schalken, J. A. An in vitro model for preclinical testing of endocrine therapy combinations for prostate cancer. Prostate (2010). , 70, 1524-1532.

[81] Conte, P, Campone, M, & Pronzato, P. Phase I trial of panobinostat (LBH589) in combination with trastuzumab in pretreated HERpositive metastatic breast cancer (MBC): preliminary safety and tolerability results. Journal Clinical Oncology (2009). , 2.

[82] Witta, S. E, Dziadziuszko, R, Yoshida, K, Hedman, K, & Varella-garcia, M. Bunn PA Jr, Hirsch FR. ErbB-3 expression is associated with E-cadherin and their coexpression restores response to gefitinib in non-small-cell lung cancer (NSCLC). Annals of Oncology (2009). , 20, 989-695.

[83] Baradari, V, Höpfner, M, Huether, A, Schuppan, D, & Scherübl, H. Histone deacetylase inhibitor MS-275 alone or combined with bortezomib or sorafenib exhibits strong antiproliferative action in human cholangiocarcinoma cells. World Journal of Gastroenterology (2007). , 13, 4458-4466.

[84] Wedel, S, Hudak, L, Seibel, J. M, Juengel, E, Tsaur, I, Wiesner, C, Haferkamp, A, & Blaheta, R. A. Inhibitory effects of the HDAC inhibitor valproic acid on prostate cancer growth are enhanced by simultaneous application of the mTOR inhibitor RAD001. Life Science (2011). , 88, 418-424.

[85] Nguyen, T, Dai, Y, Attkisson, E, Kramer, L, Jordan, N, Nguyen, N, Kolluri, N, Muschen, M, & Grant, S. HDAC inhibitors potentiate the activity of the BCR/ABL kinase inhibitor KW-2449 in imatinib-sensitive or-resistant BCR/ABL+ leukemia cells in vitro and in vivo. Clinical Cancer Research (2011). , 17, 3219-3232.

[86] Rahmani, M, Reese, E, Dai, Y, Bauer, C, Kramer, L. B, Huang, M, Jove, R, Dent, P, & Grant, S. Cotreatment with suberanoylanilide hydroxamic acid and 17-allylamino 17-demethoxygeldanamycin synergistically induces apoptosis in Bcr-Abl+ Cells sensitive and resistant to STI571 (imatinib mesylate) in association with down-regulation of Bcr-Abl, abrogation of signal transducer and activator of transcription 5 activity, and Bax conformational change. Molecular Pharmacology (2005). , 67, 1166-1176.

[87] Yu, C, Rahmani, M, Conrad, D, Subler, M, Dent, P, & Grant, S. The proteasome inhibitor bortezomib interacts synergistically with histone deacetylase inhibitors to induce apoptosis in Bcr/Abl+ cells sensitive and resistant to STI571. Blood (2003). , 102, 3765-3774.

[88] Zaremba, T, & Curtin, N. J. PARP inhibitor development for systemic cancer targetings. Anti- Cancer Agents in Medicinal Chemistry (2007). , 7(5), 515-523.

[89] Chambon, P, Weill, J. D, & Mandel, P. Nicotinamide mononucleotide activations of new DNA-dependent polyadenylic acid synthesizing nuclear enzyme. Biochemical and Biophysical Research Communications (1963). , 11, 39-43.

[90] Malanga, M, & Althaus, F. R. The role of poly(ADP-ribose) in the DNA damage signaling network. Biochemistry and Cell Biology (2005). , 83, 354-364.

[91] Schreiber, V, Dantzer, F, Ame, J. C, & De Murcia, G. Poly(ADP-ribose): novel functions for an old molecule. Nature Reviews Molecular Cell Biology (2006). , 7(7), 517-528.

[92] Sevrioukova, I. F. Apoptosis-inducing factor: structure, function, andredox regulation. Antioxid.Redox. Signal (2011). , 14, 2545-2579.

[93] Durkacz, B. W, Omidiji, O, Gray, D. A, & Shall, S. ADP-ribose)n participates in DNA excision repair. Nature (1980). , 283(5747), 593-596.

[94] Roesner, J. P, Mersmann, J, Bergt, S, Bohnenberg, K, Barthuber, C, Szabo, C, Nöldgeschomburg, G. E, & Zacharowsi, K. Therapeutic injection of PARP inhibitor INO-1001 preserves cardiac function in porcine myocardial ischemia and reperfusion without reducing infarct size. Shock (2010). , 33, 507-512.

[95] Petrilli, V, Herceg, Z, Hassa, P. O, & Patel, N. S. Di Paola R, Cortes U, Dugo L, Filipe HM, Thiemermann C, Hottiger MO, Cuzzodrea S, Wang ZQ. Noncleavablepoly(ADP-ribose) polymerase-1 regulates the inflammation response in mice. Journal of Clinical Investigation (2004). , 114, 1072-1081.

[96] Drel, V. R, Pacher, P, Stevens, M. J, & Obrosova, I. G. Aldose reductase inhibition counteracts nitrosative stress and poly(ADP-ribose) polymerase activation in diabetic rat kidney and high-glucose-exposed human mesangial cells. Free Radical Biology & Medicine (2006). , 40, 1454-1465.

[97] Suzuki, Y, Masini, E, Mazzocca, C, Cuzzocrea, S, Ciampa, A, Suzuki, H, & Bani, D. Inhibition of poly(ADP-ribose) polymerase prevents allergen-induced asthmalike reaction in sensitized Guinea pigs. Journal of Pharmacology and Experimental Therapeutics (2004). , 311, 1241-1248.

[98] Cosi, C, Suzuki, H, Skaper, S. D, Milani, D, Facci, L, Menegazzi, M, Vantini, G, Kanai, Y, Degryse, A, Colpaert, F, Koek, W, & Marien, M. R. Poly(ADP-ribose) polymerase (PARP) revisited. A new role for na old enzyme: PARP involvement in neurodegen-

eration and PARP inhibitors as possible neuroprotectiveagentes. Annals of the New York Academy of Sciences (1997). , 825, 366-379.

[99] Yasar, M, Uysal, B, Kaldirim, U, Oztas, Y, Sadir, S, Ozler, M, Topal, T, Coskun, O, Kilic, A, Cayci, T, Poyrazoglu, Y, Oter, S, Korkmaz, A, & Guven, A. Poly(ADP-ribose) polymerase inhibition modulates experimental acute necrotizing pancreatitis induced oxidative stress, bacterial translocation and neopterin concentrations in rats. Experimental Biology and Medicine (2010). , 235, 1126-1133.

[100] Kaelin, W. G. The concept of synthetic lethality in the context of anticancer therapy. Nature Reviews Cancer (2005). , 5, 689-698.

[101] Satoh, M. S, Poirier, G. G, & Lindahl, T. Dual function for poly(ADP-ribose) synthesis in response to DNA strand breakage. Biochemistry (1994). , 33(23), 7099-7106.

[102] Bryant, H. E, Schultz, N, Thomas, H. D, Parker, K. M, Flower, D, Lopez, E, Kyle, S, Meuth, M, Curtin, N. J, & Helleday, T. Specific killing of BRCA2-deficient tumours with inhibitors of poly(ADP-ribose) polymerase. Nature (2005). , 434, 913-917.

[103] Farmer, H, Mccabe, N, & Lord, C. J. Tutt ANJ, Johnson DA, Richardson TB, Santarosa M, Dillon KJ, Hickson I, Knights C., Martin NMB, Jackson SP, Smith GCM, Ashworth A. Targeting the DNA repair defect in BRCA mutant cells as a therapeutic strategy. Nature (2005). , 434, 917-921.

[104] Audeh, M. W, Carmichael, J, Penson, R. T, Friedlander, M, & Powell, B. Bell-McGuinn KM, Scott C, Weitzel JN, Oaknin A, Loman N, Lu K, Schmutzler RK, Matulonis U, Wickens M, Tutt A. Oral poly(ADPribose) polymerase inhibitor olaparib in patiens with BRCA1 or BRCA2 mutations and recurrent ovarian cancer: a proof-of-concept trial. Lancet (2010). , 376, 245-251.

[105] Fong, P. C, Boss, D. S, Yap, T. A, Tutt, A. N, Wu, P, Mergui-roelvink, M, Mortimer, P, Swaisland, H, Lau, A, Connor, O, Ashworth, M. J, Carmichael, A, Kaye, J, Schellens, S. B, & De Bono, J. H. JS. Inhibition of poly(ADP-ribose) polymerase in tumors from BRCA mutation carriers. The New England Journal of Medicine (2009). , 361, 123-134.

[106] Tutt, A. N, Robson, M, Garber, J. E, Domchek, S. M, Audeh, M. W, Weitzel, J. N, Friedlander, M, Arun, B, Loman, N, Schmutzler, R. K, Wardley, A, Mitchell, G, Earl, H, Wickens, M, & Carmichael, J. Oral poly(ADPribose) polymerase inhibitor olaparib in patients with BRCA1 or BRCA2 mutations and advanced breast cancer: a proof-of-concept trial. Lancet (2010). , 376, 235-244.

[107] Guha, M. PARP inhibitors stumble in breast cancer. Nature Biotechnology (2011). , 29, 373-374.

[108] Shaughnessy, O, Osborne, J, Pippen, C, Yoffe, J. E, Patt, M, Rocha, D, Koo, C, Sherman, I. C, & Bradley, B. M. C. Iniparib plus chemotherapy in metastatic triple-negative breast cancer. The New England Journal of Medicine (2011). , 364, 205-214.

[109] Hirschhom, R. In vivo reversion to normal of inherited mutation in humans. Journal of Medical Genetics (2003). , 40(10), 721-728.

[110] Ihnem, M. Therapeutic advantage of chemotherapy drugs in combination with PARP inhitor PF-01367338 (AG-014699) in human ovarian cancer cells [abstract]. European Organization for Research and Treatment of Cancer (2010).

[111] Plummer, R. First and final report of a phase II study of the poly(ADP-ribose) polymerase (PARP) inhibitor, AG014699, in combination with temozolomide (TMZ) in patiens with metastatic malignant melanoma (MM). Journal of Clinical Oncology (2006). s): ASCO abst8013.

[112] Rajan, A. A phase I combination study of olaparib (AZD 2208; KU-0059436) and cisplatin plus gemcitabine in adults with solid tumors [Abstract]. Target Anticancer Therapies (2010).

[113] Kopetz, S. First in human phase I study of BSI-201, a small molecule inhibitor of poly ADP-ribose polymerase (PARP) in subjects with advanced solid tumors [ASCO Abstract 3577]. Journal of Clinical Oncology (2008).

[114] Donawho, C. K, Luo, Y, Penning, T. D, Bauch, J. L, Bouska, J. J, Bontcheva-diaz, V. D, Cox, B. F, Deweese, T. L, Dillehay, L. E, Ferguson, D. C, Ghoreishi-haack, N. S, Grimm, D. R, Guan, R, Han, E. K, Holley-shanks, R. R, Hristov, B, Idler, K. B, Jarvis, K, Johnson, E. F, Kleinberg, L. R, Klinghofer, V, Lasko, L. M, Liu, X, Marsh, K. C, Mcgonigal, T. P, Meulbroek, J. A, Olson, A. M, Palma, J. P, Rodriguez, L. E, Shi, Y, Stavropoulos, J. A, Tsurutani, A. C, Zhu, G. D, Rosenberg, S. H, Giranda, V. L, & Frost, D. J. ABT-888, an orally active poly(ADPribose) polymerase inhibitor that potentiates DNA-damaging agents in preclinical tumor models. Clinical Cancer Research (2007). , 13(9), 2728-2737.

[115] Kummar, S, Chen, A. P, Zhang, R, Putvana, R. J, Kinders, L, Rubinstein, L, Parchment, R. E, Tomazewski, J. E, Doroshow, J. H, & Bethesda, M. D. Pharmacodynamic response in phase I combination study of ABT-888 and topotecan in adults with refractory solid tumors and lymphomas [ASCO Abstract]. Journal of Clinical Oncology (2010). s).

[116] Bunting, S. F, Callen, E, Wong, N, Chen, H. T, Polato, F, Gunn, A, Bothmer, A, Feldhahn, N, Fernandez-capetillo, O, Cao, L, Xu, X, Deng, C. X, Finkel, T, Nussenzweig, M, Stark, J. M, & Nussenzweig, A. BP1 inhibits homologous recombination in BRCA1-deficient cells by blocking resection of DNA breaks. Cell (2010). , 141(2), 243-254.

[117] Issaeva, N, Thomas, H. D, Djurenovic, T, Jaspers, J. E, Stoimenov, I, Kyle, S, Pedley, N, Gottipati, P, Zur, R, Sleeth, K, Chatzakos, V, Mulligan, E. A, Lundin, C, Gubanova, E, Kerbergen, A, Harris, A. L, Sharma, R. A, Rottenberg, S, Curtin, N. J, & Helleday, T. Thioguanine selectively kills BRAC2-defective tumors and overcomes PARP inhibitor resistance. Cancer Research (2010). , 70(15), 6268-6276.

Chapter 3

Anticancer Properties of Cardiac Glycosides

Varisa Pongrakhananon

Additional information is available at the end of the chapter

http://dx.doi.org/10.5772/55381

1. Introduction

Cardiac glycosides comprise a large family of naturally derived compounds, the core structures of which contain a steroid nucleus with a five-membered lactone ring (cardenolides) or a six-membered lactone ring (bufadienolides) and sugar moieties [1]. A few widely recognized examples of cardiac glycosides are digoxin, digitoxin, ouabain, and oleandrin. The cardenolides digitoxin and digoxin, two well-known cardiac glycosides, are inhibitors of the plasma membrane Na^+/K^+-ATPase that are clinically used for the treatment of heart failure. Their positive inotropic effects help suppress the active counter-transportation of Na^+ and K^+ across the cell membrane, leading to an increase in the intracellular Na^+ concentration, a decrease in the intracellular K^+ concentration, and a consequent increase in cardiac contraction [2]. Epidemiologic evidence suggests that breast cancer patients who were treated with digitalis have a significantly lower mortality rate, and their cancer cells had more benign characteristics than those from patients not treated with digitalis [3,4]. Interestingly, the concentrations of cardiac glycosides used for cancer treatment are extremely close to those found in the plasma of cardiac patients treated with the same drugs, suggesting that the anticancer effects of these drugs are exerted at non-toxic concentrations [5]. Furthermore, studies have suggested that cardiac glycosides target cancer cells selectively [6]. These encouraging findings have gained considerable attention in the field of anticancer research, and subsequent studies on the anticancer properties of these compounds have been conducted. These studies investigated not only digoxin and digitoxin but also other related cardiac glycosides, such as ouabain, oleandrin, proscillaridin A, and bufalin [7-10]. Several mechanisms of action, including the inhibition of cancer cell proliferation, the induction of apoptosis, and chemotherapy sensitization, have been reported in a large number of published articles that support the potential use of these compounds for cancer treatment [11-14]. However, further clinical studies are still ongoing to better characterize the pharmacological and safety issues associated with these compounds. This chapter provides an overview of the anticancer activities of cardiac glycosides and describes the selectivity of these compounds, which could prove to be promising treatments in cancer therapy.

2. The chemistry of cardiac glycosides and their biological activities

Cardiac glycosides from both plants and animals have been known for over one hundred years [14]. Major plant-derived cardiac glycosides include digitoxin, digoxin, ouabain, oleandrin and proscillaridin, which are extracted from the plant families Scrophulariaceae, Apocynaceae, and Asparagaceae (*Digitalis purpurea, Digitalis lanata, Strophanthus gratus, Nerium oleander* and *Urginea maritima*). These compounds consist of a steroidal nucleus linked with a sugar at position 3 (C3) and a lactone ring at position 17 (C17) (Fig 1) [15]. The various types of sugar moieties and lactones provide a large number of cardiac glycosides that, based on their lactone moieties, can be divided into two sub-groups: cardenolides, which contain a five-membered unsaturated butyrolactone ring, and bufadienolides, which contain a six-membered unsaturated pyrone ring. The core steroidal portion of each molecule has an A/B and C/D cis-conformation, which has significant pharmacological relevance. The attached sugars, such as glucose, galactose, mannose, rhamnose, and digitalose, determine the pharmacodynamic and pharmacokinetic activities of each cardiac glycoside.

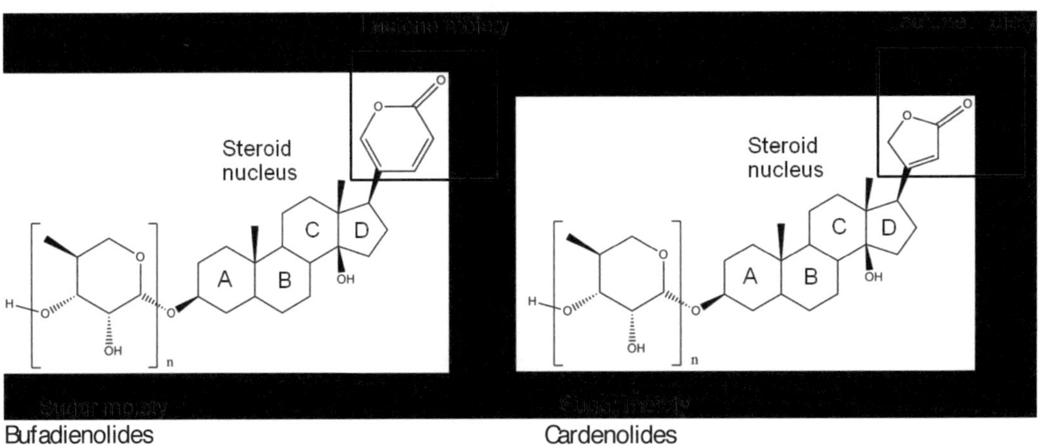

Figure 1. Structural characteristics of cardiac glycosides

Cardiac glycosides have been found in animals as well as plants; for example, bufadienolide was isolated from the venom of a toad species [16], and endogenous digitalis-like compounds have been found in mammalian tissues [17,18]. Several studies have reported that ouabain and proscillaridin A are found in human plasma, that digoxin and marinobufagenin are present in human urine, and that 19-norbufalin exists in cataractous human lenses [18-22]. Table 1 presents a list of the cardiac glycosides found in plants and animals along with their chemical structures.

http://dx.doi.org/10.5772/55381

A digitalis preparation from *Digitalis purpurea* was first used for the treatment of congestive heart failure by William Withering in 1785 [23]. Currently, digoxin is recognized as a primary treatment for patients with heart failure. Its mode of action has been identified as the potent inhibition of Na^+/K^+-ATPase. Na^+/K^+-ATPase, a ubiquitous transmembrane enzyme, is a p-type cation transporter that actively drives two K^+ ions into the cell and drives three Na^+ ions out of the cell using ATP as an energy source. This pump plays a vital role, acting as a secondary transporter of nutrients such as glucose and amino acids and helping to maintain the electrochemical gradient by keeping the intracellular Na^+ concentration low [24]. The elevation of the intracellular Na^+ level in response to cardiac glycosides stimulates the Na^+/Ca^{2+} exchanger mechanism. As a result, the intracellular Ca^{2+} concentration is increased, consequently promoting cellular events such as myocardial contractibility, accounting for the positive inotropic effects of the cardiac glycosides.

Accumulating evidence has established that the Na^+/K^+-ATPase acts as a scaffold for signaling molecules or for the formation of a signalosome complex that activates various signaling cascades. Several signaling molecules, such as caveolin, SRC kinase, epidermal growth factor receptor (EGFR), and the inositol 1,4,5-triphosphate (IP3) receptor, have been investigated [25-27]. The inhibitory effects of cardiac glycosides on Na^+/K^+-ATPase activity might lead to alterations in these downstream transduction pathways, which could account for the biological properties of these compounds, including their anticancer activities.

Name	**Structure**
• Digoxin (Cardenolide) • From *Digitalis purpurea* • Family: Scrophulariaceae	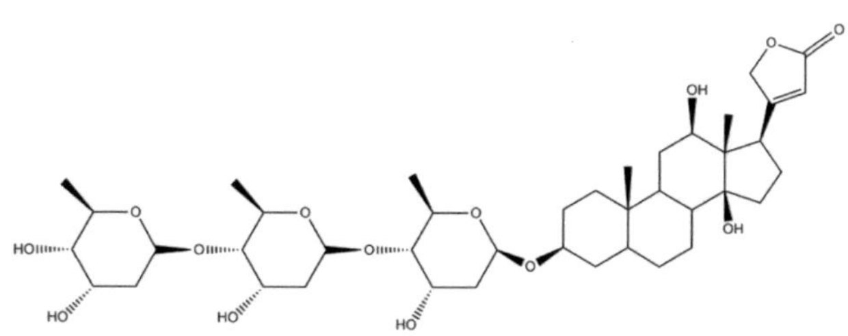
• Digitoxin (Cardenolide) • From *Digitalis purpurea* • Family: Scrophulariaceae	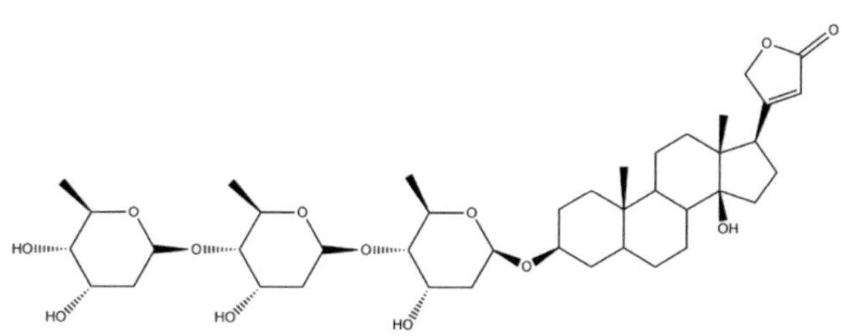

Name	Structure
Ouabain (Cardenolide) From *Nerium oleander* Family: Apocynaceae	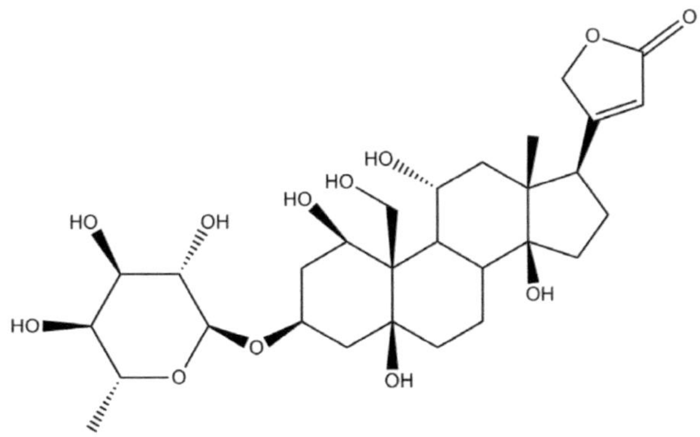
• Oleandrin (Cardenolide) • From *Nerium oleander* • Family: Apocynaceae	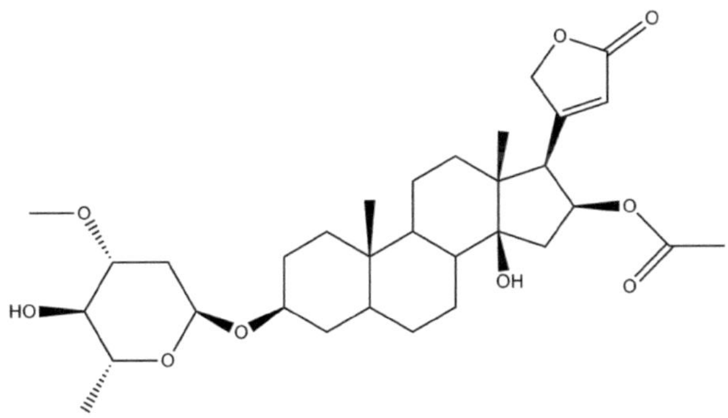
• Proscillaridin (Bufadienolide) • From *Urginea maritima* • Family: Liliaceae	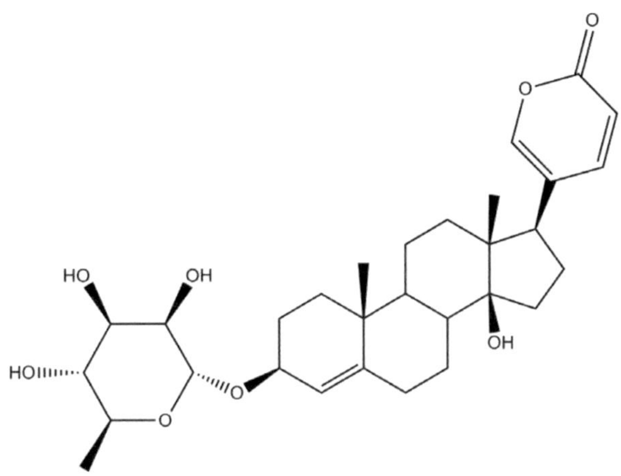

Name	Structure
• Cinobufagin (Bufadienolide) • From *Bufo bufo gargarizans* • Family: Bufonidae	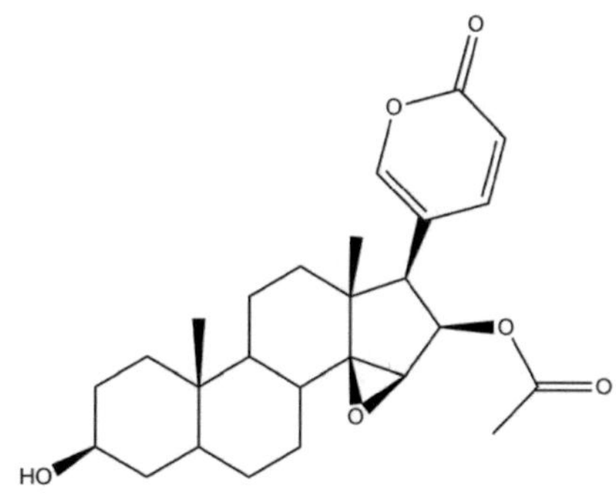
• Bufalin (Bufadienolide) • From Bufo gargarizans • Family: Bufonidae	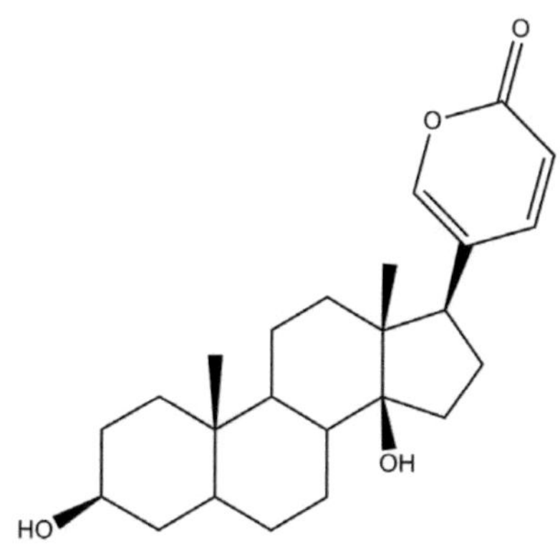
• Marinobufagenin (Bufadienolide) • From Bufo marinus • Family: Bufonidae	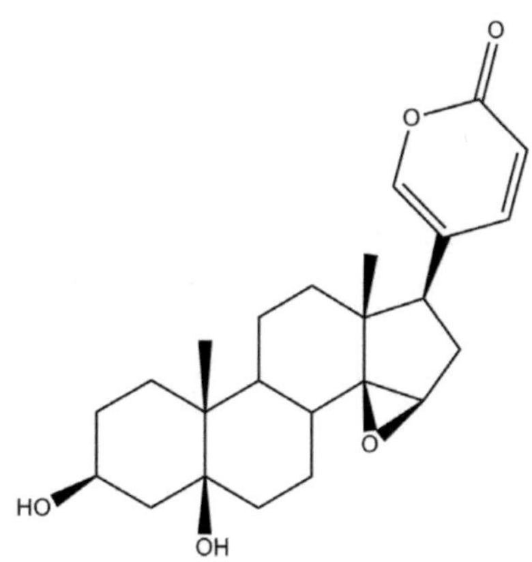

Table 1. The chemical structures of cardiac glycosides

3. Clinical analysis of the effects of cardiac glycosides on cancers

Epidemiologic evidence for the anticancer effects of digitalis was first reported in 1980 by Stenkvist and colleagues. Their study indicated that breast cancer tissue samples from congestive heart failure patients treated with cardiac glycoside therapy exhibited more benign characteristics than cancer tissue samples from control patients who were not treated with the cardiac glycoside regimen [28]. In addition, 5 years after undergoing mastectomy, the recurrence rate for the cardiac glycoside treated-group was 9.6 times lower than that for the control group [28-29]. Four years later, Glodin and colleagues investigated the mortality in 127 cancer patients who received digitalis therapy. These researchers reported that up to 21 patients in the control group died from cancer, whereas only one member of the digitalis-treated group died [30]. Interestingly, the long-term observations of Stenkvist and colleagues also supported the previous finding that digitalis therapy significantly reduces the mortality rate of breast cancer. Among 32 breast cancer patients treated with digitoxin, only two (6%) died, whereas the control group of 143 patients had 48 cancer-related deaths (34%) [4]. Several types of cancer other than breast cancer have also been examined. Recently, Haux and colleagues published an analytical descriptive study on the antineoplastic effects of cardiac glycosides on leukemia and cancers of the kidney/urinary tract [31]. This study indicated that the doses of cardiac glycosides that are active against cancers are similar to the therapeutic plasma concentrations found in cardiac patients treated with these drugs. These clinical observations have established the benificial outcome of cardiac glycosides for cancer therapy. Although these agents seem to be safe at the doses used for the treatment of cardiac disorders, further supporting evidence is still needed before these compounds can be used clinically.

4. Anticancer properties and their mechanisms

At present, cancer is one of the major causes of death worldwide. Extensive research has been conducted over the last decade in an attempt to identify promising compounds that have anticancer effects. Cardiac glycosides are natural compounds that have been previously documented to be antiarrhythmic agents, and their potential anticancer properties were identified thereafter. Cardiac glycosides have been shown to have anticancer activities during various stages of carcinogenesis. These activities include antiproliferative, pro-apoptotic, and chemotherapy sensitization effects.

4.1. Antiproliferative effects

Aberrant cell growth is recognized as one hallmark of cancer [32]. Excessive cell replication is the basic characteristic of cancer progression that facilitates tumor formation and expansion. Defects in normal growth signals result in the inadequate regulation of cell division, which drives quiescent cells to proliferate [33]. Cardiac glycosides have been demonstrated to have antiproliferative activities via their regulation of the cell cycle. The extract from the skin glands of *Bufo bufo gargarizans*, which contains bufalin, is able to induce arrest in human malignant melanoma cells in the G2/M phase of the cell cycle [34]. In lung cancer cells, bufalin upregulates p21 WAF1 and suppresses cyclin D expression in response to the activation of p53 [35]. Because the tumor suppressor p21 WAF1 acts as a potent inhibitor of cell cycle progression [36] and because cyclin D1 is a subunit of cyclin dependent kinase (Cdk)-4 and Cdk-6, which are responsible for cell cycle progression from G1 to S phase [37], these changes prevent cells from entering the next phase of the cycle.

Likewise, digitoxin causes cell cycle arrest in G2/M in a dose-dependent manner, resulting in a large increase in the number of cells in the sub-G0 phase [38]. A synthetic monosaccharide analog of digitoxin, D6-MA, has 5-fold greater potency than digitoxin. The mode of action of D6-MA has been reported to involve the downregulation of key elements required for cell replication, including cyclin B1, cdc2 and survivin. It has been suggested that these events might be downstream signaling events resulting from the modulation of second messengers, such as tyrosine kinase Src, PI3K, phospholipase C and Ras/MAPK pathway components, by cardiac glycoside-bound Na^+/K^+-ATPase [25-27].

An antiproliferative effect of ouabain against human breast and prostate cancer cells has also been reported [39]. Ouabain mediates the depletion of the Na^+/K^+-ATPase through endocytosis and a degradation-dependent pathway, which in turn elevates the level of the cell cycle inhibitor p21. It has been suggested that the cellular level of Na^+/K^+-ATPase plays an important role in determining the rate of cell growth. Additional mechanistic studies have demonstrated that an increase in the intracellular Ca^{2+} concentration following treatment with digoxin, digitoxin, or ouabain is associated with the antiproliferative effects of these compounds in androgen-dependent and androgen-independent prostate cancer cell lines [40]. Because Ca^{2+} serves as a mediator in several signaling pathways, the elevation of the Ca^{2+} concentration may stimulate cellular processes that switch the cells into a growth-retarded state. Several of the antiproliferative effects of cardiac glycosides are summarized in Table 2.

4.2. Induction of apoptosis

Resistance to apoptosis in response to stress conditions is a basic feature of cancer cells and results from the overactivation of survival pathways or the attenuation of cell death mechanisms. The primary readout for screens of anticancer agents is thus usually an apoptosis-inducing effect. Cardiac glycosides have been established as cytotoxic agents that are active against various types of cancers. As mentioned above, the inhibition of Na^+/K^+-ATPase by cardiac glycosides triggers the formation of the signalosome complex, contributing to the initiation of signaling cascades that favor cell death [25-27].

It is well documented that apoptosis generally occurs through two main pathways: the mitochondrial-dependent and death receptor-dependent pathways [46]. Gan and colleagues have reported that oleandrin induces cervical cell apoptosis through the mitochondrial cell death mechanism [47]. This compound significantly stimulates the caspase-dependent pathway by triggering the cleavage of caspase-3/7, -6, and -9 and by upregulating the proapoptotic factor Bim. Similarly, data reported by Elbaz and colleagues support the hypothesis that digitoxin mediates the induction of the mitochondrial apoptotic pathway via caspase-9

Cardiac glycoside	Mechanism
Digitoxin	Induction of cell cycle arrest in G2/M phase through the downregulation of cyclin B1, cdc2 and survivin [38] Increase in the intracellular Ca^{2+} concentration [40]
Digoxin	Increase in the intracellular Ca^{2+} concentration [40] Inhibition of DNA topoisomerases I and II and an increase in the intracellular Ca^{2+} concentration [41] Induction of cell cycle arrest through the upregulation of HIF-1α [42]
Ouabain	Depletion of Na^+/K^+-ATPase and upregulation of p21 [39] Increase in the intracellular Ca^{2+} concentration [40] Inhibition of DNA topoisomerases I and II and increase in the intracellular Ca2+ concentration [41]
Oleandrin	Attenuation of NF-kB, JNK and AP-1 (nuclear transcription factors) activation [43,44]
Bufalin	Induction of cell cycle arrest in G2/M phase through the upregulation of p21 WAF1 and p53 and the downregulation of cyclin D [34,35] Inhibition of DNA topoisomerases I and II [45]
Proscillaridin A	Inhibition of DNA topoisomerases I and II and an increase in the intracellular Ca^{2+} concentration [41]

Table 2. Antiproliferative effects of cardiac glycosides

activation [38]. This study demonstrated not only a cell growth inhibitory effect but also an apoptotic induction effect for digitoxin.

Fas and TNF-related apoptosis-inducing ligand (TRAIL) are important mediators of the death receptor pathway, and the deregulation of their expression is a major cause of chemoresistance and immune escape in cancers [48]. Recently, Sreenivasna and colleagues investigated whether oleandrin triggers the expression of the Fas receptor to potentiate apoptosis in cancer cells without affecting normal primary cells [49]. Additionally, oleandrin has been found to be able to attenuate the NF-kB pathway, which is a key pathway with antiapoptosis and pro-proliferative effects. Cardiac glycosides including oleandrin, bufalin, digitoxin, and digoxin also initiate apoptosis through Apo2L/TRAIL by elevating the levels of death receptors 4 and 5 in non-small cell lung cancer cells [50]. Interestingly, both Fas and Apo2L/TRAIL induce apoptosis in cancer cells but have little to no effect on normal cells. Furthermore, our recent work has demonstrated that ouabain was able to increse TRAIL-mediated lung cancer cell death through anti-apoptosis Mcl-1 down-regulation [51]. Because of these results, cardiac glycosides are of great interest in the field of cancer research.

A growing number of studies have indicated that the disruption of the oxidative state inside cancer cells, due to either the suppression of the antioxidant system or the introduction of reactive oxygen species, can lead to cell death [52]. In androgen-independent prostate cancer cells, ouabain triggers apoptosis by interfering with mitochondrial function [53]. Because the mitochondria are a major source of reactive oxygen species, the application of ouabain causes a steady increase in the level of these species, which leads to apoptosis. This study also indicated that a low dose of ouabain was able to upregulate prostate apoptosis response 4, which is required to reach the desired level of apoptotic cell death.

Other mechanisms of cardiac glycoside-induced apoptosis have also been reported (Fig 2). Mitogen-activated protein kinases (MAPKs) have been reported to be targeted in bufulin-induced human leukemia cell apoptosis [54]. JNK and AP-1 are transcription factors that activate the transcription of various genes, including apoptosis-related genes [55,56]. In response to bufalin treatment, the MAPK signaling pathway is triggered, leading to a notable elevation in the activities of c-Jun N-terminal protein kinase (JNK) and AP-1.

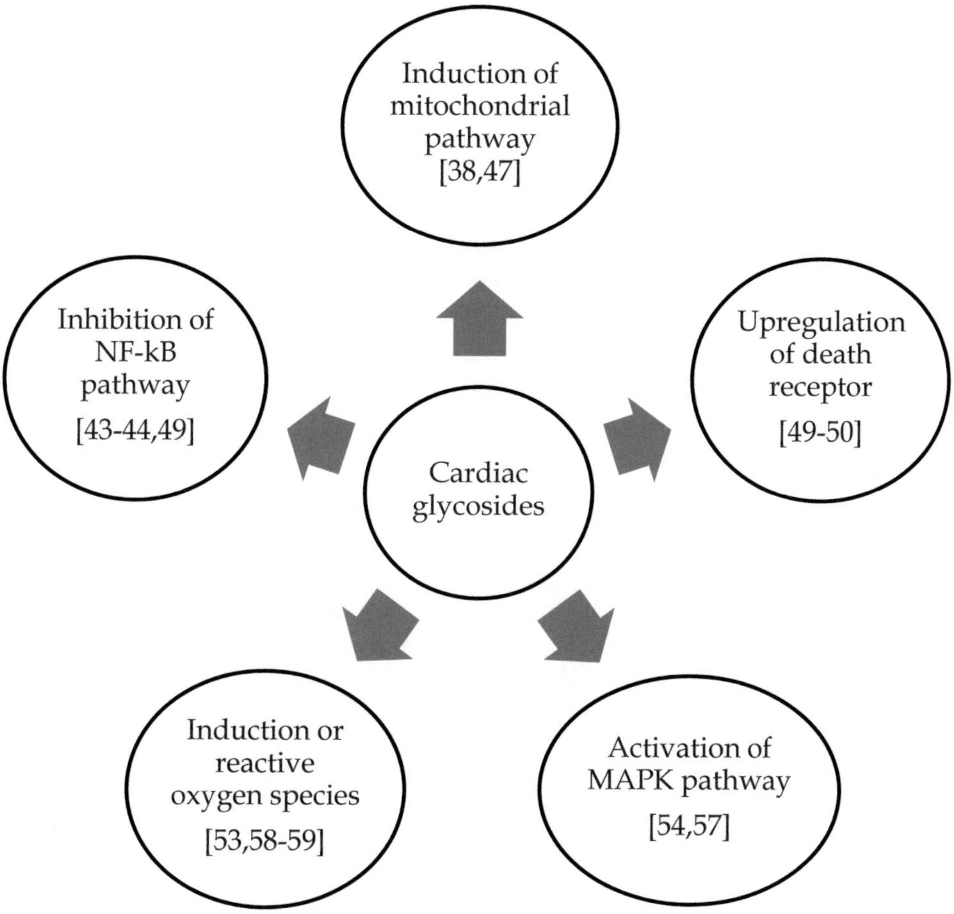

Figure 2. Molecular mechanisms of cardiac glycoside-induced apoptosis

4.3. Sensitization to chemotherapy and enhancement of radiotherapy sensitivity

The susceptibility of a given cancer to chemotherapy often appears to decrease after several rounds of chemotherapy. Resistance to drug-induced cell death is therefore a critical problem in cancer therapy. Combination therapy may be initiated as an alternative approach to overcome this problem. Furthermore, the use of combination therapy increases the cytotoxicity of anticancer agents and reduces their serious side effects on normal cells by reducing the dosage required for each individual agent. Cardiac glycosides have beneficial effects when used as part of combination therapies. Felth and colleagues have investigated the cytotoxicities of cardiac glycosides alone and in combination with various clinically relevant anticancer drugs [60]. Of the glycosides tested, convallatoxin, oleandrin, and proscillaridin A have been shown to be the most potent inducers of colon cancer cell death. Furthermore, co-treatment with cardiac glycosides, including digoxin, digitoxin, oleandrin, and digitonin, and other anticancer drugs, namely 5-fluorouracil, oxaliplatin, cisplatin, and irinotecan, was shown to result in a substantial increase in cancer cell death. However, this study was only a primary screen of the effects of these compounds, and the mechanisms responsible for these effects have not been elucidated.

It is significant that the members of the ATP binding cassette family of transporters, including ABCC7 (CFTR), ABCB1 (P-glycoprotein), and ABCC1 (MRP1), play critical roles in pumping a broad range of drugs out of cells and that these transporters are obviously overexpressed in several tumors [61]. Ouabain has been identified in a recent study to be able to regulate both the expression and activity of ABCC1 in an embryonic kidney cell line. The impairment of ABCC1 following ouabain treatment suggests that this compound might be able to prevent the reduction of the therapeutic concentration inside target cells.

Radiotherapy is a traditional approach used to destroy localized and unresectable tumor cells and to prevent these cells from metastasizing. The combination of chemotherapy and radiation limits the aggressiveness of cancers and increases the patient survival rate. The basic concept underlying chemoradiation is that chemotherapeutics are administered to make cancer cells more susceptible to radiation. Unfortunately, most cancers develop chemoresistance, and anticancer agents have serious side effects in normal cells. The administration of potent anticancer agents with less toxicity against normal cells to sensitize the tumor cells to readio-therapy is a promising strategy. Cardiac glycosides are substances that exhibit selectivity and significant activity against cancer cell lines; thus, the addition of these compounds to existing chemoradiation regimens has been investigated. Huachansu, which is extracted from the skin glands of *Bufo bufo gargarizans,* exhibits a radiosensitizing effect on human lung cancer cells [62]. This Chinese medicine contains a group of steroidal cardiac glycosides and substantially increases radiation-mediated cell death via a p53-dependent pathway. The underlying mechanism involves the cleavage of caspase-3 and poly-(ADP-ribose) polymerase (PARP) concurrent with the downregulation of the antiapoptotic protein Bcl-2 and the inhibition of DNA repair.

The ability of ouabain to sensitize cancer cells to radiotherapy has also been established. Transformed fibroblasts and tumor cells exposed to gamma radiation undergo apoptosis in the presence of ouabain [63-65]. In addition, the recovery of cells is clearly delayed when the cells are exposed to ouabain after irradiation. These events are the results of the inhibitory effect of ouabain on the G2/M phase of the cell cycle.

4.4. The selectivity and sensitivity of cardiac glycosides for cancer cells

The ideal anticancer agent would not only be effective but also selective against tumor cells. As emphasized above, cardiac glycosides have beneficial anticancer effects but do not affect normal cells. Oleandrin attenuates the activation of nuclear transcription factor-kB and activator protein-1 and mediates ceramide-induced apoptosis [43]. These effects are apparently specific to human tumor cells. Consistent with the above findings, bufalin selectively kills leukemia cells, whereas normal leukocytes remain largely unharmed [66, 67]. Furthermore, cardiac glycosides have also been shown to exhibit selectivity in sensitizing cancer cells to apoptosis during radiation treatment. Large numbers of tumor cells and transformed cells die in response to radiation following ouabain pretreatment, but normal cells do not [63, 65]. These studies support the hypothesis that cardiac glycosides have selective anticancer effects, suggesting that these compounds have potential clinical uses.

This selective killing effect has received attention in the search for the fundamental differences between cancer cells and normal cells that modulate the survival pathway. One attempt to identify such differences demonstrated that the subunit composition of Na^+/K^+-ATPase is dissimilar in rodent and human cancer cells, affecting the sensitivity to apoptosis induced by cardiac glycosides [68]. The Na^+/K^+-ATPase consists of two main subunits, the catalytic α subunit and the glycosylated β subunit. It is well known that the α subunit serves as a binding site for cardiac glycosides, Na^+, K^+ and ATP, whereas the β subunit plays a role in the regulation of heterodimer assembly and insertion into the plasma membrane [69, 70]. Recent data indicate that the $\alpha1$ and $\alpha3$ subunits are commonly expressed in human tumor cells, whereas only $\alpha1$ can be found in rodent tumor cell lines [71,72]. It has also been suggested that the lack of the $\alpha3$ subunit in rodent cancer cells causes resistance to apoptosis mediated by cardiac glycosides. This finding strengthens the hypothesis that normal cells might have lower $\alpha3$ subunit expression levels than cancer cells, accounting for the selective anticancer effects of cardiac glycosides. Furthermore, it has been demonstrated that the biological activity of cardiac glycosides results from the binding of these compounds with all α subunits, but the $\alpha3$ subunit is a favorable target [73]. Ouabain, for example, has a 1000-fold stronger interaction with the $\alpha3$ isoform than the $\alpha1$ isoform [74].

Expanding on the above findings, that the expression of the $\alpha3$ subunit has been shown to increase concurrent with the decrease in $\alpha1$ subunit expression in human colorectal cancer and colon adenoma cell lines, whereas no significant alteration of $\alpha3$ subunit expression is detected in normal kidney and renal cells [75]. These results indicate that the overexpression of the $\alpha3$ subunit is associated with responsiveness to cardiac glycosides. Because all α subunits are commonly expressed at a basal level in cancers, the $\alpha3/\alpha1$ ratio might be a marker of cell sensitivity to cardiac glycosides, and this ratio could be determined in tumor biopsy samples taken prior to treatment with cardiac glycosides [76]. A lower $\alpha3/\alpha1$ ratio may indicate unresponsiveness to cardiac glycosides; conversely, cardiac glycoside treatment may improve the clinical outcomes of patients who have tumor tissues with higher ratios.

It has been established that the $\alpha 1$ isoform of the Na^+/K^+-ATPase plays a critical role in the progression of non-small cell lung cancer. The suppression of $\alpha 1$ subunit expression by RNA interference attenuates the invasiveness of cancer, reducing both migration and proliferation [77]. In addition, an increase the $\alpha 1$ subunit level enhances sensitivity to cardiac glycosides. In more than half of glioblastoma samples, the level of Na^+/K^+-ATPase $\alpha 1$ mRNA was markedly elevated, up to 10 times greater than that in normal samples [78]. Similarly, significant upregulation of the $\alpha 1$ isoform was observed in metastatic melanoma cell lines and melanoma tissue samples [79, 80]. These results indicate that the responsiveness of either cancer cells or normal cells to cardiac glycosides based on the $\alpha 3/\alpha 1$ ratio is tissue specific. It is important to determine the differences in the expression levels of the α subunits between cancer cells and normal cells. Furthermore, the characterization of the specificity of each cardiac glycoside for each enzyme subunit is necessary to identify cancers with the appropriate $\alpha 3/\alpha 1$ expression pattern for treatment and to reduce the effect on normal cells, thus optimizing the effectiveness of cardiac glycosides as potent anticancer drugs.

5. Conclusion

Cancer remains a life-threating disease that is typically characterized by frequently related to dysregulated cell growth and resistance to apoptosis. Within the past decade, cancer research has provided interesting insights with the potential to define the exact causes of cancer and to aid in the development of anticancer agents with enhanced effectiveness against and selectivity for cancer. Several plant-derived compounds were once used as ingredients of treatments for diseases without any established scientific evidence to support the claimed effects. Later, these compounds were found to exhibit relevant biological activities. Numerous studies have screened medicinal plants for compounds with anticancer activity, including cardiac glycosides. Generally, cardiac glycosides are recognized as antiarrhythmic drugs that function by inhibiting Na^+/K^+-ATPase. These compounds have been reported to be therapeutically beneficial for the treatment of various tumor types because of their antiproliferative effects, ability to induce apoptosis, and ability to sensitize cells to chemo/radiotherapy-induced cell death.

As already emphasized, cardiac glycosides have a narrow therapeutic index, which could cause serious cardiovascular toxicity. Interestingly, it has been observed that the concentration required to treat cancer was lower than of that used to treat cardiac disorders. Furthermore, cardiac glycosides appear to exert a cancer-specific killing activity by targeting the Na^+/K^+-ATPase α subunit in tumor cells. However, the expression pattern of the enzyme subunits and the target specificity of cardiac glycosides must be optimized. Synthetic cardiac glycosides have been designed to achieve the desired effects; these compounds include UNBS-1450 [81,82] and D6-MA [38 ,83]. Although cardiac glycosides have potential effects on cancer, at present, evidence supporting their usefulness is still needed, and the safety profile of cardiac glycosides as anticancer agents must be determined.

http://dx.doi.org/10.5772/55381

Acknowledgements

This work was supported by a Grant for Development of New Faculty Staff, Chulalongkorn University, and the Thailand Research Fund. The author wishes to thank Dr. Yon Rojanasakul and Dr. Pithi Chanvorachote.

Author details

Varisa Pongrakhananon

Cell-based Drug and Health Product Development Research Unit, Department of Pharmacology and Physiology, Faculty of Pharmaceutical Sciences, Chulalongkorn University, Bangkok, Thailand

References

[1] Mijatovic T, Ingrassia L, Facchini V, Kiss R. Na^+/K^+-ATPase alpha subunits as new targets in anticancer therapy. Expert Opinion on Therapeutic Targets 2008;12 1403-1417.

[2] Böhm M. Digoxin in patients with heart failure. The New England Journal of Medicine. 1997;337 129-130.

[3] Stenkvist B. Cardenolides and cancer. Anticancer Drugs 2001;12 635-638.

[4] Stenkvist B. Is digitalis a therapy for breast carcinoma? Oncology Report 1999;6 493-496.

[5] Gupta RS, Chopra A, Stetsko DK. Cellular basis for the species differences in sensitivity to cardiac glycosides (digitalis). Journal of cellular physiology 1986;127 197-206.

[6] López-Lázaro M. Digitoxin as an anticancer agent with selectivity for cancer cells: possible mechanisms involved. Expert Opinion on Therapeutic Targets 2007;11 1043-1053.

[7] Huang YT, Chueh SC, Teng CM, Guh JH. Investigation of ouabain-induced anticancer effect in human androgen-independent prostate cancer PC-3 cells. Biochemical Pharmacology 2004;67 727-733.

[8] Yang P, Menter DG, Cartwright C, Chan D, Dixon S, Suraokar M, Mendoza G, Llansa N, Newman RA. Oleandrin-mediated inhibition of human tumor cell proliferation: importance of Na,K-ATPase alpha subunits as drug targets. Molecular Cancer Therapeutic 2009;8 2319-2328.

[9] Winnicka K, Bielawski K, Bielawska A, Miltyk W. Apoptosis-mediated cytotoxicity of ouabain, digoxin and proscillaridin A in the estrogen independent MDA-MB-231 breast cancer cells. Archives of pharmacal research 2007;30 1216-1224.

[10] Jiang Y, Zhang Y, Luan J, Duan H, Zhang F, Yagasaki K, Zhang G. Effects of bufalin on the proliferation of human lung cancer cells and its molecular mechanisms of action. Cytotechnology 2010;62 573-83.

[11] Haux J. Digitoxin is a potential anticancer agent for several types of cancer. Medical Hypotheses 1999;53 543-548.

[12] Mijatovic T, Dufrasne F, Kiss R. Cardiotonic steroids-mediated targeting of the Na^+/K^+-ATPase to combat chemoresistant cancers. Current Medical Chemistry 2012;19 627-646.

[13] Newman RA, Yang P, Pawlus AD, Block KI. Cardiac glycosides as novel cancer therapeutic agents. Molecular Intervention 2008;8 36-49.

[14] Prassas I, Diamandis EP. Novel therapeutic applications of cardiac glycosides. Nature reviews. Drug discovery 2008;7 926-95.

[15] Schönfeld W, Weiland J, Lindig C, Masnyk M, Kabat MM, Kurek A, Wicha J, Repke KR. The lead structure in cardiac glycosides is 5a,14a-androstane-3a14-diol. Naunyn-Schmiedeberg's Archives of Pharmacology 1985;329 414-426.

[16] Steyn PS, van Heerden FR. Bufadienolides of plant and animal origin. Natural Product Reports 1998;15 397-413.

[17] Mathews WR, DuCharme DW, Hamlyn JM, Harris DW, Mandel F, Clark MA, Ludens JH. Mass spectral characterization of an endogenous digitalislike factor from human plasma. Hypertension 1991;17 930-935.

[18] Hamlyn JM, Blaustein MP, Bova S, DuCharme DW, Harris DW, Mandel F, Mathews WR, Ludens JH. Identification and characterization of a ouabain-like compound from human plasma. Proceedings of the National Academy of Sciences of the United States of America 1991;88 6259-6263.

[19] Schneider R, Antolovic R, Kost H, Sich B, Kirch U, Tepel M, Zidek W, Schoner W. Proscillaridin A immunoreactivity: its purification, transport in blood by a specific binding protein and its correlation with blood pressure. Clinical and Experimental Hypertension 1998;20 593-599.

[20] Goto A, Yamada K, Ishii M, Sugimoto T. Digitalis-like activity in human plasma: relation to blood pressure and sodium balance. The American Journal of Medicine 1990;89 420-426.

[21] Bagrov AY, Fedorova OV, Dmitrieva RI, Howald WN, Hunter AP, Kuznetsova EA, Shpen VM. Characterization of a urinary bufodienolide Na^+, K^+-ATPase inhibitor in patients after acute myocardial infarction. Hypertension 1998;31 1097-1103.

[22] Schoner W, Scheiner-Bobis G. Endogenous and exogenous cardiac glycosides: their roles in hypertension, salt metabolism, and cell growth. American Journal of Physiology Cell Physiology 2007;293 C509-36.

[23] Aronson JK. (1986) An account of the foxglove and its medical uses 1785-1985. Oxford University Press.

[24] Kaplan JH. Biochemistry of Na,K-ATPase. Annual Review of Biochemistry 2002;71 511-35.

[25] Xie Z, Cai T. Na^{+}/K^{+} ATPase-mediated signal transduction: from protein interaction to cellular function. Molecular Intervention 2003;3 157-168.

[26] Haas M, Wang H, Tian J, Xie Z. Src-mediated inter-receptor cross-talk between the Na^{+}/K^{+}-ATPase and the epidermal growth factor receptor relays the signal from ouabain to mitogen-activated protein kinases. Journal of Biological Chemistry 2002;277 18694-702.

[27] Aperia A. New roles for an old enzyme: Na,K-ATPase emerges as an interesting drug target. Journal of Internal Medicine 2007;261 44-52.

[28] Stenkvist B. Cardiac glycosides and breast cancer. Lancet 1979;1 563.

[29] Stenkvist B: Evidence of a modifying influence of heart glucosides on the development of breast cancer. Analytical and Quantitative Cytology 1980;2 49-54.

[30] Goldin AG, Safa AR: Digitalis and cancer. Lancet 1984;1 1134.

[31] Haux J, Klepp O, Spigset O, Tretli S. Digitoxin medication and cancer; case control and internal dose-response studies. BMC Cancer 2001;1 11.

[32] Hanahan D, Weinberg RA. The Hallmarks of cancer. Cell 2000:1 57-70.

[33] Evan GI, Vousden KH. Proliferation, cell cycle and apoptosis in cancer. Nature 2001;6835 342-348.

[34] Yang P, Chan D, Vijjeswarapu M, Cartwright C, Cohen L, Meng Z, Liu L, Newman RA. Anti-proliferative activity of Huachansu, a Bufo toad skin extract, against human malignant melanoma cells. Proceeding of American Association Cancer Research 2006; 47

[35] Jiang Y, Zhang Y, Luan J, Duan H, Zhang F, Yagasaki K, Zhang G. Effects of bufalin on the proliferation of human lung cancer cells and its molecular mechanisms of action. Cytotechnology 2010;62 573-83.

[36] Pestell RG, Albanese C, Reutens AT, Segall JE, Lee RJ, Arnold A. The cyclins and cyclin-dependent kinase inhibitors in hormonal regulation of proliferation and differentiation. Endocrine Review 1999;20 501-534.

[37] Baldin V, Lukas J, Marcote MJ, Pagano M, Draetta G. Cyclin D1 is a nuclear protein required for cell cycle progression in G1. Genes & Development 1993;7 812-21.

[38] Elbaz HA, Stueckle TA, Wang HY, O'Doherty GA, Lowry DT, Sargent LM, Wang L, Dinu CZ, Rojanasakul Y. Digitoxin and a synthetic monosaccharide analog inhibit cell viability in lung cancer cells. Toxicology and Applied Pharmacology 2012;258 51-60.

[39] Tian J, Li X, Liang M, Liu L, Xie JX, Ye Q, Kometiani P, Tillekeratne M, Jin R, Xie Z. Changes in sodium pump expression dictate the effects of ouabain on cell growth. Journal of Biological Chemistry 2009;284 14921-14929.

[40] Yeh JY, Huang WJ, Kan SF, Wang PS. Inhibitory effects of digitalis on the proliferation of androgen dependent and independent prostate cancercells. Journal of Urology 2001;166 1937-42.

[41] Winnicka K, Bielawski K, Bielawska A, Surazyński A. Antiproliferative activity of derivatives of ouabain, digoxin and proscillaridin A in human MCF-7 and MDA-MB-231 breast cancer cells. Biological and Pharmaceutical Bulletin 2008;31 1131-1140.

[42] Zhang H, Qian DZ, Tan YS, Lee K, Gao P, Ren YR, Rey S, Hammers H, Chang D, Pili R, Dang CV, Liu JO, Semenza GL. Digoxin and other cardiac glycosides inhibit HIF-1alpha synthesis and block tumor growth. Proceedings of the National Academy of Sciences of the United States of America 2008;105 19579-19586.

[43] Sreenivasan Y, Sarkar A, Manna SK. Oleandrin suppresses activation of nuclear transcription factor-kB and activator protein-1 and potentiates apoptosis induced by ceramide. Biochemical Pharmacology 2003;66 2223–2239.

[44] Manna SK, Sah NK, Newman RA, Cisneros A, Aggarwal BB. Oleandrin suppresses activation of nuclear transcription factor-kappaB, activator protein-1, and c-Jun NH2 terminal kinase. Cancer Research 2000;60 3838-3847.

[45] Hashimoto S, Jing Y, Kawazoe N, Masuda Y, Nakajo S, Yoshida T, Kuroiwa Y, Nakaya K. Bufain reduces the level of topoisomerase II in human leukemia cells and affects the cytotoxicity of anticancer drugs. Leukemia Research 1997;21 875-883.

[46] Lavrik IN, Golks A, and Krammer PH. Caspases: pharmacological manipulation of cell death. The Journal of Clinical Investigation 2005;115 2665-2672.

[47] Gan N, Chen G, Zhang W, Zhou J. Oleanen induces apoptosis of cervical cancer cells by up-regulation of Bim. International Journal of Gynecological Cancer 2012;22 38-42.

[48] Toillon RA, Descamps S, Adriaenssens E, Ricort JM, Bernard D, Boilly B, Le Bourhis X. Normal breast epithelial cells induce apoptosis of breast cancer cells via Fas signaling. Experimental Cell Research 2002;275 31-43.

[49] Sreenivasan Y, Raghavendra PB, Manna SK. Oleandrin-mediated expression of Fas potentiates apoptosis in tumor cells. Journal of Clinical Immunology 2006;26 308-322.

[50] Frese S, Frese-Schaper M, Anne-Catherine A, Miescher D, Zumkehr B, Schmid RA. Cardiac glycosides initiate Apo2L/TRAIL induced apoptosis in non-small cell lung

cancer cells by up-regulation of death receptors 4 and 5. Cancer Research 2006;66 6867–5874.

[51] Chanvorachote P, Pongrakhananon V. Ouabain down-regulates Mcl-1 and sensitizes lung cancer cells to TRAIL-induced apoptosis. American Journal of Physiology-Cell Physiology 2012; doi:10.1152/ajpcell.00225.2012.

[52] Simon HU, Haj-Yehia A, Levi-Schaffer F. Role of reactive oxygen species (ROS) in apoptosis induction. Apoptosis 2000;5 415-418.

[53] Huang YT, Chueh SC, Teng CM, Guh JH. Investigation of ouabain-induced anticancer effect in human androgen-independent prostate cancer PC-3 cells. Biochemical Pharmacology 2004;67 727-733.

[54] Watabe M, Ito K, Masuda Y, Nakajo S, Nakaya K. Activation of AP-1 is required for bufalin-induced apoptosis in human leukemia U937cells. Oncogene 1998;16 779-787.

[55] Ameyar M, Wisniewska M, Weitzman JB. A role for AP-1 in apoptosis: the case for and against. Biochimie 2003;85 747-52.

[56] Okamoto K, Fujisawa K, Hasunuma T, Kobata T, Sumida T, Nishioka K. Selective activation of the JNK/AP-1 pathway in Fas-mediated apoptosis of rheumatoid arthritis synoviocytes. Arthritis & Rheumatism 1997;40 919-926.

[57] Wang Z, Zheng M, Li Z, Li R, Jia L. Xiong X, Southall N, Wang S, Xia M, Austin CP, Zheng W, Xie Z, Sun Y. Cardiac glycosides inhibit p53 synthesis by a mechanism relieved by Src or MAPK inhibition. Cancer Research 2009;69 6556-6564.

[58] Liu J, Tian J, Haas M, Shapiro JI, Askari A, Xie Z. Ouabain interaction with cardiac Na^+/K^+-ATPase initiates signal cascades independent of changes in intracellular Na^+ and Ca^{2+} concentrations. Journal of Biological Chemistry 2000; 275 27838–27844.

[59] Newman RA, Yang P, Hittelman WN, Lu T, Ho DH, Ni D, Chan D, Vijjeswarapu M, Cartwright C, Dixon S, Felix E, Addington C. Oleandrin-mediated oxidative stress in human melanoma cells. Journal of Experimental Therapeutics & Oncology 2006;5 167-181.

[60] Felth J, Rickardson L, Rosén J, Wickström M, Fryknäs M, Lindskog M, Bohlin L, Gullbo J. Cytotoxic effects of cardiac glycosides in colon cancer cells, alone and in combination with standard chemotherapeutic drugs. Journal of Natural Products 2009;72 1969-1974.

[61] Kunta JR, Sinko PJ. Intestinal drug transporters: in vivo function and clinical importance. Current Drug Metabolism 2004;5 109-24.

[62] Wang L, Raju U, Milas L, Molkentine D, Zhang Z, Yang P, Cohen L, Meng Z, Liao Z. Huachansu, containing cardiac glycosides, enhances radiosensitivity of human lung cancer cells. Anticancer Research 2011;31 2141-2148.

[63] Verheye-Dua FA, Böhm L. Na^+, K^+-ATPase inhibitor, ouabain accentuates irradiation damage in human tumour cell lines. Radiation Oncology Investigations 1998;6 109-119.

[64] Verheye-Dua FA, Böhm L. Influence of ouabain on cell inactivation by irradiation. Strahlentherapie und Onkologie 1996;172 156-161.

[65] Lawrence T.S. Ouabain sensitizes tumor cells but not normal cells to radiation. International Journal of Radiation Oncology, Biology, Physics 1998;15 953-958.

[66] Numazawa S, Honna Y, Yamamoto T, Yoshida T, Kuroiwa YA. cardiotonic steroid bufalin-like factor in human plasma induces leukemia cell differentiation. Leukemia Research 1995;19 945-953.

[67] Zhang L, Nakaya K, Yoshida T, Kuroiwa Y. Induction by bufalin of differentiation of human leukemia cells HL60, U937 and ML1 toward macrophage/monocyte-like cells and its potent synergistic effect on the differentiation of human leukemia cells in combination with other inducers. Cancer Research 1992;52 4634-4641.

[68] Pathak S, Multani AS, Narayan S, Kumar V, Newman RA. Anvirzel, an extract of Nerium oleander, induces cell death in human but not murine cancer cells. Anticancer Drugs 2000;11 455-63.

[69] Blanco G. Na,K-ATPase subunit heterogeneity as a mechanism for tissue-specifi c ion regulation. Seminar in Nephrology 2005;25 292-303.

[70] Mobasheri A, Avila J, Cózar-Castellano I, Brownleader MD, Trevan M, Francis MJ, Lamb JF, Martín-Vasallo P. Na/K-ATPase isozyme diversity; comparative biochemistry and physiological implications of novel functional interactions. Bioscience Report 2000;20 51-91.

[71] Lin Y, Dubinsky WP, Ho DH, Felix E, Newman RA. Determinants of human and mouse melanoma cell sensitivities to oleandrin. Journal of Experimental Therapeutics & Oncology. 2008;7 195-205.

[72] Lucchesi PA, Sweadner KJ. Postnatal changes in Na, K-ATPase isoforms expression in rat cardiac ventricle. conservation of biphasic ouabain affinity. Journal of Biological Chemistry 1991;266 9327-9331.

[73] Noel F, Fagoo M, Godfraind T. A comparison of the affinities of rat (Na^+,K^+)-ATPase isozymes for cardioactive steroids, role of lactone ring, sugar moiety ad KCl concentration. Biochemical Pharmacology 1990;40 2611-2616.

[74] O'Brien WJ, Lingrel JB, Wallick ET. Ouabain binding kinetics of the rat alpha two and alpha 3 isoforms of the sodium-potassium adenosine triphosphate. Archives of Biochemistry and Biophysics 1994;310 32-39.

[75] Sakai H, Suzuki T, Maeda M, Takahashi Y, Horikawa N, Minamimura T, Tsukada K, Takeguchi N. Up-regulation of Na(+),K(+)-ATPase alpha 3-isoform and down-regulation of the alpha1-isoform in human colorectal cancer. FEBS Letters 2004;563 151-154.

[76] Yang P, Menter DG, Cartwright C, Chan D, Dixon S, Suraokar M, Mendoza G, Llansa N, Newman RA. Oleandrin-mediated inhibition of human tumor cell proliferation: importance of Na,K-ATPase alpha subunits as drug targets. Molecular Cancer Therapeutics 2009;8 2319-2328.

[77] Mijatovic T, Roland I, Van Quaquebek, Nilsson EB, Mathieu A, Van Vynckt F, Darro F, Blanco G, Facchini V, Kiss R. The $\alpha 1$ subunit of the sodium pump could represent a novel target to combat non-small cell lung cancers. Journal of Pathology 2007;212 170-179.

[78] Lefranc F, Mijatovic T, Kondo Y, Sauvage S, Roland I, Debeir O, Krstic D, Vasic V, Gailly P, Kondo S, Blanco G, Kiss R. Targeting the á 1 subunit of the sodium pump to combat glioblastoma cells. Neurosurgery 2008;62 211-221.

[79] Boukerche H, Su ZZ, Kang DC, Fisher PB. Identification and cloning of genes displaying elevated expression as a consequence of metastatic progression in human melanoma cells by rapid subtraction hybridization. Gene 2004;343 191-201.

[80] Mathieu V, Pirker C, Vernier M, Mijatovic T, Berger W, Kiss R. New cardenolides, binders of the sodium pump, could represent interesting chemotherapeutical agents for melanoma treatment. American Association for Cancer Research (AACR) Annual Meeting, April 12-16, San Diego, USA; 2008.

[81] Juncker T, Cerella C, Teiten MH, Morceau F, Schumacher M, Ghelfi J, Gaascht F, Schnekenburger M, Henry E, Dicato M, Diederich M. UNBS1450, a steroid cardiac glycoside inducing apoptotic cell death in humanleukemia cells. Biochemical Pharmacology 2011;81 13-23.

[82] Juncker T, Schumacher M, Dicato M, Diederich M. UNBS1450 from Calotropis procera as a regulator of signaling pathways involved in proliferation and cell death. Biochemical Pharmacology 2009;78 1-10.

[83] Elbaz HA, Stueckle TA, Tse W, Rojanasakul Y, Dinu CZ. Digitoxin and its analogs as novel cancer therapeutics. Experimental Hematology & Oncology 2012; 1 4.

Chapter 4

Liposomes as Carriers of Anticancer Drugs

Sávia Caldeira de Araújo Lopes,
Cristiane dos Santos Giuberti,
Talita Guieiro Ribeiro Rocha,
Diêgo dos Santos Ferreira, Elaine Amaral Leite and
Mônica Cristina Oliveira

Additional information is available at the end of the chapter

http://dx.doi.org/10.5772/55290

1. Introduction

Nanotechnology and nanoscience present a highly positive prospective of bringing benefits to many research areas and applications. Nanosized vehicles have received considerable attention over the past 30 years as pharmaceutical carriers with a wide range of applications, including drug delivery vehicles, adjuvants in vaccinations, signal enhancers/carriers in medical diagnostics and analytical biochemistry, solubilizers for various materials, as well as their role as a support matrix for chemical ingredients and as penetration enhancers in cosmetic products. More recent developments have reported on the field of liposomal drugs, from the viewpoint of clinically approved products, with cancer therapy representing the main area of interest [1-3]. In this context, liposomes can be used to improve current cancer treatment regimens due to their capacity to increase the solubility of poorly water-soluble antitumor drugs. Moreover, these also act to decrease the mononuclear phagocyte system's (MPS) uptake by using long-circulating liposomes which promote a passive directing toward the tumor region and can lead to an active directing toward the tumor site by connecting specific ligands to the liposome surface [4,5]. These strategies minimize drug degradation and inactivation upon administration, as well as increase the drug's bioavailability and the fraction of drug delivered within the pathological area, thus improving efficacy and/or minimizing drug toxicity.

2. Definition, structure, and classification of liposomes

Liposomes are spherical vesicles composed of one or more lipid bilayers, involving an aqueous compartment (Figure 1). These are formed spontaneously when the lipids are dispersed in an aqueous medium by stirring, in turn giving rise to a population of vesicles which may reach a size range from dozens of nanometers to dozens of microns in diameter [6]. The lipid molecules possess head groups which are attracted to water molecules and organize themselves in such a way as to point toward the aqueous cavity, whereas the hydrocarbon tails are repelled by the water molecules and point in the opposite direction.

The head groups of the inner layer point in the direction of the intravesicular fluid, with the tails pointing away from it. As such, the hydrocarbon tails of one layer point toward the hydrocarbon tails of the outer layer, in turn forming the normal bilipid membrane [3]. Once the liposomes have reached both the aqueous and lipid phases, they can encapsulate drugs with widely varying lipophilicities in the lipid bilayer, in the entrapped aqueous volume, or at the bilayer interface [7,8].

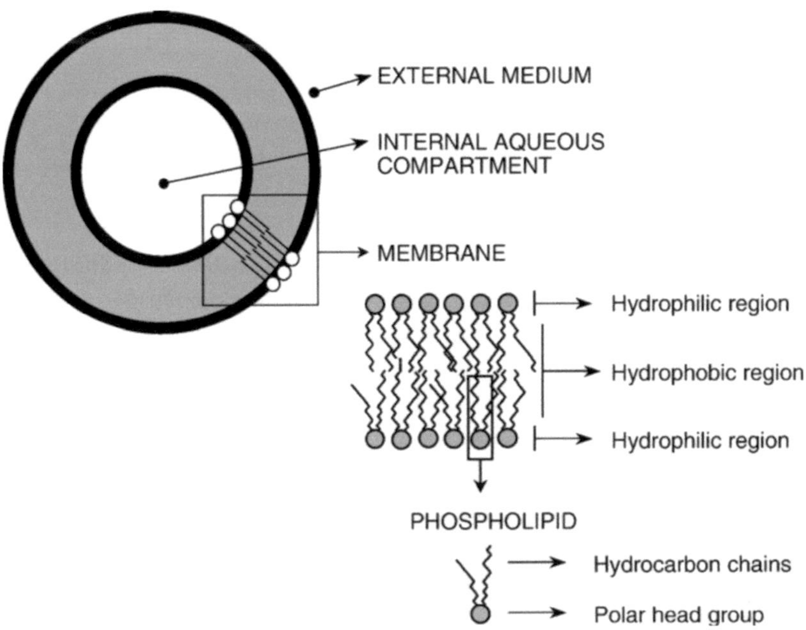

Figure 1. Basic structure and composition of liposomes. See [9].

Biodegradable and biocompatible phospholipids and sphingolipids are the lipids that are most commonly used to prepare liposomes (Table 1 and Figure 2). These structural lipids can be of

http://dx.doi.org/10.5772/55290

either natural or synthetic origin, given that those of natural origin consist of a mixture of various lipids. In general, cylindrical molecular-shape lipids, such as phosphatidylcholine, phosphatidylserine, phosphatidylglycerol, and sphingomyelin, are chosen for liposome formulations, as they organize into stable bilayers in aqueous solutions. Among these lipids, phosphatidylcholines are the most widely used due to their appropriate stability and their ability to act against changes in pH or salt concentrations in the product or/and biological environment [10].

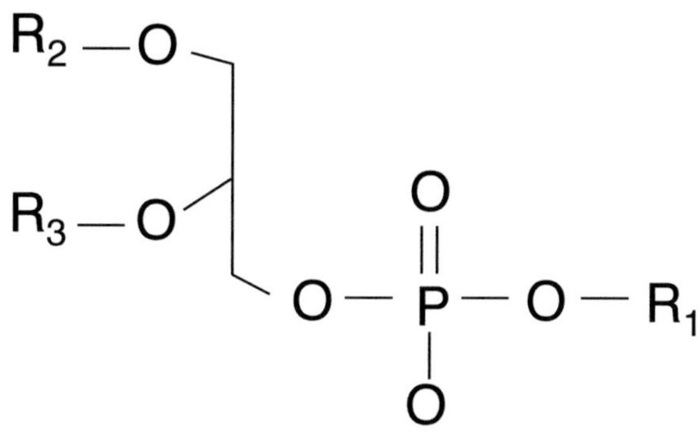

Phospholipid structural formula

Phospholipid (R_1)	Hydrophobic chains (R_2,R_3) (name)	Lipid Name (Abbreviation)
Phosphatidylcholine $CH_2CH_2N^+(CH_3)_3$	$CH_3(CH_2)_7CH{=}CH(CH_2)_7C(O)$- (oleyl)	Dioleylphosphatidylcholine (DOPC)
	$CH_3(CH_2)_{12}C(O)$- (myristoyl)	Dimyristoylphosphatidylcholine (DMPC)
	$CH_3(CH_2)_{14}C(O)$- (palmitoyl)	Dipalmitoylphosphatidylcholine (DPPC)
	$CH_3(CH_2)_{16}C(O)$- (stearoyl)	Distearoylphosphatidylcholine (DSPC)
Phosphatidylethanolamine $CH_2CH_2NH_3^+$	$CH_3(CH_2)_7CH{=}CH(CH_2)_7C(O)$- (oleyl)	Dioleoylphosphatidylethanolamine (DOPE)
	$CH_3(CH_2)_{16}C(O)$- (stearoyl)	Distearoylphosphatidylethanolamine (DSPE)
Phosphatidylglycerol $CH_2CHOHCH_2OH$	$CH_3(CH_2)_{12}C(O)$- (myristoyl)	Dimyristoylphosphatidylglycerol (DMPG)
	$CH_3(CH_2)_{14}C(O)$- (palmitoyl)	Dipalmitoylphosphatidylglycerol (DPPG)
Phosphatidylserine $CH_2CHNH_3^+COO^-$	$CH_3(CH_2)_{14}C(O)$- (palmitoyl)	Dipalmitoylphosphatidylserine (DPPS)
	$CH_3(CH_2)_{16}C(O)$- (stearoyl)	Distearoylphosphatidylserine (DSPS)

Table 1. Examples of phospholipids used in liposome preparation.

Liposomes are mainly classified in terms of size (small, intermediate, or large), number of bilayers (uni- and multi-lamellar), composition and mechanism of drug delivery. Small unilamellar vesicles (SUV) consist of a single lipid bilayer with an average diameter ranging

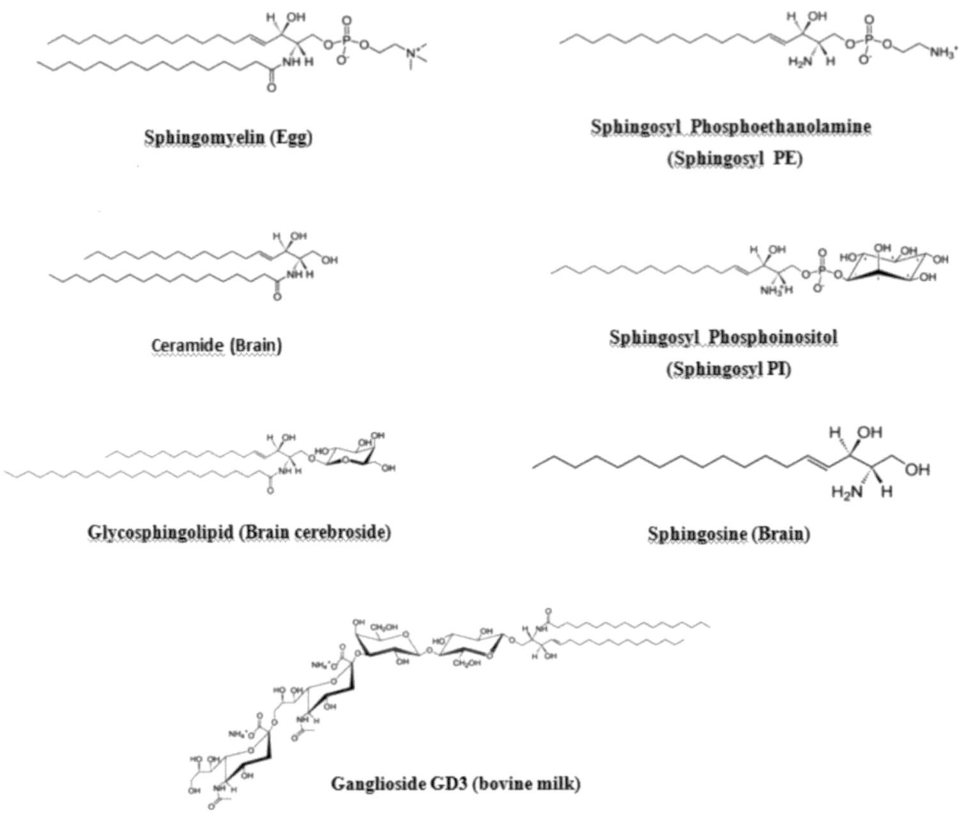

Figure 2. Chemical structures of some classes of sphingolipids. The length and saturation grade of the carbon chain can vary in each class of sphingolipid.

from 25 to 100 nm. Large unilamellar vesicles (LUV) also consist of one lipid bilayer and are greater than 100 nm, whereas multilamellar vesicles (MLV) are made up of several concentric lipid bilayers and measure of 1- 5 μm [7,11] (Figure 3). As regards the composition and mechanism of drug delivery, the liposomes can be classified as conventional liposomes, long-circulating liposomes, polymorphic liposomes (pH-sensitive, thermo-sensitive, and cationic liposomes), and decorated liposomes (surface-modified liposomes and immunoliposomes) (Figure 4).

Conventional liposomes can possess different lipid compositions; however, the most commonly used lipids are phosphatidylcholines and cholesterol (CHOL). A major drawback of conventional liposomes is their rapid uptake by MPS after systemic administration [8]. In the 1980s, the development of long-circulating liposomes boosted interest in the clinical application of liposomes as a drug delivery system for cancer treatment. Prior studies have shown that the presence of a dense glycocalyx with a high sialic acid content, used to produce a hydrophilic layer around the erythrocytes, prevented their destruction by MPS macrophages [12]. Allen and Chonn [13] applied this same concept to liposome development, incorpo-

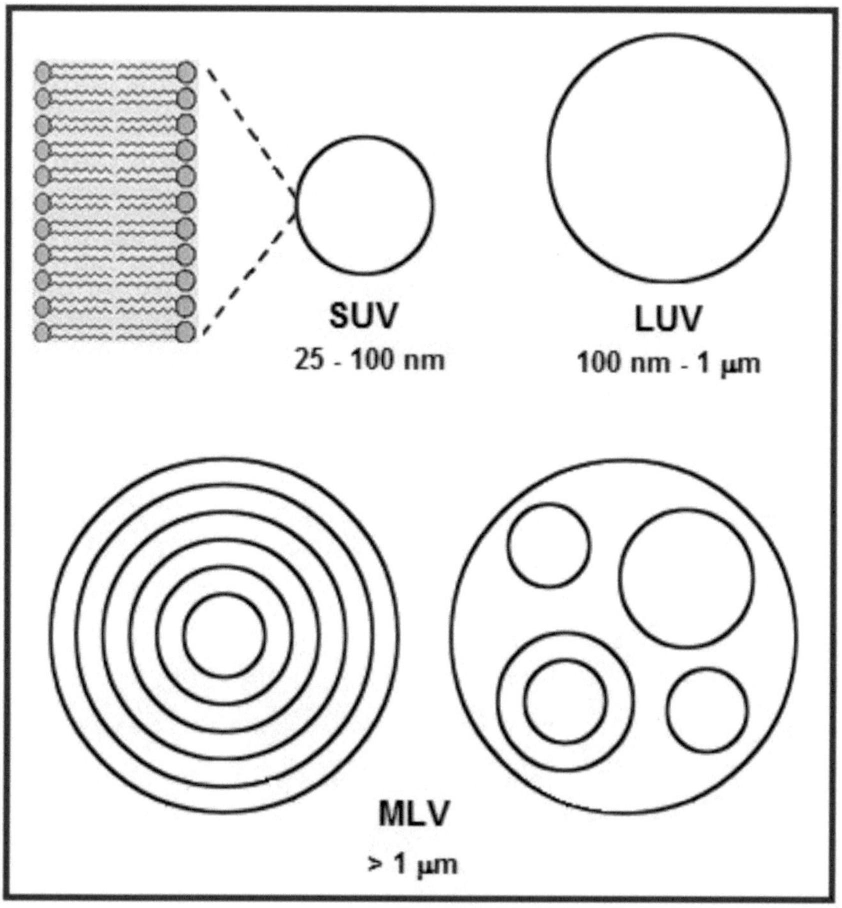

Figure 3. Classification of liposomes according to average diameter and number of bilayers.

rating purified glycolipids in the membranes of liposomes and testing their stability in mice. The results showed that the incorporation of monosialoganglioside GM1 and sphingomyelin acted synergistically to diminish the rate and extent of uptake of liposomes by macrophages *in vivo*. However, monosialoganglioside GM1 did present some inconveniences, such as the expensive extraction process and the brain, as a prime source, which was considered unsuitable for use in pharmaceutical products. Klibanov and coworkers [14] were the first to show that the incorporation in the bilayer membrane of polyethylene glycol (PEG) lipid derivatives, significantly prolonged the circulation half-life of liposomes. It could be observed that the introduction of five to ten percent of PEG lipid-derivatives prevents opsonization through the induction of a fixed aqueous layer on the liposome surface, which shields surface charges, increases surface hydrophilicity, enhances repulsive interactions between polymer-coated liposomes and blood components, and forms a polymeric layer which is impermeable for large opsonin molecules even at relatively low polymer concentrations [15-18]. This

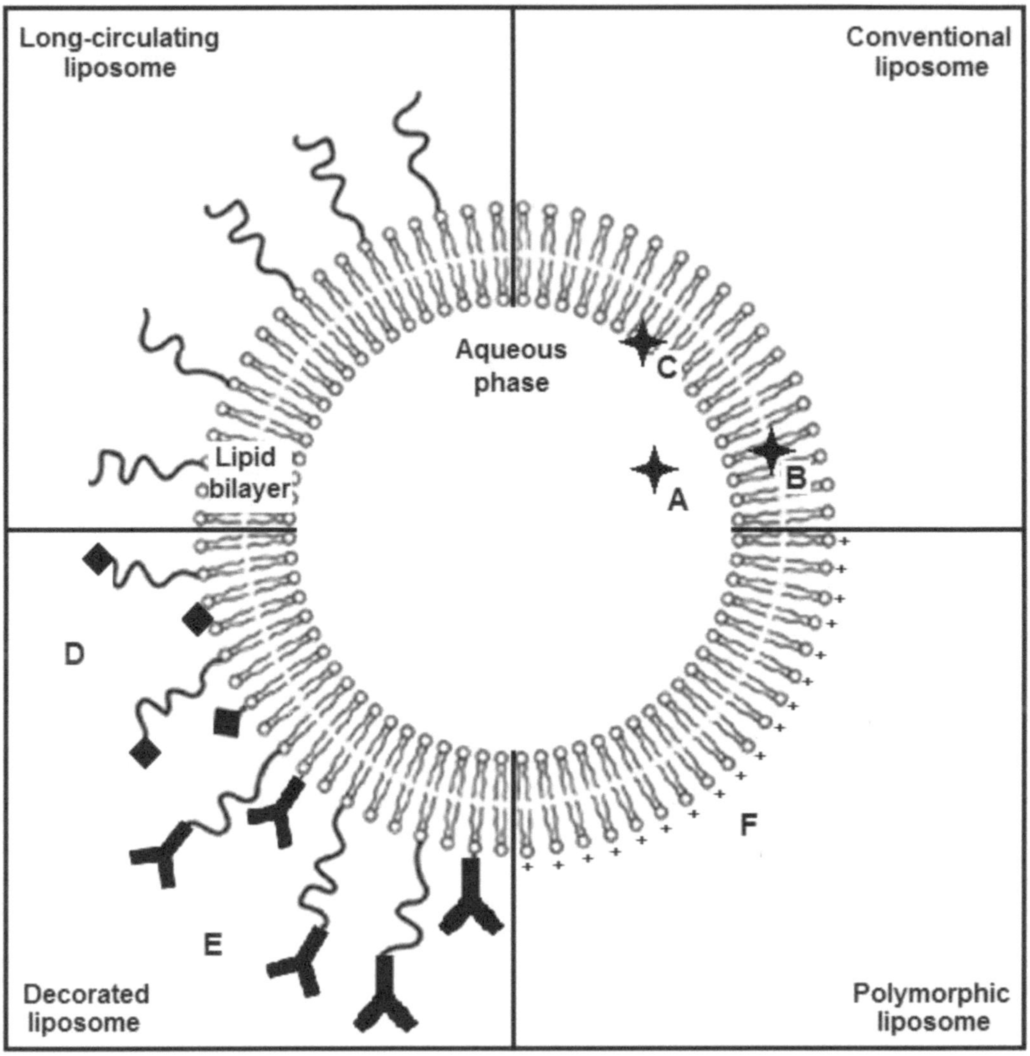

Figure 4. Structural composition of different liposomes. Hydrophilic drugs (A) are incorporated in the inner aqueous phase of liposomes; lipophilic drugs (B) are incorporated in the liposome bilayer; amphifilic drugs (C) can be found in the interface lipid bilayer-inner aqueous phase. Conventional liposomes are exclusively made up of lipids. Long-circulating liposomes present a hydrophilic polymer attached to the liposome surface. The decorated liposomes can be subdivided as surface-modified liposomes (D) or immunoliposomes (E). Ligands can be directly attached to the liposome surface or to the extremity of a hydrophilic polymer. The cationic liposomes (F) are a type of polymorphic liposome used in the intracellular delivery of DNA.

discovery was a major breakthrough in liposome field research, supplying a safe synthetic compound that can be easily produced in mass scale.

Regardless of the strategies mentioned above, conventional and long-circulating liposomes may present a slow release of the active substance or may be unable to fuse with the endosome after internalization. As such, polymorphic liposomes have been developed to overcome these problems, mainly due to the fact that these liposomes become reactive when submitted to membrane changes triggered by pH, variations in temperature, or surface charge alterations.

A pH-sensitive liposome is generally stable at physiological pH but can undergo destabilization and acquires fusogenic properties under acidic conditions, thus leading to the release of its aqueous contents [19,20]. The development of this kind of liposome was proposed after the observation that some pathological tissues, including tumors or areas of inflammation and infection, as compared to normal tissues, reveal an acidic environment [21]. The endosome formed during the cellular internalization of liposomes also presents an acidic pH. The pH-sensitive liposomes consist mainly of phosphatidylethanolamine (PE) or its derivatives combined with amphiphilic compounds containing an acid group (e.g. carboxylic group) that acts as a stabilizer of the bilayer at neutral pH (Figure 5). The PE presents a conic geometry, since it contains a less bulky polar group, as compared to its hydrocarbon chain. This fact allows for strong intermolecular interaction between amine and phosphate groups in the polar moiety of PE. The molecules organize in a structure, called the inverted hexagonal phase, in which the polar head of the phospholipid points toward the inner cavity, while the carbon chains point toward the outer areas. The introduction of carboxylated compounds among phospholipid molecules promotes the repulsion of the phosphate groups with the carboxylate groups, which is deprotonated at neutral pH, favoring the formation of the bilayer (lamellar phase). The exposure of pH-sensitive liposomes to acidic pH leads to the protonation of carboxylate groups, removing the repulsion with phosphates, in turn destabilizing the bilayer and releasing the encapsulated substances [19, 22]. Hong and coworkers [23] showed that pH-sensitive liposomes made up of DOPE/distearoylphosphatidylglycerol (DSPG)/distearoylphosphatidylethanolaminepolyethyleneglycol$_{2000}$ (DSPE-PEG$_{2000}$), as compared to non-pH-sensitive liposomes made up of DPPC/CHOL/DSPE-PEG$_{2000}$ are stable in plasma and are able to release an entrapped marker more rapidly within tumor tissues.

Lipid molecules are able to organize at the lamellar phase, depending on the temperature, molecular shape of the lipids, and the conditions in the lipid-water mixture (concentration and ionic strength). Lamellar phases are classified in crystalline lamellar (L_C), lamellar gel (L_β), and lamellar liquid-crystalline (L_α). Lipid phase-transitions occur at certain temperatures according to the conditions of the medium. The main phase transition occurs at the temperature in which the lipid membrane passes from a tightly ordered gel (L_β) to a fluid lamellar (L_α), where the freedom of movement of individual molecules is high.

Thermo-sensitive liposomes, another kind of polymorphic liposome, are vesicles that present a bilayer composition in which the phase-transition temperature is slightly above 37°C, as can be seen in DPPC or lipids attached to thermosensitive copolymers (N-isopropylacrylamide and N-acryloylpyrrolidine). The local release of drugs entrapped in these liposomes is triggered by hyperthermia. Cationic liposomes present a positive surface charge, due to the presence of cationic lipids; can fuse with cell or endosome membranes; and are suitable for the delivery of negatively charged macromolecules (DNA, RNA, and oligonucleotides) [10].

In an attempt to improve the specificity of liposomes for injured organs or tissues and to prevent their uptake by the healthy tissues, liposomes with a functionalized surface, called *"decorated"* liposomes, have been developed by binding specific ligands. These ligands are

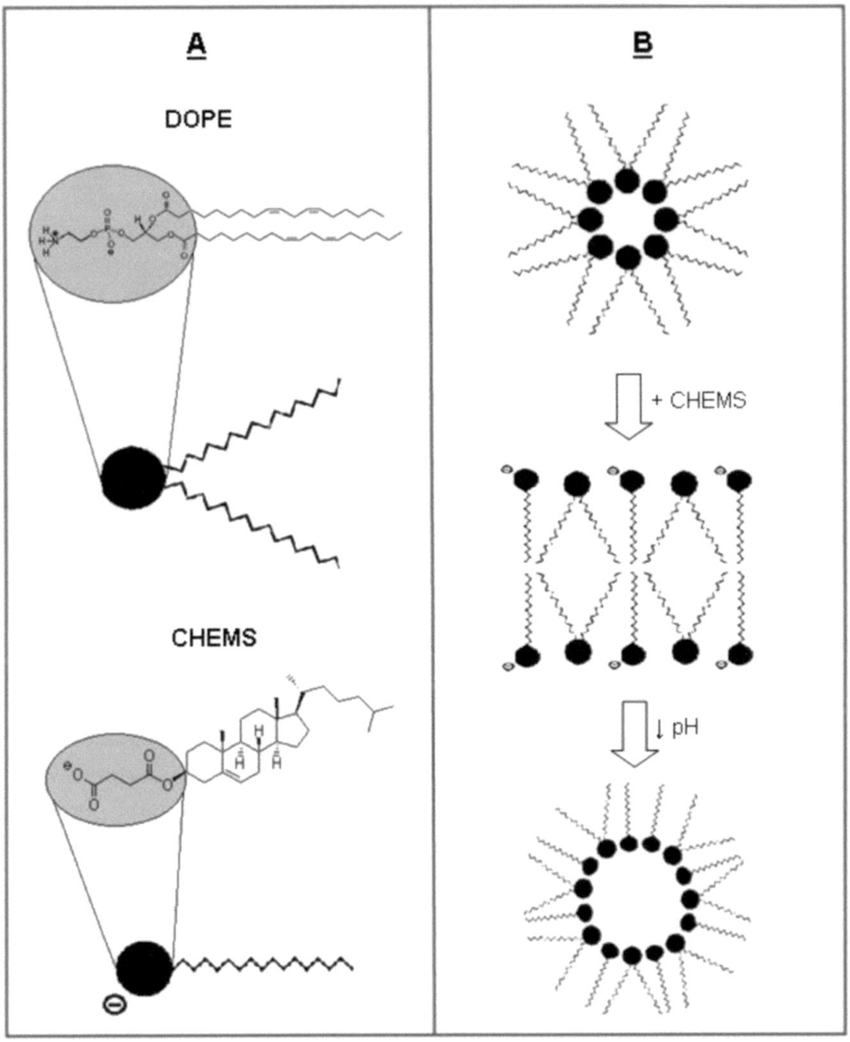

Figure 5. Main constituents of pH-sensitive liposomes and their structural representation (A) - DOPE and cholesteryl hemisuccinate (CHEMS); DOPE molecules alone will form the inverted hexagonal phase (B, upper). The introduction of CHEMS allows for the formation of the lamellar phase, which corresponds to the formation of liposomes (B, mid). When in contact with acidic pH, the liposomes undergo destabilization and return to the inverted hexagonal phase (B, low).

substances with a high affinity for receptors or other substances overexpressed by injured cells or tissues. These are also either absent or minimally present in healthy tissues [24] and are capable of directing the liposomes to the region of interest in a process called *active targeting*. The ligand can be introduced by covalent binding to the liposome surface or by electrostatic and hydrophobic insertion into the liposomal membrane [10]. Some examples of ligands are listed in Table 2.

Immunoliposomes			
Ligand	Target	Some types of cancer that overexpress the target (cell lines)	References
mAb 2C5	Surface-bound nucleosomes	Brain cancer (U-87)	[25]
mAb C225 (Cetuximab)	EGFR	Several types of tumor	[26]
scFv C10 (derived from mAb anti-human EGFR)	EGFR	Several types of tumor	[26]
mAb αCD19	CD19	Lymphomas and leukemias (B Cells)	[27]
mAb αCD20 (rituximab)	CD20	Lymphomas and leukemias (B Cells)	[27]
rhu-mAbHER2-Fab (Fab′ of trastuzumab)	HER2	Some types of breast cancer (BT-474 or MCF-7)	[28]
scFv F5 (derived from mAb anti-human HER2)	HER2	Some types of breast cancer (BT-474 or MCF-7)	[28]
Fab′222-1D8 (Fab′ of mAb anti-human MT1-MMP)	MT1-MMP	Several types of tumor	[29]
anti-TfR scFv	TfR	Several types of tumor	[30]
Surface modified liposomes with small molecules or peptides			
Ligand	Target	Some types of cancer that overexpress the target (cell lines)	References
RGD	Integrins	Melanoma (A375 and B16)	[31]
Transferrin	TfR	Several types of tumor	[32]
Estrone	ER	Some types of breast cancer (BT-474 or MCF-7)	[33]
Folate	FR	Ovarian carcinoma (KB)	[34]

mAb = monoclonal antibody; scFv = single chain variable fragment; RGD = Arginine-Glycine-Aspartic acid peptide; EGFR = Epidermal growth factor receptor; CD 19 = B-lymphocyte antigen CD19; CD 20 = B-lymphocyte antigen CD20; HER2 = Human epidermal growth factor receptor 2; MT1-MMP = membrane type-1 matrix metalloproteinase; TfR = Transferrin receptor; ER = estrogen receptor; FR = Folate receptor.

Table 2. Some examples of ligands of "*decorated*" liposomes for active tumoral targeting

3. Methods of liposome preparation

As aforementioned, liposomes are spontaneously formed when phospholipids are hydrated. Additional steps are often necessary to modify the size distribution and lamellarity of liposomes. Liposome preparation involves three major steps: vesicle formation, vesicle size reduction, and purification. Several preparation methods have been established based on the scale of the production and other considerations, such as drug encapsulation efficiency, the drug's physicochemical characteristics, and the administration route (Table 3).

VESICLES FORMATION	**LIPOSOMES' TYPES**
Lipid hydration followed by vortex or manual stirring	MLV
Reverse-phase evaporation	MLV, LUV
Organic solvent injection	MLV, LUV, SUV
Freeze-thawing	MLV, LUV
pH gradient	LUV, SUV
Dehydration-rehydration	MLV
Detergent dialysis	MLV, LUV
VESICLE SIZE REDUCTION	
Extrusion through polycarbonate membranes	LUV, SUV
High-pressure homogenization	LUV, SUV
Microfluidization	Mainly SUV
Sonication	Mainly SUV
PURIFICATION	
Centrifugation	-
Dialysis	-
Column chromatography separation	-
Ultrafiltration	-

Table 3. Methods of liposomes preparation. For more details see [6, 11, 35].

The most commonly used methods for liposome preparation are lipid hydration and the replacement of organic solvents by an aqueous media (reverse-phase evaporation and organic-solvent injection). The lipid hydration followed by vortex or manual stirring, also known as Bangham's method, consists of dissolving the lipids in a suitable organic solvent, such as chloroform or methanol. This process is then followed by removing the solvent under reduced pressure, by rotary evaporation, until a thin film has been formed. After, the thin film is hydrated in an aqueous medium, above the phase-transition temperature, resulting in the formation of MLV liposomes (Figure 6). This is the simplest method of vesicle formation; however, it is limited in use due to its low encapsulation ability [36,37].

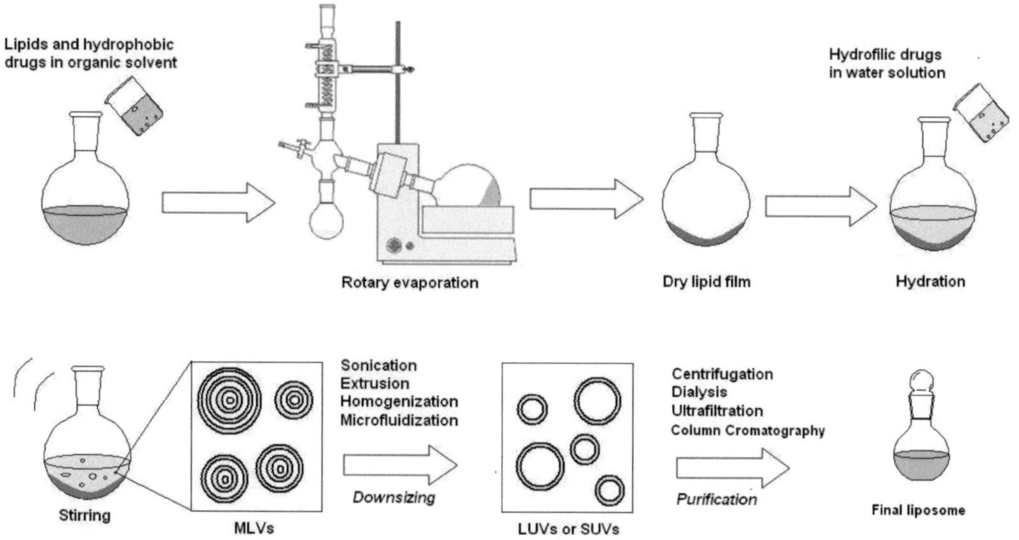

Figure 6. Representation of liposome production by lipid hydration followed by vortex or manual stirring.

All methods based on the replacement of an organic solvent by an aqueous media show that the solvents, whether miscible or immiscible with water, are replaced by an aqueous solution. First, the water-immiscible organic solution containing lipids is injected into the aqueous phase (reverse-phase method), or the stepwise addition of the organic phase (specifically, ethanol) is injected into the aqueous phase (organic solvent injection method), followed by the removal of the solvent. These methods are able to form liposomes with a high encapsulation percentage of both hydrophilic and lipophilic substances. Generally, the incorporation of lipophilic drugs is performed through their codissolution with the lipids [37]. Hydrophilic drugs are dissolved in the aqueous medium, whereas amphiphilic drugs can be dissolved in both mediums. The processes of liposome preparation can result in the formation of large vesicles (MLV) with heterogeneous size distribution; therefore, it is important to calibrate the formulation using a vesicle size reduction method (Table 3).

4. Liposome characterization

The behavior of liposomes in storage conditions and biological mediums is determined by specific factors, such as the size and surface charge of vesicles, chemical composition, membrane permeability, quantity of entrapped solutes, as well as the quality and purity of raw materials. Thus, it is of utmost importance to have as much information as possible regarding these parameters [6].

Bilayer constituents are responsible for the shelf-life; interactions with biological components, such as specific tissues, cells, and proteins; as well as the kinetics of the release of the entrapped drug in liposomes. The size of the liposomes influences their *in vivo* distribution, as this factor can determine the amount of time that the liposomes will remain in the bloodstream before being removed. By contrast, the surface charge of vesicles influences their physical stability due to the possible occurrence of fusion and/or aggregation phenomena [6]. Therefore, detailed chemical, physical, and physicochemical characterizations are important in an attempt to ensure the efficacy and stabilization of the liposome formulation.

Chemical analyses include the quantification of phospholipids and lysophospholipids, the evaluation of lipid oxidation, and the determination of the encapsulation percentage. As phospholipids represent the main constituents of the lipid bilayer, their quantification is important in evaluating the efficiency of the preparation method. Two degradation pathways have been described for phospholipids in aqueous liposomal dispersions: oxidative and hydrolytic degradation. The ester groups of the phospholipids can be hydrolyzed in the presence of water, producing lysophospholipids, a high concentration of which commonly leads to an increased permeability of the lipid bilayer and a destabilization of the system [38]. The oxidative pathway mainly involves phospholipids with unsaturated fatty acyl chains and tends to occur through the free radical mechanism. Lipid oxidation changes the bilayer's integrity, commonly resulting in drug leakage, in turn inducing aggregation and/or fusion phenomena. Another important chemical characterization is the encapsulation percentage, which is the ratio between the amount of drug already contained within the liposomes and the amount of drug added to the liposome at the beginning of the preparation. *In vivo* efficacy of the liposomes, as well as their physical and physicochemical properties, depends on the total amount of drug encapsulated within the liposome.

Physical characterization consists of determining the size, surface charge, and lamellarity of the liposomes. As the performance of liposomes *in vivo* and physical stability strongly depend on the vesicle size, liposome size distribution should be determined during the preparation process and storage. On the other hand, the nature and density of the charge on the liposome surface are important parameters that influence the mechanism and extent of liposome-cell interaction. Furthermore, the retention of the superficial charge for long periods during storage contributes to the high physical stability of the formulation.

Concerning the physicochemical characterization, the main evaluated parameters include the lipid phase and the phase-transition temperature. The determination of phase transitions and the fluidity of the bilayer are important in the production and application of liposomes, since the behavior of the liposome membrane determines the permeability, fusion/aggregation, and protein binding, thus influencing the stability of liposomes and their kinetics in biological systems.

The methods most commonly used for liposome characterization, according to the parameters described above, are listed in Table 4.

CHARACTERISTICS	METHODOLOGY
Phospholipids quantification	Lipid phosphorus content (Bartlett method)
Lysophospholipids quantification	Liquid chromatography combined with Bartlett method
Lipid oxidation	Spectroscopy, thin layer chromatography (TLC), high-performance liquid chromatography (HPLC), gas-liquid chromatography (GC)
Determination of the encapsulation percentage	Spectrophotometry, fluorescence spectroscopy, enzyme-based methods, electrochemical techniques and HPLC
Size	Static and dynamic light scattering, microscopy techniques (light, electronic and atomic force), size-exclusion chromatography, field-flow fractionation and analytical centrifugation
Surface charge	Photon correlation spectroscopy associated with the electrophoretic mobility
Lamellarity	Nuclear magnetic resonance (^{31}P-NMR), electron microscopy, small angle X-ray scattering
Lipid phase	X-ray diffraction, differential scanning calorimetry
Phase-transition temperature	Differential scanning calorimetry and nuclear magnetic resonance (^{31}P-NMR or ^{1}H-NMR)

Table 4. Major methods of liposomes characterization. Based on [39, 40].

5. Strategies to optimize liposome stability: Focus on freeze-drying

As for any new high-tech product, the transfer from academic research to an industrial enterprise is crucial. Any commercial product involving a liposome formulation must contain well-defined stability characteristics and a shelf-life of more than one year. In this context, it is currently possible to obtain a reproducible preparation of large volumes of stable liposomes, and, in most cases, long-term stability problems have also been successfully solved [7].

The stability of liposomes is of major concern in their development for pharmaceutical applications. However, the potential application of liposomes as therapeutic tools is challenged by their inherent physical and chemical instability in aqueous mediums, which can result in an increased bilayer permeability and subsequent drug leakage, vesicle aggregation/ fusion, and precipitation [41]. These instabilities can be stimulated by bilayer defects induced by chemical degradation (e.g. lipid oxidation and hydrolysis); by physical factors, such as heating or freezing; or due to phase transitions that occur when these aqueous dispersions are stored for extended periods [42,43]

The major approach to increase liposome stability is to establish an appropriate formulation, which requires the selection of the appropriate lipid composition and concentration, as well as the addition of other substances to improve its shelf-life. For example, the inclusion of cholesterol and its derivatives can reduce the permeability of the lipid bilayer. As unsaturated lipids commonly suffer peroxidation, the use of antioxidants and metal chelators may be necessary. Furthermore, it is of utmost importance to avoid the presence of oxygen both in the form of dissolved oxygen and in the headspace of the container. Liposomes in an aqueous dispersion can also be hydrolyzed to form lysophospholipids and fatty acids. This process is catalyzed by hydroxyl and hydrogen ions and can be diminished by pH control, i.e., by adding a neutral buffer [44].

Beyond formulation optimization, many methods available for the stabilization of liposomes have been investigated, such as freeze-drying and spray-drying. Freeze-drying is the main approach used to extend the shelf-life of liposomes, especially for thermosensitive drugs encapsulated within liposomes [43].

Freeze drying, also known as lyophilization, is a complex drying process employed to convert solutions of labile materials into solids of sufficient stability for distribution and storage. Freeze-drying is an industrial process which consists of removing the water from a frozen sample by sublimation and desorption through a vacuum process. Nevertheless, this process generates a wide range of stress, including fusion and drug loss, during the freezing and drying steps when conducted without the proper stabilizers [42,45]. To promote the stability of the vesicles during freeze-drying, cryoprotectants, such as saccharides and their derivates (e.g. sucrose, trehalose, hydroxypropyl-β-cyclodextrin (HP--CD), are employed [46,47].

It is generally accepted that sugars can depress the main phase transition temperature (T_m) from the lamellar gel (L_β) to the lamellar liquid-crystalline (L_α) phase during drying. Two main hypotheses were proposed to explain this depression effect of sugars: water replacement and vitrification.

Water replacement is the earliest established and the most widely accepted mechanism of membrane stabilization by sugars. It has been proposed that specific and particular interactions between phospholipids and sugars are required to produce the protective effect. Water is generally found around the polar head groups, with a slight penetration within the ester region between the glycerol backbone and the fatty acid residues. Accordingly, studies have shown that the interactions occur through the hydrogen bond between hydroxyl groups of the sugars and the phosphate groups on the bilayer surface. In summary, the sugars reduce the interactions between the water and phospholipids, and then the water is replaced [43,48]. It could be observed that trehalose, which has been considered an anomalous sugar in some studies, can also penetrate deeply into the membrane and form hydrogen bonds with the carbonyl groups of the phospholipids [49,50,51]. Therefore, trehalose seems to have a higher affinity for bonding with phospholipids.

The vitrification hypothesis is based on the effect of the hydration's repulsive force, which separates the membrane phospholipids when there is an excess of water. During drying, when the water content, or the hydration repulse, is lowered, the compressive stress will increase. Vitrification states that sugars limit the close approach of phospholipids in the lamellar liquid-crystalline-to-lamellar gel phase transition through their nonspecific effects (no particular sugar-lipid interaction is required), namely, osmotic and volumetric properties as well as vitrification. The increase in the osmotic pressure of the solution, due to the presence of sugars, confines the water removal from the interface of the membranes. A high osmotic pressure leads to a low suction of any water molecules; therefore, less water is removed. Furthermore, the molecular volume of moderately large sugars will maintain the phospholipids molecules separate. A further reduction of the stress levels occurs when the sugars do not crystallize, but rather vitrify in the membrane space during drying. It has been proposed that the rigidity or mechanical resistance of the glassy solid makes it more difficult for the membranes to reduce their spatial distance under compressive stress [52].

It should be noted that mechanisms of water replacement and vitrification are not mutually exclusive. The more important issue is the determining factor for T_m depression. According to the former hypothesis, it has been reported that vitrification is often required for the stabilization of the membrane but is not sufficient on its own [53]. Alternatively, it has also been proposed that specific sugar/lipid interaction may well exist but contributes little to the effect of preventing an increase in T_m without the vitrification of sugars [48].

In addition to stability, discussed above, other criteria must also be fulfilled to provide the acceptance of liposomes as pharmaceuticals. An efficient and adequate process for the preparation of sterile, pryrogen-free liposomes, by parenteral route, should be developed on an industrial scale. Furthermore, the final product must contain high and reproducible levels of drug entrapment, with minimal amounts of free drugs.

6. Liposomes in cancer therapy: A review of pharmacodynamic, pharmacokinetic, and toxicological studies

To develop pharmaceutical products, preclinical studies of pharmacodynamic, pharmacokinetic, and toxicological properties are required by regulatory agencies as part of procedures that must be followed prior to beginning clinical trials [54]. The Food and Drug Administration (FDA) requires that animal studies be reasonable predictors of the pharmacological activity of the investigated agent. In addition, toxicity studies should also be used to reveal adverse events that could be relevant to humans [55].

Pharmacodynamic studies include the characterization of action mechanisms, resistance, and treatment schedules, as well as the evaluation of the pharmacological activity *in vivo*. Although many drugs do act strongly against cancer, their use is commonly limited due to their toxic effects. Consequently, the definition of a toxicity profile is essential for the development of new drugs.

Concerning antitumor therapy, the primary role of preclinical toxicology is to identify a safe starting dose for Phase I trials, in addition to a potential for toxicity and its reversibility. The evaluation of toxicity includes pharmacological safety studies; single and repeated dose toxicity studies; as well as genotoxicity/carcinogenicity, reproductive toxicity, and local tolerance studies. Furthermore, wherever possible, pharmacokinetic/toxicokinetic studies should be included to define pharmacological endpoints related to both toxicity and efficacy for their use in the design of Phase I trials [54].

Liposomes have been used as carriers of platinum compounds (cisplatin and oxaplatin), anthracyclines (doxorubicin and daunorubicin), paclitaxel, camptothecin derivatives, antimetabolites (methotrexate, cytarabine), and Vinca alkaloids (vincristine, vinblastine and vinorelbine), aimed at reducing the toxic side-effects of cytostatic drugs without hampering their efficacy [56]. Their applications are based on the ability of liposomes to modify the tissue distribution of the entrapped drug, which becomes dependent on the physicochemical features of the liposomes and not the encapsulated content [57-59]. In addition, in cancer chemotherapy, the passive targeting of liposomes takes advantage of the inherent size of nanoparticles and the unique properties of tumor vasculature. As tumors grow and begin to outstrip the available supply of oxygen and nutrients, they release molecules that recruit new blood vessels to the tumor in a process called angiogenesis. Unlike the tight blood vessels in normal tissues, angiogenic blood vessels in tumor tissues contain gaps as large as 600 to 800 nm between adjacent endothelial cells. This dysregulated nature of tumor angiogenesis, coupled with poor lymphatic drainage, induces an enhanced permeability and a retention effect (EPR). Therefore, long-circulating liposomes will preferentially extravasate from these abnormal vessels and can selectively accumulate within the tumor interstitium [8,60-62].

6.1. Platinum compounds

Cisplatin (CDDP) (Figure 7) is one of the most effective chemotherapeutic agents used by intravenous route in the treatment of ovary, lung, testicle, head, and neck carcinomas [63-69]. Furthermore, CDDP has been widely used in the treatment of peritoneal carcinomatosis by intraperitoneal route. However, the administration of CDDP by both routes is still hindered by toxicity, mainly nephrotoxicity. Conventional liposomes composed of phosphatidylcholine/phosphatidylserine/CHOL containing CDDP were evaluated in IgM immunocytoma-bearing LOU/M rats. The results showed a lower incidence and severity of renal lesions after the liposomal formulation injection as compared to the free CDDP formulation. By contrast, the antitumor activity of this liposomal CDDP was similar to that of free CDDP, and the encapsulation of CDDP within this liposome formulation was unable to overcome drug resistance [70]. Newman and coworkers [71] developed a long-circulating formulation composed by hydrogenated soy phosphatidylcholine/DSPE-PEG$_{2000}$/CHOL (SPI-077) and performed *in vivo* studies using both C26 colon carcinoma and the Lewis lung tumor model. SPI-077 exhibited a 55-fold lower distribution volume and a 60-fold larger plasma area under the concentration–time curve (AUC). An increased tumor platinum uptake and a significantly improved antitumor effect could be observed with the use of SPI-077, as compared to free CDDP [72]. The experience from several clinical trials (phase I/II) with SPI-077® indicated a promising toxicity profile; however, the therapeutic efficacy might be hampered by an unsatisfactory release of CDDP from the liposomes. In a phase I study performed with 27 adult patients, no antitumor efficacy after SPI-077® treatment, along with relatively low levels of platinum-DNA adducts in tumor samples, could be observed [73].

Another long-circulating liposomal formulation containing CDDP made up of soy phosphatidylcholine (SPC)/ DPPG /CHOL/DSPE-PEG$_{2000}$ is called Lipoplatin®. This formulation was developed to reduce the systemic toxicity of CDDP while simultaneously improving the targeting of the drug to the primary tumor and metastasis by enhancing the circulation time in body fluids and tissues [74]. Cytotoxicity studies of this formulation were performed in cell

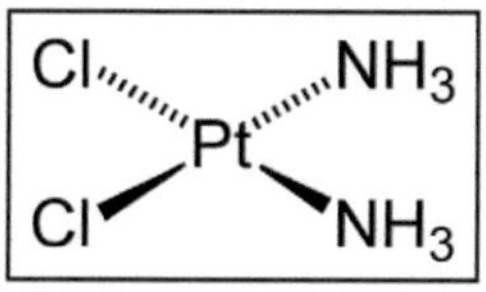

Figure 7. Chemical structure of CDDP

lines derived from non-small cell lung cancer, renal cell carcinoma, and in normal hematopoietic cell precursors. Lipoplatin®, when compared to CDDP, produced a stronger cytotoxic effect in both evaluated tumor cells lines and a lower toxicity in normal bone marrow stem cells [75]. Fielder and coworkers [76] investigated whether the cytotoxic effect of Lipoplatin® is dependent on the function integrity of DNA mismatch repair and concluded that this function is a key determining factor accounting for the cytotoxicity of lipoplatin. Antitumor efficacy of Lipoplatin® was assessed in xenografts of human breast, prostate, and pancreatic cancer, where a reduction in tumor size could be observed. Histopathological analyses of the tumors showed apoptosis in the tumor cells in a mechanism similar to that of CDDP [77]. Concerning toxicity, mice and rats treated with CDDP developed renal insufficiency with clear evidence of tubular damage, but those treated with the same dose of Lipoplatin® were completely free of kidney injury [78]. In addition, Lipoplatin® was safely administered to normal dogs at doses of up to 150 mg/m^2 without the need for concurrent hydration protocols [79]. As regards clinical trials, Stathopoulos and coworkers [74] investigated the pharmacokinetics and toxicity of Lipoplatin® (25-125 mg/m^2) in patients with pretreated advanced malignant tumors. Measurement of platinum levels in the plasma of patients as a function of time showed that a maximum platinum level is attained at 6-8 h. The half-life of Lipoplatin® was 60-117 h, depending on the dose. Urine excretion reached approximately 40% of the infused dose in 3 days. Grades 1 and 2 gastrointestinal tract and hematological toxicities were detected after the administration of the highest dose. No nephrotoxicity could be observed. Boulikas and coworkers [80] explored the hypothesis that intravenous infusion of Lipoplatin® can result in preferential tumor uptake in clinical trials. The determining of platinum levels in excised tumors and normal tissues showed that Lipoplatin® has the ability to preferentially concentrate on the malignant tissue (10-50 fold) of both primary and metastatic origin, as compared to adjacent normal tissue, following intravenous infusion in patients. Two phase I and I-II studies were carried out to investigate the maximum tolerated dose (MTD) as well as the dose-limiting toxicity (DLT). The first trial was conducted using a combination of Lipoplatin® and gemcitabine in patients with pretreated advanced pancreatic cancer, refractory to prior chemotherapy with gemcitabine. The results showed an absence of nephrotoxicity after administration of Lipoplatin® at doses of 100 and 125 mg/m^2. However, grade 2 neutropenia and grade 1 nausea/vomiting, fatigue, diarrhea, neurotoxicity, and thrombotic episodes could be observed after the administration of Lipoplatin® at similar doses. Thus, the DLT and MTD to Lipoplatin, established in combination with 1000 mg/m^2 of gemcitabine, were 125 and 100 mg/m^2, respectively.

The combination achieved a partial response in 8.33% of the patients, disease stability in 58.3%, and clinical benefit in 33.3% [81]. In the second study, similar DLT and MTD were defined in patients with refractory or resistant non-small cell lung carcinoma [82]. However, as lipoplatin was combined with gemcitabine, the latter can be responsible for the toxicity observed. In this context, the administration of single Lipoplatin® was also tested and nephrotoxicity, gastro-intestinal toxicity, and myelotoxicity were investigated as the main adverse reactions. From this study, DLT and MTD values were found for Lipoplatin® at 350 mg/m^2 and 300 mg/m^2, respectively. The dose of 350 mg/m^2 was not accompanied by nephrotoxicity, only by gastro-intestinal side effects and grade 1-2 myelotoxicity. It seems that the dose of Lipoplatin® can reach a level that is double or even higher than that of CDDP without increasing toxicity [83]. A phase II study combining Lipoplatin® and vinorelbine in the first-line treatment of HER2/neu-negative metastatic breast cancer was also conducted [84]. The results showed complete response in 9.4% of the patients, partial response in 43.8%, stable disease in 37.5%, and progressive disease in 9.4%. In addition, this regimen was well tolerated and no grade 3/4 nephrotoxicity and neurotoxicity could be detected. In another phase II trial, Lipoplatin® (120 mg/m^2 given on days 1, 8, 15), administered in association with gemcitabine (1000 mg/m^2 given on days 1, 8) in inoperable (stage IIIB/IV) non-small cell lung cancer, showed a better response rate (31.7%) than those treated with CDDP associated with gemcitabine (25.6%). Furthermore, lower nephrotoxicity after Lipoplatin® treatment, as compared to CDDP treatment, could be observed [85]. The first phase III clinical trial reported is a randomized, multicenter safety and efficacy study in patients with advanced squamous cell carcinoma of the head and neck. The pharmacokinetic profile of Lipoplatin® in combination with 5-fluorouracil showed that the liposomal formulation has a greater body clearance and a shorter half-life than does free CDDP, which confirms the clinical observation of decreased toxicity, especially nephrotoxicity [86]. The efficacy results showed 38.8% and 19% objective partial remission after treatment with free CDDP and lipoplatin, respectively. On the other hand, 64% of the patients achieved a stable disease after Lipoplatin® treatment, as compared to 50% of the patients that received CDDP [87]. In a second phase III trial, Lipoplatin® was much more well-tolerated than was CDDP in non-small cell lung cancer. Chemotherapy-naive patients received either 200 mg/m^2 of liposomal CDDP and 135 mg/m^2 paclitaxel (arm A) or 75 mg/m^2 of liposomal CDDP and 135 mg/m^2 of paclitaxel (arm B), once every 2 weeks. Arm A patients showed statistically significant lower nephrotoxicity, grade 3 and 4 leucopenia, grade 2 and 3 neuropathy, nausea, vomiting, and fatigue. There was no significant difference in the median and overall survival and in time to tumor progression (TTP) between the two arms; the median survival was 9 and 10 months in arms A and B, respectively, while TTP was 6.5 and 6 months in arms A and B, respectively [88]. Therefore, phase I, II, and III trials have shown that Lipoplatin® presents similar antitumor efficacy to CDDP in pancreatic, head and neck, breast cancers, and non-small cell lung carcinoma, as well as reduced toxicity, mainly nephrotoxicity. Preliminary studies have shown that Lipoplatin® is a candidate to be used in patients with renal failure [89].

Hirai and coworkers [68] encapsulated CDDP into liposomes and further conjugated the CDDP liposomes (CDDP-Lip) with a tetrasaccharide carbohydrate, Sialyl Lewis^X (CDDP-SLX-Lip). These liposomes consisted of DPPC/CHOL/ganglioside/dicetylphosphate/dipalmitoyl-phosphatidylethanolamine (DPPE) at the molar ratio of 35:40:5:15:5, respectively. A549 tumor-bearing mice treated with CDDP-SLX-Lip showed a survival rate of 75% at 14 days, even when a lethal level of CDDP was injected. Loss of body weight was negligible, and no histological abnormality could be found in many of the normal tissues. Accumulation of CDDP-SLX-Lip was approximately 6 times more than that of CDDP-Lip or CDDP. Therefore, a better antitumor activity could be observed for CDDP-SLX-Lip than for CDDP-Lip, with significantly less toxic effects in normal tissues.

Although CDDP is one of the most widely used chemotherapeutic agents, the development of tumor cell resistance against CDDP is a limitation in the clinical application of this drug. In this context, Krieger and coworkers [69] performed *in vitro* studies which demonstrated that liposomes have the potential to overcome the chemoresistance of tumor cells. The lipid composition of liposomes contained SPC/CHOL/distearoylphosphatidylethanolaminepolyethyleneglycol (DSPE-PEG) in a 65/30/5 molar ratio, respectively. In these studies, PEGylated CDDP-containing liposomes were prepared, and the targetability of transferrin receptors (TfR) to correlate CDDP cell uptake with cytotoxicity in sensitive and CDDP resistant ovarian cancer cells (A2780), as compared to the free drug, was analyzed. Cytotoxicity proved to be even higher for liposomes, as compared to free CDDP, in the resistant cells after 24, 48, and 72 h, and slightly lower in the sensitive cells.

Júnior and coworkers [90] developed long-circulating and pH-sensitive liposomes containing CDDP (SpHL-CDDP), which were made up of DOPE/CHEMS/DSPE-PEG_{2000} at a molar ratio of 5.7:3.8:0.5, respectively. In an acid medium, such as tumor sites, CHEMS molecules undergo protonation, followed by the destabilization of liposomes and the release of CDDP. Thus, it is expected that the released CDDP in this specific site can improve the antitumor effect and reduce, or even eliminate, the side effects. Studies were carried out concerning the stability, cytotoxicity, and accumulation of this new formulation in a human small-cell lung carcinoma cell line (GLC4), as well as in its resistant subline. These liposomes were stable in plasma, circumvented the preclinical resistance to treatment with CDDP, and were able to introduce the same level of CDDP within resistant and sensitive cells. Biodistribution studies have demonstrated the ability of SpHL-CDDP, as compared to the injection of free CDDP, to promote a higher concentration and affinity of CDDP in Ehrlich solid tumors, as well as a lower renal perfusion of the anticancer agent after intravenous administration [90]. CDDP has also been widely used in the treatment of peritoneal carcinomatosis by the intraperitoneal (i.p.) route. However, CDDP, a low-molecular-weight compound, is rapidly absorbed by the capillaries in the i.p. serosa and transferred to the bloodstream, inducing the appearance of systemic side-effects, such as nephrotoxicity. Furthermore, i.p. CDDP chemotherapy is limited to patients whose residual tumor nodules are less than 0.5 cm in diameter after surgical debulking [91]. The failure of i.p. therapy is attributed to the poor penetration of CDDP within larger tumor masses. To achieve an optimal drug penetration within the tumor, the use of a high concentration and a longer time of contact with the tumor are required. In this context, Araújo and coworkers [92] evaluated the tissue distribution of SpHL-CDDP after their i.p. administration in Ehrlich ascitic tumor-bearing mice. The CDDP AUC obtained for ascitic fluid and blood after SpHL-CDDP administration was 3.3-fold larger and 1.3-fold lower, respectively, when compared with free CDDP treatment, thus indicating its high retention within the peritoneal cavity.

In addition, MTD values obtained after i.v. and i.p. administration of SpHL-CDDP in healthy mice were approximately three times higher than those obtained using free CDDP. Hematological investigations revealed no alterations in red and white blood cell counts upon i.v. and i.p. administration of SpHL-CDDP at a dose corresponding to the MTD in mice. In addition, SpHL-CDDP treatment caused no pronounced alterations in the blood urea and creatinine levels, nor did it induce morphological alterations in the kidneys of the mice [93, 94]. These findings indicate that the use of SpHL-CDDP as a drug delivery system can increase the safety of the drug and improve the therapeutic efficacy of the CDDP-based treatment. Thus, antitumor activity studies were conducted, and the results showed a significant reduction in the tumor volume, a higher tumor growth inhibition ratio, and the complete remission of the tumor in 18.2% of the Ehrlich solid tumor-bearing mice treated with SpHL-CDDP by intravenous route, as compared to the free CDDP treatment [94, 95]. In addition, the survival of animals treated with SpH-CDDP was higher than those treated with free CDDP after i.p. administration in initial or disseminated Ehrlich ascitic tumor-bearing mice [96]. These findings strongly indicate the potential of SpHL-CDDP for future clinical studies.

Oxaliplatin (Figure 8), an analoge of CDDP, has shown a good *in vitro* and *in vivo* antitumor effect and a better safety profile than cisplatin. However, the use of oxaliplatin is associated with side-effects which include neurotoxicity, hematologic toxicity and gastrointestinal tract toxicity. In addition, there is a significant risk of grade 3/4 neutropenia to the patients, and the occurrence of nausea and vomiting were generally mild to moderate. Nephrotoxicity is mild, allowing for the administration of oxaliplatin without hydration. Often, severe side effects can be observed, such as tubular necrosis. Furthermore, cellular resistance to free oxaliplatin has been observed, preventing the potential efficacy of free oxaliplatin [97]. Lipoxal® is a liposomal formulation of oxaliplatin made up of hydrogenated soy phospahatidylcholine (HSPC)/DPPG/CHOL/DSPE-PEG. This liposomal formulation containing oxaliplatin has also proven to induce the complete disappearance of human breast cancers in mice after 6 intravenous injections with 4 days intervals at a dose of 16 mg/Kg. On the other hand, the free oxaliplatin at its MTD could only cause shrinkage, not the disappearance of tumors. To estimate the adverse reactions and detect the dose limiting toxicity (DLT), as well as the MTD of Lipoxal®, a Phase I clinical study was conducted. Twenty-seven patients with advanced disease of the gastrointestinal system (stage IV gastrointestinal cancers, including colorectal, gastric, and pancreatic), who had failed previous standard chemotherapy, were treated with escalating doses of Lipoxal® once weekly for 8 weeks. No serious side effects were observed at doses of 100-250 mg/m^2, whereas at doses of 300 and 350 mg/m^2 of Lipoxal® monotherapy mild myelotoxicity, nausea and peripheral neuropathy were observed. Gastrointestinal tract toxicity after treatment with Lipoxal® was negligible. Nausea or mild vomiting was observed, but it was eliminated by administering ondansetron. The most common toxicity is peripheral neuropathy at the 300 and 350 mg/m^2 dose levels. Lipoxal® is well-tolerated and reduces significantly all other side effects of free oxaliplatin, especially myelotoxicity and gastrointes-

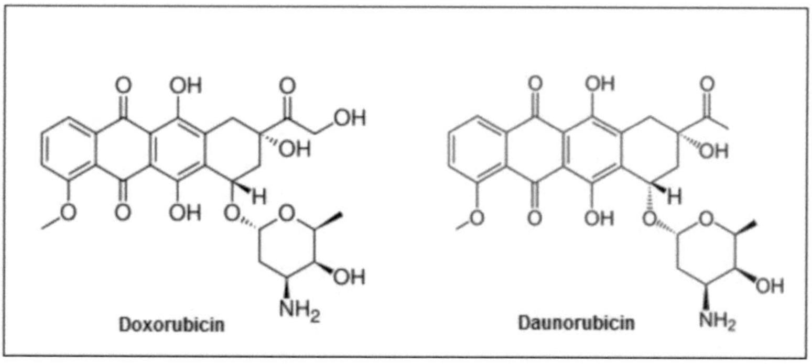

Figure 9. Chemical structures of principal anthracyclines.

tinal tract toxicity. These preliminary results showed adequate effectiveness in pretreated patients [98,99].

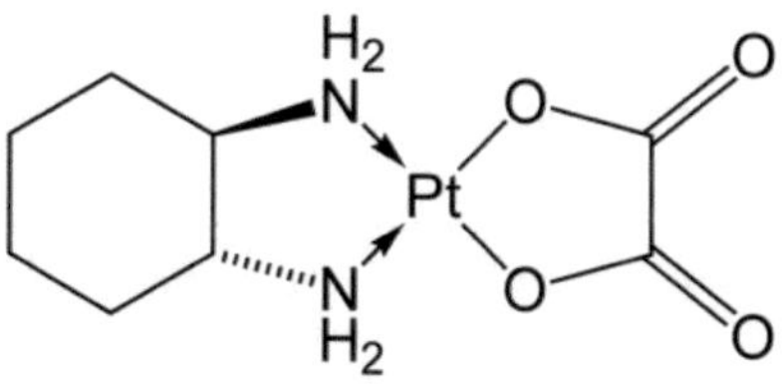

Figure 8. Chemical structure of oxaliplatin.

6.2. Anthracyclines

The anthracyclines, represented by doxorubicin, daunorubicin, and their derivatives (Figure 9), are widely used in the treatment of several hematological and solid tumors and are considered to be a first-line therapy for advanced breast cancer [100]. Although conventional anthracyclines have been extensively used for the treatment of a variety of cancers, they can be associated with the development of substantial cardiotoxicity, which is both cumulative and irreversible. Furthermore, cardiotoxicity can be increased nearly four-fold when these drugs are administered in association with other chemotherapeutic drugs [101]. In this case, the preclinical and clinical studies have focused on the development of liposomal formulations, aimed at decreasing the acute and cumulative cardiotoxicity, in addition to attenuating other drug-related events (e.g. bone marrow depression, alopecia, and nausea) [102].

Forssen and coworkers [103] reported the ability of liposomes containing daunorubicin (DNR), made up of DSPC/CHOL, to accumulate within the P-1798 murine lymphosarcoma and MA16C mammary adenocarcinona tumor model. The maximum levels of liposome uptake exceeded those achieved by the free drug between 2.5 and 20-fold, which was translated into a 10-fold increase in AUC of tumor exposure to DNR in the P-1798 system. Other investigations also significantly demonstrated increased efficacy and decreased toxicity of liposomes containing daunorubicin (DaunoXome®), as compared to free drug in the treatment of acute leukemia and advanced cutaneous T-cell lymphoma [104, 105]. In phase I/II clinical trials, DaunoXome® administration produced a 35-fold increase in the plasma AUC, higher peak plasma concentrations, a smaller distribution volume, and a lower total body clearance, when compared to free DNR [106]. Safety results from the combined phase I and II studies showed DaunoXome® to be especially well-tolerated with minimal myelosuppression, no evidence of cardiac toxicity, and a decrease in the frequency and severity of chemotherapy-related side effects when compared with free DNR. The MTD of liposomal DNR was set at 90 mg/m^2.

A randomized phase III trial was conducted to compare the safety and efficacy of DaunoXome® with that of a reference regimen of doxorubicin, bleomycin, and vincristine (ABV) as a primary therapy in advanced AIDS-related Kaposi's sarcoma. DaunoXome® presented an efficacy that was comparable to ABV, presented significantly less alopecia and neuropathy, and showed no evidence of cardiac toxicity [107]. In 1996, DaunoXome® was approved as a first-line therapy for HIV-related Kaposi's sarcoma by the FDA and the EMA. A European Phase IV study, carried out over a one year period after DaunoXome® had been approved for commercialization, demonstrated the treatment's good tolerability (absence of cardiotoxicity) and effectiveness. Furthermore, the concomitant administration of highly active antiretroviral treatment (HAART) also proved to be safe [108].

Another commercial product of conventional liposome (Myocet®), in combination with cyclophosphamide, has been approved in Europe as a first-line treatment of breast cancer. This liposome consists of egg phosphatidilcholine (EPC)/ CHOL and encapsulated doxorubicin (DXR). Preclinical toxicity studies performed on Beagles demonstrated a better toxicity profile of Myocet®, as compared to free DXR [109]. The ability of Myocet® to locate tumors could be observed in ascitic (L1210 ascitic lymphoma) and solid tumor (murine Lewis lung cancer and B16/BL6 melanoma) models, as reported in findings from Harasym and coworkers [110]. In the case of the solid tumor models, the maximum tumor concentrations were two to three-fold higher for liposomal DXR, as compared to free DXR. For the ascitic model, the maximal level in tumor drug exposure was ten-fold higher for liposomal DXR, as compared to free DXR. These findings supported the choice of Myocet® for clinical studies.

Some studies have shown that the replacement of free DXR by Myocet®, combined with cyclophosphamide, does not result in decreased efficacy parameters, but rather in a significantly reduced risk of cardiotoxicity [56]. A phase III comparison of free DXR with Myocet® in patients with metastatic breast cancer, for instance, demonstrated that, at comparable response rates (RR: 26% for both) and progression-free survival times (PFS: 4 months for both), the incidence of cardiac events (29% vs. 13%) and of congestive heart failure (8% vs. 2%) were significantly lower for Myocet® [102].

Cowens and coworkers [111] carried out a phase I study in 38 patients with refractory solid tumors and demonstrated diminished myelosupression and gastrointestinal toxicity after the intravenous injection of Myocet®, as compared to findings for free DXR at the same dose. The MTD for Myocet® was established as 90 mg/m^2. A multicentric study including 297 patients with metastatic breast cancer, carried out by Batist and coworkers [112], demonstrated that the combination of Myocet® (60 mg/m^2) with cyclophosphamide (600 mg/m^2) presents a similar efficacy and a lower toxicity than does the association of free DXR and cyclophosphamide at the same dose. The cardiotoxicity was dramatically reduced (21% vs. 6%).

The tissue distribution, efficacy, and toxicity of DXR encapsulated in a long-circulating liposomal formulation made up of HSPC/DSPE-PEG$_{2000}$/CHOL (Doxil®/Caelyx®) were also investigated. Therapeutic efficacy studies performed in different animal models demonstrated that Doxil®/Caelyx® was significantly more active than free DXR [113, 114]. A tissue distribution study of this formulation indicated a preferential accumulation within various implanted tumors and human tumor xenografts, with an enhancement of drug concentrations, when compared with free drug, in the tumors. In addition, the cardiac toxicity of Doxil®, as compared to free DXR, was significantly reduced [115].

Doxil®/Caelix® was the first and is still the only long-circulating liposome formulation to be approved in both the USA and Europe to treat Kaposi's sarcoma and recurrent ovarian cancer [116, 117]. In association with Velcade®(Bortezomib), this drug is approved by the FDA for the treatment of multiple myeloma. In Europe, this drug is still approved for the treatment of metastatic breast cancer. When compared to free DXR, Doxil® presents a lower plasma clearance (0.1 vs. 25 L/hour for Doxil® and free DXR, respectively) and a small distribuition volume (4 vs. 200 L). Doxil® presents two distribution phases: an initial phase with a half-life of 1-3 hours and a second phase with a half-life of 30-90 hours. Its half-life is longer than the free DXR (0.2 hours). Due to this, its cardiotoxicity, myelosuppression, alopecia, and nausea are significantly reduced when compared with an equieffective dose of free DXR. It has also been demonstrated that nearly all circulating drugs (>98%) are used in liposome-encapsulated form, indicating that the pharmacokinetics of liposomal DXR is governed by the liposome carrier and that most of the drug is delivered to the tissues in liposome-associated form [115]. Several studies are currently in progress using Doxil®/Caelix® to treat other malignancies, such as breast cancer and recurrent high-grade glioma [118-120].

6.3. Other chemotherapeutic agents

Another important drug in cancer therapy is paclitaxel. This is an alkaloid which stabilizes microtubules and inhibits endothelial cell proliferation, motility, and tube formation [121]. Some studies have presented difficulties in the development of liposomes containing paclitaxel due to its hydrophobic nature. Zhang and coworkers [122] developed a liposomal formulation of paclitaxel consisting of 1,2-dioleyl-sn-glycero-3-phosphocholine/ CHOL /cardiolipin (LEP-ETU). Therapeutic efficacy studies performed in a mouse xenograft model of human ovarian (OVCAR-3), human lung (A-549), breast (MX-1), and prostate (PC-3) cancer, as compared to the administration of free drugs, demonstrated greater tumor growth inhibition after the administration of liposomal paclitaxel. In addition, toxicology studies have shown that liposomal paclitaxel is less toxic than free paclitaxel. An improved pegylated liposomal formulation of paclitaxel was developed, demonstrating that cytotoxicity in human breast cancer cell lines (MDA-MB-231 and SK-BR-3) of the tested paclitaxel formulation was equipotent after 72 h of incubation, when compared to Taxol®. The pegylated liposomes, as compared to the conventional liposomes, increased the biological half-life of paclitaxel from 5.05 ± 1.52 h to 17.8 ± 2.35 h in rats. Biodistribution studies in a breast cancer xenograft nude mouse model demonstrated that the uptake of these liposomes significantly increased in tumor tissues after their injection, as compared to Taxol® or the conventional liposomal formulation. Moreover, the pegylated liposome showed a greater tumor growth inhibition effect in *in vivo* studies [123]. In a study by Strieth et al. (2008) [124], paclitaxel was encapsulated in cationic liposomes composed of dioleytrimethylammoniumpropane (DOTAP)/DOPC (EndoTAG-1) as a vascular targeting formulation to treat solid tumors and quantified the therapeutic combination with conventional CDDP chemotherapy. This study showed that vascular targeting with EndoTAG-1 increased tumor microvessel leakage, most likely due to vascular damage, and concluded that manipulating the blood-tumor barrier by repeated tumor microvessel targeting using EndoTAG-1 can effectively be combined with tumor cell directed conventional cisplatin chemotherapy.

In a study by Strieth and coworkers, paclitaxel was encapsulated in cationic liposomes composed of dioleytrimethylammoniumpropane (DOTAP)/dioleoylphosphatidylcholine (DOPC) (EndoTAG-1) as a vascular targeting formulation to treat solid tumors and quantified the therapeutic combination with conventional cisplatin chemotherapy. This study showed that vascular targeting with EndoTAG-1 increased tumor microvessel leakage, most likely due to vascular damage, and concluded that manipulating the blood-tumor barrier by repeated tumor microvessel targeting using EndoTAG-1 can effectively be combined with tumor cell directed conventional cisplatin chemotherapy [124].

Another formulation approved in Europe for lymphomatous meningitis is DepoCyte®, a sustained-release formulation of cytarabine. A randomized study to evaluate the efficacy and safety of this liposomal formulation, in comparison with free drug, was performed in 28 patients with lymphomatous meningitis. While the reference treatment required the administration of free cytarabine biweekly, it could be observed that the administration of Depocyte® intrathecal maintains cytotoxic concentrations of the drug in the cerebrospinal fluid of most patients for more than 14 days. Response rates (i.e. clearing of cerebrospinal fluid and absence of neurological progression) were significantly higher in Depocyte®. In addition, the less demanding injection schedule is favorable to the patients' quality of life. The major adverse events were headache and arachnoiditis, which were often caused by the underlying disease [125]. Another randomized trial compared DepoCyte® with methotrexate in patients with solid tumor neoplastic meningitis. The results showed that median survival was not different, but a greater median time to neurological progression was obtained with DepoCyte®. The frequency and grade of adverse events were comparable between treatments [126]. More recently, a phase II study of intrathecal liposomal cytarabine was performed at the dose of 50 mg in 30 patients with human immunodeficiency virus–non-Hodgkin lymphoma (HIV-NHL) to evaluate the feasibility and activity of prophylaxis. In this study, liposomal cytarabine was well-tolerated, with a headache of grade I to III being the most frequent side effect in 40% of the patients. With a median follow-up of 10.5 months, only 1 (3%) patient developed a combined systemic and meningeal recurrence. The use of liposomal cytarabine allowed for a significant reduction in the number of lumbar injections, as compared to the standard schedules (approximately 50%), improving the patients' quality of life and reducing their risk of professional exposure [127]

Marqibo®, a DSPC/CHOL encapsulation of vincristine sulfate has targeted, increased, and sustained the delivery of vincristine to tumor tissues. A phase II study evaluated the efficacy and tolerability of Marqibo® as a single agent in patients with multiple relapsed or refractory aggressive non-Hodgkin lymphoma (NHL). In this study, eligible patients again presented relapsed, refractory, or transformed aggressive NHL and prior treatment with at least 2 multiagent chemotherapy regimens. Marqibo® was administered at 2 mg/m^2, every 2 weeks, for a maximum of 12 cycles or until toxicity or disease progression had been resolved. Marqibo® proved to be an active agent in patients with heavily pretreated aggressive NHL and to be tolerated at approximately twice the dose intensity of standard vincristine [128].

6.4. Recent advances in targeted liposomes

Considering that tumor cells are often characterized by a specific expression pattern of membrane associated proteins, such as receptors, membrane transport systems, or adhesion molecules, cancer therapies that exploit targeting ligands to deliver attached cytotoxic drugs selectively to malignant cells are currently receiving significant attention and are being recognized as an effective strategy for increasing the therapeutic indices of anticancer drugs. In an attempt to improve the binding and cellular internalization of liposomes in the tumor area, several ligands were attached to the liposome surface, including monoclonal antibodies, folate, transferrin, vasoactive intestinal peptide (VIP), epidermal growth factor (EGF), hyaluronan, galactosides, and condroitin sulphate [129, 130].

The majority of research in this area is related to cancer targeting, which uses a variety of monoclonal antibodies. To target HER2-overexpressing tumors, it was suggested that anti-HER2 long-circulating liposomes be used. Antibody CC52 against rat colon adenocarcinoma CC531 attached to pegylated liposomes provided a specific accumulation of liposomes in rat model of metastatic CC531. A nucleosome-specific monoclonal antibody (mAb 2C5) capable of recognizing various tumor cells through the tumor cell surface-bound nucleosomes significantly improved Doxil®, by targeting to tumor cells, and increased its cytotoxicity both *in vitro* and *in vivo* in different testing systems, including the intracranial human brain U-87 tumor xenograft in nude mice. The same antibody was also used to effectively target long-circulating liposomes loaded with an agent for tumor photodynamic therapy (PDT) for both multiple cancer cells *in vitro* and experimental tumors *in vivo*, and provided a significantly enhanced elimination of tumor cells under PDT conditions [5].

Previous studies have demonstrated that DXR-loaded long-circulating liposomes prolong circulation in the blood but create a steric barrier that could cause a reduction in the interaction of liposomes with the target cells [131]. In this light, XueMing Li and coworkers [132] prepared DXR-loaded long-circulating liposomes conjugated with transferrin (Tf) and observed that Tf-modified liposomes could be used to enhance the intracellular delivery of anticancer agents, such as cytotoxic drugs, antisense nucleic acids, ribozymes, or imaging agents.

Saccharide molecules represent good models for tumor targeting molecules, as many malignant cells express the lectin, sugar-binding protein. In this context, Song and coworkers [133] investigated the *in vitro* characteristics of liposomes consisting of HSPC/CHOL/DSPE-PEG$_{2000}$-disaccharide whose surface had been modified with a disaccharide molecule, sucrose, or maltose and that were then loaded with DXR. They concluded that disaccharide-modified liposomes may be promising cancer targeting carriers which can enhance intracellular uptake and cytotoxicity of the drug-loaded liposomes by means of lectin-mediated endocytosis.

One approach that has received considerable attention has been the use of folic acid to deliver drugs selectively to folate receptor-expressing cancer cells [130]. Studies of folate-conjugated liposomes containing DNR or DXR showed an increased cytotoxicity of the encapsulated anticancer drugs in various tumor cells [134, 135]. The i.v. administration of anti-tumor-associated glycoprotein (TAG)-72 Polyethyleneglycol (PEG)-immunoliposomes showed that they were more effectively located in LS174 T human colon cancer cells than conventional liposomes [136]. It is worth noting that the co-immobilization of PEG and ligands on the same surface liposome can in fact lead to poor target recognition due to a steric hindrance by the hydrophilic corona [137]. Thus, it has been suggested that targeting vectors be attached to the distal end of pegylated phospholipids [138].

Several liposomal formulations of anticancer drugs have also been investigated in preclinical tumor models and many liposomal preparations of anticancer drugs have been approved for cancer chemotherapy or are in advanced stages of clinical development. Some of these products are listed in Table 5.

Product	Entrapped Drug	Lipid composition	Company	Therapeutic Indication	Status[a]
Doxil®/ Caelyx®	Doxorubicin	HSPC/CHOL/ DSPE-PEG_{2000}	Janssen-Cilag	Kaposi's sarcoma, recurrent ovarian, multiple myeloma, and metastatic breast cancer	A
Myocet®	Doxorubicin	EPC/CHOL	Cephalon	Metastatic breast cancer	A[b]
DaunoXome®	Daunorubicin	DSPC/CHOL	Galen US	Kaposi's sarcoma	A
DepoCyte®	Cytarabine	DOPC/DPPG/CHOL/ TRIOLEIN	Pacira	Lymphomatous meningitis	A
SPI-077®	Cisplatin	HSPC/CHOL/DSPE-PEG_{2000}	Sequus	Ovarian cancer	P II
Lipoplatin®	Cisplatin	DPPG/SPC/CHOL/ DSPE-PEG_{2000}	Regulon	Lung cancer	P III
Aroplatin®	bis-neodecanoate diaminocyclohexane platinum	DMPC/DMPG	Aronex	Colorectal, lung, and pancreatic cancer	P II
LEP-ETU®	Paclitaxel	DOPC/CHOL/ CARDIOLIPIN	Insys Therapeutics	Breast, lung, ovarian cancer	P II
EndoTAG-1®	Paclitaxel	DOPC/DOTAP	MediGene	Breast, pancreatic, and hepatic cancer	P II
ThermoDox®	Doxorubicin	DPPC/MSPC/DSPE-PEG_{2000}	Celsion	Bone metastasis, breast, and hepatocelular cancer	P II

Product	Entrapped Drug	Lipid composition	Company	Therapeutic Indication	Status[a]
Marqibo®	Vincristine	DSPC/CHOL	Talonn Therapeutics	Non-Hodgkin's lymphoma, acute lymphoblastic leukemia, and Hodgkin's lymphoma	P III
OSI-211® (NX211)	Lurtotecan	HSPC/CHOL	OSI	Ovarian cancer and small cell lung cancer	P III
LE-SN38®	Irinotecan metabolite SN38	DSPC/CHOL	NeoPharm	Colorectal and lung cancer	P II
INX-0076®	Topotecan	Sphingomyelin/CHOL	Inex	Ovarian and small lung cancer	P II
Alocrest®	vinorelbine	Sphingomyelin/CHOL	Inex	Non-small cell lung cancer and breast cancer	P I
Oncolipin®	Interleukin 2	DMPC	Biomirma USA Inc	kidney cancer	P II
OSI-7904L®	Thimidylate synthase inhibitor	HSPC/CHOL	OSI	Colorectal cancer	P II
CPX-351	Cytarabine and Daunorubicin	DSPC/DSPG/CHOL	Celator Pharmaceuticals	Acute myeloid leukemia	P II
CPX-1	Irinotecan and floxuridine	DSPC/DSPG/CHOL	Celator Pharmaceuticals	Advanced colorectal cancer	P II

[a] A = approved, PI = phase I study, PII = phase II study, PIII = phase III study; [b]approved by EMA

HSPC, hydrogenated soy phosphatidylcholine; CHOL, cholesterol; DSPE-PEG_{2000}, distearoylphosphatidylethanolamine-$polyethyleneglycol_{2000}$; EPC, egg phosphatidylcholine; DSPC, distearoylphosphatidylcholine; SPC, soy phosphatidylcholine; DOPC, dioleylphosphatidylcholine; DOTAP, dioleytrimethylammoniumpropane; DMPC, dimyristoyl phophatidylcholine; DSPG, Distearoylphosphatidylglycerol; MSPC, Myristoylstearoylphosphatidylcholine

Table 5. Approved and emerging liposome encapsulated anticancer drugs.

7. Future perspectives and challenges

This chapter focused on liposome-based drug delivery systems, which are the most widely used drug nanoparticles in cancer treatments. Basic concepts were presented concerning liposomes and an overview of the clinically used and tested liposomes for the treatment of cancer. It has been demonstrated, based on prior studies, that liposomes offer safety and effectiveness as compared to other conventional treatments.

The greater interest in the development of these sophisticated drug delivery systems is to improve the efficacy and decrease the side effects of new and old anti-cancer drugs. In this context, the optimized pharmacokinetic properties of liposomes, resulting in an improved toxicity profile, is still the main argument for the use of liposomal carriers.

Other new strategies in the biology and pharmacokinetic behavior of liposomes, such as the anti-angiogenic properties of cationic liposomes, as well as the development of immunoliposomes or antisense oligonucleotides, also offer a great therapeutic repertoire for these drug delivery systems.

However, despite all progress achieved to date, it is still important to discuss not only the benefits, but also the problems, which remain as a challenge in liposome-based drug delivery systems. As reviewed by Ruenraroengsak and coworkers [139], there are many issues regarding the instability of particles through flocculation and aggregation, their complex flow, and adhesion patterns in the capillary network, the heterogeneity of the access of drugs to specific tumor sites, the diffusion of free drugs, and nanoparticles in tumor tissues as well as in single cells.

The "passive" form of encapsulated drug delivery today is still mostly based on leakage in the tumor microenvironment, followed by the possibility of the cellular uptake of the free drug at the tumor site. As a result, many research groups are working on more "active" therapies that exploit targeting ligands to deliver attached cytotoxic drugs selectively to malignant cells. These ligands specifically recognize and preferentially bind receptors found on the cells of interest, thereby allowing for a more precise delivery method [140].

Although current studies have shown that the use of these targeted nanoparticles as a drug delivery system is a promising strategy to treat human cancers, it is still in its early stage of development. Clinical data using targeted nanoparticles are limited, since most targeted nanoparticles have not yet reached the clinical level. Only a few targeted nanoparticles are currently under clinical investigation. In addition, advanced imaging techniques are essential, especially in small animals, to verify the true extent of tumor and target localization [139].

In sum, liposomes provide many targeting strategies and have shown a promising future as a new generation of cancer therapeutics. Certain critical questions and many obstacles still remain, which present specific limitations to their overall efficacy. However, as soon as more clinical data becomes available, further understanding will certainly lead to a more rational design of optimized liposomes with improved selectivity, efficacy, and safety in cancer treatment [140].

Author details

Sávia Caldeira de Araújo Lopes[1], Cristiane dos Santos Giuberti[1,2], Talita Guieiro Ribeiro Rocha[1], Diêgo dos Santos Ferreira[1], Elaine Amaral Leite[3] and Mônica Cristina Oliveira[1]

1 Department of Pharmaceutical Products, School of Pharmacy, Federal University of Minas Gerais, Belo Horizonte, Minas Gerais, Brazil

2 Department of Pharmaceutical Sciences, Health Sciences Center, Federal University of Espirito Santo, Vitória, Brazil

3 Department of Pharmacy, School of Biological and Health Sciences, Federal University of Vales do Jequitinhonha e Mucuri, Diamantina, Minas Gerais, Brazil

References

[1] Thassu D, Pathak Y, Dellers M., editors. Nanoparticles Drug Delivery System. Drugs and Pharmaceuticals Sciences. London: Informa Healthcare; 2007.

[2] Malam Y, Loizidou M, Seifalian AM. Liposomes and nanoparticles: nanosized vehicles for drug delivery in cancer. Trends in Pharmacological Sciences 2009;30(11) 592-599.

[3] Raffa V, Vittorio O, Riggio C, Cuschieri A. Progress in nanotechnology for healthcare, Minimally Invasive Therapy 2010;19(3) 127–135.

[4] Tran MA, Watts RJ, Robertson GP. Use of liposomes as drug delivery vehicles for treatment of melanoma. Pigment cell melanoma Research 2009;22(4) 388-399.

[5] Torchilin V. Multifunctional and stimuli-sensitive pharmaceutical nanocarriers. European Journal of Pharmaceutics and Biopharmaceutics 2009;71(3) 431–444.

[6] New, RRC. Liposomes: a pratical approach. New York: Oxford University Press; 1990.

[7] Lasic, DD. Novel application of liposomes. Trends in Biotechnology 1998;16(7) 307-321.

[8] Huwyler J, Drewe J, Krähenbühl S. Tumor targeting using liposomal antineoplastic drugs. International Journal of Nanomedicine 2008;3(1) 21–29.

[9] Frezard F, Silva-Barcelos NM, Santos, RAS. A novel approach based on nanotechnology for investigating the chronic actions of short-lived peptides in specific sites of the brain. Regulatory Peptides 2007;138(2-3) 59–65.

[10] Batista, CM, Carvalho, CMB, Magalhães, NSS. Lipossomas e suas aplicações terapêuticas: Estado da arte. Brazilian Journal of Pharmaceutical Sciences 2007;43(2) 167-179.

[11] Vemuri S, Rhodes CT. Preparation and characterization of liposomes as therapeutic delivery systems: a review. Pharmaceutica Acta Helvetiae 1995;70(2) 95-111.

[12] Durocher JR, Payne RC, Conrad ME. Role of sialic acid in erythrocyte survival. Blood 1975;45(1) 11-20.

[13] Allen TM, Chonn A. Large unilamellar liposomes with low uptake into the reticuloendothelial system. FEBS Letters 1987;23(1) 42-46.

[14] Klibanov AL, Maruyama K, Torchilin VP, Huang L. Amphipathic polyethyleneglycols effectively prolong the circulation time of liposomes. FEBS Letters 1990;268(1) 235-237.

[15] Needham D, McIntosh TJ, Lasic DD. Repulsive interactions and mechanical stability of polymer-grafted lipid membranes. Biochimica et Biophysica Acta 1992;1108(1) 40-48.

[16] Torchilin VP, Omelyanenko VG, Papisov MI, Bogdanov AA Jr, Trubetskoy VS, Herron JN, Gentry CA. Poly(ethyleneglycol) on the liposome surface: on the mechanism of polymer-coated liposome longevity. Biochimica et Biophysica 1994;1195(1) 11-20.

[17] Zeisig R, Shimada K, Hirota S, Arndt D. Effect of sterical stabilization on macrophage uptake in vitro and on thickness of the fixed aqueous layer of liposomes made from alkylphosphocholines. Biochimica et Biophysica Acta 1996;1285(2) 237-45.

[18] Ulrich AS. Biophysical aspects of using liposomes as delivery vehicles. Bioscience Reports 2002;22(2) 129-150.

[19] Simões S, Moreira JN, Fonseca C, Düzgüneş N, de Lima MC. On the formulation of pH-sensitive liposomes with long circulation times. Advanced Drug Delivery Reviews 2004;56(7) 947-965.

[20] Carvalho-Júnior AD, Vieira FP, Melo VJM, Lopes MTP, Silveira JN, Ramaldes GA, Garnier-Suillerot A, Pereira-Maia EC, Oliveira MC. Preparation and cytotoxicity of cisplatin loaded liposomes. Brazilian Journal of Medical and Biological Research 2007;40(8) 1149-1157.

[21] Gulino PM, Grantham FH, Smith SH, Haggerty AC. Modification of the acid-basic status of the internal milieu of tumors. Journal of the National Cancer Institute 1967;34(6) 857-869.

[22] Bergstrand N, Arfvidsson MC, Kim JM, Thompson DH, Edwards K. Interactions between pH-sensitive liposomes and model membranes. Biophysical Chemistry 2003;104(1) 361-79.

[23] Hong MS, Lim SJ, Oh YK, Kim CK. pH-sensitive, serum-stable and long-circulating liposomes as a new drug delivery system. Journal of Pharmacy and Pharmacology 2002;54(1) 51-58.

[24] Wang M, Thanou M. Targeting nanoparticles to cancer. Pharmacological Research 2010;62(2) 90-99.

[25] Sawant RR, Torchilin VP. Challenges in Development of Targeted Liposomal Therapeutics. The AAPS Journal 2012;14(2) 303-315.

[26] Mamot C, Drummond DC, Noble CO, Kallab V, Guo Z, Hong K, Kirpotin DB, Park JW. Epidermal Growth Factor Receptor–Targeted Immunoliposomes Significantly Enhance the Efficacy of Multiple Anticancer Drugs In vivo. Cancer Research 2005;65(24) 11631-11638.

[27] Sapra P, Allen TM. Improved outcome when B-cell lymphoma is treated with combinations of immunoliposomal anticancer drugs targeted to both the CD19 and CD20 epitopes. Clinical Cancer Research 2004;10(7) 2530 – 2537.

[28] Kirpotin DB, Drummond DC, Shao Y, Shalaby MR, Hong K, Nielsen UB, Marks JD, Benz CC, Park JW. Antibody targeting of long-circulating lipidic nanoparticles does

not increase tumor localization but does increase internalization in animal models. Cancer Research 2006;66(13) 6732-6740.

[29] Hatakeyama H, Akita H, Ishida E, Hashimoto K, Kobayashi H, Aoki T, Yasuda J, Obata K, Kikuchi I, Ishida T, Kiwada H, Harashima H. Tumor targeting of doxorubicin by anti-MT1-MMP antibody-modified PEG liposomes. International Journal of Pharmaceutics 2007;342(1-2) 194–200.

[30] Xu L, Huang CC, Huang W, Tang WH, Rait A, Yin YZ, Cruz I, Xiang LM, Pirollo KF, Chang EH. Systemic tumor-targeted gene delivery by anti-transferrin receptor scFv-immunoliposomes. Mollecular Cancer Therapy 2002,1(5) 337–346.

[31] Xiong XB, Huang Y, Lü WL, Zhang X, Zhang H, Zhang Q. Preparation of doxorubicin-loaded stealth liposomes modified with RGD mimetic and cellular association in vitro. Acta Pharmaceutica Sinica 2005;40(12) 1085-1990.

[32] Li X, Ding L, Xu Y, Wang Y, Ping Q. Targeted delivery of doxorubicin using stealth liposomes modified with transferrin. International Journal of Pharmaceutics 2009;373(1-2) 116-123.

[33] Paliwal SR, Paliwal R, Mishra N, Mehta A, Vyas SP. A novel cancer targeting approach based on estrone anchored stealth liposome for site-specific breast cancer therapy. Current Cancer Drug Targets 2010;10(3) 343-353.

[34] Yamada A, Taniguchi Y, Kawano K, Honda T, Hattori Y, Maitani Y. Design of folate-linked liposomal doxorubicin to its antitumor effect in mice. Clinical Cancer Research 2008;14(24) 8161-8168.

[35] Lasch J., Weissing V., Brandl M. Preparation of liposomes. In: Torchilin VP., Weissig V. (2 ed) Liposomes: a pratical approach. New York: Oxford Universty Press; 2003, p3-27.

[36] Bangham AD, Standish MM, Watkins JC. Diffusion of univalent ions the lamellae of swollen phospholipids. Journal of Molecular Biology 1965;13(1) 238-252.

[37] Wagner A, Vorauer-Uhl K. Liposome technology for industrial purposes. Journal of Drug Delivery 2011;2011 (Article ID 591325) 1-9.

[38] Zuidam NJ, Gouw HK, Barenholz Y, Crommelin DJ. Physical (in) stability of liposomes upon chemical hydrolyxis: the role of lysophospholipids and fatty acids. Biochimica et Biophysica Acta 1995;1240(1) 101-110.

[39] Swarbrick, J., Boylan, J.C. Liposome as Pharmaceutical Dosage Forms. In: Dekker M. Encyclopedia of Pharmaceutical Technology. New York:Oxford Universty Press; 1994 p1-39

[40] Edwards KA, Baeumner AJ. Analysis of liposomes. Talanta 2006;68(5) 1432–1441.

[41] Plessis JD, Ramachandran C, Weiner N, Muller G. The influence of lipid composition and lamellarity of liposomes on the physical stability of liposomes upon storage. International Journal of Pharmaceutics 1996;127(2) 273-278.

[42] Abdelwahed W, Degobert G, Stainmesse S, Fessi H. Freeze-drying of nanoparticles: Formulation, process and storage considerations. Advanced Drug Delivery Reviews 2006;58(15) 1688–1713.

[43] Chen C, Han D, Cai C. Tang, X. An overview of liposome lyophilization and its future potential. Journal of Controlled Release 2010;142(3) 299–311.

[44] Zhang JA, Pawelchak J. Effect of pH, ionic strength and oxygen burden on the chemical stability of EPC/cholesterol liposomes under accelerated conditions. Part 1: Lipid hydrolysis. European Journal of Pharmaceutics and Biopharmaceutics 2000;50(3) 357-364.

[45] Abdelwahed W, Degobert G, Fessi H. Investigation of nanocapsules stabilization by amorphous excipients during freeze-drying and storage 2006;63(2) 87-94.

[46] Bendas G, Wilhen F, Nuhm P. Synthetic glycolipids as membrane bound cryoprotectants in the freeze-drying process of liposomes. European Journal of Pharmaceutical Sciences1996;4(4) 211-222.

[47] Mohammed AR, Bramwell VW, Coombes AGA, Perrie Y. Lyophilisation and sterilisation of liposomal vaccines to produce stable and sterile products. Methods 2006;40(1) 30–38.

[48] Santivarangkna C, Higl B, Foerst P. Protection mechanisms of sugars during different stages of preparation process of dried lactic acid starter cultures. Food Microbiology 2008;25(3) 429-441.

[49] Diaz S, Amalfa F, De Lopez B, Disalvo EA. Effect of water polarized at the carbonyl groups of phosphatidylcholines on the dipole potential of lipid bilayers. Langmuir 1999;15(15) 5179-5182.

[50] Luzardo MC, Amalfa F, Nunez AM, Diaz, S, De Lopez ACB, Disalvo EA. Effect of trehalose and sucrose on the hydration and dipole potential of lipid bilayers. Byophysical Journal 2000;78(5) 2452-2458.

[51] Villarreal MA, Diaz SB, Disalvo EA, Montich GG. Molecular dynamics simulation study of the interaction of trehalose with lipids membranes. Langmuir 2004;20(18) 7844-7851.

[52] Koster KL, Lei YP, Anderson M, Martin S, Bryant, G. Effects of vitrified and nonvitrified sugars on phosphatidylcholine fluid-to-gel phase transitions. Byophysical Journal 2000;78(4) 1932–1946.

[53] Crowe JH, Hoekstra FA, Nguyen KHN, Crowe LM. Is vitrification involved in depression of the phase transition temperature in dry phospholipids? Biochimica et Biophysica Acta – Biomembranes 1996;1280(2) 187-196

[54] European Medicines Agency - EMA. Note for Guidance on the Pre-Clinical Evaluation of Anticancer Medicinal Products - CPMP/SWP/997/96. 1998; http:www.emea.europa.eu/pdfs/human/swp/099796en.pdf (accessed 06 May 2009).

[55] Mcelvany, KD. FDA Requirements for Preclinical Studies. Clinical Trials in the Neurosciences 2009;25 46–49.

[56] Hofheinz RD, Gnad-Vogt SU, Beyer U, Hochhaus A. Liposomal encapsulated anticancer drugs. Anti-Cancer Drugs 2005;16(7) 691-707

[57] Harrington KJ, Lewanski CR, Stewart JSW. Liposomes as vehicles for targeted therapy of cancer. Part 1: preclinical development. Clinical Oncology (Royal College of Radiologists – Great Britain) 2000;12(1) 2–15.

[58] Harrington KJ, Lewanski CR, Stewart JSW. Liposomes as vehicles for targeted therapy of cancer. Part 2: clinical development. Clinical Oncology (Royal College of Radiologists – Great Britain) 2000;12(1) 16–24.

[59] Ferrari, M. Cancer nanotechnology: opportunities and challenges. Nature Reviews Cancer 2005;5(3) 161-171.

[60] Park, JW. Liposome-based drug delivery in breast cancer treatment. Breast Cancer Research 2002; 4(3)95-99

[61] Wong HL, Bendayan R, Rauth AM, Li Y, Wu XY. Chemotherapy with anticancer drugs encapsulated in solid lipid nanoparticles. Advanced Drug Delivery Reviews 2007;59(6) 491-504.

[62] Wang X, Wang Y, Chen Z, Shin DM. Advances of Cancer Therapy by Nanotechnology. Cancer Research Treatment 2009;41(1) 1-11.

[63] Kondagunta GV, Bacik J, Donadio A, Bajorin D, Marion S, Sheinfeld J, Bosl GJ, Motzer RJ. Combination of paclitaxel, ifosfamide and cisplatin is an effective second-line therapy for patients with relapsed testicular germ cell tumors. Journal of Clinical Oncology 2005;23(27) 6549-6555.

[64] Guillot T, Spielmann M, Kac J, Luboinski B, Tellez-Bernal E, Munck JN, Bachouchi M, Armand JP, Cvitkovic E. Neoadjuvant chemotherapy in multiple synchronous head and neck and esophagus squamous cell carcinomas. Laryngoscope 1992;102(3) 311–319.

[65] Le Chevalier T, Brisgand D, Douillard JY, Pujol JL, Alberola V, Monnier A, Riviere A, Lianes P, Chomy P, Cigolari S. Randomized study of vinorelbine and cisplatin versus vindesine and cisplatin versus vinorelbine alone in advanced non-small-cell lung

cancer: results of a European multicenter trial including 612 patients. Journal of Clinical Oncology 1994;12(2) 360-367.

[66] Shirazi FH, Molepo JM, Stewart DJ, Ng CE, Raaphorst GP, Goel R. Cytotoxicity, accumulation, and efflux of cisplatin and its metabolites in human ovarian carcinoma cells. Toxicology and Applied Pharmacology 1996;140(2):211-218.

[67] Muggia FM, Fojo T. Platinums: extending their therapeutic spectrum. Journal of Chemotherapy 2004;16 (Suppl 4) 77-82.

[68] Hirai M, Minematsu H, Hiramatsu Y, Kitagawa H, Otani T, Iwashita S, Kudoh T, Chen L, Li Y, Okada M, Salomon DS, Igarashi K, Chikuma M, Seno M. Novel and simple loading procedure of cisplatin into liposomes and targeting tumor endothelial cells. International Journal of Pharmaceutics 2010;391(1-2) 274–283.

[69] Krieger M, Eckstein N, Schneider V, Koch M, Royer, HD, Jaehde U, Bendas G. Overcoming cisplatin resistance of ovarian cancer cells by targeted liposomes in vitro. International Journal of Pharmaceutics 2010;389(1-2) 10-17.

[70] Steerenberg PA, Storm G, de Groot G, Claessen A, Bergers JJ, Franken MA, van Hoesel QG, Wubs KL, de Jong WH. Liposomes as drug carrier system for cis-diamminedichloroplatinum (II). II. Antitumor activity in vivo, induction of drug resistance, nephrotoxicity and Pt distribution. Cancer Chemotherapy and Pharmacology 1988;21(4) 299-307.

[71] Newman MS, Colbern GT, Working PK, Engbers C, Amantea MA. Comparative pharmacokinetics, tissue distribution, and therapeutic effectiveness of cisplatin encapsulated in long-circulating, pegylated liposomes (SPI-077) in tumor-bearing mice. Cancer Chemotherapy and Pharmacology 1999;43(1) 1-7.

[72] Vaage J, Donovan D, Wipff E, Abra R, Colbern G, Uster P, Working P. Therapy of a xenografted human colonic carcinoma using cisplatin or doxorubicin encapsulated in long-circulating pegylated stealth liposomes. International Journal of Cancer 1999;80(1) 134-137.

[73] Meerum Terwogt JM, Groenewegen G, Pluim D, Maliepaard M, Tibben MM, Huisman A, ten Bokkel Huinink WW, Schot M, Welbank H, Voest EE, Beijnen JH, Schellens JM. Phase I and pharmacokinetic study of SPI-77, a liposomal encapsulated dosage form of cisplatin. Cancer Chemotherapy and Pharmacology 2002;49(3) 201-210.

[74] Stathopoulos GP, Boulikas T, Vougiouka M, Deliconstantinos G, Rigatos S, Darli E, Viliotou V and Stathopoulos JG. Pharmacokinetics and adverse reactions of a new liposomal cisplatin (Lipoplatin): phase I study. Oncology Reports 2005;13(4) 589-595.

[75] Arienti C, Tesei A, Ravaioli A, Ratta M, Carloni S, Mangianti S, Ulivi P, Nicoletti S, Amadori D, Zoli W. Activity of lipoplatin in tumor and in normal cells in vitro. Anticancer Drugs. 2008;19(10) 983-990.

[76] Fedier A, Poyet C, Perucchini D, Boulikas T, Fink D. MLH1-deficient tumor cells are resistant to lipoplatin, but retain sensitivity to lipoxal. Anticancer Drugs. 2006;17(3) 315-323.

[77] Boulikas T. Low toxicity and anticancer activity of a novel liposomal cisplatin (Lipoplatin) in mouse xenografts. Oncology Report 2004;12(1) 3-12.

[78] Devarajan P, Tarabishi R, Mishra J, Ma K, Kourvetaris A, Vougiouka M, Boulikas T. Low renal toxicity of Lipoplatin compared to cisplatin in animals. Anticancer Research, 2004; 24 (4) 2193-2200.

[79] Marr AK, Kurzman ID, Vail DM. Preclinical evaluation of a liposome-encapsulated formulation of cisplatin in clinically normal dogs. American Journal of Veterinary Research 2004;65(11) 1474-1478.

[80] Boulikas T, Stathopoulos GP, Volakakis N, Vougiouka M. Systemic Lipoplatin infusion results in preferential tumor uptake in human studies. Anticancer Research 2005;25(4) 3031-3039.

[81] Stathopoulos GP, Boulikas T, Vougiouka M, Rigatos SK, Stathopoulos JG. Liposomal cisplatin combined with gemcitabine in pretreated advanced pancreatic cancer patients: a phase I-II study. Oncology Reports 2006;15(5) 1201-1204.

[82] Froudarakis ME, Pataka A, Pappas P, Anevlavis S, Argiana E, Nikolaidou M, Kouliatis G, Pozova S, Marselos M, Bouros D. Phase 1 trial of lipoplatin and gemcitabine as a second-line chemotherapy in patients with nonsmall cell lung carcinoma. Cancer 2008;113(10) 2752-2760.

[83] Stathopoulos GP, Rigatos SK, Stathopoulos J. Liposomal cisplatin dose escalation for determining the maximum tolerated dose and dose-limiting toxicity: a phase I study. Anticancer Research 2010;30(4) 1317-1321.

[84] Farhat FS, Temraz S, Kattan J, Ibrahim K, Bitar N, Haddad N, Jalloul R, Hatoum HA, Nsouli G, Shamseddine AI. A phase II study of lipoplatin (liposomal cisplatin)/vinorelbine combination in HER-2/neu-negative metastatic breast cancer. Clinical Breast Cancer 2011;11(6) 384-389.

[85] Mylonakis N, Athanasiou A, Ziras N, Angel J, Rapti A, Lampaki S, Politis N, Karanikas C, Kosmas C. Phase II study of liposomal cisplatin (Lipoplatin) plus gemcitabine versus cisplatin plus gemcitabine as first line treatment in inoperable (stage IIIB/IV) non-small cell lung cancer. Lung Cancer 2010;68(2) 240-247.

[86] Jehn CF, Boulikas T, Kourvetaris A, Possinger K, Lüftner D. Pharmacokinetics of liposomal cisplatin (lipoplatin) in combination with 5-FU in patients with advanced head and neck cancer: first results of a phase III study. Anticancer Research 2007;27(1A) 471-475.

[87] Jehn CF, Boulikas T, Kourvetaris A, Kofla G, Possinger K, Lüftner D. First safety and response results of a randomized phase III study with liposomal platin in the treat-

ment of advanced squamous cell carcinoma of the head and neck (SCCHN). Anticancer Research 2008;28(6B) 3961-3964.

[88] Stathopoulos GP, Antoniu D, Dimitroulis J, Michalopoulou P, Bastas A, Marosis K, Stathopoulos J, Provata A, Yiamboudakis P, Veldekis D, Lolis N, Georgatou N, Toubis M, Pappas Ch, Tsoukalas G. Liposomal cisplatin combined with paclitaxel versus cisplatin and paclitaxel in non-small-cell lung cancer: a randomized phase III multicenter trial. Annals of Oncology 2010;21(11) 2227-2232.

[89] Stathopoulos GP, Boulikas T. Lipoplatin formulation review article. Journal of Drug Delivery 2012;2012 581363.

[90] Júnior ADC, Mota LG, Nunan EA, Wainstein AJA, Wainstein APDL, Leal AL, Cardoso VN, Oliveira MC. Tissue distribution evaluation of stealth pH-sensitive liposomal cisplatin versus free cisplatin in Erlich tumor-bearing mice. Life Sciences 2007;80(7) 659-664.

[91] Chauffert B, Favoulet P, Polycarpe E, Duvillard C, Beltramo JL, Bichat F, Rat P, Genne P, Benoit L. Rationale supporting the use of vasoconstrictors for intraperitoneal chemotherapy with platinum derivatives. Surgeon Oncology Clinics of North America 2003;12:835–48.

[92] Araújo JG, Mota LG, Leite EA, Maroni Lde C, Wainstein AJ, Coelho LG, Savassi-Rocha PR, Pereira MT, de Carvalho AT, Cardoso VN, De Oliveira MC. Biodistribution and antitumoral effect of long-circulating and pH-sensitive liposomal cisplatin administered in Ehrlich tumor-bearing mice. Experimental Biology and Medicine (Maywood) 2011;236(7) 808-815.

[93] Leite EA, Giuberti CS, Wainstein AJ, Wainstein AP, Coelho LG, Lana AM, Savassi-Rocha PR, De Oliveira MC. Acute toxicity of long-circulating and pH-sensitive liposomes containing cisplatin in mice after intraperitoneal administration. Life Sciences 2009;84(19-20) 641-649.

[94] Leite EA, Lana AM, Junior AD, Coelho LG, De Oliveira MC. Acute toxicity study of cisplatin loaded long-circulating and pH-sensitive liposomes administered in mice. Journal of Biomedical Nanotechnology 2012;8(2) 229-239.

[95] Leite EA. Avaliação da Toxicidade Aguda e Atividade Antitumoral de Lipossomas pH-sensíveis de circulação prolongada contendo cisplatina. PhD Thesis. Universidade Federal de Minas Gerais; 2010.

[96] Maroni, LC, Silveira ACO, Leite EA, Melo MM, Ribeiro AFC, Cassali GD, Souza CM, Fagundes EMS, Caldas IR, Araújo MSS, Filho OAM, Oliveira MC, Carvalho AT. Antitumor effectiveness and toxicity of cisplatin loaded long-circulating and pH-sensitive liposomes against Ehrlich ascitic tumor. Experimental Biology and Medicine 2012;DOI:10.1258/ebm.2012.011432.

[97] Stathopoulos GP, Boulikas T, Kourvetaris A, Stathopoulos J. Liposomal oxaliplatin in the treatment of advanced cancer: a phase I study. Anticancer Research. 2006:26(2B) 1489-93.

[98] Boulikas P. Cancer Treatments. C.I. 424/450; 514/492; 424; 649 US, 3 mar. 2006, 26 feb. 2009.

[99] Boulikas T, Pantos A, Bellis E, Christofis P. Designing platinum compounds in cancer: structures and mechanisms. Cancer Therapy 2007;5 537-583.

[100] Leonard RCF, Williams S, Tulpule A, Levine AM, Oliveros S. Improving the therapeutic index of anthracycline chemotherapy: Focus on liposomal doxorubicin (Myocet®). The Breast 2009;18(4) 218–224.

[101] Safra T. Cardiac safety of liposomal anthracyclines, The oncologist 2003;8(suppl 2) 17-24.

[102] Harris L, Batist G, Belt R, Rovira D, Navari R, Azarnia N, Welles L, Winer E. Liposome-Encapsulated Doxorubicin Compared with Conventional Doxorubicin in a Randomized Multicenter Trial as First-Line Therapy of Metastatic Breast Carcinoma. Cancer 2002;94(1) 25-36.

[103] Forssen EA, Coulter DM, Proffitt RT. Selective in vivo localisation of daunorubicin small unilamellar vesicles in solid tumours. Cancer Research 1992;52(12) 3255-3261.

[104] Forssen EA, Ross ME. DaunoxomeTM treatment of solid tumors: Preclinical and clinical investigations, Journal of Liposome Research 1994;4(1) 481–512.

[105] Pea F, Russo D, Michieli M, Baraldo M, Ermacora A, Damiani D, Baccarani M, Furlanut M.Liposomal daunorubicin plasmatic and renal disposition in patients with acute leukemia. Cancer Chemotherapy and Pharmacology 2000;46(4) 279-286.

[106] Gill PS, Espina BM, Muggia F, Cabriales S, Tulpule A, Esplin JA, Liebman HA, Forssen E, Ross ME, Levine AM. Phase I/II clinical and pharmacokinetic evaluation of liposomal daunorubicin. Journal of Clinical Oncology 1995;13(4) 996-1003.

[107] Gill PS, Wernz J, Scadden DT, Cohen P, Mukwaya GM, Von Roenn JH, Jacobs M, Kempin S, Silverberg I, Gonzales G, Rarick MU, Myers AM, Shepherd F, Sawka C, Pike MC, Ross ME. Randomized phase III trial of liposomal daunorubicin versus doxorubicin, bleomycin, and vincristine in AIDS-related Kaposi's sarcoma. Journal of Clinical Oncology 1996;14(8) 2353-2364.

[108] Rosenthal E, Poizot-Martin I, Saint-Marc T, Spano JP, Cacoub P. Phase IV study of liposomal daunorubicin (DaunoXome) in AIDS-related Kaposi sarcoma. American Journal of Clinical Oncology 2002;25(1) 57-59.

[109] Kanter PM, Bullard GA, Pilkiewicz FG, Mayer LD, Cullis PR, Pavelic ZP. Preclinical toxicology study of liposome encapsulated doxorubicin (TLC D-99): comparison with doxorubicin and empty liposomes in mice and dogs. In Vivo 1993;7(1):85-95.

[110] Harasym TO, Cullis PR, Bally MB. Intratumour distribution of doxorubicin following i.v. administration of drug encapsulated in egg phosphatidylcholine/cholesterol liposomes. Cancer Chemotherapy and Pharmacology 1997;40(4) 309–317.

[111] Cowens JW, Creaven PJ, Greco WR, Brenner DE, Tung Y, Ostro M, Pilkiewicz F, Ginsberg R, Petrelli N. Initial clinical (phase I) trial of TLC D-99 (doxorubicin encapsulated in liposomes). Cancer Research 1993;53(12) 2796-2802.

[112] Batist G, Ramakrishnan G, Rao CS, Chandrasekharan A, Gutheil J, Guthrie T, Shah P, Khojasteh A, Nair MK, Hoelzer K, Tkaczuk K, Park YC, Lee LW. Reduced cardiotoxicity and preserved antitumor efficacy of liposome-encapsulated doxorubicin and cyclophosphamide compared with conventional doxorubicin and cyclophosphamide in a randomized, multicenter trial of metastatic breast cancer. Journal of Clinical Oncology 2001;19(5) 1444-1454.

[113] Vaage J, Donovan D, Mayhew E, Uster P, Woodle M. Therapy of mouse mammary carcinomas with vincristine and doxorubicin encapsulated in sterically stabilized liposomes. International Journal of Cancer 1993;54(6) 959-964.

[114] Vaage J, Donovan D, Mayhew E, Abra R, Huang A. Therapy of human ovarian carcinoma xenografts using doxorubicin encapsulated in sterically stabilized liposomes. Cancer 1993;72(12) 3671-3675.

[115] Gabizon A, Shmeeda H, Barenholz Y. Pharmacokinetics of pegylated liposomal doxorubicin. Clinical Pharmacokinetic 2003;42(5) 419-436.

[116] Krown SE, Northfelt DW, Osoba D, Stewart JS. Use of liposomal anthracyclines in Kaposi's sarcoma. Seminars in Oncology 2004;31(6 Suppl 13) 36-52.

[117] Rose PG. Pegylated liposomal doxorubicin: optimizing the dosing schedule in ovarian cancer. Oncologist 2005;10(3) 205-214.

[118] Hussein MA, Anderson KC. Role of liposomal anthracyclines in the treatment of multiple myeloma. Seminars in Oncology 2004; 31(6 Supplement 13) 147–160.

[119] Robert NJ, Vogel CL, Henderson IC, Sparano JA, Moore MR, Silverman P, Overmoyer BA, Shapiro CL, Park JW, Colbern GT, Winer EP, Gabizon AA. The role of the liposomal anthracyclines and other systemic therapies in the management of advanced breast cancer. Seminars in Oncology 2004;31(6 Suppl 13) 106-146.

[120] Hau P, Fabel K, Baumgart U, Rümmele P, Grauer O, Bock A, Dietmaier C, Dietmaier W, Dietrich J, Dudel C, Hübner F, Jauch T, Drechsel E, Kleiter I, Wismeth C, Zellner A, Brawanski A, Steinbrecher A, Marienhagen J, Bogdahn U. Pegylated liposomal doxorubicin efficacy in patients with recurrent high-grade glioma. Cancer 2004;100(6) 1199–207.

[121] Zhang Q, Huang XE, Gao LL. A clinical study on the premedication of paclitaxel liposome in the treatment of solid tumors. Biomedicine & Pharmacotherapy 2009; 63(8) 603-607.

[122] Zhang JA, Anyarambhatla G, Ma L, Ugwu S, Xuan T, Sardone T, Ahmad I. Development and characterisation of a novel Cremophor EL free liposome based paclitaxel (LEP-ETU) formulation. European Journal of Pharmaceutics and Biopharmaceutics 2005;59(1) 177-187.

[123] Yang T, Cui FD, Choi MK, Cho JW, Chung SJ, Shim CK, Kim DD. Enhanced solubility and stability of PEGylated liposomal paclitaxel: In vitro and in vivo evaluation. International Journal of Pharmaceutics 2007; 338(1-2) 317–326.

[124] Strieth S, Eichhirn ME, Werner A, Sauer B, Teifeil M, Michaelis U, Berghaus A, Dellian M. Paclitaxel encapsulated in cationic liposomes increases tumor microvessel leakiness and improves therapeutic efficacy in combination with cisplatin. Clinical Cancer Research 2008; 14(14) 4603-4611.

[125] Glantz MJ, Lafollette S, Jaeckle KA, Shapiro W, Swinnen L, Rozental JR, Phuphanich S, Rogers LR, Gutheil JC, Batchelor T, Lyter D, Chamberlain M, Maria BL, Schiffer C, Bashir R, Thomas D, Cowens W, Howell SB. Randomized trial of a slow-release versus a standard formulation of cytarabine for the intrathecal treatment of lymphomatous meningitis. Journal of Clinical Oncology 1999;17(10) 3110–3116.

[126] Glantz MJ, Jaeckle KA, Chamberlain MC, Phuphanich S, Recht L, Swinnen LJ, Maria B, Lafollette S, Schumann GB, Cole BF, Howell SB. A randomized controlled trial comparing intrathecal sustained release cytarabine (DepoCyte) to intrathecal methotrexate in patients with neoplastic meningitis from solid tumours. Clinical Cancer Research 1999;5(11) 3394–3402.

[127] Spina M, Chimienti E, Martellotta F, Vaccher E, Berretta M, Zanet E, Lleshi A, Canzonieri V, Bulian P, Tirelli U. Phase 2 study of intrathecal, long-acting liposomal cytarabine in the prophylaxis of lymphomatous meningitis in human immunodeficiency virus-related non-Hodgkin lymphoma. Cancer 2010; 116(6) 1495-1501.

[128] Rodriguez MA, Pytlik R, Kozak T, Chhanabhai M, Gascoyne R, Lu B, Deitcher SR, Winter JN. Vincristine sulfate liposomes injection (Marqibo) in heavily pretreated patients with refractory aggressive non-Hodgkin lymphoma: report of the pivotal phase 2 study. Cancer 2009; 115(15) 3475-3482.

[129] Sapra P, Allen TM. Ligand-targeted liposomal anticancer drugs. Progress in Lipid Research 2003; 42(5) 439–462.

[130] Low PS, Kularatne SA. Folate-targeted therapeutic and imaging agents for cancer. Current Opinion in Chemical Biology 2009; 13(3) 256–262.

[131] Takeuchi H, Kojima H, Toyoda T, Yamamoto H, Hino T, Kawashima Y. Prolonged circulation time of doxorubicin-loaded liposomes coated with amodified polyvinyl alcohol after intravenous injection in rats. European Journal of Pharmaceutics and Biopharmaceutics 1999; 48(2)123–129.

[132] Li X, Ding L, Xu Y, Wang Y, Ping Q. Targeted delivery of doxorubicin using stealth liposomes modified with transferring. International Journal of Pharmaceutics 2009; 373(1-2) 116-23.

[133] Song CK, Jung SH, Kim DD, Jeong KS, Shin BC, Seong, H. Disaccharide-modified liposomes and their in vitro intracellular uptake. International Journal of Pharmaceutics 2009; 380(1-2) 161–169.

[134] Pan XQ, Lee RJ. In vivo antitumor activity of folate receptor-targeted liposomal daunorubicin in a murine leukemia model. Anticancer Research 2005;25(1A) 343-346.

[135] Shmeeda H, Mak L, Tzemach D, Astrahan P, Tarshish M, Gabizon A. Intracellular uptake and intracavitary targeting of folate-conjugated liposomes in a mouse lymphoma model with up-regulated folate receptors. Molecular Cancer Therapeutics 2006;5(4) 818-824.

[136] Kim KS, Lee YK, Kim JS, Koo KH, Hong HJ, Park YS. Targeted gene therapy of LS174 T human colon carcinoma by anti-TAG-72 immunoliposomes. Cancer Gene Therapy 2008;15(5) 331-340.

[137] Schnyder A, Huwyler J. Drug transport to brain with targeted liposomes. NeuroRx: The Journal of the American Society for Experimental NeuroTherapeutics 2005;2(1) 99-107.

[138] Huwyler J, Drewe J, Krähenbühl S. Tumor targeting using liposomal antineoplastic drugs. International Journal of Nanomedicine 2008;3(1) 21–29.

[139] Ruenraroengsak P, Cook JM, Florence AT. Nanosystem drug targeting: Facing up to complex realities. Journal of Controlled Release 2010; 141(3) 265–276.

[140] Cukierman E, Khan DR. The benefits and challenges associated with the use of drug delivery systems in cancer therapy. Biochemical Pharmacology 2010; 80(5) 762-70.

Section 2

Combinatorial Strategies to Fight Cancer: Surgery, Radiotherpay, Backytherapy, Chemotherapy, and Hyperthermia

Chapter 5

The Role of Surgery in the Treatment of Hepatocellular Carcinoma

Georgios Tsoulfas and Polyxeni Agorastou

Additional information is available at the end of the chapter

http://dx.doi.org/10.5772/55341

1. Introduction

Hepatocellular carcinoma (HCC) is the sixth most common cancer world-wide with approximately 700,000 new cases a year, with increasing numbers in Europe and the United States [1]. The various risk factors are reflected in the worldwide heterogeneous incidence. The majority of cases of HCC develop in eastern Asia and sub-Saharan Africa due to chronic infection with hepatitis B virus (HBV), as well as aflatoxin. In other parts of the world such as Northern America, Europe and Japan, the prevailing risk factor is chronic infection with hepatitis C virus (HCV) and alcohol use [2]. Additional or synergistic factors include non-alcoholic steatohepatitis (NASH), diabetes, obesity and tobacco, with their high prevalence in Northern America offering a partial explanation for the continuously increasing incidence of HCC [3-6].

HCC develops in cirrhotic livers in 80% of cases, as cirrhosis is one of the strongest risk factors given its role as a preneoplastic condition [7]. The mechanism itself is not fully known, although it may be secondary to the disorderly architectural changes seen in the hepatic parenchyma of the cirrhotic liver providing a signal for malignant transformation. Additionally, there could be a role for DNA damage caused by viral integration, as incidence of HCC increases with viral load and duration of infection, thus raising the possibility of a cumulative effect of long-term viral damage [8-9].

There has been major progress in understanding the nature of the disease, as well as the available therapies. Although the full range of treatment options has increased over time, especially with the advent of new surgical and molecular technologies, the mainstay of treatment remains surgery, as the only truly therapeutic option. This chapter will discuss the evaluation of the patient with HCC, the two main surgical treatments, liver resection and orthotopic liver transplantation (OLT), as well as future prospects which include the molecular classification of HCC and the efforts for targeted molecular therapies, which in turn will have a great impact on any therapeutic decision.

2. Evaluation of patients with hepatocellular carcinoma

In order for surgical treatment for HCC to be successful, patients need to be chosen very carefully. It is essential that the evaluation, selection and treatment are performed by multi-disciplinary teams that include hepatologists, surgeons, oncologists, radiologists, pathologists and anesthesiologists. The reason is that we have to remember that we are dealing with more than one problem in the same setting. Specifically, the patient's HCC needs to be addressed, but it has to be done in the setting of the possible cirrhosis. The degree that the patient's liver function is affected can have a direct impact on several other organ systems (cardiopulmonary, renal) and thus directly influence any therapeutic decisions. It is interesting that, in contrast to several other cancers, there are not many randomized controlled trials to compare the treatments seen as curative for HCC, something which underscores the need for these patients to be followed in protocols whenever possible, so that evidence-based decisions can be made.

The first question that has to answered is whether the patient is an operative candidate, meaning whether the patient is in a position to undergo a major surgery from the standpoint of his overall health. It is essential that this evaluation is performed by physicians who are intimately aware of the challenges of liver resection or transplantation. For example, the anesthesiologist has to be aware that this will be an operation with potential significant blood loss and periods of hypotension, all of which will stress the cardiovascular system. This should help determine the kind of preoperative testing that is needed, although there is to-date no universally agreed upon preoperative protocol for patients undergoing liver resection. The importance of this can be seen even more clearly if we consider that given the improvements in surveillance and surgical technique and the general ageing of the population, older patients belonging to a higher risk group are being increasingly evaluated for liver surgery. Once the question of the patient as an operative candidate has been answered satisfactorily, the next one is whether the HCC is resectable. The answer to this question depends on identifying the stage of the disease, as well as the hepatic reserve of the patient.

2.1. Staging of patients with hepatocellular carcinoma

Regarding the stage, there is a lack of a common language as there is no consensus on a universal staging system. There are different ones, each one taking slightly different aspects of the disease into consideration. Some depend on clinical and radiological findings prior to the treatment, whereas others are based on the histopathological findings. Ideally, clinically-applicable staging for HCC should assess the tumor stage, the underlying liver function and the patient's biological status. Some of the staging systems, such as The American Joint Committee on Cancer/Union Internationale Contre le Cancer Tumor-Node-Metastasis staging system (AJCC/UICC TNM) stratifying patients into prognostic groups, are best suited to only patients undergoing resection or transplantation, without taking into consideration the underlying liver disease [10]. In an effort to consider tumor features and hepatic function, the Okuda system and the Cancer of the Liver Italian Program (CLIP) classifications were proposed [11-12]. Both of them have the ability to identify end stage disease but are not as accurate with early stage disease. A step towards solving this problem has been the Japan

http://dx.doi.org/10.5772/55341

Integrated Staging score, which combines the Child-Turcotte-Pugh (CTP) classification with the simplified TNM system by the Liver Cancer Study Group of Japan (LCSGJ) [13].

The most widely accepted system appears to be the Barcelona Clinic Liver Cancer (BCLC) system, which was introduced in 1999 as an attempt to improve on the Okuda system, so as to include the functional aspect of the disease. It was developed based on a combination of data from a variety of studies looking into different types of treatment for different stages of the disease [14-16]. The BCLC takes into account the total cancer load, the stage of the cirrhosis and the patient's functional status, in an effort to determine the type of treatment necessary and the expected survival (Figure 1). It is the staging system most widely (but not universally) accepted, as it has been externally validated and it offers a pathway between staging and the different treatment modalities with an estimation of life expectancy [17]. It provides suggested treatments for the different stages of the disease, including early stage HCC where the aim is a cure, as opposed to advanced HCC where palliative treatments are proposed. In addition to providing proper patient care, universally-accepted staging for HCC is critical in allowing the comparison between results from different studies in order to draw the appropriate conclusions. A system such as the BCLC, which is a clinical system with predictive abilities, can offer a solid platform for the initial staging. Other systems, such as the simplified TNM, which includes pathological findings such as microvascular invasion, can be of more value in those patients undergoing resection or OLT.

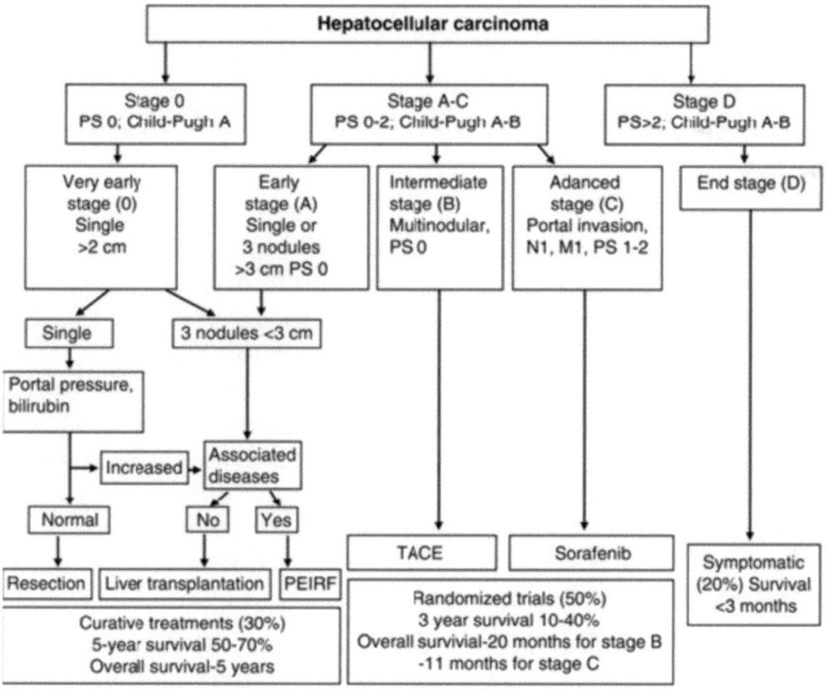

Figure 1.

2.2. Evaluation of hepatic reserve of patients with hepatocellular carcinoma

As far as evaluating the hepatic reserve of the patient is concerned, that is a determination of both quantity and quality. This is a major change from the past when there were multiple exclusion criteria, as the only ones that have been consistently validated over time are the postoperative remnant liver volume and hepatic function [18-20]. It has been shown that if 3 or more hepatic segments are left behind after a resection, or an adequate hepatic remnant, which is 25% for a normal liver and 40% for a cirrhotic one, then postoperative liver dysfunction can be avoided [21-22]. This means that it is essential to be able to accurately estimate the liver remnant and the future remaining liver volume preoperatively, especially in the case of extended resections. The most reliable way to do this has been CT volumetry, which with the advent of the Digital Imaging and Communications in Medicine (DICOM) standard has enabled volumetry to be performed even by the surgeon on a personal computer. Quality can be assessed either directly (liver biopsy) or indirectly, through assessment of the synthetic function of the liver (INR, platelets, albumin) or other marks of portal hypertension and cirrhosis, such as esophagogastroduodenoscopy (EGD) looking for varices. The underlying chronic liver disease, including its duration and whether the patient has received any treatment, are also important pieces of information.

By fully evaluating the patient with HCC, one can proceed more safely into determining whether the patient is a candidate for surgical treatment and which one: resection versus transplantation. Frequently, it may be necessary for the patient to be evaluated for both, as a patient undergoing a liver resection could show signs of hepatic failure postoperatively, leading to a discussion of whether transplantation is an option. It is wise for these decisions to be made beforehand, rather than during emotionally-charged times.

3. Hepatectomy

The first question one has to consider when discussing the issue of hepatic resection for HCC is the presence or not of cirrhosis. In non-cirrhotic patients, hepatic resection represents the preferred treatment, as the lack of cirrhosis means that the patient can tolerate even an extended resection, and the non-cirrhotic liver will allow future re-resection, although it has a lower chance of de novo recurrence. Unfortunately, these patients without cirrhosis represent only 5% of cases in the West [23]. Even so, in these patients without cirrhosis, surgical resection for HCC can lead to 3-year survival of 46-76% and 5-year survivals of 30-50%, depending on the selection criteria and on whether fibrolamellar HCC cases are included in the study [24-26]. A high recurrence rate at 5 years of around 60% remains, even after potentially curative resections, possibly owing to intrahepatic metastases rather than existing disease, as the effect of the underlying chronic liver disease and the cirrhosis is not present [27].

In patients with cirrhosis, using proper selection criteria to avoid postoperative hepatic failure is critical. That set of criteria was originally based on the Child-Pugh classification, which however was not shown to have a consistent predictive value, as patients may show signs of hepatic dysfunction even at a stage of Child-Pugh A, thus making a resection a high-risk one [28]. The best candidates for liver resection, and those who could achieve 5-year survivals of up to 70%, are those patients with single lesion, asymptomatic HCC, and most importantly with preserved liver function [29-31]. The definition of preserved liver function includes the absence of clinically significant portal hypertension (hepatic vein wedge pressure difference less than 10mmHg, absence of varices or splenomegaly, and platelets over 100,000/mm^3) and normal bilirubin values [32]. In patients with significant portal hypertension, 5-year survival after resection goes down to 50%, whereas in those with combined portal hypertension and increased bilirubin levels it can be as low as 25% [33]. In order to predict the risk of postoperative hepatic insufficiency other groups have used the Model for End-stage Liver Disease (MELD) score, which is based on the values of the patient's creatinine, bilirubin and prothrombin time. Several studies have shown that when the MELD score is 9 or less, then hepatic resection can be safe with almost minimal chances of postoperative patient destabilization [33-35].

The preference for patients with a single lesion has to do with the fact that in most cases multifocal HCC is associated with decreased survival and increased recurrence, potentially as an indication of already existing intrahepatic metastases. Although not prohibitive for resection, the presence of multiple lesions should alert the surgeon to the possibility of using treatments such as radiofrequency ablation and chemoembolization in combination with resection to obtain optimal results. Similar to multifocality, an increased tumor size is not necessarily prohibitive, but can serve as an indication of possible vascular invasion, which can in turn negatively affect the prognosis. When all of this is considered, the percentage of patients that can undergo hepatic resection under ideal conditions is less than 10%. However, even in this group of patients with cirrhosis, it is possible to achieve moderate long-term results [36-38].

3.1. Considerations in liver resection

When considering liver resection for HCC apart from the main question of the presence or absence of cirrhosis, there are other key issues to be addressed, such as ways to increase resectability, the differences between anatomic and non-anatomic resection and the use of laparoscopic surgery among others.

3.1.1. The role of portal vein embolization

In an effort to treat large HCC with hepatic resection or in those patients with inadequate liver remnant, there are certain preoperative manoeuvres that can help increase resectability in these challenging patients. Preoperative portal vein embolization (PVE) was introduced in 1986 by Kinoshita to prevent postoperative hepatic insufficiency, whereas Makuuchi had first introduced the concept to clinical practice in 1982 for the treatment of hepatic cholangiocarcinoma [39-40]. The main principle is to occlude the portal venous flow to the side of the tumor, and cause ipsilateral atrophy and, more importantly, contralateral hypertrophy of the part of the liver that will be the future remnant after the resection. This can lead to an increase in the future remnant by about 20-40% within 4-6 weeks, thus potentially increasing the pool of candidates for resection [41-43]. Although there are no absolute contraindications, especially as experience with the procedure continues to grow, there are some relative ones, including uncorrectable coagulopathy, tumor invasion of the portal vein, biliary dilatation and renal failure. Bilobar disease used to be a contraindication, however in light of the increased use of the two-stage hepatectomy, PVE can play a significant role in these patients [42,44]. Although there are two methods to access the portal vein for PVE, the transileocolic and the percutaneous transhepatic one, with both being equally effective, the percutaneous procedure has the distinct advantage of avoiding a minilaparotomy and general anesthesia. Regarding the choice of embolic agents, there is a great variety with similar results. However, since it is not an exact science how much embolic material or what size particles are needed to cause a specific amount of hypertrophy and regeneration, we need to understand that this procedure is very much operator-dependent. Certain principles need to be closely adhered to, such as embolizing till stasis is achieved, and also avoiding reflux of the embolic material into the veins that will supply the future liver remnant.

There are some remaining concerns regarding PVE, such as whether PVE may stimulate the growth of hepatic tumor (of more interest in the case of hepatic metastases from colorectal or other cancers), or whether it is a safe procedure in patients with high-grade varices. The difficulty in answering these questions is the fact that we lack an understanding of the mechanism involved in the contralateral hypertrophy caused by the PVE. It is probably a combination of hepatic and extrahepatic factors, including cytokines (such as IL-6), growth factors (such as hepatocyte growth factor) and nutrient factors (insulin and glucagon), although the details are not yet clear [45]. Either way, PVE provides the surgical team with an important tool that if properly applied can lead to increased resectability of HCC.

3.1.2. Anatomic versus non-anatomic hepatic resection

Hepatic resection for malignant tumors can be anatomic or nonanatomic. The anatomic approach involves a resection of liver segments based on the segmental anatomy, whereas the nonanatomical approach involves a resection of the tumor with negative margins. The main argument in favour of the anatomic resection was made by Makuuchi and the Japanese school of thought, where based on the fact that HCC tends to metastasize via the portal venous system, it is believed that removing the tumor along the lines of hepatic segments, which would include the portal flow to the tumor, is the more oncologically sound approach [46-47]. Using a nationwide Japanese database of 72,744 patients to compare the outcome of anatomic versus nonanatomic resection for HCC, it was shown that there was no difference in overall survival, although with anatomic resection there was an improved disease-free survival [48]. The beneficial effect of anatomic resection was most prominent for HCC lesions 2 to 5 cm, something which was explained by the fact that in smaller tumors there is very little chance of vascular invasion, whereas in bigger ones the high probability of vascular invasion and satellite lesions negates any advantage of an anatomic resection. Despite this, the extent of the hepatectomy should be primarily dictated by the extent of the existing chronic liver disease and the future liver remnant.

This type of argument has given impetus to the use of nonanatomic resection for HCC, as in the vast majority of cases the HCC occurs in the background of cirrhosis. Even so, the question remains of what the proper margin for the nonanatomic resection is. Specifically, there is an ongoing debate as to whether a margin of 1cm or more is necessary to obtain disease-free survival, or whether less than 1cm is sufficient [49-51]. A prospective, randomized trial comparing narrow (1cm) to wide (2cm) resection margins identified a significant 5-year survival benefit (75% versus 49%) for the wide margin group, especially in patients with small HCC of 2cm or less [52]. Even so, a report by the Japan Society of Hepatology in 2010 states that "it is acceptable to resect a tumor with a minimum width so as to avoid exposing the tumor during hepatectomy for HCC" [53].

3.1.3. Laparoscopic liver resection

Although the first laparoscopic liver resection (LLR) was performed in 1992 by Gagner, it has been somewhat of an uphill struggle because of several reasons [54]. Potential difficulties of LLR include a significant learning curve, the perceived difficulty in controlling hepatic bleeding should it occur, the lack of tactile sense which could affect the margins obtained and thus the oncological result of the procedure, the fear of port site metastases and that of gas embolism. To all of these we should add the lack of randomized trials with LLR. Improvements in hepatic surgery, as well as in laparoscopic surgery, advances in the laparoscopic instruments used, and patient interest in minimally invasive procedures, have all led to a significant increase in the number and type of LLRs. There has also been increased use of LLRs for hepatic malignancies, as currently more than half of all LLRs are for primary or metastatic hepatic malignancies, including anatomic lobectomies and liver resections in cirrhotic patients [55-58]. The key factor is surgeon experience and the learning curve, as in one paper it was shown that the learning curve for minor laparoscopic hepatectomy could be overcome with 60 cases [59]. The surgeon needs to be a liver surgeon with knowledge of hepatic anatomy, as well as someone with experience in advanced laparoscopic surgery, so that issues such as control of vascular or biliary structures can be dealt with laparoscopically. Additionally, experience with laparoscopic ultrasound is mandatory, as it counterbalances the lack of tactile sense. Common sense dictates that at least the earliest laparoscopic procedures performed by a surgical team should include smaller, peripheral lesions away from major vascular structures or the hilum that can be approached with a laparoscopic wedge or segmental procedure.

In the case of HCC, several series have shown a good long-term outcome without jeopardizing patient safety [60-62]. Some of the findings in these studies included decreased blood loss and transfusion requirements for LLR, as well as a shorter length of stay. Although the latter may come as no surprise given the minimally invasive nature of the procedure, the former could be potentially attributed to new and improved coagulation and transection devices used in LLR. Another advantage of LLR is the possible decreased risk of hepatic function destabilization, if we consider that most of these patients have cirrhosis. It is believed that the lack of the big abdominal incisions, can cause less of an effect on the portal pressure, thus decreasing the risk of postoperative hepatic decompensation [63-64]. The result of the decreased biological and surgical stress for the patient could also be part of the reason why it was shown that prior

LLR for HCC facilitated salvage liver transplantation with improved results compared to prior open liver resection [65].

3.1.4. HCC recurrence after resection

HCC recurrence after hepatic resection is a significant concern with reported rates between 60-70% at 5 years [66-68]. The challenge lies in deciding what the best treatment for these patients is. The options include a second resection versus radiofrequency ablation versus salvage liver transplantation. Evaluating radiofrequency ablation has not been easy as there are significant variations in the inclusion criteria used in the various studies. Regarding OLT, an analysis of the UNOS database by Pelletier et al. reported a 61% 5-year intention to treat survival of patients with tumors within Milan criteria [69]. However, there have been studies advocating the use of a second resection in properly selected patients. In the largest study in the Western world a 5-year 67% overall survival was reported from a second resection after HCC recurrence, with the two main risk factors being gross vascular invasion and time to recurrence from primary resection less than a year [70]. It should be noted though that when these strict criteria were used, only 15% of patients with recurrence were candidates for a second resection.

3.1.5. Liver resection as a bridge to OLT

The issue of HCC recurrence raises an important question. When discussing the different surgical treatments of HCC, it is imperative to stress the fact that liver resection and OLT are not necessarily competitive surgical options, but can very frequently be seen as complimentary. Specifically, the cirrhotic patient who undergoes a hepatectomy for a HCC, no matter how stable the liver function is, certainly runs the risk of peri- or post-operative liver failure, thus necessitating an urgent evaluation and referral for OLT. The implication here is that patients with HCC and cirrhosis should be evaluated for both liver resection and OLT and preferably be treated at a center where both options are available.

4. Orthotopic liver transplantation for HCC

Patients suffering from cirrhosis and HCC that are not candidates for resection, either because of the degree of liver disease or the location or anatomy of the tumor, are best treated by OLT. The main advantage is that OLT provides a solution for both the cirrhosis and the HCC. The problem arises from the fact that there is a limited organ supply, and for that reason there have been criteria established for patients to enter the waiting list. The most frequently used ones are the Milan criteria (single lesion less or equal to 5 cm in size or three or no more than three lesions, none of which are over 3cm in size), which can lead to 5-year survival of 70% [9]. There has been an effort to expand these criteria, as it has been shown that moderate expansion in terms of number and/or size of the lesions can lead to comparable survival.

This chapter will analyze the following issues having to do with OLT and HCC: a) results for OLT for HCC and criteria used to prioritize these patients, b) the practice of bridging therapies to OLT and downstaging prior to OLT, and c) the role of living donor liver transplantation (LDLT) for OLT.

4.1. Results and criteria for OLT for HCC

As mentioned above the most consistent prognostic factors regarding OLT for HCC are derived from the characteristics originating from the Milan criteria having to do with the size and number of the lesions, in addition to no macrovascular involvement and no extrahepatic metastatic disease to lymph nodes, lungs, bones, or other abdominal organs. These criteria can lead to 5-year survival of around 70% and recurrence-free survival of 70-80% [70-71]. In properly selected patients, it is possible to achieve even long-term results that are more than satisfactory with 9-year survival of 52% [72]. Getting to this point however has been challenging, as there is a continuous need to reevaluate the listing and priority criteria for OLT for HCC.

Originally, HCC was considered a contraindication for OLT given the dismal patient survival rates that were the result of patients being transplanted at a very late stage of their cancer, as the technique was still considered experimental. The combined work of Bismuth in 1993 and the subsequent Milan criteria by Mazzaferro showed that if patients were carefully chosen, so that the lesions were within a certain number and size, then it was possible to achieve these excellent results with OLT for HCC [70, 73]. Recently, however, several groups have argued that the Milan criteria are too restrictive and that more patients with HCC could benefit from OLT. The strongest argument along these lines is based on the University of California San Francisco (UCSF) criteria (single HCC lesion up to 6.5cm diameter or up to three lesions, none larger than 4.5cm, with a cumulative diameter of 8cm) [74]. Another retrospective study with the largest number of patients outside the Milan criteria has shown encouraging outcomes by using the "up-to-seven" rule [75]. This approach uses the sum of the combination of size and number covariates equal to seven or less. Although it appears as a strong proposal to expand the existing criteria, it does have the disadvantage of being based on post-transplant pathology. All of this has led many to discuss the "metroticket" theory, which is based on the belief that the further you go (the more you expand the existing criteria), the higher is the price you will be forced to pay (decreased survival and increased recurrence) [76]. In the United States, where the MELD score is used for listing, patients within the Milan criteria receive 22 MELD exception points for transplantation priority [77]. Despite an additional 10% increase in MELD every 3 months, patients may end up waiting 6 months to a year, depending on the region that they are [77].

4.2. Bridging therapy to OLT for HCC

The fact that, despite receiving extra priority points on the waiting list, patients with HCC may still have to wait significantly and risk falling outside the Milan criteria, makes the issue of bridging therapy all the more important. Bridging therapy is mainly aimed towards patients that are already within Milan criteria and thus eligible for OLT, and for whom the goal is to avoid tumor progression while on the waiting list. Although it is hard to clarify the usefulness of bridging therapy for patients with HCC, mainly because of the retrospective nature of most studies on the topic, it has been shown that the drop-out rate while on the waiting list increases as waiting time progresses, especially in the case of HCC [78]. Based on the estimates that have formed the basis of the UNOS MELD score exception policy, it is suggested to use bridging therapies for T2 patients, even if the estimated waiting time is less than 3 months [79].

Regarding the question of which therapy is best for bridging, the most promising therapy appears to be radiofrequency ablation, as several studies have shown decreased drop-out in radiofrequency ablation pretreated patients with a single HCC nodule [80-81]. Additionally, there may be a role for transarterial chemoembolization (TACE) for patients with lesions larger than 3cm or with a multinodular pattern, although this has not been verified in prospective studies. Another possibility, which is currently under investigation, is the use of transarterial radioembolization with Uttrium-90 microspheres, with promising results to this point [82-83].

4.3. Downstaging therapy for HCC prior to OLT

Downstaging refers to the effort made in patients that find themselves outside the Milan or UCSF criteria for transplantability, to decrease their tumor burden to the extent that they fall within these criteria again. This way, these patients become candidates for OLT. Additionally, it is thought that the response to downstaging and the maintenance of this response represent a surrogate marker of the aggressiveness of the tumor, which in itself could help guide any decisions regarding the transplantability of a patient [84]. As to which the best method for downstaging is, TACE appears to have the advantage for single treatment, especially for multifocal tumors [84]. Even so, the combination of TACE, radiofrequency ablation and resection seems to be an even more effective method of downstaging compared to TACE alone (70% success versus 40%) [83, 85].

4.4. The role of living donor liver transplantation in the management of HCC

For many, LDLT represents a possible solution to the organ shortage problem and the long waiting list; for others it presents an opportunity for an aggressive approach in dealing with HCC patients whose tumors are outside the accepted criteria (such as the Milan and UCSF ones), if a suitable living donor exists. Currently in the US, LDLT represents about 5% of all liver transplantations. Despite the fact that the experience with LDLT is still being accumulated, there appears to be significant optimism. In one of the bigger studies from Japan with 316 patients undergoing LDLT for HCC, one- and three-year survivals were 78% and 69% respectively, whereas recurrence-free one- and three-year survivals were 73% and 65% [86]. Although these results may not seem as impressive at first, it should be noted that 54% of these patients were outside the Milan criteria, thus representing a higher risk group. Some studies have shown improved survival for patients undergoing LDLT compared to those undergoing OLT from deceased donors, with 1-year survival of 86% for LDLT versus 71% for deceased donor recipients [87]. Despite these encouraging results, there remains a lot of concern. The main reason is the consideration that the health of the living donor is placed at risk, as living donors are in the unique situation of undergoing a major surgical procedure without any health benefit to themselves. Additionally, regarding the argument of expanding HCC criteria for patients undergoing LDLT, since they have their own living donor, the question remains of what should happen if these recipients suffer hepatic dysfunction or nonfunction of the liver graft. That is, should they be listed in the deceased donor waiting list, something which would not have been possible before, given the size or number of their lesions. The answer at this point appears in most cases to be "no" and thus these are all considerations that should be carefully addressed by the surgical and medical teams before proceeding with a LDLT for HCC. Finally, as it has been seen in one of the bigger, multicenter trials in the US, the Adult-to-Adult Living Donor Liver Transplantation Cohort Study (A2ALL), although the survival results between recipients of deceased donor and living donor transplantation are similar, there appears to be a higher chance of recurrence after the LDLT of 29% versus 0%, despite the much shorter waiting time (160 days for LDLT versus 469 days for deceased donor OLT) [88]. However, this could also be because of the shorter waiting time, as some would argue that by being able to proceed to transplantation quickly, one loses the "opportunity" to evaluate the biological behavior of the HCC.

5. Future challenges

Given the significant developments and progress in surgical technique, the biggest challenge in the treatment of HCC is identifying the biological behavior of a given tumor, so that a patient-tailored, or rather a tumor-targeted, treatment can be applied. To do this, it is necessary to identify those factors, other than tumor size and number, that determine tumor aggressiveness. Several studies have identified a variety of parameters, such as the response to chemoembolization, the presence of microvascular invasion, the degree of differentiation and the combination of total tumor volume (TTV) together with AFP as surrogate markers for the tumor's biological behavior [89-93]. Regarding the latter, in an overview of the Scientific Registry of Transplant Recipients data from March 2002 to January 2008, it was shown that AFP>400 ng/ml or TTV>115 cm^3 led to a three-year survival of less than 50% [94]. Essentially, this represents a novel approach, where the issue is not necessary the number or size of the HCC lesions per se, but rather the total tumor load.

The most promising area in terms of defining the nature and behavior of HCC is that of molecular biology, with the use of genetic markers. Currently, identification of targets such as vascular endothelial growth factor (VEGF) and platelet-derived growth factor receptor (PDGFR) has led to medications being used in clinical practice for advanced HCC, such as sorafenib and imatinib [95-98]. More importantly, the identification of microRNAs (miRNAs), which are a non-protein coding family of genes regulating gene expression, has opened a new window to the future. Specifically, they have been shown to function as oncogenes and tumor suppressor genes, making this a very useful screening tool for potential resection or liver transplantation candidates [99-100]. Several miRNA targets have been identified, with prominent among them miR-122a and miR-21, with the former being down-regulated and the latter up-regulated in HCC [101-102]. Advances in understanding the multistep process that is hepatic carcinogenesis, as well as beginning to identify the different signaling cascades involved, has provided researchers and clinicians with the opportunity to proceed with molecular classification of HCC [103-104]. This will provide critical information in terms of assessing the biological behavior of different HCCs, which in turn can help improve the therapeutic decision-making process.

6. Conclusion

Hepatocellular carcinoma is a disease with a far-reaching effect globally. The main therapeutic treatment method remains surgery, with the two options being liver resection or orthotopic liver transplantation. This chapter has discussed patient evaluation and selection for the different therapies, the advantages and disadvantages of liver resection and transplantation (with special emphasis on the fact that they both have a role in the continuum of care for these patients), and the future challenges and opportunities provided by the molecular tools available to today's surgeon.

Author details

Georgios Tsoulfas[1*] and Polyxeni Agorastou[2]

*Address all correspondence to: tsoulfasg@gmail.com

1 Department of Surgery, Aristotle University of Thessaloniki, Greece

2 Department of Gastroenterology, Aristotle University of Thessaloniki, Greece

References

[1] Parkin DM, Bray F, Ferlay J, Pisani P. Global cancer statistics 2002. CA Cancer J Clin 2005; 55: 74-108.

[2] El-Serag HB. Hepatocellular carcinoma. N Engl J Med 2011; 365: 118-127.

[3] Tanaka Y. Kurbanov F, Mano S, et al. Molecular tracing of the global hepatitis C virus epidemic predicts regional patterns of hepatocellular carcinoma mortality. Gastroenterology 2006; 130: 703-714.

[4] El-Serag HB, Tran T, Everhart JE. Diabetes increases the risk of chronic liver disease and hepatocellular carcinoma. Gastroenterology 2004; 126: 460-468.

[5] Calle EE, Rodriguez C, Walker-Thurmond K, Thun MJ. Overweight, obesity, and mortality from cancer in a prospectively studied cohort of US adults. N Engl J Med 2003; 348: 1625-1638.

[6] Marrero JA, Fontana RJ, Fu S, Conjeevaram HS, Su GL, Lok AS. Alcohol, tobacco and obesity are synergistic risk factors for hepatocellular carcinoma. J Hepatol 2005; 42: 218-224.

[7] Sangiovanni A, Del Ninno E, Fasani P, et al. Increased survival of cirrhotic patients with a hepatocellular carcinoma detected during surveillance. Gastroenterology 2004; 126: 1005-1014.

[8] Brechot C, Thiers V, Kremsdorf D, Nalpas B, Pol S, Paterlinin-Brechot P. Persistent hepatitis B virus infection in subjects without hepatitis B surface antigen: clinically significant or purely "occult"? Hepatology 2001; 34: 194-203.

[9] Chen JD, Yang HI, Iloeje UH, et al. Carriers of inactive hepatitis B virus are still at risk for hepatocellular carcinoma and liver-related death. Gastroenterology 2010; 138: 1747-1754.

[10] Minagawa M, Ikai I, Matsuyama Y, et al. Staging of hepatocellular carcinoma: assessment of the Japanese TNM and AJCC/UICC TNM systems in a cohort of 13,772 patients in Japan. Ann Surg 2007; 245: 909-922.

[11] Okuda K, Ohtsuki T, Obata H, et al. Natural history of hepatocellular carcinoma and prognosis in relation to treatment. Study of 850 patients. Cancer 1985; 56: 918-928.

[12] Prospective validation of the CLIP score: a new prognostic system for patients with cirrhosis and hepatocellular carcinoma. The Cancer of the Liver Italian Program (CLIP) Investigators. Hepatology 2003; 31: 840-845.

[13] Kudo M, Chung H, Osaki Y. Prognostic staging system for hepatocellular carcinoma (CLIP score): its value and limitations, and a proposal for a new staging system, the Japan Integrated Staging Score (JIS score). J Gastroenterol 2003; 38: 207-215.

[14] Grieco A, Pompili M, Caminiti G, et al. Prognostic factors for survival in patients with early-intermediate hepatocellular carcinoma undergoing non-surgical therapy: comparison of Okuda, CLIP, and BCLC staging systems in a single Italian centre. Gut 2005; 54: 411-418.

[15] Sorensen JB, Klee M, Palshof T, Hansen HH. Performance status assessment in cancer patients. AN inter-observer variability study. Br J Cancer 1993; 67: 773-775.

[16] Verger E, Salamero M, Conill C. Can Karnofsky performance status be transformed to the Eastern Cooperative Oncology Group scoring scale and vice versa? Eur J Cancer 1992; 28: 1328-1330.

[17] Llovet JM, Fuster J, Bruix H. The Barcelona approach: diagnosis, staging and treatment of hepatocellular carcinoma. Liver Transpl 2004; 10: S115-S120.

[18] Shah SA, Haddad R, Al-Sukhni W, et al. Surgical resection of hepatic and pulmonary metastases from colorectal carcinoma. J Am Coll Surg 2006; 202: 468-475.

[19] Fusai G, Davidson BR. Management of colorectal liver metastases. Colorectal Dis 2003; 5: 2-23.

[20] Scheele J, Altendorf-Hofmann A, Grube T, et al. Resection of colorectal liver metastases: what prognostic factors determine patient selection? Chirurg 2001; 72: 547-560.

[21] Schindl MJ, Redhead DN, Fearon KC, et al. The value of residual liver volume as a predictor of hepatic dysfunction and infection after major liver resection. Gut 2005; 54: 289-296.

[22] Shoup M, Gonen M, D'Angelica M, et al. Volumetric analysis predicts hepatic dysfunction in patients undergoing major liver resection. J Gastrointest Surg 2003; 7: 325-330.

[23] Bismuth H, Mjno P. Hepatobiliary surgery. J Hepatol 2000; 32: 208-224

[24] Chang CH, Chau GY, Lui WY, et al. Long-term results of hepatic resection for hepatocellular carcinoma originating from the noncirrhotic liver. Arch Surg 2004; 139: 320-325.

[25] Laurent C, Blanc JF, Nobili S, et al. Prognostic factors and long-term survival after hepatic resection for hepatocellular carcinoma originating from noncirrhotic liver. J Am Coll Surg 2005; 201: 656-662.

[26] Verhoef C, de Man RA, Zondervan PE, et al. Good outcomes after resection of large hepatocellular carcinoma in the noncirrhotic liver. Dig Surg 2004; 21: 380-386.

[27] Lang H, Sotiropoulos GC, Brokalaki EI, et al. Survival and recurrence rates after resection for hepatocellular carcinoma in noncirrhotic livers. J Am Coll Surg 2007; 205: 27-36.

[28] Pugh RN, Murray-Lyon IM, Dawson JL, Pietroni MC, Williams R. Transection of the esophagus for bleeding esophageal varices. Br J Surg 1973; 60: 646-649.

[29] Llovet JM, Burroughs A, Bruix J. Hepatocellular carcinoma. Lancet 2003; 362: 1907-1917.

[30] Bruix J, Castells A, Bosch J, et al. Surgical resection of hepatocellular carcinoma in cirrhotic patients: prognostic value of preoperative portal pressure. Gastroenterology 1996; 111: 1018-1022.

[31] Llovet JM, Fuster J, Bruix J. Intention-to-treat analysis of surgical treatment for early hepatocellular carcinoma: resection versus transplantation. Hepatology 1999; 39: 1434-1440.

[32] Bruix J, Sherman M. Management of hepatocellular carcinoma: an update. Hepatology 2011; 53: 1020-1022.

[33] Ishizawa T, Hasegawa K, Aoki T, et al. Neither multiple tumors nor portal hypertension are surgical contraindications for hepatocellular carcinoma. Gastroenterology 2008; 134: 1908-1916.

[34] Cucchetti A, Ercolani G, Vivarelli M, et al. Impact of model for end-stage liver disease (MELD) score on prognosis after hepatectomy for hepatocellular carcinoma on cirrhosis. Liver Transpl 2006; 12: 966-971.

[35] The SH, Christein J, Donohue J, et al. Hepatic resection of hepatocellular carcinoma in patients with cirrhosis: Model of End-Stage Liver Disease (MELD) score predicts perioperative mortality. J Gastrointest Surg 2005; 9: 1207-1215.

[36] Grazi GL, Ercolani G, Pierangeli F, et al. Improved results of liver resection for hepatocellular carcinoma on cirrhosis give the procedure added value. Ann Surg 2001; 234: 71-78.

[37] Fong Y, Sun RL, Jarnagin W, et al. An analysis of 412 cases of hepatocellular carcinoma at a Western center. Ann Surg 1999; 229: 790-799.

[38] Ercolani G, Grazi GL, Ravaioli M, et al. Liver resection for hepatocellular carcinoma on cirrhosis: univariate and multivariate analysis of risk factors for intrahepatic recurrence. Ann Surg 2003; 237: 536-543.

[39] Kinoshita H, Sakai K, Hirohashi K, et al. Preoperative portal vein embolization for hepatocellular carcinoma. World J Surg 1986; 10: 803-808.

[40] Makuuchi M, Thai BL, Takayasu K, et al. Preoperative portal vein embolization to increase safety of major hepatectomy for hilar bile duct carcinoma: a preliminary report. Surgery 1990; 107: 521-527.

[41] Farges O, Belghiti J, Kianmanesh R, et al. Portal vein embolization before right hepatectomy: prospective clinical trial. Ann Surg 2003; 237: 208-217.

[42] Jaeck D, Bachellier P, Nakano H, et al. One or two-stage hepatectomy combined with portal vein embolization for initially nonresectable colorectal liver metastases. Am J Surg 2003; 185: 221-229.

[43] Kaneko T, Nakao A, Takagi H. Clinical studies of new material for portal vein embolization: comparison of embolic effect with different agents. Hepatogastroenterology 2002; 49: 472-477.

[44] Madoff DC, Hicks ME, Vauthey JN, et al. Transhepatic portal vein embolization: anatomy, indications, and technical considerations. Radiographics 2002; 22: 1063-1076.

[45] Michalopoulos GK, DeFrances MC. Liver regeneration. Science 1997; 276: 60-66.

[46] Hasegawa K, Kokudo N, Imamura H, et al. Prognostic impact of anatomic resection for hepatocellular carcinoma. Ann Surg 2005; 242: 252-259.

[47] Vauthey JN, Klimstra D, Franceschi D, et al. Factors affecting long-term outcome after hepatic resection for hepatocellular carcinoma. Am J Surg 1995; 169: 28-34.

[48] Eguchi S, Kanematsu T, Arii S, et al. Liver Cancer Study group of Japan. Comparison of the outcomes between an anatomical subsegmentectomy and a non-anatomical minor hepatectomy for single hepatocellular carcinomas based on a Japanese nationwide survey. Surgery 2008; 143: 469-475.

[49] Lise M, Bacchetti S, Da Pian P, et al. Prognostic factors affecting long term outcome after liver resection for hepatocellular carcinoma: results in a series of 100 Italian patients. Cancer 1998; 82: 1028-1036.

[50] Poon RT, Fan ST, Ng IO, et al. Significance of resection margin in hepatectomy for hepatocellular carcinoma: a critical reappraisal. Ann Surg 2000; 231: 544-551.

[51] Matsui Y, Terakawa N, Satoi S, et al. Postoperative outcomes in patients with hepatocellular carcinomas resected with exposure of the tumor surface: clinical role of the no-margin resection. Arch Surg 2007; 142: 596-602.

[52] Shi M, Guo RP, Lin XJ, et al. Partial hepatectomy with wide versus narrow resection margin for solitary hepatocellular carcinoma: a prospective randomized trial. Ann Surg 2007; 245: 36-43.

[53] The Japan Society of Hepatology. Does width of the surgical margin contribute to prognosis? Hepatology Research 2010; 40 (Suppl 1): 48-73.

[54] Gagner M, Rheault M, Dubuc J. Laparoscopic partial hepatectomy for liver tumor. Surg Endosc 1992; 6: 99.

[55] Nguyen KT, Gamblin TC, Geller DA. Laparoscopic liver resection for cancer. Futur Oncol 2008; 4: 661-670.

[56] Sasaki A, Nitta H, Otsuka K, et al. Ten-year experience of totally laparoscopic liver resection in a single institution. Br J Surg 2009; 96: 274-279.

[57] Gigot JF, Glineur D, Santiago Azagra J, et al. Laparoscopic liver resection for malignant liver tumors: preliminary results of a multicenter European study. Ann Surg 2002; 236: 90-97.

[58] Kazaryan AM, Mavango IP, Rosok BI, et al. Laparoscopic resection of colorectal liver metastases: surgical and long-term outcomes. Ann Surg 2010; 252: 1005-1012.

[59] Vigano L, Laurent A, Tayar C, et al. the learning curve in laparoscopic liver resection: improved feasibility and reproducibility. Ann Surg 2009; 250: 772-782.

[60] Cherqui D, Laurent A, Tayar C, et al. Laparoscopic liver resection for peripheral hepatocellular carcinoma in patients with chronic liver disease: midterm results and perspectives. Ann Surg 2006; 243: 499-506.

[61] Dagher I, Belli G, Fantini C, et al. Laparoscopic hepatectomy for hepatocellular carcinoma: a European experience. J Am Coll Surg 2010; 211: 16-23.

[62] Zhou YM, Shao WY, Zhao YF, Xu DH, Li B. Meta-analysis of laparoscopic versus open resection for hepatocellular carcinoma. Dig Dis Sci 2011; 56: 1937-1943.

[63] Laurent A, Cherqui D, Lesurtel M, Brunetti F, Tayar C, Fagniez PL. Laparoscopic liver resection for subcapsular hepatocellular carcinoma complicating chronic liver disease. Arch Surg 2003; 138: 763-769.

[64] Cai XJ, Yang J, Yu H, et al. Clinical study of laparoscopic versus open hepatectomy for malignant liver tumors. Surg Endosc 2008; 22: 2350-2356.

[65] Laurent A, Tayar C, Andreoletti M, et al. Laparoscopic liver resection facilitates salvage liver transplantation for hepatocellular carcinoma. J Hepatobiliary Pancreat Surg 2009; 16: 310-314.

[66] Roayaie S, Blume IN, Thung S, et al. A system of classifying microvascular invasion to predict outcome after resection in patients with hepatocellular carcinoma. Gastroenterology 2009; 137: 850-855.

[67] Imamura H, Matsuyama Y, Tanaka E, et al. Risk factors contributing to early and late phase intrahepatic recurrence of hepatocellular carcinoma after hepatectomy. J Hepatol 2003; 38: 200-207.

[68] Mazzaferro M, Romito R, Schiavo M, et al. Prevention of hepatocellular carcinoma recurrence with alpha-interferon after liver resection in HCV cirrhosis. Hepatology 2006; 44: 1543-1554.

[69] Pelletier SJ, Fu S, Thyagarajan V, et al. An intention-to-treat analysis of liver transplantation for hepatocellular carcinoma using organ procurement transplant network data. Liver Transpl 2009; 15: 859-868.

[70] Mazzaferro V, Regalia E, Doci R, et al. Liver transplantation for the treatment of small hepatocellular carcinoma in patients with cirrhosis. N Engl J Med 1996; 334: 693-699.

[71] Llovet JM, Bruix J, Fuster J, et al. Liver transplantation for small hepatocellular carcinoma: the tumor-node-metastasis classification does not have prognostic power. Hepatology 1998; 27:1572-1577.

[72] Majella Doyle MB, Vachharajani N, Maynard E, et al. Liver transplantation for hepatocellular carcinoma: long-term results suggest excellent outcomes. J Am Coll Surg 2012; 215: 19-28.

[73] Bismuth H, Cliché L, Adam R, Castaing D, Diamond T, Dennison A. Liver resection versus transplantation in cirrhotic patients with hepatocellular carcinoma in cirrhosis. Ann Surg 1993; 218: 145-151.

[74] Yao FY, Roberts JP. Applying expanded criteria to liver transplantation for hepatocellular carcinoma: too much, too soon, or is now the time? Liver Transpl 2004; 10: 919-921.

[75] Mazzaferro V, Llovet JM, Miceli R, et al. Predicting survival after liver transplantation in patients with hepatocellular carcinoma beyond the Milan criteria: a retrospective, exploratory analysis. Lancet Oncol 2009; 10: 35-43.

[76] Bhoori S, Sposito C, Germini A, Coppa J, Mazzaferro V. The challenges of liver transplantation for hepatocellular carcinoma. Transpl Int 2010; 23: 712-722.

[77] Pomfret EA, Washburn K, Wald, et al. Report of a national conference on liver allocation in patients with hepatocellular carcinoma in the United States. Liver Transpl 2010; 16: 262-278.

[78] Freeman RB, Edwards EB, Harper AM. Waiting list removal rates among patients with chronic and malignant liver diseases. Am J Transplant 2006; 6: 1416-1421.

[79] Llovet JM, Mas X, Aponte JJ, et al. Cost effectiveness of adjuvant therapy for hepatocellular carcinoma during the waiting list for liver transplantation. Gut 2002; 50: 123-128.

[80] Mazzaferro V, Battiston C, Perrone S, et al. Radiofrequency ablation of small hepatocellular carcinoma in cirrhotic patients awaiting liver transplantation: a prospective study. Ann Surg 2004; 240: 900-909.

[81] Fontana RJ, Hamidullah H, Nghiem H, et al. Percutaneous radiofrequency thermal ablation of hepatocellular carcinoma: a safe and effective bridge to liver transplantation. Liver Transpl 2002; 8: 1165-1174.

[82] Geschwind JF, Salem R, Carr BI, et al. Yttrium-90 microspheres for the treatment of hepatocellular carcinoma. Gastroenterology 2004; 127: S194-S205.

[83] Lewandowski RJ, Kulik LM, Riaz A, et al. A comparative analysis of transarterial downstaging for hepatocellular carcinoma: chemoembolization versus Radioembolization. Am J Transplant 2009; 9: 1920-1928.

[84] Yao FY, Kerlan RK Jr, Hirose R, et al. Excellent outcome following down-staging of hepatocellular carcinoma prior to liver transplantation: an intention-to-treat analysis. Hepatology 2008; 48: 819-827.

[85] Chapman WC, Majella Doyle MB, Stuart JE, et al. Outcomes of neoadjuvant transarterial chemoembolization to downstage hepatocellular carcinoma before liver transplantation. Ann Surg 2008; 248: 617-625.

[86] Todo S, Furukawa H. Living donor liver transplantation for adult patients with hepatocellular carcinoma: experience in Japan. Ann Surg 2004; 240: 451-459.

[87] Cheng SJ, Pratt DS, Freeman RB, et al. Living-donor versus cadaveric liver transplantation for non-resectable small hepatocellular carcinoma and compensated cirrhosis: a decision analysis. Transplantation 2001; 72: 861-868.

[88] Fisher RA, Kulik LM, Freise CE, et al. Hepatocellular carcinoma recurrence and death following living and deceased donor liver transplantation. Am J Transplant 2007; 7: 1601-1608.

[89] Otto G, Herber S, Heise M, et al. Response to transarterial chemoembolization as a biological selection criteria for liver transplantation in hepatocellular carcinoma. Liver Transpl 2006; 12: 1260-1267.

[90] Cillo U, Vitale A, Bassanello M, et al. Liver transplantation for the treatment of moderately or well-differentiated hepatocellular carcinoma. Ann Surg 2004; 239: 150-159.

[91] Shirabe K, Itoh S, Yoshizumi T, et al. The predictors of microvascular invasion in candidates for liver transplantation with hepatocellular carcinoma; with special reference to the serum levels of des-gamma-carboxy Prothrombin. J Surg Oncol 2007; 95: 235-240.

[92] Jonas S, Bechstein WO, Steinmmuler T, et al. Vascular invasion and histopathologic grading determine outcome after liver transplantation for hepatocellular carcinoma in cirrhosis. Hepatology 2001; 33: 1080-1086.

[93] Sotiropoulos GC, Malago M, Bockhorn M, et al. Liver transplantation for hepatocellular carcinoma and cirrhosis in candidates with undetectable or very low alpha-fetoprotein levels: is an expansion of listing criteria justified? Hepatogastroenterology 2008; 55: 1671-1677.

[94] Toso C, Asthana S, Bigam DL, Shapiro MJ, Kneteman NM. Reassessing selection criteria prior to liver transplantation for hepatocellular carcinoma utilizing the scientific registry of transplant recipients database. Hepatology 2009; 49: 832-838.

[95] Chiang DY, Villanueva A, Hoshida Y, et al. Focal gains of VEGFA and molecular classification of hepatocellular carcinoma. Cancer Res 2008; 68: 6779-6788.

[96] Liu L, Cao Y, Chen C, et al. Sorafenib blocks the RAF/MEK/ERK pathway, inhibits tumor angiogenesis, and induces tumor cell apoptosis in hepatocellular carcinoma model PLC/PRF/5. Cancer Res 2006; 66: 11851-11858.

[97] Stock P, Monga D, Tan X, Micsenyi A, Loizos N, Monga SP. Platelet-derived growth factor receptor-alpha: a novel therapeutic target in human hepatocellular cancer. Mol Cancer Ther 2007; 6: 1932-1941.

[98] Eckel F, von Delius S, Mayr M, et al. Pharmacokinetic and clinical phase II trial of imatinib in patients with impaired liver function and advanced hepatocellular carcinoma. Oncology 2005; 69: 363-371.

[99] Esquela-Kerscher A, Slack FJ. Oncomirs-microRNAs with a role in cancer. Nat Rev Cancer 2006; 6: 259-269.

[100] He L, Hannon GJ. MicroRNAs: small RNAs with a big role in gene regulation. Nat Rev Genet 2004; 5: 522-531.

[101] Gramantieri L, Ferracin M, Fornari F, et al. Cyclin G1 is a target of miR-122a, a microRNA frequently down-regulated in human hepatocellular carcinoma. Cancer Res 2007; 67: 6092-6099/

[102] Meng F, Henson R, Wehbe-Janek H, Ghoshal K, Jacob ST, Patel T. MicroRNA-21 regulates expression of the PTEN tumor suppressor gene in human hepatocellular cancer. Gastroenterology 2007; 133: 647-658.

[103] Farazi PA, De Pinho RA. Hepatocellular carcinoma pathogenesis: from genes to environment. Nat Rec Cancer 2006; 6: 674-687.

[104] Villanueva A, Newell P, Chiang DY, Friedman SL, Llovet JM. Genomics and signalling pathways in hepatocellular carcinoma. Semin Liver Dis 2007; 27: 55-76.

Chapter 6

Laparoscopic Surgery in Genitourinary Cancer Treatment

March Villalba José Antonio

Additional information is available at the end of the chapter

http://dx.doi.org/10.5772/55448

1. Introduction

Genitourinary cancer comprises kidney, prostate, bladder, upper urinary tract and testis neoplasms. The incidence rates of them vary between 15 and 1.5% in developed countries.

The epidemiology of genitourinary cancer varies depend on the organ. Prostate cancer is the most common solid neoplasm in males (15%) and renal cell neoplasm involves since 3% of all adult cancers. Urothelial carcinomas are the fourth most common tumors, after prostate, breast (females), lung and colorectal cancer. In particular, bladder cancer is the 9th most common cancer diagnosis worldwide. Testicular cancer is the less common genitourinary cancer that represents between 1% and 1.5% of male neoplasms [1].

The wide range of treatments against these diseases comprises surgery, radiotherapy and chemotherapy. Radiotherapy is used to treat localized and locally-advanced prostate cancer even with curative intent. Also radiotherapy is used to prophylactic treatment in seminomatous testis cancer to avoid para-aortic or iliac lymphatic relapses. In bladder cancer, radiotherapy is used as a palliative treatment against hematuria. Radiotherapy does not play an important role in kidney cancer, only it is used to treat selected metastasis cases.

Chemoteraphy in prostate cancer (Taxanes) is reserved for the treatment of metastatic castration refractory prostate cancer. At renal cell carcinoma, Tyrosine kinase inhibitors or Mammalian target of rapamycin (mTOR) inhibitors should be considered as first- or second-line treatment for metastatic disease. Cisplatin-based chemoteraphy in bladder cancer is considered as a neoadyuvant or adyuvant treatment before and after cystectomy if there is suspicion or evidence of lymph node metastasis. Carboplatin-based chemoteraphy is used to treat several seminomatous testis neoplasms stages after orchiectomy. Cisplatin, eposide and bleomycin or eposide and cisplatin combinations are used to treat non-seminomatous testis neoplasm combined or not to retroperitoneal lymph node nerve-sparring surgery and also in metastatic cases.

More and more genitourinary cancers are diagnosed in localized stages, making surgical treatment possible [1]. Since Bill Schuessler performed the first laparoscopic lymphadenectomy in a patient with localized prostate cancer (October 1989), Urologists have acquired technology advances applied to laparoscopic surgery. In the last decades, those advances have made a minimally invasive approach to treat these cancers easier. That has caused that today laparoscopy approach is the technique of choice in the surgical treatment of some localized genitourinary cancers [2].

According the PUBMED database, there is an increase in the publication of articles dealing with the laparoscopic treatment. In the last 5 years almost 10% of those articles referring specifically to laparoscopic surgery. (Graphic 1).

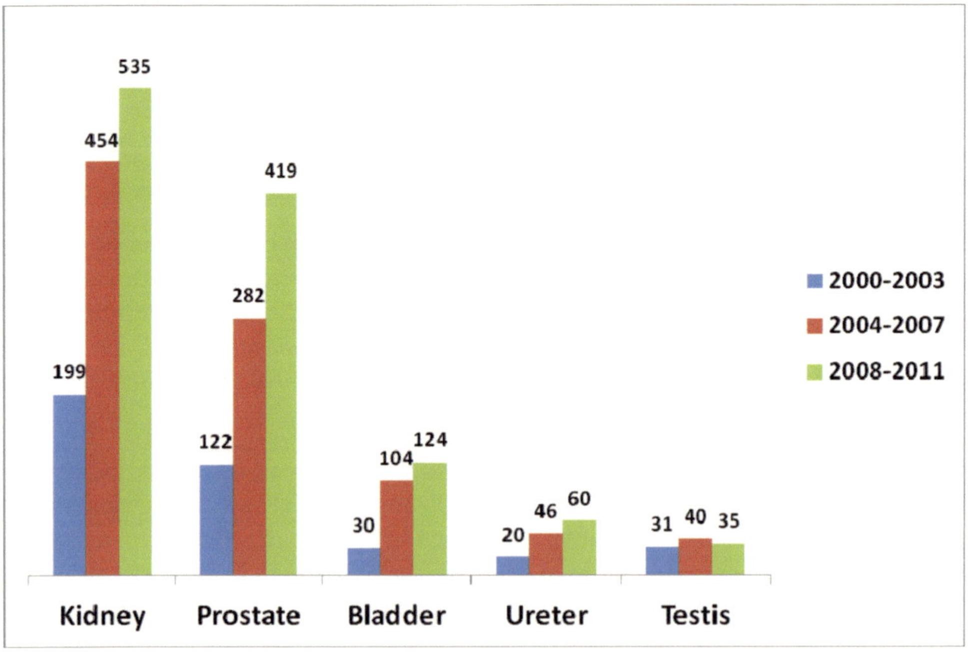

Figure 1. Evolution of published articles on laparoscopic surgery in PUBMED (MESH database).

Today there is a trend towards minimally invasive surgery but it is necessary to establish whether the outcomes of competing treatment options (open Vs laparoscopy) are comparable, focusing in postoperative morbidity and oncologic outcomes.

This chapter gives a summary of laparoscopic treatment reviewing the indication, morbidity and oncologic and functional results compared to conventional surgery for each of the listed cancers, providing a general overview.

T1	Tumor ≤ 7 cm in greatest dimension limited to the kidney
T1a	<4 cm
T1b	4-7 cm
T2	Tumor > 7 cm in greatest dimension limited to the kidney
T2a	7-10 cm
T2b	> 10 cm
T3	Tumor extends into major veins or perinephric tissues but not into the ipsilateral adrenal gland and not beyond Gerota´s fascia.
T3a	Renal vein/ perirenal or renal sinus.
T3b	Vena cava below diaphragm.
T3c	Vena cava wall / beyond diaphragm.
T4	Tumor extends beyond Gerota´s fascia.

Table 1. Kidney. Primary tumor stage (T) [41].

2. Renal cancer

Renal cell carcinoma (RCC) accounts for 2-3% of all adult cancers. More than 50% are diagnosed at a localized stage (pT1-pT2) (Table 2). Open radical or partial nephrectomy has been the standard curative intervention for localized RCC for the past five decades, laparoscopy also being an alternative in RCC with renal vein tumor thrombus (pT3a) (Table 2). With the new minimally invasive approaches, laparoscopic radical or partial nephrectomy has become an acceptable alternative to open surgery [3,4]

pT2	Organ-confined.
pT2a	Unilateral, one-half of one side or less
pT2b	Unilateral involving more than one-half of side but not both sides
pT2c	Bilateral disease
pT3	Extraprostatic extension
pT3a	Prostate capsule or microscopic invasion of bladder neck
pT3b	Seminal vesicle invasion
pT4	Invasion of rectum, levator muscles and/or pelvic wall

Table 2. Prostate. Pathologic tumor stage (pT) [42].

2.1. Morbidity and functional outcomes

In comparison with open radical nephrectomy, laparoscopic procedure offers less morbidity (back pain and postoperative blood loss) and hospital stay [3].

Nephron-sparing surgery offers better preservation of renal function than radical nephrectomy and lower risk of cardiac death but efforts should be made to limit the renal function loss associated with surgery for localized renal masses regarding transient ischemia at surgery, because warm ischemia time seems to be the most important independent variable for predicting renal damage. This damage occurs within the third postoperative month [5,6].

Laparoscopic nephron-sparing surgery provides less blood loss, median operative time, median analgesic requirement, hospital stay and median convalescence time, compared to open partial nephrectomy. But it means more major intra-operative complications (5% Vs 0%), renal / urological complications (11% Vs 2%) and warmer ischemia time [7].

2.2. Oncologic outcomes

2.2.1. Localised renal cell carcinoma

There are no randomised studies assessing oncological outcomes. Papers published found similar oncological outcomes; the 5 year overall survival for laparoscopic versus open radical nephrectomy was 87.8% and 88.7%, respectively. There was no evidence of any difference in cancer-specific and recurrence-free survival at 5 year reported in the studies [4].

With respect to the approach at localized RCC, few randomized studies compared retroperitoneal with transperitoneal radical nephrectomy. Both of them were found to have a similar oncological outcomes and no incidences of positive surgical margins were reported [4,8].

When laparoscopic partial nephrectomy was compared to open partial nephrectomy, a database review of Lane *et al.* noted an overall survival benefit increase in laparoscopic versus open partial nephrectomy when adjusting for age, gender, race, Charlson index, tumor size, hypertension and the predicted risk of recurrence at 5 year in those patients with a minimum of 1 year follow-up, but there were no differences in 3 year cancer-specific survival, 5 year overall survival and 7 year follow-up (92.7% Vs 95.6% in cancer-specific survival respectively). This study described a lower risk of all-cause death in the laparoscopic group [9]. The same results were described by Gill *et al.* and Marszalek et al; both of them did not find differences in the recurrence patterns between both groups [10,11].

There has been controversy about the suitable tumor size to perform a laparoscopy nephron-sparing intervention. A cut-off of 4cm has been recommended but some authors have argued that partial nephrectomy is feasible up to 7cm with no reduction in oncologic outcomes. In this view Simmons *et al.* published a database review for tumors larger than 4cm treated by laparoscopic partial nephrectomy versus laparoscopic radical nephrectomy. There was no difference in estimated overall survival (74% versus qué), cancer-specific survival and recurrence-free survival rates (both 81% versus qué) [4,12].

In addition to size, other factors about renal mass anatomy such as growth pattern (endo-/ meso-/exophytic) and location (central/hilar/peripheral, anterior/posterior, lateral/medial, polar) are important to consider a nephron-sparing surgery. It is more feasible if tumor is placed in a peripheral/polar/posterior site, for example [13].

2.2.2. *Locally-advanced renal cell carcinoma*

Laparoscopic surgery has been extended to patients with renal cell carcinoma associated with limited local invasion and lymph node metastases or in the presence of renal vein and inferior vena cava thrombi. In well-selected patients with metastatic renal cell carcinoma, laparoscopic cytoreductive nephrectomy can be performed safely, with less morbidity than open nephrectomy [14]. Laparoscopic nephrectomy in metastatic RCC should be recommended to those patients with a good performance status before oncological treatment. The expanding indications for laparoscopic radical nephrectomy are: larger tumors (>7cm), renal vein tumor thrombus, cytoreductive nephrectomy and limited locally invasive tumors into psoas or diaphragm muscle. This technique must be performed in selected patients [8,15]..

2.3. Conclusions

For localized renal cancer, laparoscopic radical nephrectomy is the approach of choice because it offers less morbidity than open nephrectomy and both of them achieve similar oncological outcomes, such as survival and recurrence rates. There are no differences between transperitoneal and retroperitoneal approach.

When renal tumors are ≤ 4cm laparoscopic partial nephrectomy is a good choice but location of tumor is also important to perform surgery. In these cases, partial nephrectomy improves survival.

Laparoscopic partial nephrectomy shows no improvement than laparoscopic radical nephrectomy when renal tumors are > 4cm but laparoscopic approach is a correct choice depending on surgeon skill and renal mass anatomy.

For locally-advanced renal cancer, laparoscopic radical nephrectomy is a technically feasible approach in carefully selected patients with a good performance status. Optimal patient selection, large laparoscopic experience and multidisciplinary support are the more important elements for a safe application of this approach.

Additional data are needed because most of the studies are retrospective and is necessary to improve methodological quality.

3. Prostate cancer

Prostate cancer (PCa) is one of the most common solid neoplasm in male. In Europe it has an incidence rate of 214 cases per 1000 men, outnumbering lung and colorectal cancer. PCa is currently the second most common cause of cancer death in men [16].

Currently, there is an increase in the diagnosis of PCa, concretely clinically localized prostate cancer (table 3). Radical prostatectomy is a common treatment for these patients, who have also life expectancy more than 10 years [17]. Radical prostatectomy has been associated with complications and sequel, including intraoperative blood loss, postoperative urinary incontinence and erectile dysfunction. With the intent of reducing the invasiveness of traditional open retropubic approach and complications, urologists have developed the laparoscopic technique, which represents a different perspective of surgical anatomy that implies an important learning curve [17].

Tis	Carcinoma in situ (Cis) "flat tumor"
T1	Tumor invades subepithelial connective tissue
T2	Tumor invades muscularis propia
T2a	superficial muscularis propia (inner half)
T2b	deep muscularis propia (outer half)
T3	Tumor invades: perivesical tissue (bladder: T3a microscopically and T3b extravesical mass), peripelvic fat or renal parenchyma (pelvis), periureteric fat (ureter).
T4	Tumor extends to adjacent organs: perinephric fat (ureter/pelvis), prostatic stroma,uterus vagina (T4a in bladder), pelvic wall or abdominal wall (T4b in bladder).

Urothelium. Histologic grade (WHO/SIUP 1993)[43,44].

Grade 1 well differenciated
Grade 2 Moderately differenciated
Grade 3 poorly differenciated

Table 3. Urothelium. Primary tumor stage (T) [43,44].

3.1. Morbidity and functional outcomes

Several studies demonstrate that operative time of laparoscopic approach was significantly longer than open retropubic approach, but laparoscopic approach showed less blood loss and lower transfusion rates than the open procedure [17,18]. The overall complications rate was significantly lower in those patients undergoing laparoscopy radical prostatectomy [17,18].

A single, nonrandomized prospective trial compared retropubic radical prostatectomy with laparoscopy prostatectomy, demonstrating that tissue damage was significantly lower in laparoscopic approach. Specifically, plasmatic levels of IL-6 and C-reactive protein were lower at the end of procedure, 12 hours later and 24 hours later [17].

In relation to postoperative pain (measured by validated 10-point visual analogue scale), laparoscopic radical prostatectomy with retroperitoneal approach seems to be the best tolerated technique during the first five postoperative days, compared with transperitoneal and open approaches [19]. Considering the studies reporting the requirements of morphine sulfate equivalent during the postoperative course, it seems to be no differences between open and laparoscopic approach [17].

In the published comparative studies, catheterization times and hospital stay were lower in laparoscopic approach [17]. Full recovery was faster in laparoscopic than open approach [18]. Laparoscopic radical prostatectomy had a lower rate of anastomotic strictures compared to open retropubic prostatectomy [17].

About urinary incontinence and erectile function, cumulative analysis of the available data suggest that continence rates and erectile function after open or laparoscopic approach are similar [17,18]. The same occurs when quality of life after surgery was analyzed in both groups [17].

3.2. Oncologic outcomes

With regard to the oncologic outcomes, in the published comparative studies, the main item evaluated was the surgical margins. Guazzoni et al published the study with the highest level of evidence, demonstrating that the positive surgical margins rates obtained after open retropubic radical prostatectomy and laparoscopic radical prostatectomy were overlapping [20]. In addition, when the data were stratified by the pathologic stages, there were no differences between the two procedures [17,21].

3.3. Conclusions

Laparoscopy radical prostatectomy implies an important learning curve to achieve good functional and oncologic outcomes. Currently, laparoscopy approach is better than open approach in terms of perioperative and early postoperative outcomes such as: blood loss, transfusion requirements, tissue damage, postoperative pain (only the first few days), hospital stay, and full recovery time.

Several studies showed a lower rate of anastomotic stricture after laparoscopic approach.

At laparoscopic approach, the surgeon skill is very important to perform good bladder neck preservation, paraurethral dissection and nerve sparing surgery (when it is possible), to obtain good functional results. In general, laparoscopic approach does not offer more advantages in urinary continence or erectile function after surgery and the oncologic outcomes, compared to open approach, are similar.

There were no differences between retroperitoneal and transperitoneal approach [22].

It is necessary more prospective studies, as well randomised series to analyze oncologic outcomes and morbidity comparing more than retroperitoneal or transperitoneal approach at the laparoscopic procedure, as well as the addition of lymphadenectomy.

It is likely that the most critical issue in surgical treatment of localized prostate cancer is the selection of the best surgical technique fitted to the surgeon, rather than only the surgical approach.

4. Urothelial cancer: Bladder and upper urinary tract

4.1. Bladder cancer

Bladder cancer is the 9th most common cancer diagnosis worldwide, with an estimated male: female ratio of 3.8:1.0. At the initial diagnosis of bladder cancer approximately 30% has muscle-invasive disease [23].

Muscle invasive urothelial bladder cancer is a highly aggressive disease in which surgical treatment is essential for survival. Although open radical cystectomy is the gold standard treatment for muscle-invasive, organ-confined bladder carcinoma, there is increasing interest in laparoscopic radical cystectomy [24,25].

Radical cystectomy is also an optional or recommended treatment in high grade tumors like T1G3 or Cis (table3) with high risk of progression and/or multiple recurrences after immunotherapy (intravesical BCG) treatment [23].

Laparoscopic radical cystectomy could be divided in three times: 1, cystoprostatectomy in males or cystectomy plus hysterectomy and ooforectomy in females; 2, lymphadenectomy and 3, urinary device reconstruction (intra or extracorporeal).

At this surgery it is necessary to have performed a correct selection criteria, including organ-confined disease (≤T3), nonbulky limphadenopathy, absence of uncorrected coagulopathy, body mass index < 35 kg/m^2, non severe cardiorespiratory compromise and absence of prior abdominal surgery or prior pelvic radiation therapy, because it has been shown that the patients who do not meet these criteria have higher complication rates and poor profit of lymphadenectomy [24].

About lymphadenectomy, there is strong evidence that the more nodes removed at cystectomy, the better long-term survival time, so it is very important the extent of the lympadenectomy and the number of nodes removed. At laparosopic approach, it requires high-level laparoscopic skills [24].

4.1.1. Morbidity and functional outcomes

General postoperative complications rate of open radical cystectomy vary between 30%-60% of patients and the mortality is about 1.5%. At laparoscopic cystectomy the reported rates fall between 8%-42% and 1% of mortality, but these reports do not define blood transfusion as a complication [24]. Nix *et al.* performed the only randomized controlled trial and reported no difference in complications between open and laparoscopic approach, but the groups were too small [26]. Haber *et al.* in their retrospectively series (n=50 in each group) showed an important benefit for the laparoscopic approach and extracorporeal urinary diversion. These cases were associated with reduced blood loss, decreased ileus, shorter hospital stay and no differences in operating time and post-operative complications, and appear to have less postoperative analgesic requirements [27].

The indications or nerve-sparing cystectomy are limited to selected young patients with organ-confined low-volume of tumor and extratrigonal location who are keen to maintain their sexual potency. This preservation has rarely been analyzed and the series published lacked potency data. Prostate-sparing radical cystectomy, another way to preserve erection, is controversial, and there are no data about long-term oncological outcomes to validate their safety [27].

Regarding to urinary diversion, Haber *et al.* showed that the laparoscopic assisted urinary diversion technique provides decreases in operating time, blood loss, transfusion rate, and more rapid postoperative return to oral intake and ambulation, although major complications requiring re-operation occurred more in this group than in the extracorporeal reconstruction [27].

4.1.2. Oncologic outcomes

About surgical margins, both approaches obtained equivalent rates. The international Laparoscopic Cystectomy Registry has been established a surgical margins rate of 2%, compared to 1.6% for patients with organ-confined disease after open radical cystectomy [24, 27]. Chade *et al.* published an incidence of positive surgical margins ranged from 4-5% and 0-5% in open and laparoscopic approach respectively [25].

Lymphadenectomy plays an important role in oncological outcome. Published reports showed an inferior average of nodal retrieval in laparoscopic procedure than in open approach. This procedure strongly depends on the surgeon skills [25].

Local recurrence rates also appeared similar in both groups, around 7-10% [24]. Overall survival published in the laparoscopic series was 90-100% at 1-2 years and 63-79% at 2-3 years (selected cases), compared to open radical cystectomy series showing 62-68% at 5 years [25]. It is important to consider that the majority of published series had inadequate follow-up periods or/and the laparoscopic and open cohorts were no identical (strong selection bias) [28].

Port-site recurrence seems rare with current laparoscopic techniques for placement of the specimens into a laparoscopic bag, although there are few papers published on this topic. Tanaka *et al.*, for example, described one case of recurrence in a patient with a locally-advanced stage (0.3%) [29].

4.1.3. Conclusions

Laparoscopic radical cystectomy is a difficult surgical technique specially to perform a correct pelvic lymphadenectomy. Today it cannot be considered an alternative to open approach because the postoperative series failed in selection criteria and follow-up period (not more than 5 years). Multicentre prospective trials are needed.

Hand-assisted laparoscopic radical cystectomy has a less period of learning curve but it decreases the advantages of a minimally invasive technique like pure laparoscopic cystectomy.

The extirpative component of laparoscopic cystectomy is well established. However laparoscopic lymphadenectomy and reconstruction remains challenging, time-consuming, and could be associated with major complications. Shorter number of cases demonstrated that it is preferable to perform intracorporeal construction of the urinary diversion.

In conclusion, laparoscopic radical cystectomy with urinary diversion is a difficult procedure that should be reserved for selected cases (localized bladder cancer) and performed by experienced laparoscopic surgeons in selected centers.

4.2. Upper urinary tract urothelial cell cancer

Urothelial carcinomas are the fourth most common tumors after prostate (males) or breast (females) cancer, lung cancer and colorectal cancer. They can be located in the upper urinary tract (pyelocaliceal cavities and ureter). Upper urinary tract carcinomas are uncommon and account for only 5-10% of urothelial carcinomas. In 8-13% of patients, concurrent bladder cancer is present [30].

Laparoscopic radical nephroureterectomy is reserved for localized disease (the tumor not invades beyond peripelvic or periureteric fat or renal parenchyma). This technique must comply with oncologic principles, which consists on preventing tumour seeding by avoiding drilling the upper urinary tract during resection. The excision includes the distal ureter to avoid recurrence. In the first experience there were reports of retroperitoneal metastatic or trocar dissemination when locally-advanced tumors are manipulated [30]. Laparoscopic nephroureterectomy must take a place in a closed system, tumor morcelation should be avoided and an endobag is necessary to extract the specimen (kidney and ureter removed en bloc with the bladder cuff) [30].

Open and laparoscopic access seems to be equivalent in terms of efficacy and oncologic results, but regarding to functional outcomes laparoscopy approach is superior to open surgery (as in the laparoscopy nephrectomy). Laparoscopic approach resulted in less blood loss, shorter hospital stay, decreased analgesic use, a shorter interval to oral intake, a decreased analgesic use and a decrease interval to convalescence, with no significant difference in the rate of perioperative complications [30,31].

Laparoscopy lymph node dissection associated with nephroureterectomy allows for optimal staging and has a therapeutic purpose. However, the anatomic areas to perform it have not yet clearly defined and it is not possible to standardize the indications to perform an extended lymphadenectomy because the published data are retrospective [30].

Several reports analyzed retroperitoneoscopic nephroureterectomy; most of them found that this approach was associated with longer operative times. However, blood loss, analgesic use, and length of hospital stay were decreased in comparison to open approach [31].

In conclusion, laparoscopic nephroureterectomy is a feasible approach at localized upper urinary tract tumors when it is impossible to perform a conservative treatment.

5. Testicular cancer

Testicular cancer represents between 1% and 1.5% of male neoplasms and 5% of urological tumors in general. About 15-20% of stage I (no clinical node metastasis) seminoma and up to 30% of nonseminomatous germ cells cancer patients have subclinical metastases. Surgical resection is the gold standard for managing postchemotherapy residual retroperitoneal tumor mass cases [32,33].

Laparoscopic surgery in testicular cancer is focused on the treatment of residual retroperitoneal mass or lymph node metastasis after chemotherapy. Retroperitoneal lymph node dissection is still a diagnostic and therapeutic option mainly in stage I disease [34,33].

5.1. Morbidity and functional outcomes

Compared with open retroperitoneal lymph node dissection, laparoscopic approach, done by expert hands, showed improvements in terms of analgesic requirements, complication rate (15.6% Vs 33%), re-do surgery rate (1.4% Vs 6.6%) and hospital stay but laparoscopic approach was associated with longer operating time [34-36].

Complication rates about laparoscopic approach varied between 5.6% and 46.7%. Major intraoperative complications included bleeding and ureteral, duodenal and gallbladder injury. In expert hands the vast of complications could be managed laparoscopically as low conversion rates reported (1-5.4%). About retrograde ejaculation, a late complication, reports showed a 2-3% [34-36].

Retroperitoneal laparoscopic lymph node dissection was described by some authors. Results showed its equivalence compared to conventional transperitoneal laparoscopic approach [37].

5.2. Oncologic outcome

Regarding stage I nonseminomatous germ cell tumor (any stage but not lymph node invasion or metastasis), there were no differences between open and laparoscopic approach in terms of retroperitoneal relapse, distant progression, biochemical failure and in-field relapse. There were three reports of port-site metastasis (0.3%) in the literature. The rate of positive lymph nodes was lower after laparoscopic approach. The need for secondary retroperitoneal surgery did not differ (1.1-1.5%) and both groups showed similar cure rates (99.6%-100%) [34].

5.3. Conclusion

To justify laparoscopic approach instead of open surgery, laparoscopic retroperitoneal lymph node dissection is a safe procedure with low complication rate and with perioperative outcomes comparable with open surgery [35].

The consensus of the authors is that open or laparoscopic retroperitoneal lymph node dissection should be concentrated in dedicated referral centers. Thus laparoscopic lymph node resection might be indicated in: low-risk stages, if primary tumor contains mature teratoma or if the primary nonseminomatous germ cell tumor is marker negative. Laparoscopic retroperitoneal lymph node dissection represents a valuable tool for selected patients with clinical stage I. Further studies should focus on the curative potential of the procedures as well as on the role of post chemotherapy [33,34].

Laparoendoscopic single-site and natural orifice transluminal endoscopic in Urology oncologic surgery. To minimize minimal invasive surgery.

Natural orifice transluminal endoscopic surgery (NOTES) and laparoendoscopic single-site surgery (LESS) have been developed to reduce morbidity and scarring. NOTES uses existing orifices of the human body to perform surgical or diagnostic techniques. The use of accessory transabdominal ports as a part of evolution of NOTES is defined as *hybrid* NOTES. LESS procedure implies only a single-port or a single-incision laparoscopy [38].

LESS surgery was performed in several oncologic procedures, such a radical nephrectomy, radical prostatectomy, nephroureterectomy and radical cystectomy. Cumulative series showing results have been published. LESS has shown to be feasible (in expert hands) offering patient satisfaction and shortened convalescence applied to nephrectomy and radical prostatectomy. Patient selection is the most important to minimizing complication and conversion rates [38].

Comparative series between conventional laparoscopy and LESS have been demonstrated that there were only differences about cosmetic results when LESS was applied to perform radical nephrectomy. Also, there were no differences concerning analgesia and hospital stay. So far, all the comparative series fall to offer large number of cases, and they were retrospective and norandomized [38].

About hybrid NOTES applied to oncologic surgery, the most commonly procedure performed was transvaginal radical nephrectomy. Vaginal access was only used to insert a deflectable camera, whereas two additional abdominal trocars were used as main working ports for instrumentation. Currently, there are few papers with short number of cases and it requires clinical and external validation [38].

LESS has proved to be immediately applicable in the clinical practicum, but requires a skilled laparoscopic surgeon and well-selected patients. The current benefits of LESS are limited to improve cosmetic results [39]. About NOTES, the question is whether women would prefer a transvaginal access; there were studies published that showed a negative / neutral opinion of nulliparous younger women, concerning about the effect of NOTES on sexual function [38,40].

In the future, it is important to perform a standard evaluation of cosmetic results, to design prospective series combining LESS and NOTES as well as improving laparoscopic ergonomics and instrumental [40].

Acknowledgements

To Katherinne Eloise, Katherine Julia, José Jr. and my parents.

Author details

March Villalba José Antonio

European Board of Urology , Hospital Clínico Universitario de Valencia, Spain

References

[1] European Association of Urology guidelines 2012ed. http://www.uroweb.org/guidelines/online-guidelines/.

[2] Bishoff, J. T. Kavoussi. Atlas of laparoscopic Urologic Surgery. Prologue. Bishoff JT, Kavoussi:Elsevier Masson;(2008). Barcelona.Spain.13.

[3] Maclennan, S, Imamura, M, Lapitan, M. C, Omar, M. I, Lam, T. B, Hilvano-cabungcal, A. M, et al. UCAN Systematic Review Reference Group. Systematic Review of Perioperative and Quality-of-life Outcomes Following Surgical Management of Localised Renal Cancer. Eur Urol. (2012). Jul 20. [Epub ahead of print]

[4] Maclennan, S, Imamura, M, Lapitan, M. C, Omar, M. I, Lam, T. B, Hilvano-cabungcal, A. M, et al. UCAN Systematic Review Reference Group. Systematic review of oncological outcomes following surgical management of localized renal cancer. Eur Urol. (2012)., 61, 972-993.

[5] Weight, C. J, Larson, B. T, Fergany, A. F, et al. Nephrectomy induced chronic renal insufficiency is associated with increased risk of cardiovascular death and death from any cause in patients with localized cT1b renal masses. J Urol (2010)., 183, 1317-23.

[6] Porpiglia, F, Fiori, C, Bertolo, R, Morra, I, Russo, R, Piccoli, G, et al. Long-term functional evaluation of the treated kidney in a prospective series of patients who underwent laparoscopic partial nephrectomy for small renal tumors. Eur Urol. (2012). Jul;, 62(1), 130-5.

[7] Gill, I. S, Matin, S. F, Desai, M. M, et al. Comparative analysis of laparoscopic versus open partial nephrectomy for renal tumors in 200 patients. J Urol. (2003)., 170, 64-8.

[8] Desai, M. M, Strzempkowski, B, Matin, S. F, Steinberg, A. P, Ng, C, Meraney, A. M, Kaouk, J. H, & Gill, I. S. Prospective randomized comparison of transperitoneal versus retroperitoneal laparoscopic radical nephrectomy. J Urol. (2005). Jan;, 173(1), 38-41.

[9] Lane, B. R, & Gill, I. S. year oncological outcomes after laparoscopic and open partial nephrectomy. J Urol. (2010). Feb;, 183(2), 473-9.

[10] Gill, I. S, Kavoussi, L. R, Lane, B. R, Blute, M. L, Babineau, D, Colombo, J. R, et al. Comparison of 1,800 laparoscopic and open partial nephrectomies for single renal tumors. J Urol. (2007). Jul;, 178(1), 41-6.

[11] Marszalek, M, Meixl, H, Polajnar, M, Rauchenwald, M, Jeschke, K, & Madersbacher, S. Laparoscopic and open partial nephrectomy: a matched-pair comparison of 200 patients. Eur Urol. (2009). May;, 55(5), 1171-8.

[12] Simmons, M. N, Chung, B. I, & Gill, I. S. Perioperative efficacy of laparoscopic partial nephrectomy for tumors larger than 4 cm. Eur Urol. (2009). Jan;, 55(1), 199-207.

[13] Tsivian, M, Ulusoy, S, Abern, M, Wandel, A, Sidi, A. A, & Tsivian, A. Renal Mass Anatomic Characteristics and Perioperative Outcomes of Laparoscopic Partial Nephrectomy: A Critical Analysis. J Endourol. (2012). Jul 30. [Epub ahead of print]

[14] Mattar, K, & Finelli, A. Expanding the indications for laparoscopic radical nephrectomy. Curr Opin Urol. (2007). Mar;, 17(2), 88-92.

[15] Canda, A. E, & Kirkali, Z. Current management of renal cell carcinoma and targeted therapy. Urol J. (2006). Winter;, 3(1), 1-14.

[16] Heidenreich, A, Bastian, P. J, Bellmunt, J, Bolla, M, Joniau, S, Mason, M. D, Matveev, V, et al. Guidelines of prostate cáncer. Avaible at: http://www.uroweb.org/gls/pdf/08%20Prostate%20Cancer_LR%20March%(2013). th%202012.pdf).

[17] Ficarra, V, Novara, G, Artibani, W, Cestari, A, Galfano, A, Graefen, M, et al. Retropubic, laparoscopic, and robot-assisted radical prostatectomy: a systematic review and cumulative analysis of comparative studies..Eur Urol. (2009). May;, 55(5), 1037-63.

[18] Ghavamian, R, Knoll, A, Boczko, J, & Melman, A. Comparison of operative and functional outcomes of laparoscopic radical prostatectomy and radical retropubic prostatectomy: single surgeon experience. Urology. (2006). Jun;, 67(6), 1241-6.

[19] Remzi, M, Klingler, H. C, Tinzl, M. V, Fong, Y. K, Lodde, M, Kiss, B, & Marberger, M. Morbidity of laparoscopic extraperitoneal versus transperitoneal radical prostatectomy verus open retropubic radical prostatectomy. Eur Urol. (2005). Jul;, 48(1), 83-9.

[20] Guazzoni, G, Cestari, A, Naspro, R, Riva, M, Centemero, A, Zanoni, M, et al. Intra- and peri-operative outcomes comparing radical retropubic and laparoscopic radical prostatectomy: results from a prospective, randomised, single-surgeon study. Eur Urol. (2006). Jul;, 50(1), 98-104.

[21] Magheli, A, Gonzalgo, M. L, Su, L. M, Guzzo, T. J, Netto, G, Humphreys, E. B, et al. Impact of surgical technique (open vs laparoscopic vs robotic-assisted) on pathological and biochemical outcomes following radical prostatectomy: an analysis using propensity score matching. BJU Int. (2011). Jun;, 107(12), 1956-62.

[22] Van Velthoven, R. F. Laparoscopic radical prostatectomy: transperitoneal versus retroperitoneal approach: is there an advantage for the patient? Curr Opin Urol. (2005). Mar;, 15(2), 83-8.

[23] Stenzl, A, Witjes, J. A, Compérat, E, Cowan, N. C, De Santis, M, Kuczyk, M, Lebret, T, Ribal, M. J, et al. European urology Guidelines on Bladder Cancer Muscle-invasive and Metastatic. Avaiable in: http://www.uroweb.org/gls/pdf/07_Bladder%20Cancer_LR%20II.pdf

[24] Challacombe, B. J, Bochner, B. H, Dasgupta, P, Gill, I, Guru, K, Herr, H, et al. The role of laparoscopic and robotic cystectomy in the management of muscle-invasive bladder cancer with special emphasis on cancer control and complications. Eur Urol. (2011). Oct;, 60(4), 767-75.

[25] Chade, D. C, Laudone, V. P, Bochner, B. H, & Parra, R. O. Oncological outcomes after radical cystectomy for bladder cancer: open versus minimally invasive approaches. J Urol. (2010). Mar;, 183(3), 862-69.

[26] Nix, J, Smith, A, Kurpad, R, Nielsen, M. E, Wallen, E. M, & Pruthi, R. S. Prospective randomized controlled trial of robotic versus open radical cystectomy for bladder cancer: perioperative and pathologic results. Eur Urol. (2010). Feb;, 57(2), 196-201.

[27] Haber, G. P, Crouzet, S, & Gill, I. S. Laparoscopic and robotic assisted radical cystectomy for bladder cancer: a critical analysis. Eur Urol. (2008). Jul;, 54(1), 54-62.

[28] Hautmann, R. E. The oncologic results of laparoscopic radical cystectomy are not (yet) equivalent to open cystectomy. Curr Opin Urol. (2009). Sep;, 19(5), 522-6.

[29] Tanaka, K, Hara, I, Takenaka, A, Kawabata, G, & Fujisawa, M. Incidence of local and port site recurrence of urologic cancer after laparoscopic surgery. Urology. (2008). Apr;, 71(4), 728-34.

[30] Rouprêt, M, Zigeuner, R, Palou, J, Boehle, A, Kaasinen, E, Sylvester, R, et al. European guidelines for the diagnosis and management of upper urinary tract urothelial cell carcinomas: (2011). update. Eur Urol. 2011;, 59, 584-94.

[31] Ristau, B. T, Tomaszewski, J. J, & Ost, M. C. Upper tract urothelial carcinoma. Current treatment and outcomes. Urology (2012). , 4, 749-56.

[32] Albers, P, Albrecht, W, Algaba, F, Bokemeyer, C, Cohn-cedermark, G, Fizazi, K, et al. Testicular cancer guidelines. European guidelines (2011). Avaiable at: http://www.uroweb.org/gls/pdf/10_Testicular_Cancer.pdf.

[33] Öztürk, Ç, Van Ginkel, R. J, Krol, R. M, Gietema, J. A, Hofker, H. S, & Hoekstra, H. J. Laparoscopic resection of a residual retroperitoneal tumor mass of nonseminomatos testicular germ cell tumors. Surg Endosc (2012). , 26, 458-67.

[34] Rassweiler, J. J, Scheitlin, W, Heidenreich, A, Laguna, M. P, & Janetschek, G. Laparoscopic retroperitoneal lymph node dissection: does it still have a role in the management of clinical stage I nonseminomatous testis cancer? A European perspective.

[35] Hyams, E. S, Pierorazio, P, Proteek, O, Sroka, M, Kavoussi, L. R, & Allaf, M. E. Laparoscopic retroperitoneal lymph node dissection for clinical stage I nonseminomatous germ cell tumor: a large single institution experience. J Urol (2012). , 487-92.

[36] Steiner, H, Zangerl, F, Stöhr, B, Granig, T, Ho, H, Bartsch, G, et al. Results of bilateral nerve sparing laparoscopic retroperitoneal lymph node dissection for testicular cancer. J Urol (2008). , 1348-53.

[37] Arai, Y, Kaiho, Y, Yamada, S, Saito, H, Mitsuzuka, K, Yamashita, S, et al. Extraperitoneal laparoscopic retroperitoneal lymph node dissection after chemotherapy for nonsemonimatous testicular germ-cell tumor:surgical and oncological outcomes. Int Urol Nephrol (2012).

[38] Autorino, R, Cadeddu, J. A, Desai, M. M, Gettman, M, Gill, I. S, Kavoussi, L. R, et al. Laparoendoscopic single-site and natural orifice transluminal endoscopic surgery in urology: a critical analysis of the literature. Eur Urol (2011). , 59, 26-45.

[39] Oh, T. H. Current status of laparoscopic single-site surgery in urologic surgery. Kor J Urol (2012). , 53, 443-50.

[40] Rassweiler, J. J. Is LESS/NOTES relay more? Eur Urol (2011). , 59, 46-50.

[41] Edge, S. B, Byrd, D. R, Compton, C. C, Fritz, A. G, Greene, F. I, & Trotti, A. Kidney.Cancer staging handbook AJCC. Seventh ed. Chicago IL: Springer; (2010). , 73-86.

[42] Edge, S. B, Byrd, D. R, Compton, C. C, Fritz, A. G, & Greene, F. I. Trotti A Prostate. Cancer staging handbook AJCC. Seventh ed. Chicago IL: Springer; (2010). , 51-64.

[43] Edge, S. B, Byrd, D. R, Compton, C. C, Fritz, A. G, Greene, F. I, & Trotti, A. Urinary Bladder Cancer staging handbook AJCC. Seventh ed. Chicago IL: Springer; (2010). , 95-103.

[44] Edge, S. B, Byrd, D. R, Compton, C. C, Fritz, A. G, Greene, F. I, & Trotti, A. Renal pelvis and Ureter Cancer staging handbook AJCC. Seventh ed. Chicago IL: Springer; (2010). , 87-93.

Chapter 7

Current Strategies in the Management of Adenocarcinoma of the Rectum

Sergio Huerta and Sean P. Dineen

Additional information is available at the end of the chapter

http://dx.doi.org/10.5772/55827

1. Introduction

In 2012, rectal cancer affected 40,290 Americans. Colon and rectal cancer resulted in a mortality of 51,690 individuals during the same year [1]. Patients affected with rectal cancer who have a clinical stage II (T3-T4, NO, MO) or III (Any T, N1-N3, M0) tumor are treated with pre-operative chemoradiation (CRT) followed by surgical intervention 5-10 weeks after the last CRT treatment. An adequate oncologic operation involves removal of the tumor and the entire mesorectum (total mesorectal excision). This has been demonstrated to decrease local recurrence substantially as the lymphatic drainage of the rectum is contained within the investing fascia (mesorectum). Distal rectal tumors involving the anorectal sphincter complex are classically treated with an abdominoperineal resection (APR); whereas, more proximal tumors might be treated with an anterior protosigmoidectomy with a primary colorectal anastomosis (LAR). There has been a substantial shift in the number of APR operations to LAR procedures over the past decade owing to the implementation of new circular stapling devices and the use of neoadjuvant CRT.

2. The rectum

In a Cochrane review of 19 clinical trials assessing preoperative radiotherapy *vs.* surgery alone, the rectum was alternatively defined as below the sacral promontory in three studies, below the pelvic brim in one study, and by the distance from the anal verge in several studies: 12 cm (one study), 13 cm (one study), 14 cm (one study), 15 cm (five studies), and 16 cm (one study) [2]. The hazard ratio for recurrence in patients receiving radiotherapy was less if tumors were located within five to 10 cm from the anal verge, but there was no difference in local recurrence in patients treated with combination radiotherapy and surgery *vs.* surgery alone in patients that had tumors 10.1 cm from the anal verge [3]. Thus, the benefit of radiotherapy appears to be for more distal tumors (0-10 cm from the anal verge). For the purpose of selecting patient to receive pre-operative CRT, practice guide lines in the United States by the National Cancer Institute (NCI) [4]and the National Comprehensive Cancer Network (NCCN) [5] have defined the rectum to be 12 cm from the anal verge.

3. Indications for neoadjuvant chemoradiation

The addition of preoperative radiation therapy to TME decreases locoregional recurrence from approximately 8% to 2%. The combination of chemotherapy and radiation (CRT) further decreases local recurrence. Chemotherapy also increases the number of patients which achieve a pathologic complete response (pCR), i.e. no detectable tumor after resection. This modality also reduces tumor burden in some patients and might allow a sphincter preserving operation (i.e. LAR) as opposed to an APR, allowing a patient to avoid a permanent colostomy. The rate of pCR is approximately 25% [6;7]. Patients who achieve pCR have better long-term outcomes compared to patients who only have a partial response or no response at all [8]. Current guide lines in the United States [4;5] dictate that patients with stage II (T3-T4) or stage III (any T with positive regional lymph nodes) should be treated with neoadjuvant CRT. Patients with stage I (T1-T2) disease or those with distant metastases (stage IV) generally do not receive neoadjuvant CRT. However, in instances of synchronous liver metastases for which liver resection is planned, neoadjuvant radiation may be considered. These recommendations emanate from the low rate of recurrence (4%) in patients with stage I tumors treated with surgery alone [9]. Further, there is no difference in the rate of locoregional recurrence in patients with stage IV tumors treated with radiotherapy and surgery compared to palliative surgery alone [3]. Similarly, there is no difference in outcomes in patients with distant metastases treated with neoadjuvant radiotherapy and surgery *vs.* palliative surgery alone [3]. Thus, the standard care of practice is to provide neoadjuvant CRT in patients with stage II and III rectal tumors.

4. Clinical staging of rectal cancer

Staging of rectal cancer begins with a thorough history and physical examination. The most common symptom of rectal cancer is bright red blood per rectum. Physical examination of the abdomen is important to identify any evidence of liver disease (ascites) or masses. A lymph node examination is important in any patient suspected of having cancer. Rectal examination will reveal distal tumors and is mandatory in the evaluation of patients with colorectal cancers. In such cases information regarding the size, degree of fixation, distance from the anal sphincters is important. In women, a rectovaginal examination may reveal extent of disease. A full colonoscopy is indicated to identify synchronous lesions (present in approximately 5% of cases). Rigid proctoscopy will define the distance of the lesion from the anus and can be critical in cases where the distance from the anus is not clear.

Because only stage II and III tumors are treated with pre-operative CRT, clinical staging is pivotal in guiding treatment options. There are currently two modalities to assess tumor stage (T stage) in the pre-operative setting: (1) endorectal ultrasound (EUS) and (2) Magnetic Resonance Imaging (MRI). The efficacy of these modalities has been assessed by two meta-analyses [10;11]. One study favors EUS [10] and the other MRI [11]. In the first analysis, 90 studies were included and assessed the accuracy of EUS, MRI, and CT in pre-operatively staging rectal cancer. The results demonstrated that EUS and MRI were similar in terms of sensitivity (Sn) with regards to tumor depth into the muscularis propia (94%). EUS was superior in determining muscularis propia invasion [specificity (Sp) of 86%] compared to MRI (Sp = 69%) and was an overall sensitive strategy (Sn = 90%) for perirectal tumor invasion compared to MRI (Sn = 82%) [10]. A second meta-analysis interrogated 84 studies. This study showed no difference in these modalities in evaluating the nodes (N-staging) [11]. In seven studies, MRI was a superior strategy in evaluating involved circumferential margins [11]. MRI seems to be emerging as a preferred modality for the assessment of rectal cancer staging in the pre-operative setting. However, the use of either of these modalities is largely based on institutional experience. The sensitivity of EUS following CRT is less compared to virgin tissue. Thus, MRI may be a preferred modality to determine response to neoadjuvant CRT.

5. Neoadjuvant chemoradiotherapy

The management of stage II and stage III rectal cancer is a tri-modality approach (Radiotherapy, Chemotherapy and Surgery) and patients are best managed following discussion at a multidisciplinary conference.

5.1. Radiotherapy

Initial studies evaluated the efficacy of radiotherapy without pre-operative chemotherapy. The data has been summarized in two meta-analyses addressing the benefit of preoperative radiation [12;13]. While the data on overall survival was not clear in these analyses, there was a clear decrease in the rate of local recurrence (46% in patients receiving preoperative radiation vs. 53% in the control group). These data established the benefits of preoperative radiotherapy followed by surgery.

5.1.1. Short course vs. long course radiotherapy

In Europe, small fractions of ionizing radiation 5.0 Grey (Gy) X 5.0 (over five days), for a total of 25.0 Gy without chemotherapy, are employed. With this strategy, the Swedish Rectal Cancer Trial found an improved rate of survival at five years with preoperative radiation [14]. In the United States, the typical IR dose is 45.0 to 50.4 Gy given in small doses (1.8 Gy/day) for five to six weeks [5]. In contrast to short course radiotherapy, in the United States, long course radiotherapy is given in combination with neoadjuvant chemotherapy. The interval between completion of radiation and subsequent operation is an area of some debate (see below) but is typically 5-10 weeks.

5.2. Neoadjuvant chemotherapy

Preoperative chemotherapy is generally used as a radiosensitizer. The EORTC group demonstrated that the addition of chemotherapy (5-FU) to the use of preoperative radiation reduced the risk of local recurrence by approximately 50%, from 17.1% to 8.7%. There was not a significant difference in overall survival in this study. Other trials have shown similar improvements in local control. Based on this data, the most established agent used in the preoperative setting in combination with radiation has been 5-fluorouracil (5-FU). The oral form of 5-FU (Capecitabine) is also being widely used in place of 5-FU with similar results [15]. Several chemotherapeutic agents used for the management of colon cancer in the adjuvant setting and for patients with metastases have been evaluated as possible radiosensitizers. These agents include: irinotecan [16], oxaliplatin [17], bevacizumab [18] and cetuximab [18]. With such strategies, there is still a wide response to ionizing radiation and these agents are not in widespread use at this time.

5.3. Pathologic complete response

A pathologic complete response (pCR) occurs in patients who undergo resection of the rectum and no residual tumor is identified. Patients who have a pCR demonstrate superior survival than those without. The EORTC 22921 showed an increased rate of pCR in patients who underwent chemoradiotherapy (13.7%) compared to patients who received radiation therapy alone (5.3%). A European trial inclusive of 762 patients receiving preoperative chemoradiation compared to radiation alone, the pCR rate was 11.4% *vs.* 3.6%, respectively [19]. A recent randomized phase II trial assessing combined chemoradiation for rectal cancer showed 28% of patients achieved a pCR. Further, 78% of patients exhibited tumor down staging [20]. Thus, chemotherapy has an additive effect to radiotherapy and has become the standard of care for patient with stage II/III tumors within 12 cm of the anal verge [5].

In the United States current guidelines recommend pre-operative radiation [50.4 Gy] in 25-28 fractions combination with 5-FU infusional or bolus with leucovorin [425 $mg/m^2/d$] or capecitibine [825 mg/m^2]. Neoadjuvant treatment is followed by surgery five to ten weeks later. While some investigators have shown that longer periods between neoadjuvant CRT and surgery might be associated with an increase rate of pCR [21], this approach is still under investigation [22].

6. Surgery

For stage II and III patients treated with CRT, surgical intervention must be planned within five to ten weeks after the last dose of chemoradiation. Although a longer window between neoadjuvant chemoradiation and operative intervention has been associated with higher rates of pCR, this must be assessed in case-to-case basis [21;22].

Transabdominal operations (LAR or APR) are the operations of choice for stage II and stage III rectal cancers. For small tumors with a good histology and for a patient with a prohibitive risk of surgical intervention, a transanal approach might be an alternative approach.

6.1. Transabdominal operations

Two operations are typically performed for rectal cancer. The abdominoperineal resection involves the removal of the distal rectum and perineum with clear tumor radial margins laterally to the pelvic sidewalls. Thus, part of this operation is the creation of a permanent colostomy. A low anterior resection involves the removal of the tumor and the creation of an anastomosis. This might require a temporary loop ileostomy especially in patients that have received neoadjuvant chemoradiation.

6.1.1. Abdominioperineal Resection (APR)

An abdominoperineal resection (Figure 1) necessitates a permanent colostomy, which frequently carries negative perception as a drastic change in quality of life for patients. Although a permanent stoma does necessitate some changes for patients, data is emerging that quality of life following an APR is not significantly less than that following an LAR [23]. This is related to the relatively high rate of complications following LAR, including sexual dysfunction, pain and fecal incontinence. However, an APR is associated with a high rate of perineal wound infections [24]. Furthermore, obtaining clear radial margins is more difficult with an APR compared to an LAR [23;25]. As a result, there is an oncologic advantage in peforming an LAR compared to an APR [25]. Thus, in patients with preserved rectal tone, the operation of choice, is an LAR provided tumor associated factors make this possible.

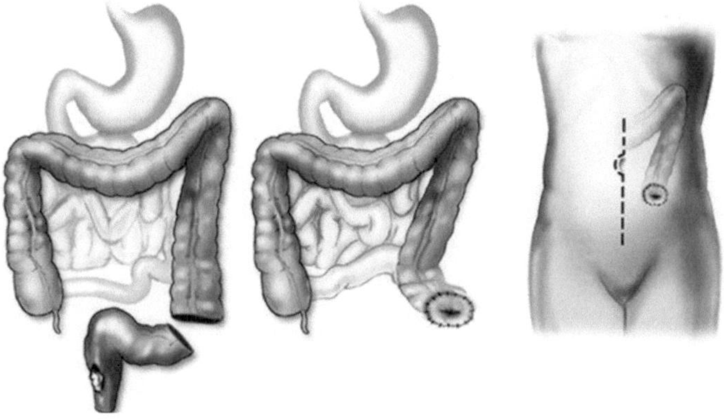

Figure 1. Abdominoperineal Resection (APR). The rectal tumor is removed, a permanent colostomy is created and the anus is obliterated.

6.1.2. Low Anterior Resection (LAR): Total Mesorectal Excision (TME)

An LAR (Figure 2) involves the creation of a primary anastomosis. The area confined within the investing fascia of the rectum and the presacral fascia involves the vascular and lymphatic

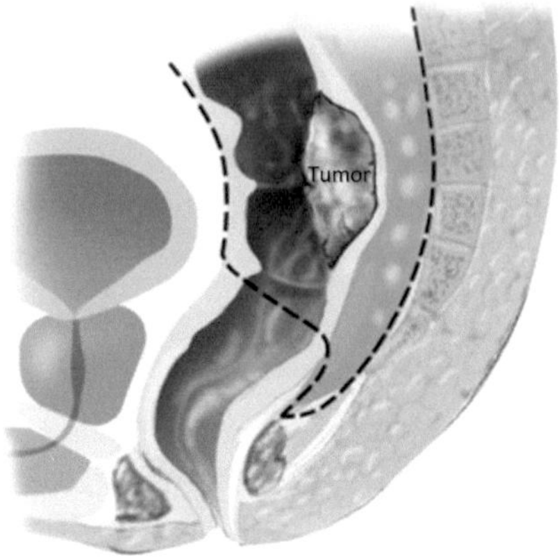

Figure 3. Total Mesorectal Excision (TIME). The dotted line represents the line of resection. The tumor is resected and a primary anastomosis is performed

structures of the mid-rectum. An en bloc resection of the rectum that circumscribes these structures is termed a TME (Figure 3). Superiorly, the mesorectum is defined at the level of the sacral promontory or the division of the right and left superior hemorrhoideal arteries. The mesorectum extends distally and reduces posteriorly at the level of the investing fasica of the levators (Waldeyer's Fascia). Prior to in the introduction of TME the rate of recurrence for rectal cancer was 25.0%. This rate has been reduced to 5.0% following the introduction of the TME [26].

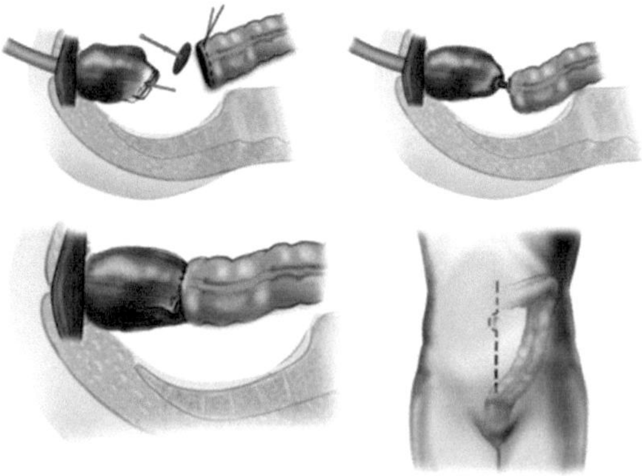

Figure 2. Low Anterior Resection (LAR). The rectum involving the tumor is resected and a primary anastomosis is created with a circular stapling device.

6.1.3. Proximal margin of resection and level of arterial ligation

No studies have interrogated the length required for proximal resection. Because of the continuity with the colon this is not such a concern. NCI guidelines recommend a 5-cm segment

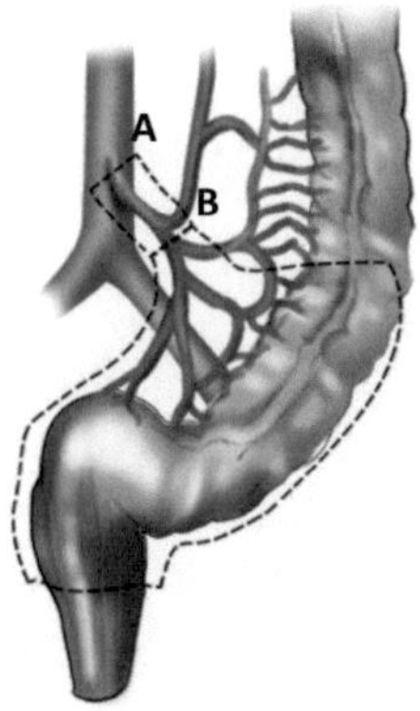

Figure 4. High ligation occurs at the root of the IMA (A). Low ligation occurs at the level of the superior rectal artery (B).

of resection proximal to the tumor [4]. While the inferior mesenteric artery (high ligation) was typically the level of arterial ligation recommended, this practice was associated with a decrease in innervation and perfusion to the anastomosis. The evidence demonstrating that this has a superior oncologic compared to ligation at the level of the superior rectal artery (low ligation) is lacking. Thus, low ligation has become the preferred strategy [27] (Figure 4).

6.2. Laparoscopic surgery for the management of adenocarcinoma of the rectum

Minimally invasive surgery has made laparoscopic resection of rectal cancer possible. However, at this juncture, this procedure remains investigational for the management of rectal cancer [5]. It is currently, recommended to include patients in study protocol to continue to address the benefits of the laparoscopic approach in rectal cancer including: oncologic efficacy, complication rates, conversion rates, patient benefit, and cost-effectiveness.

Short term outcomes have not been different in patients treated with the laparoscopic approach compared to the open techniques [28]. Multiple case series reporting laparoscopic TME have documented technical feasibility with satisfactory short term outcomes [29]. While case reports have also reported the ability of a robotic proctectomy [30], these studies need to be replicated in large series compared to the "gold-standard" to determine the general applicability of innovative approaches.

In contrast to colon cancer, where laparoscopy has been compared to the open approach [31-33], for rectal cancer these studies are currently needed. The Conventional Versus Laparoscopic-Assisted Surgery in Colorectal Cancer (CLASICC) trial specifically addressed rectal cancer [32]. In this study, the rate of complications was similar. However, the rate of positive CRM was twice in the laparoscopic approach compared to the open technique (12% *vs.* 6%; p=0.19). While this was only a trend and not correlated with an increase in the rate of recurrence, these findings need to be further investigated. Additionally, there was also a trend towards an increase in complications related to male sexual dysfunction (41% vs. 23%).

A randomized controlled trial [34] and institutional case series [35;36] indicate that the laparoscopic and the open TME have similar oncologic outcomes. More data on the long term outcomes of the laparoscopic approach will be shed with further analysis of the Colon Cancer Laparoscopic or Open Resection (COLOR) II [37] and the and the American College of Surgeons Oncology Group trial Z6051 is completed.

Thus, the current data suggest that the short-term outcomes of laparoscopic and open surgery are similar. It is crucial to analyze the current data of the available studies carefully as patient selection and the experience of the institution/surgeon are paramount in the current available literature. Long term data regarding oncologic outcome and functional status remain at large, as do data demonstrating patient benefit and cost effectiveness [38].

6.3. Transanal excision

An alternative treatment for early stage rectal cancers is a transanal excision. Candidates for this approach have small (≤ 3-cm) stage I (T1) tumors located within 8-cm from the anal verge that occupy less than 30% of the circumference of the bowel with good histological features is a transanal removal of the tumor with clear margins. There is a substantial risk for local recurrence with this approach. Local rates of recurrence with the transanal approach *vs.* similarly staged tumors treated with a transabdominal approach is 13.2% *vs.* 2.7%; respectively [39]. Twenty percent of patients with T1 tumors who undergo radical resection are discovered to have lymph node metastases [39]. Patients with rectal cancer treated exclusively by local resection show a rate of local recurrence of 9.7% for T1, 25% for T2, and 38% for T3 cancers [40]. In patients that received systemic chemotherapy after the transanal excision, the local recurrence rate was substantially decreased to: 9.5% for T1, 13.6% for T2, and 13.8% for T3 cancers [40]. This approach is, perhaps, of most benefit in patients with a high operative risk.

7. Adjuvant chemotherapy

Patients with stage II/III rectal cancer should be treated with adjuvant chemotherapy as soon as they are able. Current regimens for this approach extrapolate the experience with colon cancer such that FOLFOX (5-FU/leucovorin, and oxaliplatin) for six months is recommended. 5-FU with or without leucovorin as well as capacitibine with or without oxaliplatin are also alternative options for treatment in the adjuvant setting [5].

8. Pathological analysis of rectal cancer

8.1. Staging

In rectal cancer staging, the prefix "p" refers to pathological staging and "yp" indicates pathological staging after neoadjuvant chemoradiation.

The number of recommended nodes to be retrieved to accurately stage tumors is 12 according to the NCCN guidelines [5]. In patients treated with neoadjuvant therapy, the number of nodes resected during surgery is 3-6 less compared to patients treated with surgery alone [41-43]. Thus, care must be taken by the surgeon to remove all involved nodes and by pathology for a careful analysis of the specimen.

8.2. Pathological Inspection of the tumor

8.2.1. Circumferential Resection Margin (CRM)

The circumferential margin (CRM) is important during pathological assessment of tumors in rectal cancer [44]. The CRM refers to assessment of the non-peritonealized area (bare area) of the rectum created by subperitoneal dissection during surgery. Tumors within 1 mm of the resection margin are defined as having a positive CRM. Additionally discontinuous spread or lymph node involvement within 1mm of the CRM is defined as positive. CRM is a predictor of local recurrence in patients receiving surgery as the only modality of treatment of rectal cancer [25;45]. Patients whose CRM is less that 2 mm have a recurrence rate of 16% compared to 5.8% for patients having a CMR over 2mm. The rate of metastases is also higher in patients with less than 2mm margins vs. greater that 2mm (37.6 vs. 12.7%; respectively) [26]. This observation underscores the importance or radial margins in rectal surgery. Other studies have shown that the CRM is an important predictor of local recurrence, distant metastasis, and overall survival in patients receiving induction CRT compared to patients treated with surgery alone [25]. Thus, pathological evaluation of the resected rectal tumor must include the distance to the tumor to the closest CRM.

8.2.2. Determining response to induction chemotherapy

Pathological tumor response following neoadjuvant therapy is graded from 0 to 3. A grade of 0 indicates complete response without any viable cells; while 3 denotes minimal or no response to treatment. It is important for the pathologist and the surgeon to note the response of CRT after surgery to determine if the current regimens are adequate for the patient population and also to determine the possible aggressiveness of the tumor and plan for adjuvant therapies.

9. Clinical Complete Response (cCR)

Studies continue to accumulate that document the possibility of observing patients who achieve a clinical complete response following neoadjuvant chemoradiation [46;47]. The first study was reported by Habr-Gama's group in 2004 [46]. In this study, 8% of patients considered to have recurrence had a complete pathological response following surgery. Patients with rectal tumors within 0-7 cm from the anal verge received pre-operative radiotherapy (50.4 Gy) and chemotherapy [5-FU (425 mg/m2/d) + folinic acid (20 mg/m^2/d)]. Re-staging was performed 8 weeks after treatment and included proctoscopy with rectal biopsies. Complete clinical response was defined by the absence of any abnormalities during proctoscopy. A rectal scar or a positive biopsy was defined as an incomplete response. These patients did not receive postoperative chemotherapy unless they had recurrent disease. These findings were then reproduced by Maas et al [47].

Maas et al compared patients that achieved a cCR to patients who had a pathological complete response after surgery. Twenty-one subjects were included in the study arm and 20 in the control group. The major differences in these studies include the follow up in Maas vs. Habr-Gama's studies (24.8 *vs.* 57.3 months; respectively). While radiotherapy was similar, Maas used capecitabine rather than 5-FU. Additionally, the definition of cCR was different in these two studies. Habr-Gama used proctoscopy and rectal biopsies while Maas relied on magnetic resonance imaging (MRI), endorectal ultrasound, and biopsies. Finally, all pre-operatively staged III patients received adjuvant chemotherapy consisting of oxaliplatin and capecitabine in Maas study and none in Habr-Gama's.

While there are some differences between the studies by Habr-Gama and Maas, they provide an excellent platform to build on further prospective cohort studies. Further, two other smaller studies have replicated these observations [48;49].

10. Complications

Complications from rectal surgery are typically associated with bladder and sexual dysfunction. A TME has been associated with bladder dysfunction (17.8%), loss of erection (27.7%), and lack of ejaculation (33.9%) [50]. Up to 30% of patients with attempted curative surgical intervention will eventually develop regional (pelvic) recurrence [9]. Treatment failure is largely dependent on the cohort of patients studied and combined to patients who develop metastasis, the rate is substantially high.

11. Conclusions

The management of rectal cancer is in dynamic evolution. Drastic improvements have occurred over the past 20 years. However, the 5-year survival for these patients remains unacceptably high. The tri-modality approach has demonstrated clear advantages. In a small segment of patients (~25%) the tri-modality approach might be reduced to a bimodality treatment avoiding surgery in patients that achieve a clinical complete response. However, this strategy should be undertaken only in the setting of an Institutional Board Review protocol. Efforts to improve local control and survival in rectal cancer are continuing in multiple clinical and preclinical studies. An understanding of specific molecular pathways leading to a response in neoadjuvant modalities will refine the segment of patients who might need an operation sooner compared to patients who might be observed. Ongoing trials on the laparoscopic approach for rectal cancer will shed light into the benefits of this practice.

Author details

Sergio Huerta and Sean P. Dineen

University of Texas Southwestern Medical Center and North Texas VA Health Care System, USA

References

[1] Siegel, R, Naishadham, D, & Jemal, A. Cancer statistics, (2012). CA Cancer J Clin 2012; , 62(1), 10-29.

[2] Wong, R. K, & Tandan, V. De SS, Figueredo A. Pre-operative radiotherapy and curative surgery for the management of localized rectal carcinoma. Cochrane Database Syst Rev (2007). CD002102.

[3] Kapiteijn, E, Marijnen, C. A, Nagtegaal, I. D, Putter, H, Steup, W. H, Wiggers, T, et al. Preoperative radiotherapy combined with total mesorectal excision for resectable rectal cancer. N Engl J Med (2001). , 345(9), 638-646.

[4] Nelson, H, Petrelli, N, Carlin, A, Couture, J, Fleshman, J, Guillem, J, et al. Guidelines 2000 for colon and rectal cancer surgery. J Natl Cancer Inst (2001). , 93(8), 583-596.

[5] Engstrom, P. F, Arnoletti, J. P, & Benson, A. B. III, Chen YJ, Choti MA, Cooper HS et al. NCCN Clinical Practice Guidelines in Oncology: rectal cancer. J Natl Compr Canc Netw (2009). , 7(8), 838-881.

[6] Huerta, S. Rectal cancer and importance of chemoradiation in the treatment. Adv Exp Med Biol (2010). , 685, 124-133.

[7] Huerta, S, Hrom, J, Gao, X, Saha, D, Anthony, T, Reinhart, H, et al. Tissue microarray constructs to predict a response to chemoradiation in rectal cancer. Dig Liver Dis (2010). , 42(10), 679-684.

[8] Maas, M, Nelemans, P. J, Valentini, V, Das, P, Rodel, C, Kuo, L. J, et al. Long-term outcome in patients with a pathological complete response after chemoradiation for rectal cancer: a pooled analysis of individual patient data. Lancet Oncol (2010). , 11(9), 835-844.

[9] Rodel, C, & Sauer, R. Radiotherapy and concurrent radiochemotherapy for rectal cancer. Surg Oncol (2004).

[10] Bipat, S, Glas, A. S, Slors, F. J, Zwinderman, A. H, Bossuyt, P. M, & Stoker, J. Rectal cancer: local staging and assessment of lymph node involvement with endoluminal US, CT, and MR imaging--a meta-analysis. Radiology (2004). , 232(3), 773-783.

[11] Lahaye, M. J, Engelen, S. M, Nelemans, P. J, & Beets, G. L. van de Velde CJ, van Engelshoven JM et al. Imaging for predicting the risk factors--the circumferential resec-

tion margin and nodal disease--of local recurrence in rectal cancer: a meta-analysis. Semin Ultrasound CT MR (2005). , 26(4), 259-268.

[12] Adjuvant radiotherapy for rectal cancer: a systematic overview of 8patients from 22 randomised trials. Lancet (2001). , 358(9290), 1291-1304.

[13] Camma, C, Giunta, M, Fiorica, F, Pagliaro, L, Craxi, A, & Cottone, M. Preoperative radiotherapy for resectable rectal cancer: A meta-analysis. JAMA (2000). , 284(8), 1008-1015.

[14] Improved survival with preoperative radiotherapy in resectable rectal cancerSwedish Rectal Cancer Trial. N Engl J Med (1997). , 336(14), 980-987.

[15] Patel, P. A. Evolution of 5-fluorouracil-based chemoradiation in the management of rectal cancer. Anticancer Drugs (2011). , 22(4), 311-316.

[16] Illum, H. Irinotecan and radiosensitization in rectal cancer. Anticancer Drugs (2011). , 22(4), 324-329.

[17] Huerta, S, & Hrom, J. Oxaliplatin as a radiosensitizing agent in rectal cancer. Anticancer Drugs (2011). , 22(4), 317-323.

[18] Glynne-jones, R, Mawdsley, S, & Harrison, M. Antiepidermal growth factor receptor radiosensitizers in rectal cancer. Anticancer Drugs (2011). , 22(4), 330-340.

[19] Bosset, J. F, Collette, L, Calais, G, Mineur, L, Maingon, P, Radosevic-jelic, L, et al. Chemotherapy with preoperative radiotherapy in rectal cancer. N Engl J Med (2006). , 355(11), 1114-1123.

[20] Mohiuddin, M, Winter, K, Mitchell, E, Hanna, N, Yuen, A, Nichols, C, et al. Randomized phase II study of neoadjuvant combined-modality chemoradiation for distal rectal cancer: Radiation Therapy Oncology Group Trial 0012. J Clin Oncol (2006). , 24(4), 650-655.

[21] De Campos-lobato, L. F, & Geisler, D. P. da Luz MA, Stocchi L, Dietz D, Kalady MF. Neoadjuvant therapy for rectal cancer: the impact of longer interval between chemoradiation and surgery. J Gastrointest Surg (2011). , 15(3), 444-450.

[22] Huerta, S. Interval between neoadjuvant chemoradiation and surgery for the management of rectal cancer. J Gastrointest Surg (2011).

[23] How, P, Stelzner, S, Branagan, G, Bundy, K, Chandrakumaran, K, Heald, R. J, et al. Comparative quality of life in patients following abdominoperineal excision and low anterior resection for low rectal cancer. Dis Colon Rectum (2012). , 55(4), 400-406.

[24] MacFarlane JKRyall RD, Heald RJ. Mesorectal excision for rectal cancer. Lancet (1993). , 341(8843), 457-460.

[25] Nagtegaal, I. D, & Quirke, P. What is the role for the circumferential margin in the modern treatment of rectal cancer? J Clin Oncol (2008). , 26(2), 303-312.

[26] Machiels, J. P, Sempoux, C, Scalliet, P, Coche, J. C, Humblet, Y, et al. Phase I/II study of preoperative cetuximab, capecitabine, and external beam radiotherapy in patients with rectal cancer. Ann Oncol (2007). , 18(4), 738-744.

[27] Lange, M. M, & Buunen, M. van de Velde CJ, Lange JF. Level of arterial ligation in rectal cancer surgery: low tie preferred over high tie. A review. Dis Colon Rectum (2008). , 51(7), 1139-1145.

[28] Tjandra, J. J, Chan, M. K, & Yeh, C. H. Laparoscopic- vs. hand-assisted ultralow anterior resection: a prospective study. Dis Colon Rectum (2008). , 51(1), 26-31.

[29] Ng, K. H, Ng, D. C, Cheung, H. Y, Wong, J. C, Yau, K. K, Chung, C. C, et al. Laparoscopic resection for rectal cancers: lessons learned from 579 cases. Ann Surg (2009). , 249(1), 82-86.

[30] Luca, F, Cenciarelli, S, Valvo, M, Pozzi, S, Faso, F. L, Ravizza, D, et al. Full robotic left colon and rectal cancer resection: technique and early outcome. Ann Surg Oncol (2009). , 16(5), 1274-1278.

[31] A comparison of laparoscopically assisted and open colectomy for colon cancer. N Engl J Med 2004; 350(20):2050-2059.

[32] Guillou, P. J, Quirke, P, Thorpe, H, Walker, J, Jayne, D. G, Smith, A. M, et al. Short-term endpoints of conventional versus laparoscopic-assisted surgery in patients with colorectal cancer (MRC CLASICC trial): multicentre, randomised controlled trial. Lancet (2005). , 365(9472), 1718-1726.

[33] Veldkamp, R, Kuhry, E, Hop, W. C, Jeekel, J, Kazemier, G, Bonjer, H. J, et al. Laparoscopic surgery versus open surgery for colon cancer: short-term outcomes of a randomised trial. Lancet Oncol (2005). , 6(7), 477-484.

[34] Lujan, J, Valero, G, Hernandez, Q, Sanchez, A, Frutos, M. D, & Parrilla, P. Randomized clinical trial comparing laparoscopic and open surgery in patients with rectal cancer. Br J Surg (2009). , 96(9), 982-989.

[35] Laurent, C, Leblanc, F, Wutrich, P, Scheffler, M, & Rullier, E. Laparoscopic versus open surgery for rectal cancer: long-term oncologic results. Ann Surg (2009). , 250(1), 54-61.

[36] Milsom, J. W. de OO, Jr., Trencheva KI, Pandey S, Lee SW, Sonoda T. Long-term outcomes of patients undergoing curative laparoscopic surgery for mid and low rectal cancer. Dis Colon Rectum (2009). , 52(7), 1215-1222.

[37] Buunen, M, Bonjer, H. J, Hop, W. C, Haglind, E, Kurlberg, G, Rosenberg, J, et al. COLOR II. A randomized clinical trial comparing laparoscopic and open surgery for rectal cancer. Dan Med Bull (2009). , 56(2), 89-91.

[38] Wagman, L. D. Laparoscopic and open surgery for colorectal cancer: reaching equipoise? J Clin Oncol (2007). , 25(21), 2996-2998.

[39] Nash, G. M, Weiser, M. R, Guillem, J. G, Temple, L. K, Shia, J, Gonen, M, et al. Long-term survival after transanal excision of T1 rectal cancer. Dis Colon Rectum (2009). , 52(4), 577-582.

[40] Sengupta, S, & Tjandra, J. J. Local excision of rectal cancer: what is the evidence? Dis Colon Rectum (2001). , 44(9), 1345-1361.

[41] Baxter, N. N, Morris, A. M, Rothenberger, D. A, & Tepper, J. E. Impact of preoperative radiation for rectal cancer on subsequent lymph node evaluation: a population-based analysis. Int J Radiat Oncol Biol Phys (2005). , 61(2), 426-431.

[42] Tepper, J. E, Connell, O, Niedzwiecki, M. J, Hollis, D, Compton, D, Benson, C, & Iii, A. B. et al. Impact of number of nodes retrieved on outcome in patients with rectal cancer. J Clin Oncol (2001). , 19(1), 157-163.

[43] Wichmann, M. W, Muller, C, Meyer, G, Strauss, T, Hornung, H. M, Lau-werner, U, et al. Effect of preoperative radiochemotherapy on lymph node retrieval after resection of rectal cancer. Arch Surg (2002). , 137(2), 206-210.

[44] Compton, C. C. Key issues in reporting common cancer specimens: problems in pathologic staging of colon cancer. Arch Pathol Lab Med (2006). , 130(3), 318-324.

[45] Nagtegaal, I. D, Marijnen, C. A, Kranenbarg, E. K, Van D, V, & Van Krieken, J. H. Circumferential margin involvement is still an important predictor of local recurrence in rectal carcinoma: not one millimeter but two millimeters is the limit. Am J Surg Pathol (2002). , 26(3), 350-357.

[46] Habr-gama, A, Perez, R. O, Nadalin, W, Sabbaga, J, & Ribeiro, U. Jr., Silva e Sousa AH Jr et al. Operative versus nonoperative treatment for stage 0 distal rectal cancer following chemoradiation therapy: long-term results. Ann Surg (2004). , 240(4), 711-717.

[47] Maas, M, Beets-tan, R. G, Lambregts, D. M, Lammering, G, Nelemans, P. J, Engelen, S. M, et al. Wait-and-see policy for clinical complete responders after chemoradiation for rectal cancer. J Clin Oncol (2011). , 29(35), 4633-4640.

[48] Dalton, R. S, Velineni, R, Osborne, M. E, Thomas, R, Harries, S, Gee, A. S, et al. A single-centre experience of chemoradiotherapy for rectal cancer: is there potential for nonoperative management? Colorectal Dis (2012). , 14(5), 567-571.

[49] Smith, J. D, Ruby, J. A, Goodman, K. A, Saltz, L. B, Guillem, J. G, Weiser, M. R, et al. Nonoperative management of rectal cancer with complete clinical response after neoadjuvant therapy. Ann Surg (2012). , 256(6), 965-972.

[50] Morino, M, Parini, U, Allaix, M. E, Monasterolo, G, Brachet, C. R, & Garrone, C. Male sexual and urinary function after laparoscopic total mesorectal excision. Surg Endosc (2009). , 23(6), 1233-1240.

Chapter 8

Mesothelioma: An Evidence-Based Review

Julie Goudreault and Anne Dagnault

Additional information is available at the end of the chapter

http://dx.doi.org/10.5772/55292

1. Introduction

The initial discovery of mesothelioma can be traced back to 1767 when Dr. Joseph Lieutaud, an anatomy pathologist in France, first identified a tumour in the chest wall of a young boy [1]. Mesothelioma is a rare, aggressive form of cancer that develops from transformed cells originating in the mesothelium, which is the protective lining covering many of the body's internal organs. Mesothelioma arises in the pleura but also occurs in the peritoneum, the tunica vaginalis, and the pericardium [2]. Mesothelioma tends to have a local progression. While disseminated disease has sometimes been reported in a very late stage of the disease [3– 7], patients usually die from local progression.

2. Incidence

In Canada, there are 459 new reported cases of mesothelioma per year [8], compared to 3,000 in the United States of America. According to Connelly RR et al, the incidence of mesothelioma in the United States is 10 cases per million people per year [9]. Men are more commonly affected than women, with a male predominance of 90%. While there is a correlation between increasing age and reported cases, there is no peak and the mean age at diagnosis is 60 years.

The number of cases recorded in the Quebec Tumour Database from 1982 to 2002 (for the province of Quebec, Canada; see table 1) reveals that the incidence of pleural and peritoneal mesothelioma was higher for men than women. The overall annual rate of increase from 1982 to 2002 in Quebec was estimated to be 3.6%, which was lower than that measured from 1982 to 1996. In comparison to the international level, only Australia and Scotland showed significant increases in mesothelioma among women [10].

Type of Mesothelioma:	Pleural		Peritoneal	
Gender:	Men	Women	Men	Women
Reported Cases:	1,210	320	98	72
Rate per 100,000 people per year:	1.98	0.41	0.15	0.09

Table 1. Incidence of Pleural and Peritoneal Mesothelioma

3. Epidemiology

3.1. Asbestos

The primary risk factor for mesothelioma is asbestos exposure. Asbestos is a generic terms for a group of six naturally occurring silicate minerals classified as either serpentine or amphibole. The amphibole (rod-like) group contains five types: amosite, crocidolite, anthophyllite, tremolite, and actinolite. Serpentine (chrysotile) asbestos has a sheet or layered structure and differs from the amphibole varieties both structurally and chemically. Chrysotile, the only asbestos mineral in the serpentine group, is the main form of asbestos still mined. It is generally accepted that chrysotile asbestos is less dangerous and does less damage to the lungs than the amphiboles. Although 70% to 80% of pleural mesothelioma cases are associated with asbestos exposure, the lifetime risk of developing pleural mesothelioma among asbestos workers is thought to be 10% [11]. Furthermore, despite the lack of evidence between the relationship of asbestos exposure and peritoneal mesothelioma, one study indicates that this correlation is less significant than that between asbestos exposure and pleural mesothelioma [12].

Asbestos is still used industrially for its fire-resistance and sound-absorption properties. The association between asbestos and mesothelioma was first documented in South African miners [13]. Moreover, the Occupational Safety and Health Administration (OSHA) established that 0.2 fibres per cubic millilitre of air is the standard acceptable exposure rate for fibres longer than 5 μm [14].

Construction, boiler, and shipyard workers are at increased risk. Other sources of exposure may include a spouse or close relatives of asbestos workers. Patients from certain regions of the world (i.e. Greece, Central Turkey, California, and Bulgaria) also have endogenous environmental asbestos exposure as their soil contains high level of tremolite asbestos fibres [15–19]. Furthermore, greater environmental exposure increases incidence of mesothelioma and is also proportionate to the latency period [20–21].

In the majority of patients, the disease develops after a latency period of up to 40 years after initial exposure [22]. Fortunately, today's strict industry standards have significantly reduced asbestos exposure by 100 to 1,000 times compared to the past [23]. For example, Great Britain recorded fewer annual deaths related to mesothelioma in 1968 [153] than in 2001 [1,84,8], largely due to the latency period. The peak in mesothelioma deaths is expected to occur in 2015

(2,450 deaths) [24]. Nevertheless, the rate of deaths in Great Britain associated with mesothelioma is expected to drop significantly after 2015, most likely because of reduced asbestos exposure and stricter industry standards.

Although it was once thought that smoking could lead to mesothelioma, we now know that is not the case. It does, however, increase the risk associated with asbestos exposure [25].

3.2. Carbon nanotubes

Carbon nanotubes are stronger than steel yet lighter than aluminum. As a result, they can be found in a wide range of items such as high-performance bicycle frames, textiles (i.e. waterproofing fabrics), body armour, and concrete. Nevertheless, animal studies have demonstrated that carbon nanotubes can produce mesothelioma-like changes and may therefore cause mesothelioma [26,27]. Furthermore, it has been suggested that the mechanism involved may be either attributed to "changes in gene expression, epigenetic changes, and receptor-mediated or other intracellular signalling cascades" [28].

3.3. Radiation therapy

Ionizing radiation to supradiaphragmatic fields appears to be a risk factor for developing mesothelioma. Data from patients treated with radiation therapy for Hodgkin's lymphoma [29], non-Hodgkin's lymphoma [30], and testicular cancer [31] revealed an excess rate of mesothelioma. Although the reported number of mesotheliomas was small, the risks were statistically significant. This might be the result of broader radiation therapy for Hodgkin's and non-Hodgkin's lymphoma, since mantle-field radiation had once been the standard method of treatment. Afterwards, extended-field radiation therapy became the standard of care. Since today's preferred method of radiation therapy for lymphomas is involved-field radiation, the incidence of mesotheliomas in patients with Hodgkin's or non-Hodgkin's lymphomas should drop because the smaller radiation-therapy fields should result in fewer secondary neoplasms. Moreover, since mediastinal radiation therapy is no longer given for testicular seminomatous germ-cell tumours, such patients should evidence a decrease in radiation-induced mesothelioma.

3.4. Genetic factors

Another cause for mesothelioma may be the nuclear deubiquitinase enzyme BAP1, which plays an important role in transcriptional deregulation in the pathogenesis of mesothelioma. BAP1 deubiquitinase is known to target histones (proteins that package DNA in the cell nucleus) and HCF1 (a transcriptional co-factor involved in the cell cycle), which also affects the E2F and Polycomb (a group of genes that codifies a family of transcription factors) target genes. Inactivating mutations of BAP1 were found in about one quarter of mesothelioma tumour tissues tested [32, 33]. Common genetic changes, involving the loss of the tumour suppressor genes p14, p16 [34], NF-2 [35], and P53, have been associated with mesothelioma [2].

3.5. Viral oncogenes

Simian virus 40 (SV4 0) continues to raise controversy, as it has been suggested that SV40 may have been a contaminant in the poliomyelitis vaccine in the 1950s and 1960s. A review of mesothelioma case studies have revealed an important presence of SV40 nucleic acid in affected patients. SV40 is a DNA polyomavirus, which is thought to suppress tumour genes of the retinoblastoma family by a peptide known as SV40 large T antigen [36–40].

4. Pathology

The histopathologic subtypes of mesothelioma are epithelioid (40%), mixed or biphasic (35%), and sarcomatous or mesenchymal (25%). Needle biopsy mesothelioma can often be mistaken for adenocarcinoma. Mesothelioma under electron microscopy reveals cells with long microvilli with a needle-like shape and form. Mesothelioma is positive for calretinin, vimentin, WT1, and cytokeratin, but negative for periodic acid-shift stain, mucicarmine stain, carcinoembryonic antigen, and Leu-M1. Adenocarcinoma under electron microscopy reveals short microvilli [41].

5. Pathogenesis

Inhaled asbestos fibres create lung irritation that may lead to scarring, fibrosis, and plaques. On a cellular level, injuries caused by asbestos fibres can be followed by cell repair. Repeated cell injuries, however, may lead to DNA-strand impairment and transform into malignancy [42]. It has also been suggested that long, thin asbestos fibres are generally more carcinogenic than shorter, thicker ones and interfere more with mitosis, causing chromosome abnormalities leading to cell transformation and neoplastic progression [43]. Mesothelial cells may have increased interleukin-6 secretion, which would result in increased production of vascular endothelial growth factor (VEGF), a signal protein produced by tumour cells that stimulates angiogenesis [44].

6. Clinical presentation

Dyspnea and non-pleuritic chest pain are the most common presenting symptoms of mesothelioma. X-rays often reveal recurrent pleural effusion or pleural thickening, which should prompt the clinician to suspect mesothelioma [45].

Early malignant pleural mesothelioma presents as small pleural nodules. As the tumour progresses, the nodules increase in number and coalesce to form a thickened tumour. As the tumour replaces the pleural fluid that lies between the two pleura, the parietal and visceral pleura fuse. This results in dyspnea and hypoxemia, which are often refractory to supplemental oxygen when deoxygenated blood is shunted through the encased lung.

Mesothelioma spreads by direct extension [46] and seeding throughout the pleural space, including fissures, diaphragmatic, and pericardial surfaces; through the chest wall; and into the mediastinum and lymph nodes. The malignancy may also extend into the abdominal cavity. Metastasis, although uncommon, may occur in the opposite lung, brain, and other extrathoracic sites.

7. Physical exam

The performance status should be evaluated. Visual inspection may reveal thorax nodules or ulcers and scoliosis may be observed towards the side of the malignancy [47]. The clinician should look at all sites of previous instrumentation for evidence of tumour seeding. Unilateral dullness to percussion at the lung base may be observed. Decreased air entry on the involved side may also be perceived.

8. Lab work

Tests should include a CBC, electrolytes, creatinine, and a complete metabolic panel. Serum soluble mesothelin-related peptide and osteopontin levels could be performed, although most Canadian centres do not currently do so.

Mesothelin is a glycoprotein usually expressed on normal mesothelial cells but is overexpressed in epithelioid and mixed mesotheliomas [48, 49]. A meta-analysis showed that sensitivity ranged from 19% to 68%, depending on the criteria chosen to establish positivity [50]. The glycoprotein osteopontin is also overexpressed in mesothelioma, but a study pointed to lower diagnostic accuracy than mesothelin in patients with suspected malignant mesothelioma [51].

9. Imaging

9.1. CT scan

Thoracic, abdominal, and pelvic CT scans with contrast are useful in staging the disease. Pleural thickening is the most common finding on CT scans (92% of mesothelioma patients). Pleural thickening is defined as either extension of more than 8 cm in the craniocaudal direction or more than 5 cm of the chest wall when visualized in cross section, or when the pleural thickness exceeds 3 mm [52–54].

The second most common finding is involvement of the fissure (about 85% of cases), followed by pleural effusion (75% of patients). Other findings include contraction of a hemithorax, contralateral shift of the mediastinum, chest-wall involvement, and rib destruction [55–58]. As the disease progresses, irregular pleura-based masses are common and the interlobular fissures are often involved. CT scanning may underestimate the extent of disease.

Although CT scanning is used for tumour detection, its accuracy for detecting intrathoracic lymph-node involvement is limited [59, 60]. Mesothelioma spreads into paraesophageal nodes, pulmonary-ligament nodes, and diaphragmatic nodes more commonly than other lung cancers.

9.2. MRI

Combining magnetic resonance imaging (MRI) with CT scanning may improve evaluation of the local extent of disease. MRI helps to determine chest-wall, diaphragmatic, or apical invasion as well as transdiaphragmatic tumour growth [57].

9.3. PET–CT scan

PET–CT scanning may be useful in detecting mediastinal lymph-node involvement or extrathoracic diseases and to reclassify patients as inoperable [61–65].

10. Surgical staging

Although radiographic staging evaluation is warranted, accurate staging is only possible at the time of surgery in a substantial number of patients. Pulmonary-function tests are often performed prior to surgery. For surgical staging, mediastinoscopy or endobronchial ultrasound is used in the case of suspicious nodes. An open biopsy or CT-guided core biopsy is acceptable, but thoracenthesis or video-assisted thoracoscopic surgery (VATS) is preferred. If necessary, based on the CT scan, laparoscopy can be used to rule out transdiaphragmatic extension, and VATS to rule out contralateral disease.

11. TNM staging of mesothelioma

The TNM (Tumour, Node, Metastasis) Classification is used by both the Union for International Cancer Control (UICC) and the American Joint Committee on Cancer (AJCC). The 2010 version is the most recent.

Primary Tumour (T)

Tx: Primary tumour cannot be assessed

T0: No evidence of primary tumour

T1: Tumour limited to the ipsilateral parietal pleura, with or without mediastinal pleura and with or without diaphragmatic pleural involvement

http://dx.doi.org/10.5772/55292

T1a: No involvement of the visceral pleura

T1b: Tumour also involving the visceral pleura

T2: Tumour involves each of the ipsilateral pleural surfaces (parietal, mediastinal, diaphragmatic, and visceral pleura) with at least one of the following:

(1) Involvement of diaphragmatic muscle

(2) Extension of tumour from visceral pleura into underlying pulmonary parenchyma

T3: Locally advanced but potentially resectable tumour. Tumour involving all of the ipsilateral pleural surfaces (parietal, mediastinal, diaphragmatic, and visceral pleura) with at least one of the following:

(1) Involvement of the endothoracic fascia

(2) Extension into the mediastinal fat

(3) Solitary completely resectable focus of tumour extending into the soft tissue of the chest wall

4) Nontransmural involvement of the pericardium

T4: Locally advanced, technically unresectable tumour. Tumour involving all of the ipsilateral pleural surfaces (parietal, mediastinal, diaphragmatic, and visceral pleura) with at least one of the following:

(1) Diffuse extension or multifocal masses of tumour in the chest wall, with or without associated rib destruction

(2)Direct diaphragmatic extension of the tumour to the peritoneum

(3)Direct extension of the tumour to a mediastinal organ

(4)Direct extension of the tumour to the contralateral pleura

(5)Direct extension of the tumour into the spine

(6)Tumour extending through to the internal surface of the pericardium with or without a pericardial effusion or tumour involving the myocardium

Regional Lymph Nodes (N)

Nx: Regional lymph nodes cannot be assessed

N0: No regional lymph-node metastases

N1: Metastases in the ipsilateral bronchopulmonary and/or hilar lymph nodes

N2: Metastases in the subcarinal or ipsilateral mediastinal lymph node (including ipsilateral internal mammary and peridiaphragmatic nodes)

N3: Metastases in the contralateral mediastinal, internal, mammary, or hilar nodes and/or the ipsilateral or contralateral supraclavicular or scalene lymph nodes

Distant Metastasis (M)

Mx: Distant metastasis cannot be assessed

M0: No distant metastasis

M1: Distant metastasis

Stage Groups

I T1N0M0

IA T1aN0M0

IB	T1bN0M0
II	T2N0M0
III	T1-2N1M0
	T1-2N2M0
	T3N0-2M0
IV	T4 and any NM0
	Any T and N3M0
	Any T and any N and M1

12. Differential diagnosis

Even though most pleural tumours are malignant, the differential diagnosis also includes benign tumours and inflammatory reactions.

Primary tumours, such as fibrosarcoma and malignant fibrous histiocytoma, can present in a similar fashion and infiltrate like sarcomatous mesotheliomas. Metastatic diseases that can involve the pleura and mimic epithelioid mesothelioma include breast, lung, lymphoma, thymoma, stomach, kidney, ovarian, and prostate cancer. Finally, benign chronic organized empyema can also mimic pleural thickening.

13. Treatments

The median survival of patients with mesothelioma is poor, ranging from 7 to 17 months [66]. The overall survival (OS) rate at 5 years is 9%. Even with new therapy interventions, the overall patient survival rate has not been significantly improved. In some specific cases, in which patients were specifically chosen due to their localized disease, treatment with aggressive multimodality therapy improved their survival rates.

The first thing to consider when treating mesothelioma is whether the tumour is resectable or not. Since the tumour spreads by direct extension, only 5% of mesotheliomas are resectable at diagnosis. Usually T1 to T3 and N0-1 tumours are considered resectable. T4 and N2-3 tumours are considered unresectable. Mediastinoscopy has to be performed to rule out N2-N3 lymph nodes. In addition, patients with sarcomatoid histology have a poorer prognosis and should not be considered for extrapleural pneumonectomy [67]. Patients must be able to tolerate trimodal therapy, since it is important to ensure that they do not have postoperative morbidities without deriving the full benefits of surgery.

The treatment paradigms for resectable mesothelioma are:

Extrapleural pneumonectomy (EPP), then chemotherapy followed by hemithorax radiation therapy [7, 68–71]

Neoadjuvant chemotherapy, then EPP followed by hemithorax radiation therapy [72–73]

If the tumour is unresectable:

A combination of chemotherapy is the standard treatment. Prophylactic drain-site irradiation should be considered.

Talc pleurodesis with a pleural catheter or pleurectomy may also be considered to palliate symptoms of pleural effusion.

14. Surgery

Prior to surgery, it is important to have proper patient selection. Patients must have:

Performance status of 0–1

PaO_2 of more than 65 mm Hg

$PaCO_2$ of less than 45 mm Hg

A predicted post op FEV_1 of more than 1 L

An ejection fraction of more than 40%

A mean pulmonary arterial pressure of less than 30 mm Hg

An epithelioid histology

14.1. Extrapleural Pneumonectomy (EPP)

EPP involves the removal of parietal pleura, lung, pericardium, and ipsilateral diaphragm. Mediastinal node dissection is usually performed. Finally, a graft is inserted to prevent herniation of abdominal contents through the diaphragmatic defect. Although no survival benefit was observed from randomized trials, observational studies indicated that EPP is the only intervention that has been demonstrated to result in long-term, disease-free survival in highly selected patients with favourable prognostic indication [7]. In a review of 83 patients who underwent EPP, the observed 5-year survival rate was 15% [74].

The benefits of EPP is that it allows complete resection or at least a cytoreduction, permitting higher radiation doses to be delivered safely to the ipsilateral hemithorax. This procedure has the disadvantage of being technically complex and associated with significant perioperative morbidity and mortality. Complications include atrial fibrillation (44.2%), prolonged intubation (7.9%), vocal-cord paralysis (6.7%), deep-vein thrombosis (6.4%), technical complications (patch dehiscence, haemorrhage, or both; 6.1%), tamponade (3.6%), acute respiratory-distress syndrome (3.6%), cardiac arrest (3%), constrictive physiology (2.7%), aspiration (2.7%), renal failure (2.7%), empyema (2.4%), tracheostomy 1.8%, myocardial infarction (1.5%), pulmonary embolus (1.5%), and bronchopleural fistula (0.6%) [75]. In extensive experience, the early postoperative mortality rate approaches 7% [76] but can be as high as 30%. The mean survival (MS) rate after surgery is 4 to 20 months.

14.2. Pleurectomy/Decortication (P/D)

In case of more advanced disease, mixed histology, and medically high-risk operable patients, pleurectomy/decortication is preferred over EPP. Pleurectomy/decortication is performed in two phases. Phase 1 is pleurectomy and involves removing the pleural lining. Phase 2 is decortication, which is the removal of any tumour growing inside the lining. The procedure's perioperative mortality is 4% [76].

Retrospective studies have indicated that parietal pleurectomy and decortication may be as efficient as extrapleural pneumonectomy [76]. When comparing EPP to PD, it was observed that PD patients had a greater local recurrence of disease, while EPP patients experienced higher mortality and surgical morbidity.

15. Radiotherapy (RT)

15.1. Adjuvant radiation therapy after EPP

Radiation therapy is a local treatment that uses ionizing radiation to destroy tumour cells. As mentioned above, aggressive surgery alone does not improve survival. Observational data do not provide evidence that adjuvant RT following pleurectomy offers a survival benefit [77]. That notwithstanding, the MSKCC phase-II trial with hemithorax radiotherapy to 54 Gy following EPP showed improved mean survival rates at 34 months for stage I-II disease and at 10 months with later-stage disease compared to historical controls [78]. In addition to a small survival benefit demonstrated in the MSKCC study, the rationale for using radiation therapy is local control. The disease is of a diffuse nature and manipulating the exposed tumour during EPP puts the entire ipsilateral chest wall, diaphragm insertion, pericardium, mediastinum, and bronchial stump at a very high risk of local recurrence, as high as 80% of patients, as reported in [78]. The evaluation of high-dose radiation therapy showed that the use of adjuvant radiation decreased the risk of local recurrence to 13% [78].

Mesothelioma is considered a tumour sensitive to external-beam radiation therapy. The recommended postoperative doses are 50 Gy for negative surgical margins, 54 to 60 Gy for close or positive margins, and 60 Gy for gross tumours [79–83]. The radiation dose has to be limited, however, due to the treatment required to the entire hemithorax and the sensitivity of critical organs such as the heart, lungs, oesophagus, liver, kidneys, and spinal cord to radiation [68].

Treatment volumes include ipsilateral mediastinum even for node-negative tumours. The superior border should include the thoracic inlet. The medial border should include the trachea, subcarinal lymph nodes, and the vertebral body. The inferior border is the insertion of the diaphragm, ranging from L1 to L4. Radiation oncologists should be careful to include the anteromedial pleural reflection of the sternopericardial recess, the medial and inferior extent of the crus of the diaphragm, and the inferior insertion of the diaphragm in the treatment volume. Nowadays, radiation therapy is delivered using three-dimensional conformal radiation therapy (3DCRT) or intensity-modulated radiation therapy (IMRT) [70, 71, 84, 85].

http://dx.doi.org/10.5772/55292

IMRT can be delivered according to the method published by the MDACC experiment using 13 to 27 fields with 8 to 11 gantry angles with 100 segments/fields. The target volume was the entire hemithorax, all surgical clips, all sites of instrumentation, and the ipsilateral mediastinum with an initial dose to 45-50 Gy, with a boost to 60 Gy for a close/positive margin. The two-year survival rate was 62% and the three-year disease-free survival (DFS) rate was 45% for negative lymph nodes and epithelioid histology. Five patients with stage-I disease had a three-year DFS of 100%. IMRT has the potential to decrease pulmonary toxicity if correct treatment algorithms are applied.

In order to decrease the side effects of radiation therapy, several dose-volume restrictions are applied. The V20 (the volume receiving 20 Gy or more) of the lung must not exceed 7%, since Rice DC et al. [86] showed a relative risk of 42% for fatal pneumonitis. The oesophagus V55 should be less than 30%; the liver V30 should be less than 30%. The kidneys V15 should be less than 20%; the heart V40 less than 50%; the spinal cord V45 less than 10%; no volume should be more than 50 Gy.

15.2. Radiation therapy to the biopsy site

A debate in radiation oncology for mesothelioma remains whether to offer radiation therapy to inoperable patients following an invasive procedure or following a biopsy in order to avoid needle-tract seeding from the tumour. The incidence of tumour seeding along the biopsy tract may range from 0% to 43% and may lead to the formation of painful subcutaneous lesions [87]. Three randomized trials [88–90] evaluated RT following thoracoscopy or thoracotomy to prevent tumour seeding. The radiation-therapy regimen was generally 3 fractions of 7 Gy (total of 21 Gy). O'Rouke et al. showed, in their randomized trial with 61 patients, that prophylactic radiation therapy to drain sites did not statistically reduce the rate of seeding. Boutin's study (40 patients) revealed a clear benefit of radiation at the biopsy site with reduction of biopsy-tract metastasis from 40% to 0% ($p < 0.00$ 1). At the Hôtel-Dieu de Québec Hospital, however, Marie-Anne Froment et al. [91] reported a benefit of radiation therapy to avoid needle-tract seeding from the tumour. At 6 months, local progression-free survival for the intervention sites was 91% with prophylactic radiation therapy and 74% without irradiation ($p = 0.00$ 2). During follow-up, 6 patients (13%) in the treated group had tumour invasion of the subcutaneous tissue compared to 40 patients (33%) in the group without radiation ($p = 0.00$ 8). Because recurrence is morbid and this treatment is easily feasible, Hôtel-Dieu de Québec Hospital generally offers radiation therapy to such patients.

15.3. Side effects of radiation therapy after EPP

The side effects of radiation therapy can be classified according to time of occurrence: acute, intermediate, or late. Acute effects, if they appear, are expected to start during treatment and be resolved within 3 months following treatment. Potential acute side effects are fatigue, skin reactions, nausea, vomiting, dysphagia, odynophagia, and cough. Potential intermediate side effects include pneumonitis and Hermitte's syndrome. If intermediate side effects occur, they usually do so 3 months after treatment and resolve within 6 months.

Finally, potential late effects would occur 6 months following treatment and could include pulmonary fibrosis, pericarditis, restrictive cardiomyopathy, myocardial infarction, congestive heart failure, and radiation myelopathy.

16. Chemotherapy

Adjuvant or Neoadjuvant Chemotherapy

Anthracyclines have historically been the most commonly used pharmacologic agents, with reported response rates of 19% [92]. Recent trials using platinum in combination with folate analogues have improved cytotoxic activity against mesothelioma. The preferred treatment during these recent trials was a combination of chemotherapy incorporated with a trimodal regimen, as adjuvant or neoadjuvant chemotherapy options are either pemetrexed/cisplatin or gemcitabine/cisplatin.

16.1. Adjuvant chemotherapy

Patients treated with EPP, followed by radiation therapy and adjuvant chemotherapy, had a median survival rates of 36 % and 14% at two to five years, respectively. Historically, the chemotherapy used was doxorubicin, cyclophosphamide, and cisplatin for four to six cycles [93]. A Harvard retrospective [93] review of 183 patients treated with a trimodality approach using adjuvant chemotherapy of Cytoxan/Adriamycin/cisplatin (CAP) or carboplatin/Taxol with concurrent radiation therapy followed by adjuvant chemotherapy had an overall mean survival rate of 19 months and a 5-year overall survival (OS) rate of 15%.

16.2. Neoadjuvant chemotherapy

The rationale for using neoadjuvant chemotherapy prior to surgery is that it may increase tolerance and improve response to surgery. A multicenter phase-II trial [72] evaluated the role of neoadjuvant chemotherapy prior to EPP and RT. The chemotherapy consisted of four cycles of pemetrexed plus cisplatin. The median survival rate of the patients who completed the therapy was 29 months; the two-year survival rate was 61%. De Perrot et al. [73] reported a median survival rate of 59 months in a subgroup of patients who had completed trimodal therapy with neoadjuvant chemotherapy, EPP, and then RT. The median survival rate was less than 14 months for the patients who did not complete the treatment regimen.

Chemotherapy as a definitive treatment

16.3. Combination chemotherapy

Combination-chemotherapy regimens using pemetrexed and platinum-based agents have yielded superior outcomes than single agents. Volgezang NJ et al. [94] showed that, for unresectable tumours, cisplatin/pemetrexed improved the response rate of 17% vs. 40% and the MS rate from 9 to 12 months compared to cisplatin alone. In 2004, pemetrexed became the first agent to receive Food and Drug Administration (FDA) approval for use in combination with cisplatin. The combination of pemetrexed and carboplatin were studied in two phase-II studies, the response rates and mean survival rates were 18.6% and 12.7 months in the Ceresoli study [95] and 25% and 14 months in the Castagneto study [96].

Several trials [97, 98] have evaluated the addition of gemcitabine, a cytidine analogue. Only 38% of patients received the four cycles as prescribed and the response rate was 26% among those who completed the treatment [98]. It should be noted that the study only included early-stage mesothelioma. Vinca alkaloid-containing regimen was compared to MVP (mitomycin, vinblastine, and cisplatin) in terms of symptom control. The median survival benefit was an additional 2 months [99].

16.4. Single-agent chemotherapy

Pemetrexed as a single agent has been studied. In one phase-II trial [100], the study design was revised to incorporate folic acid and cynocobalamin in addition to dexamethasone. The median progression-free survival was 16.3 months in the pemetrexed/vitamin-supplemented group versus 9.5 months for the pemetrexed group. Other single agents such as gemcitabine, anthracyclines, and taxanes have been tested but resulted in low response rates, such as 10%

16.5. Chemotherapy side effects

Cisplatin and carboplatin are platinum analogues. The potential side effects of platinum agents include dose-limiting myelosuppression, nausea, vomiting, renal impairment, hearing impairment, and peripheral neuropathy. Pemetrexed is an antifolate compound. Potential side effects include myelosuppression, nausea, skin rash, alopecia, diarrhoea, and fatigue.

17. Molecular target therapy

Recent anticancer agents focus on molecular targets such as surface receptors and cell-signalling proteins. Although it has been shown that mesothelial cells express the vascular endothelial growth factor (VEGF) receptor, a recent study [101] failed to demonstrate survival improvement with bevacizumab. Erlotinib, a tyrosine-kinase inhibitor of the epidermal growth-factor receptor (EGFR), was tested in a phase-II trial. EGFR is expressed primarily in the epithelial subtype of mesothelioma. Of the 63 patients who were enrolled, only 29 were assessed for outcomes; no objective responses were reported [102].

18. Prognosis and overall survival

The European Organisation for Research and Treatment of Cancer (EORTC) reviewed data for 204 adults who were enrolled in five consecutive phase-II trials over nine years. The EORTC poor prognostic factors [103] for mesothelioma are:

- White-blood-cell count greater than 8.3 X 109/ dL
- Performance status (PS) 1-2
- Sarcomatous histology
- Male gender

For low risk: 1-year OS rate is 40%; 2-year OS rate is 14%. For high risk: 1-year OS rate is 12% and 2-years OS rate is 0%. The MS rates are 4 and 12 months, respectively.

19. Palliative treatment

Surgical procedures, radiation therapy, and chemotherapy can be used to palliate symptoms.

19.1. Surgery

Large pleural effusions can cause persistent dyspnea and pain. Complete drainage of the pleural effusion by tube thoracostomy or video thoracoscopy followed by the introduction of an irritative agent to obliterate the pleural space can provide palliation. There is an ongoing randomized trial in the United Kingdom comparing the palliative benefits of VATS pleurectomy to talc pleurodesis.

19.2. Radiation therapy

In the case of palliative treatments, radiation therapy can be used for pain relief. Either 30 Gy in 10 fractions or 20 Gy in 5 fractions can be delivered. Furthermore, palliative radiation therapy with daily dose of 4 Gy appears to be more effective than fractionations of less than 4 Gy for a total dose of 20 to 40 Gy to relieve pain associated with skin nodules in the CW. Radiation therapy can alleviate symptoms in 50% of patients [104].

19.3. Chemotherapy

For unresectable tumours, palliative chemotherapy with cisplatin/pemetrexed or cisplatin/ gemcitabine can be used. There are no standard second line of chemotherapy. Therefore, a combination or single agent such as gemcitabine, vinorelbine, paclitaxel, or docetaxel may be considered.

20. Conclusion

The highest risk factor for mesothelioma is exposure to asbestos. Treatment for mesothelioma involves a trimodal approach for early-stage disease, which includes surgery, radiation, and systemic chemotherapy. In the case of locally advanced disease, nonsurgical candidates, or metastatic disease, surgery, chemotherapy, or radiation therapy can be used. Mesothelioma

http://dx.doi.org/10.5772/55292

has a poor prognosis, but recent studies of pemetrexed and platinum-analogue combination therapies have demonstrated improved response rates over other treatments. Although conducting research on mesothelioma is extremely difficult, since it is an uncommon disease, further study is required to improve patient outcomes.

Nomenclature

AP Anterior-posterior field

BAP1 A gene that encodes a nuclear localizing protein with a ubiquitin carboxy-terminal hydrolase domain that gives BAP1 its deubiquitinase activity.

CAP Cytoxan/Adriamycin/cisplatin

CBC Complete blood count

CW Chest wall

DFS Disease-free survival

E2F Group of genes that codifies a family of transcription factors

EGFR Epidermal growth-factor receptor

EORTC European Organisation for Research and Treatment of Cancer

EPP Extrapleural pneumonectomy

FDA Food and Drug Administration

Gy Gray

HCF1 A transcriptional cofactor involved in the cell cycle

MS Mean survival

MVP Mitomycin, vinblastine, and cisplatin

NF-2 Neurofibromatosis type-2 gene

OS Overall survival

P14 Tumour suppressor gene

P16 Tumour suppressor gene

P53 Tumour suppressor gene

PA Posterior-anterior field

P/D: Pleurectomy/decortication

PS Performance status

RT Radiation therapy

VATS Video-assisted thoracoscopic surgery

VEGF Vascular endothelial growth factor

WT1 Wilm's tumour gene

Author details

Julie Goudreault and Anne Dagnault

Department of Radiation Oncology, Hôtel-Dieu de Québec, Laval University, Canada

References

[1] Pass HI, Carbone M. Malignant mesothelioma: Advances in pathogenesis, diagnosis, and translational therapies. Springer Verlag; 2005a.

[2] Robinson BW, Lake RA. Advances in malignant mesothelioma. N Engl J Med 2005, Oct 13;353(15):1591-603.

[3] Gordon W, Antman KH, Greenberger JS, Weichselbaum RR, Chaffey JT. Radiation therapy in the management of patients with mesothelioma. Int J Radiat Oncol Biol Phys 1982, Jan;8(1):19-25.

[4] Rusch VW. Pleurectomy/decortication and adjuvant therapy for malignant mesothelioma. Chest 1993, Apr;103(4 Suppl):382S-4S.

[5] Butchart EG, Ashcroft T, Barnsley WC, Holden MP. Pleuropneumonectomy in the management of diffuse malignant mesothelioma of the pleura. Experience with 29 patients. Thorax 1976, Feb;31(1):15-24.

[6] Jaklitsch MT, Grondin SC, Sugarbaker DJ. Treatment of malignant mesothelioma. World J Surg 2001, Feb;25(2):210-7.

[7] Rusch VW, Piantadosi S, Holmes EC. The role of extrapleural pneumonectomy in malignant pleural mesothelioma. A lung cancer study group trial. J Thorac Cardiovasc Surg 1991, Jul;102(1):1-9.

[8] Lung Tumour Group. B.C. Cancer agency; Available from: http://www.bccancer.bc.ca/PPI/TypesofCancer/Mesothelioma/default.htm. Accessed 5 May 2012.

[9] Connelly RR, Spirtas R, Myers MH, et al:Demographic patterns for mesothelioma in the United States. J Natl Cancer Inst 1987; 78:1053-1060.

[10] Institut national de santé publique Québec. Dossier amiante; Available from: http://www.inspq.qc.ca/dossiers/amiante/infos.asp?e=cp. Accessed 28 July 2012.

[11] Selikoff IJ, Hammond EC, Seidman H. Latency of asbestos disease among insulation workers in the United States and Canada. Cancer 1980, Dec 15;46(12):2736-40.

[12] Boffetta P, Epidemiology of peritoneal mesothelioma: a review. Ann Oncol. 2007;18(6):985.

[13] Wagner JC, Sleggs CA, Marchand P. Diffuse pleural mesothelioma and asbestos exposure in the north western cape province. Br J Ind Med 1960, Oct; 17: 260-71.

[14] Occupational Safety & Heath Administration. Occupational Exposure to Asbestos; Available from http://www.osha.gov/pls/oshaweb/owadisp.show_document?p_table=FEDERAL_REGISTER&p_id=12429 . Accessed November 27 2012.

[15] Metintas M, Ozdemir N, Hillerdal G, Uçgun I, Metintas S, Baykul C, et al. Environmental asbestos exposure and malignant pleural mesothelioma. Respir Med 1999, May;93(5):349-55.

[16] Senyiğit A, Babayiğit C, Gökirmak M, Topçu F, Asan E, Coşkunsel M, et al. Incidence of malignant pleural mesothelioma due to environmental asbestos fiber exposure in the southeast of turkey. Respiration 2000;67(6):610-4.

[17] Senyiğit A, Bayram H, Babayiğit C, Topçu F, Nazaroğlu H, Bilici A, Leblebici IH. Malignant pleural mesothelioma caused by environmental exposure to asbestos in the southeast of Turkey: CT findings in 117 patients. Respiration 2000;67(6):615-22.

[18] Metintas S, Metintas M, Ucgun I, Oner U. Malignant mesothelioma due to environmental exposure to asbestos: Follow-up of a turkish cohort living in a rural area. Chest 2002, Dec;122(6):2224-9

[19] Pan XL, Dan Hw, Wang W et al. Residential proximity to naturally occuring asbestos and mesothelioma risk in California. Am J Respir Crit Care Med 2005; 172: 1019.

[20] Hansen J, de Klerk NH, Musk AW, Hobbs MS. Environmental exposure to crocidolite and mesothelioma: exposure-response relationships. AM J Respi Crit care MEd 1998; 157:69.

[21] Pira E, Pelucchi C, Buffoni L et al. Cancer mortality in a cohort of asbestos textile workers. Br J Cancer 2005; 92:580.

[22] Carbone M, Kratzke RA, Testa JR. The pathogenesis of mesothelioma. Semin Oncol 2002, Feb;29(1):2-17.

[23] Health Canada. Health risks of asbestos; Available from: http://www.hc-sc.gc.ca/hl-vs/alt_formats/pacrb-dgapcr/pdf/iyh-vsv/environ/asbestos-amiante-eng.pdf. Accessed 27 July 2012.

[24] Hodgson JT, Mc Elvenny DM, Darnton AJ, et al. The expected burden of mesothelioma mortality in Great Britain from 2002 to 2050. Br J Cancer 2005; 92:587.

[25] Muscat JE, Wynder EL. Cigarette smoking, asbestos exposure, and malignant mesothelioma. Cancer Res 1991, May 1;51(9):2263-7.

[26] Takagi A, Hirose A, Nishimura T, Fukumori N, Ogata A, Ohashi N, et al. Induction of mesothelioma in p53+/- mouse by intraperitoneal application of multi-wall carbon nanotube. J Toxicol Sci 2008, Feb;33(1):105-16.

[27] Poland CA, Duffin R, Kinloch I, Maynard A, Wallace WA, Seaton A, et al. Carbon nanotubes introduced into the abdominal cavity of mice show asbestos-like pathogenicity in a pilot study. Nat Nanotechnol 2008, Jul;3(7):423-8.

[28] Mossman BT, Lippmann M, Hesterberg TW, Kelsey KT, Barchowsky A, Bonner JC. Pulmonary endpoints (lung carcinomas and asbestosis) following inhalation exposure to asbestos. J Toxicol Environ Health B Crit Rev 2011;14(1-4):76-121.

[29] Teta MJ, Lau E, Sceurman BK, Wagner ME. Therapeutic radiation for lymphoma: Risk of malignant mesothelioma. Cancer 2007, Apr 1;109(7):1432-8.

[30] Tward JD, Wendland MM, Shrieve DC, Szabo A, Gaffney DK. The risk of secondary malignancies over 30 years after the treatment of non-hodgkin lymphoma. Cancer 2006, Jul 1;107(1):108-15.

[31] Travis LB, Fosså SD, Schonfeld SJ, McMaster ML, Lynch CF, Storm H, et al. Second cancers among 40,576 testicular cancer patients: Focus on long-term survivors. J Natl Cancer Inst 2005, Sep 21;97(18):1354-65.

[32] Bott M, Brevet M, Taylor BS, Shimizu S, Ito T, Wang L, et al. The nuclear deubiquitinase BAP1 is commonly inactivated by somatic mutations and 3p21.1 losses in malignant pleural mesothelioma. Nat Genet 2011, Jul;43(7):668-72.

[33] Testa JR, Cheung M, Pei J, Below JE, Tan Y, Sementino E, et al. Germline BAP1 mutations predispose to malignant mesothelioma. Nat Genet 2011, Oct;43(10):1022-5.

[34] Altomare DA, Menges CW, Xu J, Pei J, Zhang L, Tadevosyan A, et al. Losses of both products of the cdkn2a/arf locus contribute to asbestos-induced mesothelioma development and cooperate to accelerate tumorigenesis. PLoS One 2011;6(4):e18828.

[35] Thurneysen C, Opitz I, Kurtz S, Weder W, Stahel RA, Felley-Bosco E. Functional inactivation of NF2/merlin in human mesothelioma. Lung Cancer 2009, May;64(2): 140-7.

[36] De Luca A, Baldi A, Esposito V, Howard CM, Bagella L, Rizzo P, et al. The retinoblastoma gene family prb/p105, p107, prb2/p130 and simian virus-40 large t-antigen in human mesotheliomas. Nat Med 1997, Aug;3(8):913-6.

[37] Pass HI, Donington JS, Wu P, Rizzo P, Nishimura M, Kennedy R, Carbone M. Human mesotheliomas contain the simian virus-40 regulatory region and large tumor antigen DNA sequences. J Thorac Cardiovasc Surg 1998, Nov;116(5):854-9.

[38] Ramael M, Nagels J, Heylen H, De Schepper S, Paulussen J, De Maeyer M, Van Haesendonck C. Detection of SV40 like viral DNA and viral antigens in malignant pleural mesothelioma. Eur Respir J 1999, Dec;14(6):1381-6.

[39] McLaren BR, Haenel T, Stevenson S, Mukherjee S, Robinson BW, Lake RA. Simian virus (SV) 40 like sequences in cell lines and tumour biopsies from australian malignant mesotheliomas. Aust N Z J Med 2000, Aug;30(4):450-6.

[40] Gazdar AF, Carbone M. Molecular pathogenesis of malignant mesothelioma and its relationship to simian virus 40. Clin Lung Cancer 2003, Nov;5(3):177-81.

[41] Kushitani K, Takeshima Y, Amatya VJ, Furonaka O, Sakatani A, Inai K. Immunohistochemical marker panels for distinguishing between epithelioid mesothelioma and lung adenocarcinoma. Pathol Int 2007, Apr;57(4):190-9.

[42] Kamp DW, Israbian VA, Preusen SE, Zhang CX, Weitzman SA. Asbestos causes DNA strand breaks in cultured pulmonary epithelial cells: Role of iron-catalyzed free radicals. Am J Physiol 1995, Mar;268(3 Pt 1):L471-80.

[43] Ault JG, Cole RW, Jensen CG, Jensen LC, Bachert LA, Rieder CL. Behavior of crocidolite asbestos during mitosis in living vertebrate lung epithelial cells. Cancer Res 1995, Feb 15;55(4):792-8.

[44] Adachi Y, Aoki C, Yoshio-Hoshino N, Takayama K, Curiel DT, Nishimoto N. Interleukin-6 induces both cell growth and VEGF production in malignant mesotheliomas. Int J Cancer 2006, Sep 15;119(6):1303-11.

[45] Pisani RJ, Colby TV, Williams DE. Malignant mesothelioma of the pleura. Mayo Clin Proc 1988, Dec;63(12):1234-44.

[46] Hillerdal G. Malignant mesothelioma 1982: Review of 4710 published cases. Br J Dis Chest 1983, Oct;77(4):321-43.

[47] Antman KH. Natural history and epidemiology of malignant mesothelioma. Chest 1993, Apr;103(4 Suppl):373S-6S.

[48] Chang K, Pai LH, Pass H, Pogrebniak HW, Tsao MS, Pastan I, Willingham MC. Monoclonal antibody K1 reacts with epithelial mesothelioma but not with lung adenocarcinoma. Am J Surg Pathol 1992, Mar;16(3):259-68.

[49] Ordóñez NG. Value of mesothelin immunostaining in the diagnosis of mesothelioma. Mod Pathol 2003, Mar;16(3):192-7.

[50] Hollevoet K, Reitsma JB, Creaney J, Grigoriu BD, Robinson BW, Scherpereel A, et al. Serum mesothelin for diagnosing malignant pleural mesothelioma: An individual patient data meta-analysis. J Clin Oncol 2012, May 1;30(13):1541-9.

[51] Grigoriu BD, Scherpereel A, Devos P, Chahine B, Letourneux M, Lebailly P, et al. Utility of osteopontin and serum mesothelin in malignant pleural mesothelioma diagnosis and prognosis assessment. Clin Cancer Res 2007, May 15;13(10):2928-35.

[52] McLoud TC. CT and MR in pleural disease. Clin Chest Med 1998, Jun;19(2):261-76.

[53] Leung AN, Müller NL, Miller RR. CT in differential diagnosis of diffuse pleural disease. AJR Am J Roentgenol 1990, Mar;154(3):487-92.

[54] Aberle DR, Gamsu G, Ray CS. High-resolution CT of benign asbestos-related diseases: Clinical and radiographic correlation. AJR Am J Roentgenol 1988, Nov;151(5): 883-91.

[55] Alexander E, Clark RA, Colley DP, Mitchell SE. CT of malignant pleural mesothelioma. AJR Am J Roentgenol 1981, Aug;137(2):287-91.

[56] Grant DC, Seltzer SE, Antman KH, Finberg HJ, Koster K. Computed tomography of malignant pleural mesothelioma. J Comput Assist Tomogr 1983, Aug;7(4):626-32.

[57] Miller WT, Gefter WB, Miller WT. Asbestos-related chest diseases: Plain radiographic findings. Semin Roentgenol 1992, Apr;27(2):102-20.

[58] Wang ZJ, Reddy GP, Gotway MB, Higgins CB, Jablons DM, Ramaswamy M, et al. Malignant pleural mesothelioma: Evaluation with CT, MR imaging, and PET. Radiographics 2004;24(1):105-19.

[59] Heelan RT, Rusch VW, Begg CB, Panicek DM, Caravelli JF, Eisen C. Staging of malignant pleural mesothelioma: Comparison of CT and MR imaging. AJR Am J Roentgenol 1999, Apr;172(4):1039-47.

[60] Marom EM, Erasmus JJ, Pass HI, Patz EF. The role of imaging in malignant pleural mesothelioma. Semin Oncol 2002, Feb;29(1):26-35.

[61] Sørensen JB, Ravn J, Loft A, Brenøe J, Berthelsen AK, Nordic Mesothelioma Group. Preoperative staging of mesothelioma by 18f-fluoro-2-deoxy-d-glucose positron emission tomography/computed tomography fused imaging and mediastinoscopy compared to pathological findings after extrapleural pneumonectomy. Eur J Cardiothorac Surg 2008, Nov;34(5):1090-6.

[62] Plathow C, Staab A, Schmaehl A, Aschoff P, Zuna I, Pfannenberg C, et al. Computed tomography, positron emission tomography, positron emission tomography/ computed tomography, and magnetic resonance imaging for staging of limited pleural mesothelioma: Initial results. Invest Radiol 2008, Oct;43(10):737-44.

[63] Wilcox BE, Subramaniam RM, Peller PJ, Aughenbaugh GL, Nichols Iii FC, Aubry MC, Jett JR. Utility of integrated computed tomography-positron emission tomography for selection of operable malignant pleural mesothelioma. Clin Lung Cancer 2009, Jul;10(4):244-8.

[64] Bénard F, Sterman D, Smith RJ, Kaiser LR, Albelda SM, Alavi A. Metabolic imaging of malignant pleural mesothelioma with fluorodeoxyglucose positron emission tomography. Chest 1998, Sep;114(3):713-22.

[65] Yildirim H, Metintas M, Entok E, Ak G, Ak I, Dundar E, Erginel S. Clinical value of fluorodeoxyglucose-positron emission tomography/computed tomography in differentiation of malignant mesothelioma from asbestos-related benign pleural disease: An observational pilot study. J Thorac Oncol 2009, Dec;4(12):1480-4.

[66] Curran D, Sahmoud T, Therasse P, van Meerbeeck J, Postmus PE, Giaccone G. Prognostic factors in patients with pleural mesothelioma: The european organization for research and treatment of cancer experience. J Clin Oncol 1998, Jan;16(1):145-52.

[67] Balduyck B, Trousse D, Nakas A, Martin-Ucar AE, Edwards J, Waller DA. Therapeutic surgery for nonepithelioid malignant pleural mesothelioma: Is it really worthwhile? Ann Thorac Surg 2010, Mar;89(3):907-11.

[68] Baldini EH, Recht A, Strauss GM, DeCamp MM, Swanson SJ, Liptay MJ, et al. Patterns of failure after trimodality therapy for malignant pleural mesothelioma. Ann Thorac Surg 1997, Feb;63(2):334-8.

[69] Kutcher GJ, Kestler C, Greenblatt D, Brenner H, Hilaris BS, Nori D. Technique for external beam treatment for mesothelioma. Int J Radiat Oncol Biol Phys 1987, Nov; 13(11):1747-52.

[70] Ahamad A, Stevens CW, Smythe WR, Liao Z, Vaporciyan AA, Rice D, et al. Promising early local control of malignant pleural mesothelioma following postoperative intensity modulated radiotherapy (IMRT) to the chest. Cancer J 2003;9(6):476-84.

[71] Forster KM, Smythe WR, Starkschall G, Liao Z, Takanaka T, Kelly JF, et al. Intensity-modulated radiotherapy following extrapleural pneumonectomy for the treatment of malignant mesothelioma: Clinical implementation. Int J Radiat Oncol Biol Phys 2003, Mar 1;55(3):606-16.

[72] Krug LM, Pass HI, Rusch VW, Kindler HL, Sugarbaker DJ, Rosenzweig KE, et al. Multicenter phase II trial of neoadjuvant pemetrexed plus cisplatin followed by extrapleural pneumonectomy and radiation for malignant pleural mesothelioma. J Clin Oncol 2009, Jun 20;27(18):3007-13.

[73] De Perrot M, Feld R, Cho BC, Bezjak A, Anraku M, Burkes R, et al. Trimodality therapy with induction chemotherapy followed by extrapleural pneumonectomy and adjuvant high-dose hemithoracic radiation for malignant pleural mesothelioma. J Clin Oncol 2009, Mar 20;27(9):1413-8.

[74] Trousse DS, Avaro JP, D'Journo XB, Doddoli C, Astoul P, Giudicelli R, et al. Is malignant pleural mesothelioma a surgical disease? A review of 83 consecutive extra-pleural pneumonectomies. Eur J Cardiothorac Surg 2009, Oct;36(4):759-63.

[75] Sugarbaker DJ, Jaklitsch MT, Bueno R, Richards W, Lukanich J, Mentzer SJ, et al. Prevention, early detection, and management of complications after 328 consecutive extrapleural pneumonectomies. J Thorac Cardiovasc Surg 2004, Jul;128(1):138-46.

[76] Flores RM, Pass HI, Seshan VE, Dycoco J, Zakowski M, Carbone M, et al. Extrapleural pneumonectomy versus pleurectomy/decortication in the surgical management of malignant pleural mesothelioma: Results in 663 patients. J Thorac Cardiovasc Surg 2008, Mar;135(3):620-6, 626.e1-3.

[77] Aisner J. Current approach to malignant mesothelioma of the pleura. Chest 1995, Jun; 107(6 Suppl):332S-44S.

[78] Rusch VW, Rosenzweig K, Venkatraman E, Leon L, Raben A, Harrison L, et al. A phase II trial of surgical resection and adjuvant high-dose hemithoracic radiation for malignant pleural mesothelioma. J Thorac Cardiovasc Surg 2001, Oct;122(4):788-95.

[79] Maasilta P. Deterioration in lung function following hemithorax irradiation for pleural mesothelioma. Int J Radiat Oncol Biol Phys 1991, Mar;20(3):433-8.

[80] Hilaris BS, Nori D, Kwong E, Kutcher GJ, Martini N. Pleurectomy and intraoperative brachytherapy and postoperative radiation in the treatment of malignant pleural mesothelioma. Int J Radiat Oncol Biol Phys 1984, Mar;10(3):325-31.

[81] Lee TT, Everett DL, Shu HK, Jahan TM, Roach M, Speight JL, et al. Radical pleurectomy/decortication and intraoperative radiotherapy followed by conformal radiation with or without chemotherapy for malignant pleural mesothelioma. J Thorac Cardiovasc Surg 2002, Dec;124(6):1183-9.

[82] Yajnik S, Rosenzweig KE, Mychalczak B, Krug L, Flores R, Hong L, Rusch VW. Hemithoracic radiation after extrapleural pneumonectomy for malignant pleural mesothelioma. Int J Radiat Oncol Biol Phys 2003, Aug 1;56(5):1319-26.

[83] Weder W, Kestenholz P, Taverna C, Bodis S, Lardinois D, Jerman M, Stahel RA. Neoadjuvant chemotherapy followed by extrapleural pneumonectomy in malignant pleural mesothelioma. J Clin Oncol 2004, Sep 1;22(17):3451-7.

[84] Rice DC, Stevens CW, Correa AM, Vaporciyan AA, Tsao A, Forster KM, et al. Outcomes after extrapleural pneumonectomy and intensity-modulated radiation therapy for malignant pleural mesothelioma. Ann Thorac Surg 2007, Nov;84(5):1685-92; discussion 1692-3.

[85] Miles EF, Larrier NA, Kelsey CR, Hubbs JL, Ma J, Yoo S, Marks LB. Intensity-modulated radiotherapy for resected mesothelioma: The duke experience. Int J Radiat Oncol Biol Phys 2008, Jul 15;71(4):1143-50.

[86] Rice DC, Smythe WR, Liao Z, Guerrero T, Chang JY, McAleer MF, et al. Dose-dependent pulmonary toxicity after postoperative intensity-modulated radiotherapy for malignant pleural mesothelioma. Int J Radiat Oncol Biol Phys 2007, Oct 1;69(2): 350-7.

[87] Lee C, Bayman N, Swindell R, Faivre-Finn C. Prophylactic radiotherapy to intervention sites in mesothelioma: A systematic review and survey of UK practice. Lung Cancer 2009, Nov;66(2):150-6.

[88] McAleer MF, Tsao AS, Liao Z. Radiotherapy in malignant pleural mesothelioma. Int J Radiat Oncol Biol Phys 2009, Oct 1;75(2):326-37.

[89] Boutin C, Rey F, Viallat JR. Prevention of malignant seeding after invasive diagnostic procedures in patients with pleural mesothelioma. A randomized trial of local radiotherapy. Chest 1995, Sep;108(3):754-8.

[90] O'Rourke N, Garcia JC, Paul J, Lawless C, McMenemin R, Hill J. A randomised controlled trial of intervention site radiotherapy in malignant pleural mesothelioma. Radiother Oncol 2007, Jul;84(1):18-22.

[91] Froment MA, Fréchette E, Dagnault A. Prophylactic irradiation of intervention sites in malignant pleural mesothelioma. Radiother Oncol 2011, Nov;101(2):307-10.

[92] Berghmans T, Paesmans M, Lalami Y, Louviaux I, Luce S, Mascaux C, et al. Activity of chemotherapy and immunotherapy on malignant mesothelioma: A systematic review of the literature with meta-analysis. Lung Cancer 2002, Nov;38(2):111-21.

[93] Sugarbaker DJ, Flores RM, Jaklitsch MT, Richards WG, Strauss GM, Corson JM, et al. Resection margins, extrapleural nodal status, and cell type determine postoperative long-term survival in trimodality therapy of malignant pleural mesothelioma: Results in 183 patients. J Thorac Cardiovasc Surg 1999, Jan;117(1):54-63; discussion 63-5.

[94] Vogelzang NJ, Rusthoven JJ, Symanowski J, Denham C, Kaukel E, Ruffie P, et al. Phase III study of pemetrexed in combination with cisplatin versus cisplatin alone in patients with malignant pleural mesothelioma. J Clin Oncol 2003, Jul 15;21(14): 2636-44.

[95] Ceresoli GL, Zucali PA, Favaretto AG, Grossi F, Bidoli P, Del Conte G, et al. Phase II study of pemetrexed plus carboplatin in malignant pleural mesothelioma. J Clin Oncol 2006, Mar 20;24(9):1443-8.

[96] Castagneto B, Botta M, Aitini E, Spigno F, Degiovanni D, Alabiso O, et al. Phase II study of pemetrexed in combination with carboplatin in patients with malignant pleural mesothelioma (MPM). Ann Oncol 2008, Feb;19(2):370-3.

[97] Byrne MJ, Davidson JA, Musk AW, Dewar J, van Hazel G, Buck M, et al. Cisplatin and gemcitabine treatment for malignant mesothelioma: A phase II study. J Clin Oncol 1999, Jan;17(1):25-30.

[98] Favaretto AG, Aversa SM, Paccagnella A, Manzini Vde P, Palmisano V, Oniga F, et al. Gemcitabine combined with carboplatin in patients with malignant pleural mesothelioma: A multicentric phase II study. Cancer 2003, Jun 1;97(11):2791-7.

[99] Muers MF, Stephens RJ, Fisher P, Darlison L, Higgs CM, Lowry E, et al. Active symptom control with or without chemotherapy in the treatment of patients with malig-

nant pleural mesothelioma (MS01): A multicentre randomised trial. Lancet 2008, May 17;371(9625):1685-94.

[100] Scagliotti GV, Shin DM, Kindler HL, Vasconcelles MJ, Keppler U, Manegold C, et al. Phase II study of pemetrexed with and without folic acid and vitamin B12 as front-line therapy in malignant pleural mesothelioma. J Clin Oncol 2003, Apr 15;21(8): 1556-61.

[101] Dowell JE, Dunphy FR, Taub RN, Gerber DE, Ngov L, Yan J, et al. A multicenter phase II study of cisplatin, pemetrexed, and bevacizumab in patients with advanced malignant mesothelioma. Lung Cancer 2012, Jul 4.

[102] Garland LL, Rankin C, Gandara DR, Rivkin SE, Scott KM, Nagle RB, et al. Phase II study of erlotinib in patients with malignant pleural mesothelioma: A southwest oncology group study. J Clin Oncol 2007, Jun 10;25(17):2406-13.

[103] Bottomley A, Coens C, Efficace F, Gaafar R, Manegold C, Burgers S, et al. Symptoms and patient-reported well-being: Do they predict survival in malignant pleural mesothelioma? A prognostic factor analysis of EORTC-NCIC 08983: Randomized phase III study of cisplatin with or without raltitrexed in patients with malignant pleural mesothelioma. J Clin Oncol 2007, Dec 20;25(36):5770-6.

[104] De Graaf-Strukowska L, van der Zee J, van Putten W, Senan S. Factors influencing the outcome of radiotherapy in malignant mesothelioma of the pleura--a single-institution experience with 189 patients. Int J Radiat Oncol Biol Phys 1999, Feb 1;43(3): 511-6.

Chapter 9

Definitive Chemo-Radiotherapy for Resectable Esophageal Cancer — Unresolved Problems Remain

Shouji Shimoyama

Additional information is available at the end of the chapter

http://dx.doi.org/10.5772/55501

1. Introduction

Esophageal cancer, the 8th most common cancer and 6th leading cause of cancer deaths worldwide (Jemal et al., 2010), remains an invasive disease with 5-year overall survival rates (SRs) of only 20% in the USA (Daly, et al., 1996), 13% in UK (http://info.cancerresearchuk.org/cancerstats/types/oesophagus/survival/), and less than 10% in most parts of Europe (Keighley 2003). In Japan, an updated nationwide survey (http://ganjoho.jp/public/statistics/backnumber/2011_en.html) has demonstrated 5-year SRs of 33% for all esophageal cancers and 43% for resected cases, while in the USA, the survivals have improved to 42% in the past decade (Rice et al., 2009). Still, these statistics consistently confirm that survival remains disappointing, with less than half of all patients surviving at 5 years. Where the disease appears resectable and patients are sufficiently fit, surgery remains the mainstay of curative therapy. However, the overall poor prognosis with esophagectomies has led to the investigation of multimodal therapies in order to improve the treatment results. Among these, preoperative chemoradiotherapy (CRT) (neoadjuvant CRT) has been developed and proved promising; nonetheless, morbidity and mortality have increased. What this means is that any improvement in survival rates of complete resection or local disease control by neoadjuvant CRT happens at the expense of greater toxicity. Several meta-analysis have elucidated that preoperative CRT significantly (Fiorica et al., 2004) or at least non-significantly increased (Kranzfelder et al., 2011; Urschel et al., 2003) postoperative in-hospital mortality.

On the other hand, evidence for CRT as a curative intent (definitive CRT: dCRT) has been established for patients with esophageal cancer who otherwise do not qualify for surgery due to disease extent and/or medical comorbidity. In Japan, dCRT for T4/M1(lymph) squamous cell cancer (SCC) achieved 1-, 2-, and 3-year SRs of 41%, 27-32%, and 22-23%, respectively, which compared well with SRs of T4 SCC undergoing resection (Ishida, et al., 2004; Japanese

Society of Esophageal Diseases, 2005; Y Nishimura et al., 2002; Ohtsu, et al., 1999; Kumekawa et al., 2006) [Table 1], although they were not a nonrandomized comparison. Subsequently, three pivotal RCTs demonstrated that survival results were similar between dCRT and neoadjuvant CRT followed by surgery or surgery only. A German trial revealed that dCRT with at least 65Gy for T3-4/N0-1/M0 SCC offered similar survival results with less likelihood of treatment-related mortality as compared with neoadjuvant CRT with 40Gy radiation (Stahl, et al., 2005). A French FFCD trial recruiting T3/N0-1/M0 SCC patients found no benefit of subsequent surgery following CRT for those responding to CRT (Bedenne et al., 2007). This study has established a rationale that the response to neoadjuvant CRT is a favorable prognostic sign which allows the selection of patients most likely to benefit from dCRT, thereby indicating the potential of dCRT for organ-sparing treatments. A CURE trial conducted in China compared T2-3/N1 SCC patients undergoing standard esophagectomy with those undergoing dCRT with 50-60Gy radiation and observed no survival differences between these two treatments (Chiu et al., 2005). Consequently, a very recent meta-analysis has also elucidated that there is no trend regarding differences in overall survival between surgery and dCRT (Pöttgen et al., 2012).

Author	Tumor stage	Radiation dose	Chemotherapy	Histology	Number of patients	Complete response rate	Median survival time (months)	Survival	Tretment-related death
Ohtsu, 1999	T4 and/or M1 lymph	60 Gy	Fluorouracil Cisplatin	SCC	54	33%	9	1YSR=41% 3YSR=23%	6.8%
Nishimura, 2002	T4 N0-1 M0-1	60 Gy	Fluorouracil Cisplatin	SCC	28	32%	stage III=12 stage IV=5	2YSR=27%	NA
Ishida, 2004 (JCOG9516)	T4 and/or M1 lymph	60 Gy	Fluorouracil Cisplatin	SCC	60	15%	10	2YSR=32%	1.7%
Kumekawa, 2006	T1-4 and M1lymph	60 Gy	Fluorouracil Cisplatin	SCC	81	42%	14	1YSR=62% 3YSR=22%	11.8%

YSR; year survival rate

Table 1. Treatment results of definitive chemo-radiotherapy for far advanced esophageal cancer in Japan.

Against these backgrounds and considering that surgery for esophageal cancer is a formidable procedure with significant morbidity and mortality (as discussed in section3.1) which raises concerns about its applicability in most patients, dCRT, at first investigated with palliative intent, has been further extended to resectable cases. While there was much initial enthusiasm for dCRT, notes of caution have been raised in interpreting the accumulated dCRT experience. These should be resolved for the further advancement of multimodal approaches for esophageal cancer. This chapter introduces current problems to be taken into account when performing dCRT, especially for patients with potentially resectable esophageal cancer.

2. Definitive CRT for resectable esophageal cancer is promising and could be an alternative to esophagectomy

Many chemotherapeutic agents are potential candidates that could be combined with radiation (Kleinberg et al., 2007). Among these, the most frequently used agents are fluorouracil and cisplatin, both act as radiosensitizers. Fluorouracil inhibits DNA and RNA synthesis resulting in decreasing radiation-induced DNA injury repair, which eventually enhances radiation-induced cytotoxicity. Cisplatin forms inter- and intrastrand cross-links to DNA that impede repair. This action also leads to decrease in cellular repair in response to radiation-induced damage. Therefore, besides a direct action of fluorouracil and cisplatin to DNA, these two agents and radiation act synergistically.

Several nonrandomized comparisons have been conducted to investigate whether dCRT could achieve the same impact on survival as esophagectomy for those patients deemed suitable for surgery. More important are the encouraging results of dCRT for patients with operable rather than inoperable esophageal cancer. Table 2 lists the results of dCRT for each stage of esophageal cancer; these studies of dCRT with at least 60Gy radiation have shown consistent favorable SRs, which compare favorably with the Japan nationwide 3-year SR (44%) of surgery only (Japanese Society of Esophageal diseases, 2005). Ishikura et al. (Ishikura, et al., 2003) and Hironaka et al. (Hironaka et al., 2003) respectively recruited T1-3 (70% T3) and T2-3 SCC patients, and dCRT yielded 3-year and 5-year SRs of 49-55% and 46-49%, respectively. Three other dCRT studies revealed promising 3-year SRs which were 80% for patients with stage II SCC (Morota et al., 2009), 45% for those with stage II and III SCC (K Kato et al., 2011), and 72% for those with stage 0-III SCC (Murakami et al., 1998). These results motivated the researchers to conduct dCRT studies for less progressed esophageal SCC. For T1N0M0 stage I esophageal SCC, dCRT resulted in 1-, 2-, 3-, 4-, and 5-year SRs of 98%, 93%, 79-89%, 81%, and 66-67%, respectively, which could be compared favorably with survivals of surgical cases (H Kato et al., 2009; Minashi et al., 2006; K Yamada et al., 2006; Yamamoto et al., 2011). These findings are indeed encouraging and dCRT could be an alternative to esophagectomy. In addition, since dCRT can preserve the esophagus, it could theoretically offer better posttreatment quality of life than that for patients treated by surgery. Indeed, esophagectomy resulted in worse functional, symptomatic, and global quality of life scores at 6 weeks postoperatively than before surgery (Blazeby et al., 2000). However, the recently accumulated data on dCRT has raised several issues of concern.

3. Problems remain to be resolved

3.1. Invasiveness of dCRT

When considering dCRT—especially for potentially resectable esophageal cancer, risks from the treatment, i.e., treatment-related complications or death, should be taken into account in evaluating whether dCRT could substitute for surgery. Some patients undergoing dCRT have experienced severe grade 3/4 pericarditis, pleural effusion, and radiation pneumonitis, which

Author	Tumor stage	Radiation dose	Chemotherapy	Histology	Number of patients	Complete responders (%)	Median survival time (months)	Survival
Advanced cancer								
Hironaka, 2003	T2-3 N any M0	60Gy	Fluorouracil Cisplatin	SCC	53	37(70%)	33	3YSR=49% 5YSR=46%
Ishikura, 2003	T1-3,M0 (70% T3)	60Gy	Fluorouracil Cisplatin	SCC	67	ND	44	3YSR=55% 5YSR=49%
Kato, 2011 (JCOG9906)	II and III	60Gy	Fluorouracil Cisplatin	SCC	76	46(62%)	29	3YSR=45% 5YSR=37%
Morota, 2009	I-IVB	60Gy	Fluorouracil Cisplatin	SCC	69	36(52.2%)	ND	stage I 3YSR=80% stage II 3YSR=80% stage III 3YSR=30% stage IV 3YSR=30%
Murakami, 1998	0-III	60-75Gy	Fluorouracil Cisplatin	SCC	30	16(53.3%)	not reached	2YSR=81% 3YSR=72%
T1 cancer								
Kato, 2009 (JCOG9708)	T1N0M0	30Gy	Fluorouracil Cisplatin	SCC	72	63(88%)	not reached	2YSR=93% 4YSR=81%
Minashi, 2006	T1N0M0	60Gy	Fluorouracil Cisplatin	SCC	41	36(88%)	not reached	1YSR=98% 3YSR=79% 5YSR=67%
Yamada, 2006	T1N0M0	55-66Gy	Fluorouracil Cisplatin	SCC	63	ND	ND	5YSR=66%
Yamamoto, 2011	T1N0M0	60Gy	Fluorouracil Cisplatin	SCC	54	ND	not reached	1YSR=98% 3YSR=89%

SCC; squamous cell cancer, YSR; year survival rate

ND; not described

Table 2. Treatment results of definitive chemo-radiotherapy for potentially resectable esophageal cancer.

respectively developed in 1.4-16% (Hironaka et al., 2003; Ishikura et al., 2003; K Kato et al., 2011; Kumekawa et al., 2006; Minashi et al., 2006; Morota et al., 2009; Sasamoto et al., 2007), 1.4-14% (Hironaka et al., 2003;, Ishihara et al., 2010; Ishikura et al., 2003; K Kato et al., 2011; Kumekawa et al., 2006; Li et al., 2010; Minashi et al., 2006; Morota et al., 2009; Sasamoto et al., 2007), and 1.2-14% (Hironaka et al., 2003;, Ishihara et al., 2010; Ishikura et al., 2003; K Kato et al., 2011; Kumekawa et al., 2006; Morota et al., 2009; Sai et al., 2004; Yamamoto et al., 2011; Yamashita et al., 2008) of the study population. These complications eventually caused

http://dx.doi.org/10.5772/55501

treatment-related death at a rate of 3-14% of the study population (K Kato et al., 2011; Morota et al., 2009; Sai et al., 2004; Sasamoto et al., 2007; Yamashita et al., 2008) or 8-12% of the CR patients (Ishihara et al., 2010; Ishikura et al., 2003; Kumekawa et al., 2006; Minashi et al., 2006; Sasamoto et al., 2007) [Table 3]. Especially, 8% of treatment-related death among the CR patients with stage I disease (Minashi et al., 2006) cannot be overlooked because they would be expected to survive by surgery unless fatal complications occurred.

Author	Grade 3/4 Toxicities			Tretment-related death	
	Pericarditis	Pleural effusion	Pneumonitis	of all patients	of CR patients
Hironaka, 2003	10.8%*	13.5%*	8.1%*	0.0%	ND
Ishihara, 2010	NA	0.9%**	2.7%**	ND	8.2%
Ishikura, 2003	5.8%	5.8%	2.2%	ND	10.3%
Kato, 2011 (JCOG9906)	16.0%	9.0%	4.0%	5.3%	ND
Kumekawa, 2006	3.7%	3.7%	1.2%	ND	11.8%
Li , 2010	NA	6.8%	NA	ND	ND
Minashi, 2006	2.8%*	11.1%*	0.0%	ND	8.3%
Morota, 2009	1.4%	1.4%	1.4%	2.9%	ND
Sai, 2004	NA	NA	13.8%	13.8%	ND
Sasamoto, 2007	8.9%	8.9%	NA	7.1%	7.1%
Yamamoto, 2011	0.0%	0.0%	3.7%	ND	ND
Yamashita, 2008	NA	NA	6.1%	6.1%	ND

*among the complete responders, **death rate

ND; not described, CR; complete response

Table 3. Mortality and late morbidity of definitive chemo-radiotherapy.

The heart is susceptible to radiation injury. Pericardial damage is most frequently mentioned, but all structures of the heart are at risk. Mediastinal radiation causes inflammation and progressive fibrosis of all of the structures of this organ. A worsening of clinical severity with increased radiation volume has been suggested. The risk of pericarditis has been found to rise with increased total dose and larger dose per fraction, reaching 3-fold and 2-fold greater relative risks at total doses of 41 Gy or greater, or a dose per fraction of 3.0 Gy or greater, respectively (Cosset et al., 1991). Another study also demonstrated that larger fraction size has a significant relationship with the chance of pericarditis (Martel et al., 1998). These observations suggest that dose effect as well as fractionation effect account for the increased risk of pericarditis.

Radiation pneumonitis has been reported in patients who have undergone mediastinal radiation therapy for various diseases. The risks of radiation pneumonitis rise when radiotherapy is combined with chemotherapy (McDonald et al., 1995; M Yamada et al., 1998). The risks of lung toxicity appear to be related to dose-volume parameters such as the irradiated lung volume, mean lung dose (Hernando et al., 2001), total dose (Roach et al., 1995), daily fraction dose (Roach et al., 1995), and number of daily fractions (Roach et al., 1995), —although there are some inconsistencies (Allen et al., 2003). Similarly, the percentage of lungs receiving a specified dose has also been reported to be a predictor of pneumonitis (Madani et al., 2007; Tsujino et al., 2003).

The obstruction of cardiac and mediastinal lymphatic vessels due to radiation fibrosis has been postulated as a possible etiology of radiation-induced pericardial and pleural effusions. As a result, radiation-induced cardiac or lung disease is responsible for a certain fraction of death not directly attributable to esophageal cancer itself in some patients who would survive if they could have undergone surgery without complications. Although nonsurgical approaches are appealing in trying to manage this difficult disease, it is a fact that there is a fine therapeutic window because of the significant toxicities, and the toxicity may outweigh any potential advantages.

If treatment-related morbidity and mortality of dCRT exceed those of surgery, the benefits of dCRT may be cancelled. Therefore, the risk balance between dCRT and surgery should be taken into account in consideration of dCRT; however, one should remember that the morbidity and mortality of esophagectomy differ considerably between countries. Surgical mortality was 2-4% in Japan (Fujita et al., 2010; Suzuki et al., 2011; Tachimori et al., 2009), while 4.2-7.6% in Taiwan (Lin et al., 2006), 6% in Italy (Ruol et al., 2009), 4-13% in the Netherlands (Steyerberg et al., 2006; Wouters et al., 2008), and 6-23% in the USA (Atkins et al., 2004; Bailey et al., 2003; Birkmeyer et al., 2002; Dimick et al., 2005; Finks et al., 2011; Rentz et al., 2003), suggesting that differences in surgical mortality between countries can be more than doubled or quadrupled.

However, the risk comparison between dCRT and surgery should require considerations of the hospital volume, surgeon volume, specialization, study period, and country, i.e., when and where the studies of dCRT are conducted, as well as the number of esphagectomies that each surgeon performs. With regard to hospital volume, even in the USA —where surgical mortality is generally high, hospital mortality after esophagectomy varied from 23% for institutions undertaking <2 cases per annum to 8% for those undertaking 20 or more cases per annum (Birkmeyer et al., 2002). In Japan, the average mortality was 1.8% when >51 esophagectomies per annum were undertaken, compared with 4.6% if 20 or fewer esophagectomies were performed per annum (Suzuki et al., 2011). Fujita et al. (Fujita et al., 2010) and Kazui et al. (Kazui et al., 2007) also reported a larger hospital volume with a lower 30-day or in-hospital mortality rates. The same volume-outcome relationship was also observed in Taiwan (Lin et al., 2006) and the Netherlands (Wouters et al., 2008). In addition, high volume surgeons experienced a 4.2% mortality rate, which was one-quarter of that of low volume surgeons, approaching the average in-hospital mortality in Japan (Migliore et al., 2007). Also in Japan, risk of morbidity by low volume surgeons is twice that of high volume surgeons (Yasunaga et al., 2009). Collectively, a larger experience of esophagectomies could significantly reduce the 30-day or in-hospital mortality from 18% to 5% (Metzger et al., 2004).

http://dx.doi.org/10.5772/55501

The study period is also a determinant. Single institutions in the USA (Orringer et al., 2007) or Italy (Ruol et al., 2009) experienced consistently decreased hospital mortality from 4% to 1% (Orringer et al., 2007) or from 8.2% to 2.6% (Ruol et al., 2009). Taking into account the various determinants of hospital mortality, the treatment-related death rates of 8-12% among CR patients of dCRT are undoubtedly higher than those of surgical mortality in Japan, but equal to or lower than in some countries. Considering the balance between the risks of dCRT and those of surgery, dCRT is regarded as a risky treatment as compared with surgery in some countries or in some institutions where surgery can be performed more safely.

3.2. Response evaluation is not necessarily perfect

The lack of any definitive diagnostic methods currently available for the response evaluation after dCRT remain pressing issues following dCRT. Strikingly, some segments of patients who underwent surgery following dCRT due to persistent disease proved to be complete responders postoperatively. The rates of such seemingly unnecessary salvage surgery are 10-50% (Ariga, et al., 2009; Beseth et al., 2000; Lim et al., 2003; Murakami et al., 1998; M Nishimura et al., 2007; Tachimori et al., 2009; Wilson et al., 2002). On the other hand, clinically diagnosed CR patients sometimes prove to have residual diseases and eventually exhibit relapse. The rates of overall recurrence or local recurrence after CR are substantial, being respectively 19-67% and 14-40% (Di Fiore et al., 2006; Ishihara et al., 2010; Kumekawa et al., 2006; Minashi et al., 2006; Morota et al., 2009; Murakami et al., 1998; Takeuchi et al., 2007; Tougeron et al., 2008; Wilson et al., 2000) [Table 4], suggesting that patients whose tumor response is deemed complete after dCRT could have residual diseases and that clinically CR is not always a reason to preclude further additional treatment. Such local recurrence rates do not depend on the initial tumor stage or depth. These discrepancies may be ascribed to the limitations of current imaging methods.

There are several diagnostic tools for evaluating responses to CRT. Endoscopy is an easily available means of investigation, but its accuracy is low as recurrent or residual tumors often lie beneath the mucosa [Figure 1]. Negative endoscopy findings have sometimes included microscopic foci of a residual tumor in the resected esophagus specimens. Moreover, the differentiation between tumor and radiation changes is not easy. A false negative rate of 48% for biopsy by endoscopy (Jones et al., 1997) suggests a poor correlation between endoscopic findings and pathologic status.

Endoscopic ultrasonography (EUS) also cannot reliably distinguish a residual tumor from postinflammatory changes, which is, on the other hand, a characteristic of the efficacy of dCRT. Even in earlier reports demonstrating the efficacy of EUS, (Hirata et al., 1997; Willis et al., 2002), it should be noted that a perfect discrimination between T0 and T1 tumors was not a consideration) since a certain degree of remaining tumor (<50-70%) was considered an EUS-based response, or a scattered or even a remaining degree of 1/3< viable cells was considered a pathological response. Such a cut-off value is less useful for deciding the need for salvage surgery following dCRT because only patients with no viable cells could theoretically be escaped from salvage surgery. EUS T staging accuracy after neoadjuvant CRT was only 43%,

Author	Tumor stage	Radiation dose	Histology	Number of patients	Complete responders (%)	Overall recurrence rate after CR	Local recurrence rate after CR
Di Fiore, 2006	T1-4/N0-1/M0	50 Gy or 60 Gy	SCC	116	86 (74.1%)	ND	40%
Ishihara, 2010	I-IVA	60 Gy	ND	173	110 (63.6%)	26%	12%
Kumekawa, 2006	T1-4 and M1lymph	60 Gy	SCC	81	34(42.0%)	ND	25%
Minashi, 2006	T1N0M0	60 Gy	SCC	41	36(88%)	39%	14%
Morota, 2009	I-IVB	60 Gy	SCC	69	36(52.2%)	ND	17%
Murakami, 1998	0-III	60-75 Gy	SCC	30	16(53.3%)	19%	ND
Takeuchi, 2007	II-III	60 Gy	SCC	178	113 (63.5%)	36%	ND
Tougeron, 2008	I-IV	50-55 Gy	SCC+ADC	109	63(58%)	52%	33%
Wilson, 2000	anyT, anyN, M0	50 Gy	SCC+ADC	31	24 (77.4%)	67%	21%

SCC; squamous cell cancer. ADC; adenocarcinoma

ND; not described, CR; complete response

Table 4. Overall and local recurrence rates among CR patients undergoing dCRT.

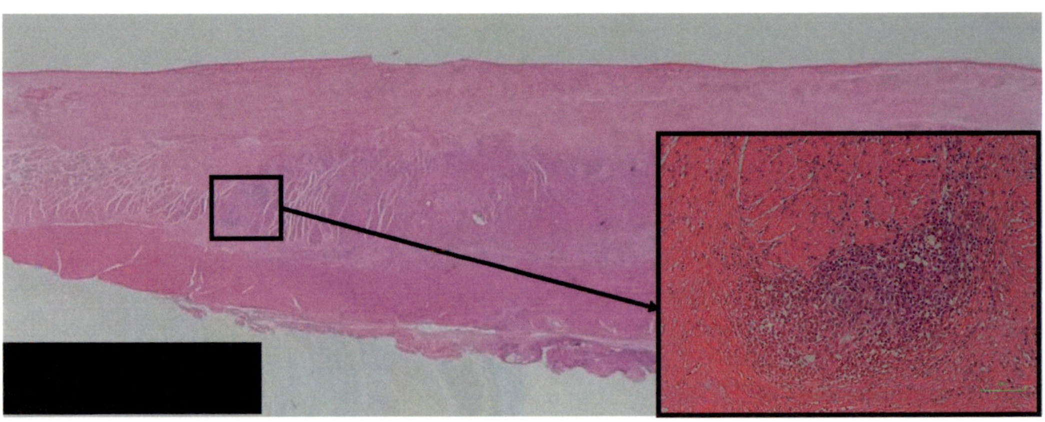

Figure 1. Low and high magnifications of a patient who was considered CR after CRT. Histological specimens revealed small foci of a residual tumor in the esophageal wall which could not be detected by endoscopically obtained biopsy specimens preoperatively.

a rate ascribed to significant fibrosis and inflammation caused by CRT (Isenberg et al., 1998). Consequently, EUS had a tendency to overstage lower pathological T stages. On the other hand, 79% of pathologically complete responders were diagnosed as having T+ disease (Zuccaro et al., 1999). These T+ patients underwent immediate post CRT surgery, but this could deem unnecessary because of pathological CR. Similarly, EUS could not detect microscopic disease, while 27% of patients with positive EUS findings proved to have no residual tumor in the resected specimens (Beseth et al., 2000). Furthermore, EUS may be suboptimal when the sonography probe cannot pass the tumor.

Researchers have reported a low accuracy of CT for the assessment of responses in patients with esophageal cancer; this accuracy was substantially worse than that of EUS and FDG-PET (fluorine18-labelled deoxyglucose in positron emission tomography). This is most likely owing to the difficulty in the differentiation between viable tumors and reactive changes, including edema, fibrosis, and inflammation at CT. CT tumor volume change was poorly correlated with pathological tumor response (Griffith et al., 1999). Some tumors exhibited marked volume regression with a poor histological response, while some tumors showed little volume regression with a considerable histological response. This means that CT by itself represents an inadequate tool in assessing those who have residual disease and those who should undergo surgery following CRT. Jones et al. reported the same results (Jones, et al., 1999).

On the other hand, PET is a useful noninvasive tool in discriminating responders from nonresponders, with the colleration between PET-based response assessment and pathology being 78% (Flamen et al., 2002). The sensitivity and specificity of PET ranged from 71-100% and 55-95%, respectively (Brücher et al., 2001; Flamen et a., 2002; Weber et al., 2001). Any false positive results are attributable to the metabolically active leukocytes or macrophages associated with post CRT inflammation. False negative phenomena can occur because PET is unable to detect perfectly the residual viable disease in the primary tumor.

3.3. Salvage surgery is highly invasive

Patients who have received dCRT should undergo subsequent surgery if the tumors exhibit strictures or subsequent relapse. Salvage surgery is a surgery for residual or recurrent disease following dCRT, but it is technically more difficult and highly invasive than primary surgery, leading to increased morbidity (50-79%) and in-hospital mortality (7-22%) due to the adverse events of predominantly respiratory complications and anastomotic leakage (Chao et al., 2009; Nakamura et al., 2004; M. Nishimura et al., 2007; Oki et al., 2007; Smithers et al., 2007; Swisher et al., 2002; Tachimori et al., 2009; Tomimaru et al., 2006). These complications are attributable to the radiation-induced injury in the thoracic cavity that causes an increase in bleeding, fibrotic masses around the tumor due to the fibrogenic pathway that makes surgical technique more difficult, and an increasingly fragile stomach, esophagus, and trachea arising from the impaired blood supply that eventually causes anastomotic leakage or conduit necrosis. Even in Japan, these hospital mortality rates are obviously higher than those for primary esophagectomy reported from specialized centers or in a nationwide survey (2-4%) (Fujita et al., 2010; Suzuki et al., 2011; Tachimori et al., 2009). Reserving surgery for patients not already cured by CRT should always be taken into account in performing dCRT, and efforts should be continuously made to reduce mortality and to select patients who stand to benefit most from this invasive treatment.

First, invasiveness undoubtedly depends on surgical procedure. The most common surgical approaches which are applicable to cancers of the upper, middle and lower esophagus are the Ivor-Lewis or McKeown esophagectomy. The Ivor-Lewis esophagectomy involves right thoracotomy with midline laparotomy and an anastomosis of the gastric conduit to the proximal mediastinal esophagus (at or above the azygos vein). The McKeown technique involves right thoracotomy, laparotomy, and cervical anastomosis, which facilitates precise surgical staging and enables more local control (van de Ven et al., 1999). The extent of lymphadenectomy is three-field (cervial thoracic, abdominal), which has traditionally been more prevalent in Japan, measuring the prevalence of positive cervical nodes (Akiyama et al., 1994; Nishihira et al., 1995). The survival benefit of three-field lymphadenectomy was suggeted in Japanese (Nishihira et al., 1998) and Western series (Altorki et al., 2002). Importantly, the risks of positive cervical nodes are substantial even at an earlier stage (Stein et al., 2005), and are seemingly independent of histological types (SCC or adenocarcinoma) or independent of tumor location within the esophagus (Akiyama et al., 1994; van de Ven et al., 1999). The McKeown technique enables this dissection to be performed under direct vision, allowing more precise dissection in cases where the tumor is large, lymphadenopathy is present, or the tumor is located in proximity to the airway (upper or middle thoracic esophagus). However, in salvage surgery, attempts have been made to reduce surgical morbidity and mortality with preservation of the blood supply to the trachea or to the main bronchus as well as to the reconstruction conduit. These include a reduced scope of lymphadenectomy with avoidance of cervical lymph node dissection or the preservation of right and left bronchial arteries (Tachimori et al., 2009).

Second, an accurate prediction of resection status prior to surgery is important at the time of completion of dCRT since resection status is one of the significant factors that affect survival after salvage surgery. Long term survivors after salvage surgery were those undergoing R0 resection, while no patients left with gross or microscopic residual tumors after salvage surgery (R1/R2 resections) survived more than 24 months in any series (Chao et al., 2009; Nakamura et al., 2004; Oki et al., 2007; Swisher et al., 2002; Tachimori et al., 2009; Tomimaru et al., 2006). Multivariate analysis also confirmed resection status correlation with patient survival (Chao et al., 2009; Tomimaru et al., 2006). However, the resection status cannot be confidently predicted before surgery or even during surgery because of the indistinct planes between a tumor and fibrotic masses within the irradiated mediastinum. In this regard, PET, which has a relatively high specificity, could identify non-responders for dCRT and may be a more useful imaging modality than CT or EUS (Swisher et al., 2004) to select patients who are absolutely unfit for salvage surgery, allowing for early modifications of the treatment strategy of such selected patients.

Third, it is imaginable that larger, more advanced cancers are more difficult to control than smaller ones and require longer doses of RT; however, higher radiation doses are associated with increased morbidity. A dose of 60Gy of radiation has been used for dCRT in Japan (Kenjo et al., 2009). In this regard, the possibility of reducing total radiation volume from 64.8Gy to

50.4Gy (Minsky et al., 2002; Nakajima et al., 2009) has recently prompted a phase II study of dCRT with a radiation dose of 50.4Gy for stage II/III esophageal SCC (JCOG0909).

4. Future perspectives

The combination of conventional CRT with molecular targeting therapies has been developing. This combination is encouraged by the findings that radiotherapy plus cetuximab, a monoclonal antibody against epidermal growth factor receptor, for loco-regionally advanced SCC of the head and neck resulted in the prolonged duration of loco-regional control, progression free survival, and overall survival as compared with radiotherapy alone (Bonner et al., 2006; Bonner et al., 2010). The feasibility of adding cetuximab to CRT for esophageal cancer is supported by the safety profiles of this combination without any increase in esophagitis or other radiation-enhanced toxicity (Safran et al., 2008). The ongoing phase III trials (NCT 00655876, NCT01107639, NCT00509561) will provide evidence whether cetuximab in combination with CRT is effective in locally advanced or resectable esophageal cancer (http://clinicaltrials.gov).

A gain in survival with a substantial increase in toxicity necessitates considerable caution that immediately draws the attention of clinicians. Diagnostic tools which can accurately evaluate tumor response early in the course of dCRT can facilitate decisions about whether this toxic therapy should be continued in responders, or stopped in non-responders. However, there are currently no modalities that can definitively confirm CR. The reason for this problem is that the tools to estimate individual patient prognosis or tumor response are unreliable, and a diagnosis of CR is possibly merely by resected specimens. This means that negative findings by these imaging methods do not rule out residual disease. Clearly, patients with residual disease would no longer be long term survivors without undergoing resection. Therefore, efforts should continue to establish diagnostic tools for the detection of residual diseases after CRT.

One challenge in this regard lies in the detection of histologic markers—such as p53, Ki67, and EGF-R—for the prediction of therapeutic response; however, neither a single marker nor a combination of markers can correctly be used to predict the response with sufficient accuracy. The small number of patients or small number of genes investigated in this field is a further limitation. In the future, gene profiling may help identify markers that can be used in combination with conventional imaging methods for the prediction of the response to dCRT.

Author details

Shouji Shimoyama

Gastrointestinal Unit, Settlement Clinic, Japan

References

[1] Akiyama, H, Tsurumaru, M, Udagawa, H, & Kajiyama, Y. (1994). Radical lymph node dissection for cancer of the thoracic esophagus. Ann Surg. , 220(3)

[2] Allen, A. M, & Henning, G. T. Ten Haken, R.K., Hayman, J.A., & Martel, M.K. ((2003). Do dose-volume metrics predict pulmonary function changes in lung irradiation? Int J Radiat Oncol Biol Phys. , 55(4), 921-929.

[3] Altorki, N, Kent, M, Ferrara, C, & Port, J. (2002). Three-field lymph node dissection for squamous cell and adenocarcinoma of the esophagus. Ann Surg. , 236(2)

[4] Ariga, H, Nemoto, K, Miyazaki, S, Yoshioka, T, Ogawa, Y, Sakayauchi, T, Jingu, K, Miyata, G, Onodera, K, Ichikawa, H, Kamei, T, Kato, S, Ishioka, C, Satomi, S, & Yamada, S. (2009). Prospective comparison of surgery alone and chemo-radiotherapy with selective surgery in resectable squamous cell carcinoma of the esophagus. Int J Radiat Oncol Biol Phys. , 75(2), 348-356.

[5] Atkins, B. Z, Shah, A. S, Hutcheson, K. A, Mangum, J. H, Pappas, T. N, & Harpole, D. H. Jr, & D'Amico, T.A. ((2004). Reducing hospital morbidity and mortality following esophagectomy. Ann Thorac Surg. , 78(4), 1170-1176.

[6] Bailey, S. H, Bull, D. A, Harpole, D. H, Rentz, J. J, Neumayer, L. A, Pappas, T. N, Daley, J, Henderson, W. G, Krasnicka, B, & Khuri, S. F. (2003). Outcomes after esophagectomy: a ten-year prospective cohort. Ann Thorac Surg. , 75(1), 217-222.

[7] Bedenne, L, Michel, P, Bouché, O, Milan, C, Mariette, C, Conroy, T, Pezet, D, Roullet, B, Seitz, J. F, Herr, J. P, Paillot, B, Arveux, P, Bonnetain, F, & Binquet, C. (2007). Chemoradiation followed by surgery compared with chemoradiation alone in squamous cancer of the esophagus: FFCD 9102. J Clin Oncol. , 25(10), 1160-1168.

[8] Beseth, B. D, Bedford, R, Isacoff, W. H, Holmes, E. C, & Cameron, R. B. (2000). Endoscopic ultrasound does not accurately assess pathologic stage of esophageal cancer after neoadjuvant chemo-radiotherapy. Am Surg. , 66(9), 827-831.

[9] Birkmeyer, J. D, Siewers, A. E, Finlayson, E. V, Stukel, T. A, Lucas, F. L, Batista, I, Welch, H. G, & Wennberg, D. E. (2002). Hospital volume and surgical mortality in the United States. N Engl J Med. , 346(15), 1128-1137.

[10] Blazeby, J. M, Farndon, J. R, Donovan, J, & Alderson, D. (2000). A prospective longitudinal study examining the quality of life of patients with esophageal carcinoma. Cancer. , 88(8), 1781-1787.

[11] Bonner, J. A, Harari, P. M, Giralt, J, Azarnia, N, Shin, D. M, Cohen, R. B, Jones, C. U, Sur, R, Raben, D, Jassem, J, Ove, R, Kies, M. S, Baselga, J, Youssoufian, H, Amellal, N, Rowinsky, E. K, & Ang, K. K. (2006). Radiotherapy plus cetuximab for squamous-cell carcinoma of the head and neck. N Engl J Med. , 354(6), 567-578.

[12] Bonner, J. A, Harari, P. M, Giralt, J, Cohen, R. B, Jones, C. U, Sur, R. K, Raben, D, Baselga, J, Spencer, S. A, Zhu, J, Youssoufian, H, Rowinsky, E. K, & Ang, K. K. (2010). Radiotherapy plus cetuximab for locoregionally advanced head and neck cancer: 5-year survival data from a phase 3 randomised trial, and relation between cetuximab-induced rash and survival. Lancet Oncol. , 11(1), 21-28.

[13] Brücher, B. L, Weber, W, Bauer, M, Fink, U, Avril, N, Stein, H. J, Werner, M, Zimmerman, F, Siewert, J. R, & Schwaiger, M. (2001). Neoadjuvant therapy of esophageal squamous cell carcinoma: response evaluation by positron emission tomography. Ann Surg. , 233(3), 300-309.

[14] Chao, Y. K, Chan, S. C, Chang, H. K, Liu, Y. H, Wu, Y. C, Hsieh, M. J, Tseng, C. K, & Liu, H. P. (2009). Salvage surgery after failed chemo-radiotherapy in squamous cell carcinoma of the esophagus. Eur J Surg Oncol. , 35(3), 289-294.

[15] Chiu, P. W, Chan, A. C, Leung, S. F, Leong, H. T, Kwong, K. H, Li, M. K, Au-yeung, A. C, Chung, S. C, & Ng, E. K. (2005). Multicenter prospective randomized trial comparing standard esophagectomy with chemo-radiotherapy for treatment of squamous esophageal cancer: early results from the Chinese University Research Group for Esophageal Cancer (CURE). J Gastrointest Surg. , 9(6), 794-802.

[16] http://clinicaltrialsgov

[17] Cosset, J. M, Henry-amar, M, Pellae-cosset, B, Carde, P, Girinski, T, Tubiana, M, & Hayat, M. (1991). Pericarditis and myocardial infarctions after Hodgkin's disease therapy. Int J Radiat Oncol Biol Phys. , 21(2), 447-449.

[18] Daly, J. M, Karnell, L. H, & Menck, H. R. (1996). National Cancer Data Base report on esophageal carcinoma. Cancer. , 78(8), 1820-1828.

[19] Di FioreF., Lecleire, S., Rigal, O., Galais, M.P., Ben Soussan, E., David, I., Paillot, B., Jacob, J.H., & Michel, P. ((2006). Predictive factors of survival in patients treated with definitive chemo-radiotherapy for squamous cell esophageal carcinoma. World J Gastroenterol. , 12(26), 4185-4190.

[20] Dimick, J. B, Wainess, R. M, & Upchurch, G. R. Jr, Iannettoni, M.D., & Orringer, M.B. ((2005). National trends in outcomes for esophageal resection. Ann Thorac Surg. , 79(1), 212-216.

[21] Finks, J. F, Osborne, N. H, & Birkmeyer, J. D. (2011). Trends in hospital volume and operative mortality for high-risk surgery. N Engl J Med. , 364(22), 2128-2137.

[22] Fiorica, F. Di Bona, D., Schepis, F., Licata, A., Shahied, L., Venturi, A., Falchi, A.M., Craxì, A., & Cammà, C. ((2004). Preoperative chemo-radiotherapy for oesophageal cancer: a systematic review and meta-analysis. Gut. , 53(7), 925-930.

[23] Flamen, P, Van Cutsem, E, Lerut, A, Cambier, J. P, Haustermans, K, Bormans, G, De Leyn, P, Van Raemdonck, D, De Wever, W, Ectors, N, Maes, A, & Mortelmans, L. (2002). Positron emission tomography for assessment of the response to induction ra-

diochemotherapy in locally advanced oesophageal cancer. Ann Oncol. , 13(3), 361-368.

[24] Fujita, H, Ozawa, S, Kuwano, H, Ueda, Y, Hattori, S, & Yanagawa, T. (2010). Esophagectomy for cancer: clinical concerns support centralizing operations within the larger hospitals. Dis Esophagus. , 23(2), 145-152.

[25] http://ganjohojp/public/statistics/backnumber/(2011). en.html

[26] Griffith, J. F, Chan, A. C, Chow, L. T, Leung, S. F, Lam, Y. H, Liang, E. Y, Chung, S. C, & Metreweli, C. (1999). Assessing chemotherapy response of squamous cell oesophageal carcinoma with spiral CT. Br J Radiol. , 72(859), 678-684.

[27] Hernando, M. L, Marks, L. B, Bentel, G. C, Zhou, S. M, Hollis, D, Das, S. K, Fan, M, Munley, M. T, Shafman, T. D, Anscher, M. S, & Lind, P. A. (2001). Radiation-induced pulmonary toxicity: a dose-volume histogram analysis in 201 patients with lung cancer. Int J Radiat Oncol Biol Phys. , 51(3), 650-659.

[28] Hirata, N, Kawamoto, K, Ueyama, T, Masuda, K, Utsunomiya, T, & Kuwano, H. (1997). Using endosonography to assess the effects of neoadjuvant therapy in patients with advanced esophageal cancer. AJR Am J Roentgenol. , 169(2), 485-491.

[29] Hironaka, S, Ohtsu, A, Boku, N, Muto, M, Nagashima, F, Saito, H, Yoshida, S, Nishimura, M, Haruno, M, Ishikura, S, Ogino, T, Yamamoto, S, & Ochiai, A. (2003). Nonrandomized comparison between definitive chemo-radiotherapy and radical surgery in patients with T(2-3)N(any) M(0) squamous cell carcinoma of the esophagus. Int J Radiat Oncol Biol Phys. , 57(2), 425-433.

[30] http://infocancerresearchuk.org/cancerstats/types/oesophagus/survival/

[31] Isenberg, G, Chak, A, Canto, M. I, Levitan, N, Clayman, J, Pollack, B. J, & Sivak, M. V. Jr. ((1998). Endoscopic ultrasound in restaging of esophageal cancer after neoadjuvant chemoradiation. Gastrointest Endosc. , 48(2), 158-163.

[32] Ishida, K, Ando, N, Yamamoto, S, Ide, H, & Shinoda, M. (2004). Phase II study of cisplatin and 5-fluorouracil with concurrent radiotherapy in advanced squamous cell carcinoma of the esophagus: a Japan Esophageal Oncology Group (JEOG)/Japan Clinical Oncology Group trial (JCOG9516). Jpn J Clin Oncol. , 34(10), 615-619.

[33] Ishihara, R, Yamamoto, S, Iishi, H, Takeuchi, Y, Sugimoto, N, Higashino, K, Uedo, N, Tatsuta, M, Yano, M, Imai, A, & Nishiyama, K. (2010). Factors predictive of tumor recurrence and survival after initial complete response of esophageal squamous cell carcinoma to definitive chemo-radiotherapy. Int J Radiat Oncol Biol Phys. , 76(1), 123-129.

[34] Ishikura, S, Nihei, K, Ohtsu, A, Boku, N, Hironaka, S, Mera, K, Muto, M, Ogino, T, & Yoshida, S. (2003). Long-term toxicity after definitive chemo-radiotherapy for squamous cell carcinoma of the thoracic esophagus. J Clin Oncol. , 21(14), 2697-2702.

[35] Japanese Society of Esophageal diseasesComprehensive registry of esophageal cancer in Japan, 1999. ((2005). Esophagus, , 2(2), 43-69.

[36] Jemal, A, Center, M. M, Desantis, C, & Ward, E. M. (2010). Global patterns of cancer incidence and mortality rates and trends. Cancer Epidemiol Biomarkers Prev. , 19(8), 1893-1907.

[37] Jones, D. R, Detterbeck, F. C, Egan, T. M, & Parker, L. A. Jr, Bernard, S.A., & Tepper, J.E. ((1997). Induction chemo-radiotherapy followed by esophagectomy in patients with carcinoma of the esophagus. Ann Thorac Surg. , 64(1), 185-191.

[38] Jones, D. R, & Parker, L. A. Jr, Detterbeck, F.C., & Egan, T.M. ((1999). Inadequacy of computed tomography in assessing patients with esophageal carcinoma after induction chemo-radiotherapy. Cancer. , 85(5)

[39] Kato, H, Sato, A, Fukuda, H, Kagami, Y, Udagawa, H, Togo, A, Ando, N, Tanaka, O, Shinoda, M, Yamana, H, & Ishikura, S. II trial of chemo-radiotherapy for stage I esophageal squamous cell carcinoma: Japan Clinical Oncology Group Study (JCOG9708). Jpn J Clin Oncol. , 39(10), 638-643.

[40] Kato, K, Muro, K, Minashi, K, Ohtsu, A, Ishikura, S, Boku, N, Takiuchi, H, Komatsu, Y, Miyata, Y, & Fukuda, H. Gastrointestinal Oncology Study Group of the Japan Clinical Oncology Group (JCOG). ((2011). Phase II Study of Chemo-radiotherapy with 5-Fluorouracil and Cisplatin for Stage II-III Esophageal Squamous Cell Carcinoma: JCOG Trial (JCOG 9906). Int J Radiat Oncol Biol Phys. , 81(3), 684-690.

[41] Kazui, T, Osada, H, & Fujita, H. Committee for Scientific Affairs. ((2007). An attempt to analyze the relation between hospital surgical volume and clinical outcome. Gen Thorac Cardiovasc Surg. , 55(12), 483-492.

[42] Keighley, M. R. (2003). Gastrointestinal cancers in Europe. Aliment Pharmacol Ther. Suppl 3, , 18, 7-30.

[43] Kenjo, M, Uno, T, Murakami, Y, Nagata, Y, Oguchi, M, Saito, S, Numasaki, H, Teshima, T, & Mitsumori, M. (2009). Radiation therapy for esophageal cancer in Japan: results of the Patterns of Care Study 1999-2001. Int J Radiat Oncol Biol Phys. , 75(2), 357-363.

[44] Kleinberg, L, Gibson, M, Forastiere, K, & Chemo-radiotherapy, A. A. for localized esophageal cancer: regimen selection and molecular mechanisms of radiosensitization. Nat Clin Pract Oncol. , 4(5), 282-294.

[45] Kranzfelder, M, Schuster, T, Geinitz, H, Friess, H, & Büchler, P. (2011). Meta-analysis of neoadjuvant treatment modalities and definitive non-surgical therapy for oesophageal squamous cell cancer. Br J Surg. , 98(6), 768-783.

[46] Kumekawa, Y, Kaneko, K, Ito, H, Kurahashi, T, Konishi, K, Katagiri, A, Yamamoto, T, Kuwahara, M, Kubota, Y, Muramoto, T, Mizutani, Y, & Imawari, M. (2006). Late

toxicity in complete response cases after definitive chemo-radiotherapy for esophageal squamous cell carcinoma. J Gastroenterol. , 41(5), 425-432.

[47] Li, Q. Q, Liu, M. Z, Hu, Y. H, Liu, H, He, Z. Y, & Lin, H. X. (2010). Definitive concomitant chemo-radiotherapy with docetaxel and cisplatin in squamous esophageal carcinoma. Dis Esophagus. , 23(3), 253-259.

[48] Lim, J. T, Truong, P. T, Berthelet, E, Pai, H, Joe, H, Wai, E, Larsson, S, Kader, H. A, Weinerman, B, Wilson, K, & Olivotto, I. A. (2003). Endoscopic response predicts for survival and organ preservation after primary chemo-radiotherapy for esophageal cancer. Int J Radiat Oncol Biol Phys. , 57(5), 1328-1335.

[49] Lin, H. C, Xirasagar, S, Lee, H. C, & Chai, C. Y. (2006). Hospital volume and inpatient mortality after cancer-related gastrointestinal resections: the experience of an Asian country. Ann Surg Oncol. , 13(9), 1182-1188.

[50] Madani, I, De Ruyck, K, Goeminne, H, De Neve, W, Thierens, H, & Van Meerbeeck, J. (2007). Predicting risk of radiation-induced lung injury. J Thorac Oncol. , 2(9), 864-874.

[51] Martel, M. K, & Sahijdak, W. M. Ten Haken, R.K., Kessler, M.L., & Turrisi, A.T. ((1998).

[52] Fraction size and dose parameters related to the incidence of pericardial effusionsInt J Radiat Oncol Biol Phys. , 40(1), 155-161.

[53] Mcdonald, S, Rubin, P, Phillips, T. L, & Marks, L. B. (1995). Injury to the lung from cancer therapy: clinical syndromes, measurable endpoints, and potential scoring systems. Int J Radiat Oncol Biol Phys. , 31(5), 1187-1203.

[54] Metzger, R, Bollschweiler, E, Vallböhmer, D, Maish, M, Demeester, T. R, & Hölscher, A. H. (2004). High volume centers for esophagectomy: what is the number needed to achieve low postoperative mortality? Dis Esophagus. , 17(4), 310-314.

[55] Migliore, M, Choong, C. K, Lim, E, Goldsmith, K. A, Ritchie, A, & Wells, F. C. s case volume of oesophagectomy for cancer strongly influences the operative mortality rate. Eur J Cardiothorac Surg. , 32(2), 375-380.

[56] Minashi, K, Doi, T, Muto, M, Mera, K, Yano, T, & Ohtsu, A. (2006). chemo-radiotherapy for superficial esophageal squamous cell carcinoma. Stomach and Intestine. , 41, 1467-1474.

[57] Minsky, B. D, Pajak, T. F, Ginsberg, R. J, Pisansky, T. M, Martenson, J, Komaki, R, Okawara, G, Rosenthal, S. A, & Kelsen, D. P. (2002). INT 0123 (Radiation Therapy Oncology Group 94-05) phase III trial of combined-modality therapy for esophageal cancer: high-dose versus standard-dose radiation therapy. J Clin Oncol. , 20(5), 1167-1174.

[58] Morota, M, Gomi, K, Kozuka, T, Chin, K, Matsuura, M, Oguchi, M, Ito, H, & Yamashita, T. (2009). Late toxicity after definitive concurrent chemo-radiotherapy for thoracic esophageal carcinoma. Int J Radiat Oncol Biol Phys. , 75(1), 122-128.

[59] Murakami, M, Kuroda, Y, Okamoto, Y, Kono, K, Yoden, E, Kusumi, F, Hajiro, K, Matsusue, S, & Takeda, H. (1998). Neoadjuvant concurrent chemo-radiotherapy followed by definitive high-dose radiotherapy or surgery for operable thoracic esophageal carcinoma. Int J Radiat Oncol Biol Phys. , 40(5), 1049-1059.

[60] Nakajima, T. E, Ura, T, Ito, Y, Kato, K, Minashi, K, Nihei, K, Hironaka, S, Boku, N, Kagami, Y, & Muro, K. I trial of 5-fluorouracil with cisplatin and concurrent standard-dose radiotherapy in Japanese patients with stage II/III esophageal cancer. Jpn J Clin Oncol. , 39(1), 37-42.

[61] Nakamura, T, Hayashi, K, Ota, M, Eguchi, R, Ide, H, Takasaki, K, & Mitsuhashi, N. (2004). Salvage esophagectomy after definitive chemotherapy and radiotherapy for advanced esophageal cancer. Am J Surg. , 188(3), 261-266.

[62] Nishihira, T, Hirayama, K, & Mori, S. (1998). A prospective randomized trial of extended cervical and superior mediastinal lymphadenectomy for carcinoma of the thoracic esophagus. Am J Surg. , 175(1)

[63] Nishihira, T, Sayama, J, Ueda, H, Sugawara, K, Takano, R, Sagawa, J, Katayama, M, Shineha, R, Hirayama, K, & Mori, S. (1995). Lymph flow and lymph node metastasis in esophageal cancer. Surg Today. , 25(4)

[64] Nishimura, M, Daiko, H, Yoshida, J, & Nagai, K. (2007). Salvage esophagectomy following definitive chemo-radiotherapy. Gen Thorac Cardiovasc Surg. , 55(11), 461-464.

[65] Nishimura, Y, Suzuki, M, Nakamatsu, K, Kanamori, S, Yagyu, Y, & Shigeoka, H. (2002). Prospective trial of concurrent chemo-radiotherapy with protracted infusion of 5-fluorouracil and cisplatin for T4 esophageal cancer with or without fistula. Int J Radiat Oncol Biol Phys. , 53(1), 134-139.

[66] Ohtsu, A, Boku, N, Muro, K, Chin, K, Muto, M, Yoshida, S, Satake, M, Ishikura, S, Ogino, T, Miyata, Y, Seki, S, Kaneko, K, & Nakamura, A. (1999). Definitive chemoradiotherapy for T4 and/or M1 lymph node squamous cell carcinoma of the esophagus. J Clin Oncol. , 17(9), 2915-2921.

[67] Oki, E, Morita, M, Kakeji, Y, Ikebe, M, Sadanaga, N, Egasira, A, Nishida, K, Koga, T, Ohata, M, Honboh, T, Yamamoto, M, Baba, H, & Maehara, Y. (2007). Salvage esophagectomy after definitive chemo-radiotherapy for esophageal cancer. Dis Esophagus. , 20(4), 301-304.

[68] Orringer, M. B, Marshall, B, Chang, A. C, Lee, J, & Pickens, A. Two thousand transhiatal esophagectomies: changing trends, lessons learned. Ann Surg. , 246(3), 363-372.

[69] Pöttgen, C, & Stuschke, M. (2012). Radiotherapy versus surgery within multimodality protocols for esophageal cancer- A meta-analysis of the randomized trials. Cancer Treat Rev. , 38(6), 599-604.

[70] Rentz, J, Bull, D, Harpole, D, Bailey, S, Neumayer, L, Pappas, T, Krasnicka, B, Henderson, W, Daley, J, & Khuri, S. (2003). Transthoracic versus transhiatal esophagectomy: a prospective study of 945 patients. J Thorac Cardiovasc Surg. , 125(5), 1114-1120.

[71] Rice, T. W, Rusch, V. W, Apperson-hansen, C, Allen, M. S, Chen, L. Q, Hunter, J. G, Kesler, K. A, Law, S, Lerut, T. E, Reed, C. E, Salo, J. A, Scott, W. J, Swisher, S. G, Watson, T. J, & Blackstone, E. H. Worldwide esophageal cancer collaboration. ((2009). Dis Esophagus. , 22(1), 1-8.

[72] Roach, M. rd,. Gandara, D.R., You, H.S., Swift, P.S., Kroll, S., Shrieve, D.C., Wara, W.M., Margolis, L., & Phillips, T.L. ((1995). Radiation pneumonitis following combined modality therapy for lung cancer: analysis of prognostic factors. J Clin Oncol. , 13(10), 2606-2612.

[73] Ruol, A, Castoro, C, Portale, G, Cavallin, F, Sileni, V. C, Cagol, M, Alfieri, R, Corti, L, Boso, C, Zaninotto, G, Peracchia, A, & Ancona, E. (2009). Trends in management and prognosis for esophageal cancer surgery: twenty-five years of experience at a single institution. Arch Surg. , 144(3), 247-254.

[74] Safran, H, Suntharalingam, M, Dipetrillo, T, Ng, T, Doyle, L. A, Krasna, M, Plette, A, Evans, D, Wanebo, H, Akerman, P, Spector, J, Kennedy, N, & Kennedy, T. (2008). Cetuximab with concurrent chemoradiation for esophagogastric cancer: assessment of toxicity. Int J Radiat Oncol Biol Phys. , 70(2), 391-395.

[75] Sai, H, Mitsumori, M, Yamauchi, C, Araki, N, Okumura, S, Nagata, Y, Nishimura, Y, & Hiraoka, M. (2004). Concurrent chemo-radiotherapy for esophageal cancer: comparison between intermittent standard-dose cisplatin with 5-fluorouracil and daily low-dose cisplatin with continuous infusion of 5-fluorouracil. Int J Clin Oncol. , 9(3), 149-153.

[76] Sasamoto, R, Sakai, K, Inakoshi, H, Sueyama, H, Saito, M, Sugita, T, Tsuchida, E, Ito, T, Matsumoto, Y, Yamanoi, T, Abe, E, Yamana, N, & Sasai, K. (2007). Long-term results of chemo-radiotherapy for locally advanced esophageal cancer, using daily low-dose 5-fluorouracil and cis-diammine-dichloro-platinum (CDDP). Int J Clin Oncol. , 12(1), 25-30.

[77] Smithers, B. M, Cullinan, M, Thomas, J. M, Martin, I, Barbour, A. P, Burmeister, B. H, Harvey, J. A, Thomson, D. B, Walpole, E. T, & Gotley, D. C. (2007). Outcomes from salvage esophagectomy post definitive chemo-radiotherapy compared with resection following preoperative neoadjuvant chemo-radiotherapy. Dis Esophagus. , 20(6), 471-477.

[78] Stahl, M, Stuschke, M, Lehmann, N, Meyer, H. J, Walz, M. K, Seeber, S, Klump, B, Budach, W, Teichmann, R, Schmitt, M, Schmitt, G, Franke, C, & Wilke, H. (2005).

Chemoradiation with and without surgery in patients with locally advanced squamous cell carcinoma of the esophagus. J Clin Oncol. , 23(10), 2310-2317.

[79] Stein, H. J, Feith, M, Bruecher, B. L, Naehrig, J, Sarbia, M, & Siewert, J. R. (2005). Early esophageal cancer: pattern of lymphatic spread and prognostic factors for long-term survival after surgical resection. Ann Surg. , 242(4)

[80] Steyerberg, E. W, Neville, B. A, Koppert, L. B, Lemmens, V. E, Tilanus, H, Coebergh, W, Weeks, J. W, & Earle, J. C. C.C. ((2006). Surgical mortality in patients with esophageal cancer: development and validation of a simple risk score. J Clin Oncol. , 24(26), 4277-4284.

[81] Suzuki, H, Gotoh, M, Sugihara, K, Kitagawa, Y, Kimura, W, Kondo, S, Shimada, M, Tomita, N, Nakagoe, T, Hashimoto, H, Baba, H, Miyata, H, & Motomura, N. (2011). Nationwide survey and establishment of a clinical database for gastrointestinal surgery in Japan: Targeting integration of a cancer registration system and improving the outcome of cancer treatment. Cancer Sci. , 102(1), 226-230.

[82] Swisher, S. G, Maish, M, Erasmus, J. J, Correa, A. M, Ajani, J. A, Bresalier, R, Komaki, R, Macapinlac, H, Munden, R. F, Putnam, J. B, Rice, D, Smythe, W. R, Vaporciyan, A. A, Walsh, G. L, Wu, T. T, & Roth, J. A. (2004). Utility of PET, CT, and EUS to identify pathologic responders in esophageal cancer. Ann Thorac Surg. , 78(4), 1152-1160.

[83] Swisher, S. G, Wynn, P, Putnam, J. B, Mosheim, M. B, Correa, A. M, Komaki, R. R, Ajani, J. A, Smythe, W. R, Vaporciyan, A. A, Roth, J. A, & Walsh, G. L. (2002). Salvage esophagectomy for recurrent tumors after definitive chemotherapy and radiotherapy. J Thorac Cardiovasc Surg. , 123(1), 175-183.

[84] Tachimori, Y, Kanamori, N, Uemura, N, Hokamura, N, Igaki, H, & Kato, H. (2009). Salvage esophagectomy after high-dose chemo-radiotherapy for esophageal squamous cell carcinoma. J Thorac Cardiovasc Surg. , 137(1), 49-54.

[85] Takeuchi, S, Ohtsu, A, Doi, T, Kojima, T, Minashi, K, Mera, K, Yano, T, Tahara, M, Muto, M, & Nihei, K. (2007). A retrospective study of definitive chemo-radiotherapy for elderly patients with esophageal cancer. Am J Clin Oncol. , 30(6), 607-611.

[86] Tomimaru, Y, Yano, M, Takachi, K, Miyashiro, I, Ishihara, R, Nishiyama, K, Sasaki, Y, Ishikawa, O, Doki, Y, & Imaoka, S. (2006). Factors affecting the prognosis of patients with esophageal cancer undergoing salvage surgery after definitive chemo-radiotherapy. J Surg Oncol. , 93(5), 422-428.

[87] Tougeron, D. Di Fiore, F., Thureau, S., Berbera, N., Iwanicki-Caron, I., Hamidou, H., Paillot, B., & Michel, P. ((2008). Safety and outcome of definitive chemo-radiotherapy in elderly patients with oesophageal cancer. Br J Cancer. , 99(10), 1586-1592.

[88] Tsujino, K, Hirota, S, Endo, M, Obayashi, K, Kotani, Y, Satouchi, M, Kado, T, & Takada, Y. (2003). Predictive value of dose-volume histogram parameters for predicting

radiation pneumonitis after concurrent chemoradiation for lung cancer. Int J Radiat Oncol Biol Phys. , 55(1), 110-115.

[89] Urschel, J. D, & Vasan, H. of randomized controlled trials that compared neoadjuvant chemoradiation and surgery to surgery alone for resectable esophageal cancer. Am J Surg. , 185(6), 538-543.

[90] van de VenC., De Leyn, P., Coosemans, W., Van Raemdonck, D., Lerut, T. ((1999). Three-field lymphadenectomy and pattern of lymph node spread in T3 adenocarcinoma of the distal esophagus and the gastro-esophageal junction. Eur J Cardiothorac Surg. , 15(6), 769-773.

[91] Weber, W. A, Ott, K, Becker, K, Dittler, H. J, Helmberger, H, Avril, N. E, Meisetschläger, G, Busch, R, Siewert, J. R, Schwaiger, M, & Fink, U. (2001). Prediction of response to preoperative chemotherapy in adenocarcinomas of the esophagogastric junction by metabolic imaging. J Clin Oncol. , 19(12), 3058-3065.

[92] Willis, J, Cooper, G. S, Isenberg, G, & Sivak, M. V. Jr, Levitan, N., Clayman, J., & Chak, A. ((2002). Correlation of EUS measurement with pathologic assessment of neoadjuvant therapy response in esophageal carcinoma. Gastrointest Endosc. , 55(6), 655-661.

[93] Wilson, K. S, & Lim, J. T. (2000). Primary chemo-radiotherapy and selective oesophagectomy for oesophageal cancer: goal of cure with organ preservation. Radiother Oncol. , 54(2), 129-134.

[94] Wilson, K. S, Wilson, A. G, & Dewar, G. J. (2002). Curative treatment for esophageal cancer: Vancouver Island Cancer Centre experience from 1993 to 1998. Can J Gastroenterol. , 16(6), 361-368.

[95] Wouters, M. W, Wijnhoven, B. P, Karim-kos, H. E, Blaauwgeers, H. G, Stassen, L. P, Steup, W. H, Tilanus, H. W, & Tollenaar, R. A. (2008). High-volume versus low-volume for esophageal resections for cancer: the essential role of case-mix adjustments based on clinical data. Ann Surg Oncol. , 15(1), 80-87.

[96] Yamada, K, Murakami, M, Okamoto, Y, Okuno, Y, Nakajima, T, Kusumi, F, Takakuwa, H, & Matsusue, S. (2006). Treatment results of chemo-radiotherapy for clinical stage I (T1N0M0) esophageal carcinoma. Int J Radiat Oncol Biol Phys. , 64(4), 1106-1111.

[97] Yamada, M, Kudoh, S, Hirata, K, Nakajima, T, & Yoshikawa, J. (1998). Risk factors of pneumonitis following chemo-radiotherapy for lung cancer. Eur J Cancer. , 34(1), 71-75.

[98] Yamamoto, S, Ishihara, R, Motoori, M, Kawaguchi, Y, Uedo, N, Takeuchi, Y, Higashino, K, Yano, M, Nakamura, S, & Iishi, H. (2011). Comparison between definitive chemo-radiotherapy and esophagectomy in patients with clinical stage I esophageal squamous cell carcinoma. Am J Gastroenterol. , 106(6), 1048-1054.

[99] Yamashita, H, Nakagawa, K, Yamada, K, Kaminishi, M, Mafune, K, & Ohtomo, K. (2008). A single institutional non-randomized retrospective comparison between definitive chemo-radiotherapy and radical surgery in 82 Japanese patients with resectable esophageal squamous cell carcinoma. Dis Esophagus. , 21(5), 430-436.

[100] Yasunaga, H, Matsuyama, Y, & Ohe, K. Japan Surgical Society. ((2009). Effects of hospital and surgeon case-volumes on postoperative complications and length of stay after esophagectomy in Japan. Surg Today. , 39(7), 566-571.

[101] Zuccaro, G. Jr, Rice, T.W., Goldblum, J., Medendorp, S.V., Becker, M., Pimentel, R., Gitlin, L., & Adelstein, D.J. ((1999). Endoscopic ultrasound cannot determine suitability for esophagectomy after aggressive chemo-radiotherapy for esophageal cancer. Am J Gastroenterol. , 94(4), 906-912.

Chapter 10

A Review of Radiation Therapy's Role in Early-Stage Breast Cancer and an Introduction to Electronic Brachytherapy

Brent Herron, Alex Herron, Kathryn Howell,
Daniel Chin and Luann Roads

Additional information is available at the end of the chapter

http://dx.doi.org/10.5772/55621

1. Introduction

With the exception of skin cancer, breast cancer is the most commonly diagnosed cancer in women in the United States and the most developed European countries [1]. Although breast cancer has been known to be a major cause of mortality in women living in affluent countries, this disease does not discriminate crossing racial, gender, geographic, and economic lines. Encouraging reports indicate there may be a trend toward decreasing breast cancer incidence in countries where there is a decline in hormone replacement therapy [31,6]. Furthermore, it has been reported that breast cancer mortality has fallen in industrialized countries in the last decade [7,36,6]. Reasons for declining mortality may include early detection and better treatment.

Treatment of breast cancer requires a multidisciplinary approach. The surgeon, medical oncologist, radiation oncologist, and pathologist play a role in developing treatment options for the patient. Radiation therapy has a significant part in the treatment of breast cancer, both for noninvasive and invasive cancers.

Breast conserving surgery includes partial mastectomy, lumpectomy, tylectomy, wide local excision, and quadrantectomy. These techniques followed by 5-7 weeks of radiation therapy have been known for over two decades as breast conservation therapy. Initially accepted as a form of breast cancer treatment in Europe, breast conservation therapy is now accepted throughout the world and has gained popularity in the United States since the early 1980s.

With the advancements in computed tomography imaging, simulation, treatment planning and delivery systems, more accurate and homogenous radiation treatment can be delivered. Radiation therapy options following breast conserving surgery include whole breast radiation, accelerated partial breast radiation with external beam treatment or brachytherapy, and hypofractionated whole breast radiation treatment. This chapter includes a review of these techniques and also introduces a relatively new option: electronic brachytherapy as the role of radiation therapy in early breast cancer management has continued to evolve.

2. Support of breast conservation treatment

Multiple international trials have demonstrated the efficacy of breast-conserving surgery followed by radiation therapy [16,47,20,21].Early detection promotions has resulted in patients presenting with even smaller and more favorable tumors than years ago [15].The improvement of mammographic imaging and screening has led to the increase incidence of patients presenting with noninvasive breast cancer from 5% to 30% [44].

Randomized trials worldwide comparing mastectomy to breast conserving surgery followed by radiation therapy have clearly shown equivalent long-term survival in both groups [20,21, 47,37,38, 9]. The Milan trial was one of the first landmark trials on this subject. From 1973 to 1980, 701 women with Stage 1 breast cancer were randomized to radical mastectomy versus breast conserving surgery with adjuvant whole breast radiation therapy (50 Gy plus a 10 Gy boost). Patients with positive lymph node metastases also received adjuvant chemotherapy. There were no significant differences between the two groups in the development of contralateral breast cancers, distant metastases, or secondary primary cancers. At a median follow-up of 20 years, survival was shown to be equivalent between the two groups.

Other landmark European trials comparing mastectomy and breast conserving surgery included the Institut Gustave-Roussy and the European Organization for Research and Treatment of Cancer (EORTC). The Institut trial randomized women with 2cm or smaller tumors to mastectomy or local excision followed by radiation therapy. 15 year survival rates and local recurrences were statistically similar in this trial as well as the EORTC trial.

In the United States, the National Surgical Adjuvant Breast and Bowel Project (NSABP) initiated the B-04 study in 1971. A total of 2163 women with 4 cm or less breast cancers were randomized to one of three treatment arms: total mastectomy, lumpectomy alone, and lumpectomy plus radiation therapy. Twenty-year follow-up analysis showed no differences in overall survival in the three arms. However, patients who underwent lumpectomy alone had a 39.2% risk of local recurrence versus 14.3% risk of recurrence in the lumpectomy plus radiation arm. Radiation therapy also showed a marginally significant decrease in breast cancer related deaths when compared to the lumpectomy alone arm [20,21].

Fortunately, the outcome for patients treated with breast conserving surgery continues to improve. There have been tremendous advancements in the last decade in surgical techniques, systemic treatment, diagnostic imaging, and radiation therapy delivery systems. Today, for patients with node negative disease, local recurrence for patients undergoing breast conserving surgery with radiation therapy and systemic chemotherapy has dropped to 0.5% annually [12, 13, 14].

3. Patient selection and factors affecting local recurrence

The American College of Radiology Practice Guidelines and the National Comprehensive Network Practice Guidelines serve as tools for selecting patients as candidates for breast conserving therapy. Most women diagnosed with localized breast cancer are candidates. However, there are contraindications to breast conserving therapy including large tumor size to size of the breast, multicentric breast cancer, diffuse malignant appearing, pregnancy, prior radiation to the chest, persistent positive margins after several re-excisions, pacemaker in radiation portal, and morbid obesity exceeding the radiation therapy table limit. Having a collagen vascular disease, such as active lupus, is a relative contraindication to breast conserving treatment.

At least two-thirds of patients are eligible for breast conserving surgery at diagnosis [6]. Several factors influence local regional recurrence. Obtaining gross negative margins at the time of surgery is no longer considered acceptable. Margins should be microscopically negative and as wide as possible. Most surgeons consider a 2-3mm clear margin as acceptable. The median rates of ipsilateral breast recurrence has been shown to be 2%, 3%, and 6% when margins of clearance were determined clear, 1mm clear, and 2mm clear respectively [41].

The presence or absence of extensive intraductal component (EIC) has traditionally been felt to affect local recurrence. Holland et al. [26] showed that the presence of EIC is associated with breast recurrence. In a series of 214 patients who underwent a mastectomy, 71% of patients with EIC had residual intraductal tumor, whereas only 28% of patients without EIC had residual disease.

In certain studies, young age, usually 40, 35 or 30 years or less, has been associated with an increase of ipsilateral tumor recurrence following breast conserving surgery. [22,50,34]. However, many of these studies also show young age to correlate with other high risk features such as high grade and the presence of EIC. A boost dose delivered to the surgical cavity following whole breast radiation therapy is particularly significant for younger patients since higher doses tend to correlate with lower recurrences.

4. External beam radiation therapy

External beam radiation therapy typically begins 3 to 6 weeks following surgery unless systemic chemotherapy is given. Treatment planning starts with the simulation process. Breast boards, wing boards, or customized cradles or molds are created or fitted to the individual patient. This allows the patient to be in a reproducible position with e ach treatment. Patients are typically placed in the supine position with their torso angled 10-15 degrees. The ipsilateral arm is abducted usually between 100-120 degrees and the shoulder is externally rotated. At this time, radio opaque wires are placed and secured along the surgical scars. The radiation oncologist then defines the treatment field borders to encompass the breast target and regional lymph nodes, if needed. CT simulation is performed. The isocenter can be selected and the daily set-up marks are placed on the patient's skin. 3–dimensional treatment planning is performed. Treatment volumes and critical structures are identified and outlined. Optimal beam arrangements are chosen. The goal is to deliver the prescribed dose to the target with a homogenous distribution, minimizing hot and cold spots, to minimize doses delivered to critical structures, such as lungs and heart, and minimize the volumes of the critical structures within the treatment fields.

For early stage breast cancer, tangential fields that include the most anterior thorax are typically used (Fig 1). These fields can include level I and II lymph node chains. Attention to tangent field borders, especially the cranial and posterior chest wall interface, is important if most of levels I and II axillary nodes are to be included [40]. Radiation therapy to the supraclavicular fossa plus or minus a posterior axillary boost is sometimes offered to patients with undissected nodes, four or more lymph node metastases or to patients with one to three positive nodes. A typical supraclavicular field is a half beam block field matched to the tangents with the beam angled 10-15 degrees away from the cord. A table kick is utilized for the tangential fields to account for the divergence of the beam into the supraclavicular field. The posterior axillary beam supplements dose to the midaxillary plane. Pierce et al. discusses several techniques to treat the internal mammary nodes [36].

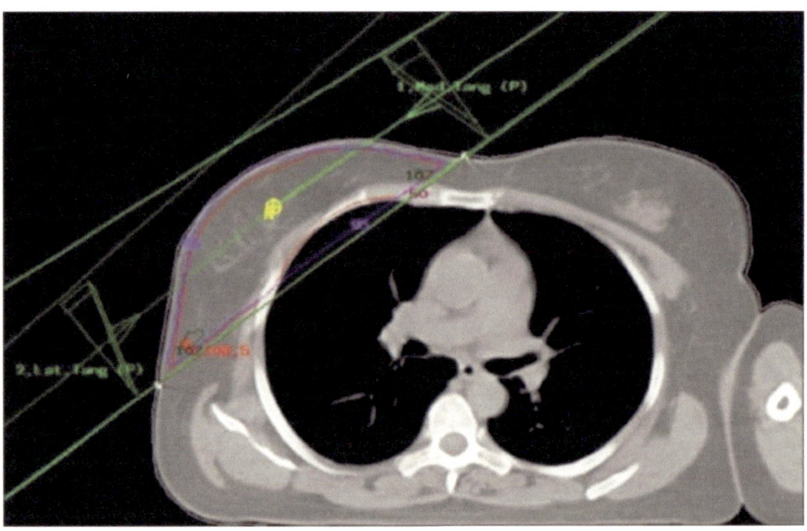

Figure 1. Depiction of tangential fields used for treatment in external beam radiation therapy.

Four to six MV photon energy is most commonly selected for treating the breast and lymph nodes. Whole breast radiation treatments are administered Monday through Friday, deliver-

http://dx.doi.org/10.5772/55621

ing approximately 50 Gy in 25 to 28 fractions. For the boost treatment, electrons typically are used. The lumpectomy cavity is boosted for another 10-16 Gy at 1.8 to 2 Gy per fraction.

New advances in radiation treatment planning and delivery have led to the development of intensity modulated radiation therapy (IMRT) or forward planning IMRT to treat the breast. The dose to the contralateral breast is reduced with IMRT [10]. By conforming doses along the breast and blocking normal structures with multi-leaf collimators, the normal structures like the lungs or heart for left sided breast cancer treatment also receive reduced doses. The dose to the breast could be more homogenous with concave isodose curves, conforming to the target. Studies have shown that forward planning IMRT when compared to standard radiotherapy, can produce homogenous plans with fewer hot spots [4,25]. This could particularly benefit large-breasted women or those with large breast separation. Whether this translates to better cosmetic outcomes is unknown until these trials mature.

In some elderly patients, particularly those over 70 years of age with early disease who receive adjuvant hormonal therapy, breast conserving surgery alone may be an option. There could be biological differences in the tumors in some elderly women. Additionally, some elderly patients tend to have more transportation, social, and other health-related issues that may affect their ability to receive daily radiation therapy. The Canadian trial [23] and the Cancer and Leukemia Group B (CALGB/Radiation Therapy Oncology Group (RTOG)/Eastern Cooperative Oncology Group (ECOG) trial [28,42,23] both randomized older women with estrogen-receptor-positive early breast cancer following breast-conserving surgery to tamoxifen with or without radiation therapy. Although both trials showed absolute benefits to women receiving radiation therapy, the benefits overall were small.

5. Breast brachytherapy for partial breast irradiation

The many trials supporting breast-conserving surgery followed by adjuvant radiation therapy have also shown that the risk of recurrence outside the tumor cavity is similar whether or not whole breast radiation was given [20,21,47,27]. This suggests that additional radiation given outside the tumor cavity may not be of additional benefit to patients.

Breast brachytherapy was historically used to treat the lumpectomy cavity as a "boost" following external whole breast radiation therapy. Many centers have now adapted the use of accelerated partial breast irradiation (APBI), either with interstitial needle implants, various applicators (i.e. Mammosite balloon, Contoura multilumen balloon, Savi), or even through the use of 3D conformal external radiation therapy as the sole radiation treatment modality following breast-conserving surgery. By irradiating less volume, higher radiation doses can be given per fraction to the tumor bed. This shortens treatment times significantly, decreasing the patient's travel time when compared to daily whole breast external beam radiation therapy.

Patients are potential candidates for APBI if they have Stage 0, 1, or II tumors, with a single tumor less than 3 cm in maximum dimension. Minimal nodal involvement and clear surgical margins are also required. Typically, partial breast radiation is delivered twice a day, with each treatment separated at least 6 hours apart, for a total of ten fractions.

Interstitial breast brachytherapy alone has been successfully used for over 10 years following breast conserving surgery (Fig 2). A trial was started by Vinci et al. in 1993 using brachytherapy as the only radiation treatment modality for patients following breast-conserving surgery [48]. By 2001, 120 patients were enrolled in this trial. Four patients developed local recurrence at a median follow-up of 82 months. During 1997-2000, 100 patients were enrolled in a Radiation Therapy Oncology Group (RTOG), prospective Phase I/II study of breast brachytherapy. Patients were either high-dose or low-dose-rate brachytherapy. For the high-dose-rate group at a median follow-up of 6.14 years; 5-year estimates of ipsilateral breast, regional, and contralateral breast failures were 3%, 5%, and 2% respectively. For patients receiving low-dose-rate brachytherapy at a median follow-up of 6.22 years; 5-year estimates of ipsilateral breast, regional, and contra-lateral breast failures were 6%, 0%, and 6%, respectively. Both groups experienced good cosmesis and local control [3]. Several institutions have shown low recurrences with brachytherapy at 5 and 10 years [2,5]

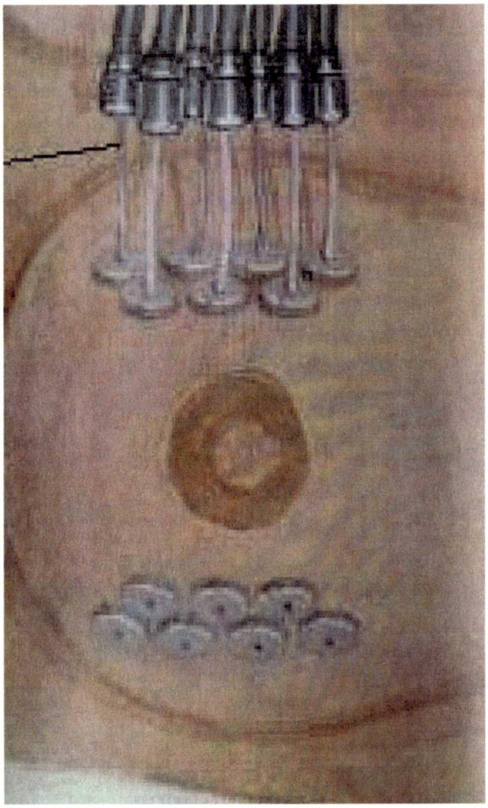

Figure 2. Tube placement for interstitial brachytherapy.

In 2002, the FDA approved Proxima Therapeutics MammoSite* balloon catheter for intracavitary high dose rate breast brachytherapy (Fig 3). Seventy patients were initially enrolled in a prospective multi-center trial evaluating the safety of the MammoSite® balloon catheter.

Subsequent evaluation of 43 patients eligible for the therapy revealed only mild to moderate self-limited side effects [30], Most recently, the American Society of Breast Surgeons reported results from their registry trial involving 1,440 women treated with the MammoSite® catheter following breast-conserving surgery. The 3-year actuarial rates of ipsilateral breast cancer and axillary recurrences were 2.15% and 0.36%, respectively. Cosmetic outcomes were reported to be acceptable and similar to patients treated with other forms of partial breast irradiation [33]. The advantages of the balloon catheter are that it is easier to place in the cavity, placement is more reproducible, and patient comfort is improved. It has become the most widely used device and has the longest track record [43]. The single catheter needs to be temporarily placed in the lumpectomy cavity, as opposed to 10-20 catheters with traditional interstitial implants. However, the balloon needs to "conform" properly to the tumor cavity and optimal dosimetry could be problematic if a large air pocket develops along the periphery of the cavity. The dose distribution is spherical or elliptical depending on the balloon chosen. Balloon-skin spacing should be at least 7 mm. The American Society of Breast Surgeons showed that skin spacing in addition to the use of chemotherapy and breast wound infection were the most important factors of cosmesis at 36 months in their MammoSite® Breast Brachytherapy Registry Trial [24].

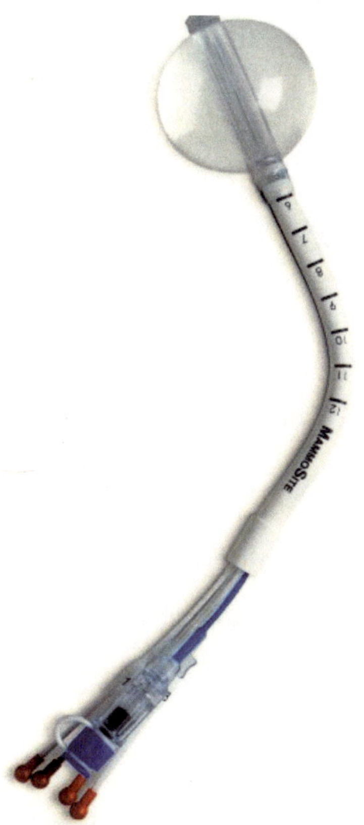

Figure 3. Hologic Mammosite balloon used for APBI treatments.

Other applicator devices have come onto the market recently, with the advantages of having the potential for improved dosimetry in select patients when compared to the MammoSite applicator. The Contura™ Multi-Lumen Balloon catheter, depicted in Figure 4, allows multiple offset lumens to provide dose shaping opportunities to reduce skin and rib doses [13]. This product may have the advantages of using a balloon type applicator, in which many surgeons and radiation oncologists are familiar and comfortable. Additionally, air and blood around the cavity could be removed with the Contura™ catheter before treatment, potentially reducing air pockets and seroma formation. However, dosimetry is still limited to the confines of a "balloon catheter."

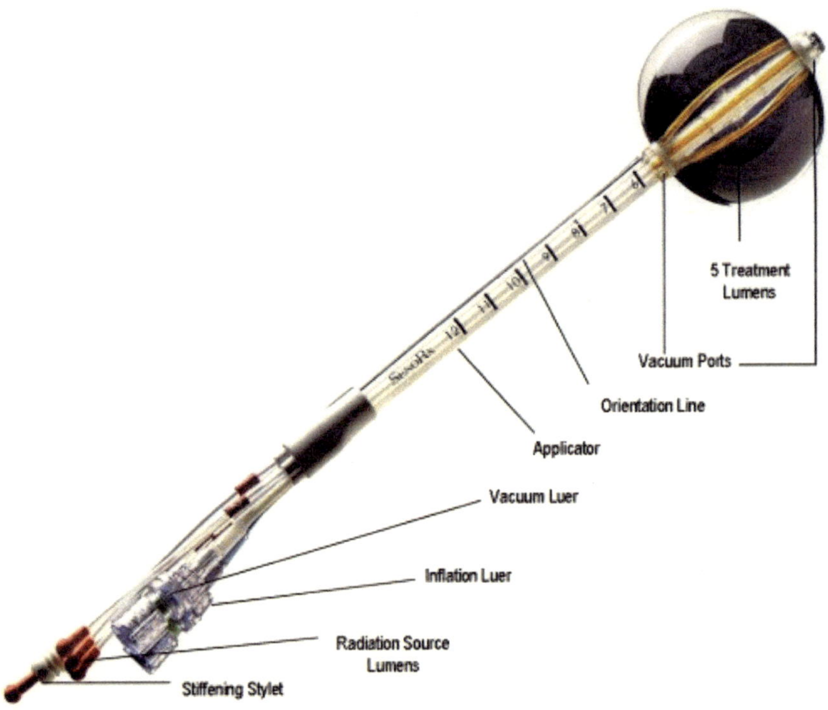

Figure 4. Bard Medical Systems Contoura Multi-lumen balloon.

The ClearPath™ multicatheter device is one of the newest brachytherapy devices available. The catheter is placed through a single entry point but without the constraints of having a single radiation source. The use of a multicatheter hybrid can reduce doses to the skin and normal tissues in the breast when compared to a single catheter system [18,19,8]. Both high-dose-rate as well as low-dose continuous release brachytherapy can be delivered. Therefore, facilities without high-rate-rate equipment can now offer brachytherapy. Additionally, patients can get continuous release treatments at home without having to make twice-daily trips to the treatment facility. Strands of I-125 seeds are inserted in the outer catheters. Patients must wear a fully shielded bra if low-dose continuous release treatment is given.

Another recent addition to the brachytherapy options is the SAVI device (Fig 5), a single-entry multicatheter applicator which allows a radiation oncologist to selectively direct radiation through up to eleven catheter channels, allowing more tailored manipulation of the isodose lines. The device is a bundle of expandable catheters around a central lumen. This applicator tries to blend in the advantages of interstitial brachytherapy with a single-entry device. Dose feathering could be done along the skin and chest. Studies have shown the device to give good tumor bed conformance with minimal normal tissue exposure [39]. Patient positioning as well as maintaining a consistent inter-fraction position is important. A potential disadvantage is that removal of the device may be more difficult when compared to the smaller balloon type catheters.

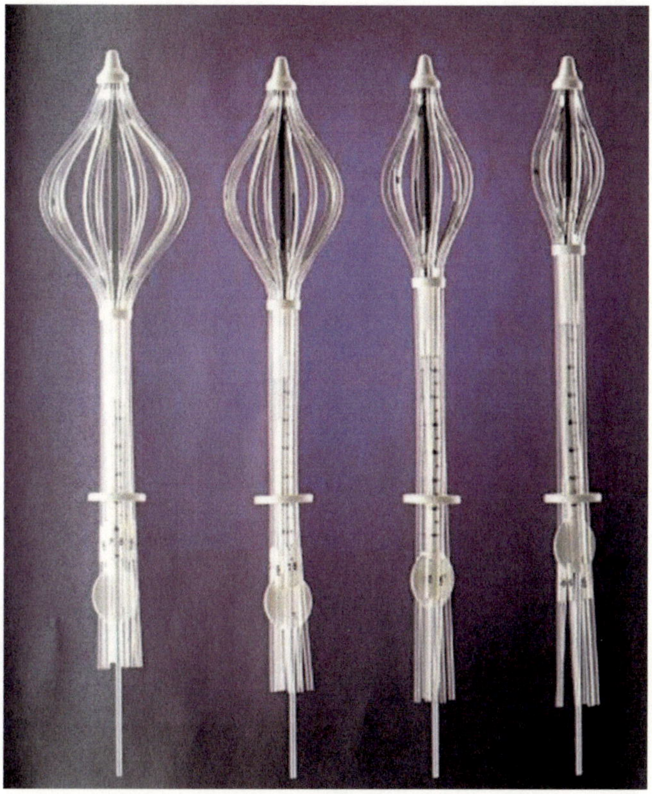

Figure 5. Cianna Medical Savi applicators.

Three-dimension (3D) conformal radiation technology has been developed in recent years. This technique of APBI has the advantage of being noninvasive, eliminating an additional procedure, allowing many medical groups that do not perform brachytherapy to offer partial breast radiation therapy. No adverse side effects were seen in 28 patients treated with 3D conformal radiation in a 1999 pilot study [49]. A potential disadvantage is that the breast is not a stationary target and there is the potential for a geographical miss with external radiation therapy to a small target.

6. Introduction to electronic brachytherapy

Alternative methods of balloon-based APBI have been explored. A modified form of balloon-based brachytherapy called Xoft Axxent Electronic Brachytherapy™ (EBX) received FDA clearance for the treatment of breast cancer in January, 2006. This device uses a unique miniaturized x-ray source (Fig 6) and a mobile controller, which generates kilovoltage (kV) x-rays. This approach to APBI requires minimal shielding and thus has the potential to increase the number of settings in which radiation treatments can be offered. In addition, EBX is not limited by rigorous radiation source regulations associated with high dose rate afterloaders used for other methods of APBI, which utilize radioisotope sources. The early results of a clinical trial to evaluate the performance and safety of EBX in the outpatient treatment of early-stage breast cancer patients were presented at the American Society of Clinical Oncology (ASCO) Breast Cancer Symposium. Treatment with EBX was found to be feasible and associated with minimal acute side effects [32].

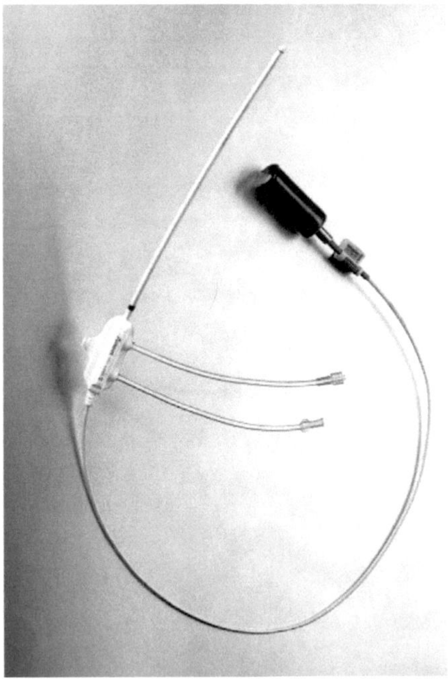

Figure 6. Xoft Accent miniature x-ray source.

Investigators have also explored delivering APBI in the operating room immediately after lumpectomy. Intraoperative radiation therapy (IORT) allows the patient to receive all her radiation in a single fraction before she awakens from surgery. Additional potential advantages include delivering the radiation before tumor cells have a chance to proliferate, performing the radiation under direct visualization at the time of surgery, and decreasing healthcare costs. Published results using IORT both as a tumor bed boost in conjunction with external beam radiation therapy and as a primary treatment in APBI have shown favorable outcomes [45,46,29].

The use of EBX in the operating room is still in its infant stages, but the acceptance of this technique is growing rapidly. The following outlines the steps of an intraoperative procedure:

1. Perform lumpectomy and sentinel node biopsy.
2. Send tumor mass and excision margins for permanent section analysis. Identified sentinel node sent for frozen section evaluation.
3. During surgery, the pathology department reviews the lymph node specimen and informs the treating physicians that the node was uninvolved by cancer.
4. Remove additional breast tissue posterior to the lumpectomy cavity down to the depth of the superficial pectoralis fascia to accommodate a chest wall shield.
5. Place a pliable piece of lead over the chest wall to shield the ribs, lung, and heart, from scatter radiation.
6. Insert a cavity evaluation device into the lumpectomy cavity through a small incision in the lateral breast and inflate with saline.
7. Evaluate the conformity of the cavity evaluation device to the surrounding breast tissue under direct visualization. Determine balloon fill volume to nearest 5cc.
8. Deflate and remove the cavity evaluation device. Based on the fill volume, choose appropriate balloon catheter kit and insert and secure with retention sutures.
9. Verify x-ray source calibration and adjust atlas plan treatment dwell times accordingly. Transfer dwell times to a control USB drive.
10. During machine calibration, perform an intraoperative ultrasound to evaluate that the minimum balloon-to-skin distance is>.6 cm.
11. Prepare for treatment by placing a sterile drape over the operative field. Add a flexible lead equivalent shield on top of the drape to decrease transmission to the patient and hospital staff.
12. The radiation oncologist connects the x-ray source into the balloon. Provide the radiation treatment.

The treatment prescription is the delivery of 20 Gy to the balloon surface. The treatment is accomplished in 10-25 minutes based on the balloon size, fill volume, and the x-ray source calibration. The duration of the entire procedure including lumpectomy, sentinel lymph node biopsy, balloon catheter placement, radiation therapy, and closing the incisions is approximately two hours.

Long-term data regarding the safety and efficacy of IORT are not available. The TARGIT trial is a phase III prospective, randomized trial comparing single fraction IORT delivered via EBX to conventional whole breast external beam radiation therapy. Sixteen international institutions are enrolling patients in the trial. Eligible patients include patients >35 years of age with T1-T3, N0 tumors eligible for breast conserving therapy. Patients with multi-focal or multi-centric lesions, clinically positive lymph nodes, extensive intraductal component, or invasive lobular cancers are not eligible for enrollment [46].

The results of the TARGIT trial will help determine whether IORT is an equivalent alternative to standard whole breast external beam radiation therapy. If IORT methods, including EBX, are established as a standard treatment option, this may allow increased access to breast conserving therapy, as well as, improved quality of life and decreased medical costs for patients with a diagnosis of early-stage breast cancer.

7. Conclusion

Early detection and treatment of breast cancer has significantly improved in recent years. Diagnostic imaging advancements have led to finer and tighter target definition for radiation therapy planning. Treatment delivery systems have changed and continue to change with a movement to shorter and less aggressive therapy. Several treatment options are available for some patients after breast conserving surgery. A 5-7 week course of whole breast external beam therapy now competes with one week of partial breast radiotherapy or a single fraction intraoperative treatment highlighted in this report. As these techniques evolve, focus remains on control, recurrence, and normal tissue response. However, the focus on treatment options also now includes patient schedules, lifestyles as well as the economic impact of the therapy. The multiple risk factors associated with the disease and the variable presentation amongst patients calls out for the need of molecular profiling to assist the oncologist possibly with information on not just who to treat, but how.

Author details

Brent Herron, Alex Herron*, Kathryn Howell, Daniel Chin and Luann Roads

*Address all correspondence to: medical.physics@hotmail.com

Radiation Oncology, PSL Medical Center, Denver, CO, USA

References

[1] American Cancer Society ((2008). Cancer facts and figures. American Cancer Society, Atlanta.

[2] Antonucci, J, Wallace, M, Goldstein, N, et al. (2009). Differences in patterns of failure in patients treated with accelerated partial breast irradiation versus whole-breast irradiation: a matched-pair analysis with 10-year follow-up. Int J Radiat Oncol Biol Phys , 74(2), 447-452.

[3] Arthur, D, Winter, K, Kuske, R, et al. (2008). A phase II trial of brachytherapy alone after lumpectomy for select breast cancer: tumor control and survival outcomes of RTOG 95-17. Int J Radiat Oncol Biol Phys , 72(2), 463-473.

[4] Bamett, G. C, Wilkinson, J, Moody, A. M, et al. (2009). A randomized controlled trial of forward-planned radiotherapy (IMRT) for early breast cancer: baseline characteristics and dosimetry results. Radiother Oncol Epub (ahead of publication)

[5] Benitez, P, Keisch, M, Vicini, F, et al. (2007). Five year results; the initial clinical trial of MammosSite balloon brachytherapy for partial breast irradiation in early-stage breast cancer. Am J Surg , 194(4), 456-462.

[6] Benson, J. R, Jotoi, I, Keisch, M, et al. (2009). Early breast cancer. Lancet , 373, 1463-1479.

[7] Beral, V, Hermon, C, Reeves, G, et al. (1995). Sudden fall in breast cancer death rates in England and Wales. Lancet , 356(8965), 1670-1674.

[8] Beriwal, S, Coon, D, Kim, H, et al. (2008). Multicatheter hybrid breast brachytherapy: a potential alternative for patients with inadequate skin distance. Brachytherapy , 7(4), 301-304.

[9] Blichert-toft, M, Nielsen, M, During, M, et al. (2008). Long-term results of breast conserving surgery vs. mastectomy for early stage breast cancer: 20-year follow-up of the Danish randomized DBCG-82TM protocol. Acta Oncol , 47(4), 672-681.

[10] Borghero, Y. O, Salehpuor, M, Mcneese, M. D, et al. (2007). Multileaf field-in-field forward-planned intensity-modulated dose compensation for whole-breast irradiation is associated with reduced contralateral breast dose: a phantom model comparison. Radiother Oncol , 82(3), 324-328.

[11] Brown, S, Mclaughlin, M, Pope, K, et al. (2009). Initial radiation experience evaluating early tolerance and toxicities in patients undergoing accelerated partial breast irradiationusing the Contura Multi-Lumen Balloon breast brachytherapy catheter. Brachytherapy , 8(2), 227-233.

[12] Buchholz, T. A. (2009). Radiation therapy for early-stage breast cancer after breast-conserving surgery. N Engl J Med , 360(1), 63-70.

[13] Buchholz, T. A, Tucker, S. L, Erwin, J, et al. (2001). Impact of systemic treatment on local control for patients with lymph node-negative breast cancer treated with breats-conservation therapy. J ClinOncol , 19(8), 2240-2246.

[14] Cabioglu, N, Hunt, K. K, Buchholz, T. A, et al. (2005). Improving local control with breast-conserving therapy: a year single institution experience. Cancer 104(l):20-29., 27.

[15] Cady, B, Stone, M. D, Schuler, J. G, et al. (1996). The new era in breast cancer: invasion, size, and nodal involvement dramatically decreasing as a result of mammographic screening. Arch Surg , 131(3), 201-308.

[16] Clarke, M, Collins, R, Darby, S, et al. (2005). Effects of radiotherapy and of differences in the extent of surgery for earl breast cancer on local recurrence and 15-year survival: an overview of the randomised trials. Lancet , 366(9503), 2087-2106.

[17] Delouche, G, Bachelot, F, Premont, M, et al. (1987). Conservation treatment of early stage breast cancer: long term results andcomplications. Int J Oncol Biol Phys 13(0:29-34.

[18] Dickler, A. (2009). Xoft Axxent electronic brachytherapy: a new device for delivering brachytherapy to the breast. Nat Clin Pract Oncol 6(3): 138 142.

[19] Dickler, A, Seif, N, Kirk, M, et al. (2009). A dosimetric comparison of MammoSite and ClearPath high-dose-rate brachytherapy devices. Brachytherapy , 8(1), 14-18.

[20] Fisher, B, Anderson, S, Bryant, J, et al. (2002). Twenty-year follow-up of a randomized trial comparing total mastectomy, lumpectomy, and lumpectomy plus irradiation for the treatment of invasive breast cancer. N Engl J Med , 347(16), 1233-1241.

[21] Fisher, B. J, Bryant, J, Dignam, J, et al. (2002). Tamoxifen, radiation therapy, or both for the prevention of ipsilateral breast tumor recurrence after lumpectomy in women with invasive breast cancers of one centimeter or less. J Clin Oncol , 20(20), 4141-4149.

[22] Fowble, B. L, Schultz, D. J, Overmoyer, B, et al. (1994). The influence of young on outcome in early stage breast cancer. Int J Radiat Oncol Biol Phys 30(l):, 23-33.

[23] Fyles, A. W, Mccready, D. R, Manchul, L. A, et al. (2004). Tamoxifen with or without breast irradiation in women 50 years of age or older with early breast cancer. N Engl J Med , 351(10), 963-970.

[24] Goyal, S, Khan, A. J, Vicini, F, et al. (2009). Factors associated with optimal cosmetic results at 36 months in patients treated with accelerated partial breast irradiation (APBI) on the American Society of Breast Surgeons (ASBrS) MammoSite ® Breast Brachytherapy Registry Trial. Ann Surg Oncol [Epub ahead of print]

[25] Harris, J. S, Neill, C. J, & Rosser, P. F. (2008). A comprehensive clinical 3-dimensional dosimetric analysis of forward planned IMRT and conventional wedge planned wedged techniques for intact breast radiotherapy. Med Dosim 33(I):62-70.

[26] Holland, R, Connolly, J. L, Gelman, R, et al. (1990). The presence of extensive intraductal component component following a limited excision correlates with prominent residual disease in the remainder of the breast. J Clin Oncol , 8(1), 113-118.

[27] Holli, K, Saaristo, R, Isalo, J, et al. (2001). Lumpectomy with or without postopertive radiotherapy for breast cancer with favorable prognostic features: results of a randomized study. Br J Cancer , 84(2), 164-169.

[28] Hughes, K. S, Schnaper, L. A, Berry, D, et al. (2004). Lupectomy plus tamoxifen with or without irradiation in women 70 years of age or older with early breast cancer. N Engl J Med , 351(10), 971-977.

[29] Intra, M, Gatti, G, Luini, A, et al. (2002). Surgical technique of intraoperative radiotherapy in conservative treatment of limited stage breast cancer. Arch Surg , 137, 737-740.

[30] Keisch, M, Vicini, F, Kuske, R, et al. (2003). Initial clinical experience with the Mammo Site breast brachytherapy applicator in women with early-stage breast cancer treated with breast-conserving therapy. Int J Radiat Oncol Biol Phys 55 (2):289 293.

[31] Kumle, M. (2008). Declining breast cancer incidence with decreased HRT use. Lancet , 372(9639), 608-610.

[32] Mehta, V. K, Dooley, W, Griem, K. L, et al. (2008). Early experience with an electronic brachytherapy for intracavitary accelerated partial breast irradiation. Proceedings of the 2008 ASCO Brest Cancer Symposium.

[33] Nelson, J, Beitsch, P, Vicini, F, et al. (2009). Four year clinical update from the American Society of Breast Surgeons MammoSite brachytherapy trial. Am J Surg , 198(1), 83-91.

[34] Nixon, A. J, Neuberg, D, Hayes, D. F, et al. (1994). Relationship of patient's age to pathologic features of the tumor and prognosis for patients with stage I or II breast cancer. J Clin Oncol , 12(5), 888-894.

[35] Peto, R, Boreham, J, Clarke, M, et al. (2000). UK and USA breast cancer deaths down 25% in year 2000 at ages years. Lancet 355(9217):1822., 29-69.

[36] Pierce, L. J, Butler, J. B, Martel, M. K, et al. (2002). Postmastectomy radiotherapy of the chest wal: dosimetric comparision of common techniques. Int J Radiat Oncol Biol Phys , 52(5), 1220-1230.

[37] Poggi, M. M, Danforth, D. N, Sciuto, L. C, et al. (2003). Eighteen-year results in the treatment of early breast carcinoma with mastectomy versus breast conservation therapy: the National Cancer Institute Randomized Trial. Cancer , 98(4), 697-702.

[38] Sarrazin, D, Le, M. G, Arriagada, R, et al. (1989). Ten-year results of a randomized trial comparing a conservative treatment to mastectomy in early breast cancer. Radiother Oncol , 14(3), 177-184.

[39] Scanderbeg, J, Yashar, C, Rice, R, et al. (2009). Clinical implementation of a new brachytherapy device for partial breast irradiation. Radiother Oncol 90(l):, 36-42.

[40] Schlembach, P. J, Buchholz, T. A, Ross, M. I, et al. (2001). Relationship of sentinel and axillary level 1 and II lymph nodes to tangential fields used in breast irradiation. Int J Radiat Oncol Biol Phys , 51(3), 671-678.

[41] Singletary, S. E. (2002). Surgical margins in patients with early stage breast cancer treated with breast conservation therapy. Am J Surg , 184, 383-393.

[42] Smith, B. D, Gross, C. P, Smith, G. L, et al. (2006). Effectiveness of radiation therapy for older women with early breast cancer. J Natl Cancer Inst , 98(10), 681-690.

[43] Streeter, O, Vicini, F, Keisch, M, et al. (2003). MammoSite ® radiation therapy system. Breast , 12(6), 491-496.

[44] Taghian, A. G, & Powel, S. N. (1999). The role of radiation therapy for primary breast cancer. Surg Clin North Am , 79(5), 1091-1115.

[45] Vaidya, J. S, Walton, L, & Dewar, J. (2006). Single dose targeted intraoperative radiotherapy (TARGIT) for breast cancer can be delivered as a second procedure under local anaesthetic. World]Surg Oncol 4:2.

[46] Vaidya, J. S, Baum, M, Tobias, J. S, et al. (2006). Targeted intraoperative radiotherapy (TARGIT) yields very low recurrence rates when given as a boost. Int] Radiat Oncol Biol Phys , 66, 1335-8.

[47] Veronesi, U, Cascinelli, N, Mariani, L, et al. (2002). Twenty-year follow-up of a randomized study comparing breast-conserving surgery with radical mastectomy for early breast cancer. N Engl J Med, 347(16), 1227-1232.

[48] Vicini, F, Baglan, K, Kestin, L, et al. (2001). Accelerated treatment of breast cancer. J Clin Oncol , 19(7), 1993-2001.

[49] Vicini, F, Remouchamps, V, Wallace, M, et al. (2003). Ongoing clinical experience utilizing 3-D conformal external beam radiotherapy to deliver partial-breast irradiation in patients with early stage breast cancer treated with breast-conserving surgery. Int J Radiat Oncol Biol Phys , 57(5), 1247-1253.

[50] Vicini, F. A, Recht, A, Abner, A, et al. (1992). Recurrence in breast following conservative surgery and radiation therapy for early stage breast cancer. J Natl Cancer Inst Monogr (11): 33-39.

Chapter 11

Radiosurgery and Hypofractionated Stereotactic Irradiation with Photons or Protons for Tumours of the Skull Base

Dante Amelio, Marco Cianchetti, Barbara Rombi,
Sabina Vennarini, Francesco Dionisi,
Maurizio Amichetti and Giuseppe Minniti

Additional information is available at the end of the chapter

http://dx.doi.org/10.5772/55692

1. Introduction

The fundamental goal of improving radiation therapy (RT) is to maximize dose to the tumour while limiting dose to normal tissues. Higher radiation dose to the tumour can result in better disease control, and possibly also in improving survival. Decreasing dose to normal tissues is desirable in order to avoid acute and late side effects.

Recent technological advances in photon-RT have allowed an improvement in targeting accuracy, dose escalation, delivery of multiple large fractions (hypofractionated stereotactic radiation therapy - HSRT) or single fraction stereotactic ablative radiation therapy (radiosurgery - SRS). Radiosurgery delivers a single large dose with very steep dose fall-off outside the lesion to very small volumes in order to be tumouricidal through DNA damage or ablative causing necrosis via a vascular endothelial damage [1]. Furthermore, it has been shown that molecular responses to radiation differ based on dose per fraction. More recently, HSRT in two to five sessions has been employed to deliver extremely hypofractionated regimens. Preliminary data suggest that HSRT may represent an effective treatment associated with lower risk of radiation-related adverse effects in patients with perioptic or large benign tumours as compared with single fraction SRS, although potential benefits remain to be demonstrated.

Different techniques are used to deliver both HSRT and SRS, enabling patient immobilization, set-up uncertainty reduction, targeting accuracy, delivery of high doses, and heterogeneous dose distribution with a steep dose gradient. Despite these enhancements in delivery with better conformality indices, photons still have a relatively high exit dose (beyond the tumour target), which can produce significant normal-tissue exposure.

Protons are positively-charged elementary particles, with similar biological effectiveness to conventional photon radiation. They have a defined range exhibited by the Bragg peak resulting in an energy deposition with no exit dose beyond the target volume. Thanks to these fundamental physics characteristics, proton radiation therapy offers superior dose distribution and reduced low-dose integral irradiated volume [2] enabling more radiation dose to be delivered to the tumour while significantly lowering the dose to the surrounding normal tissues.

The skull base (SB) is a very complex anatomical region that includes portions of the anterior cranial fossa, clivus, petrous bone, middle cranial fossa, cavernous sinus and infratemporal fossa encompassing several critical neurovascular structures. Tumours of the SB are challenging lesions because of their anatomical location and close proximity to several critical neurovascular structures. Surgical treatment is considered the first managing step and it has the aim to remove (completely or partially) the tumour. The deep location of SB tumour requires extensive experience in surgical procedures; in fact, surgical damage could severely affect vision, hearing, speech, swallowing, and could even be life-threatening.

New RT techniques allow targeting SB tumours when surgery is not feasible, macroscopic residual is left after surgical intervention or even as an alternative, definitive treatment. Most patients with lesions of the SB have a benign tumour and a long-life expectancy. They need to be treated with techniques allowing target irradiation with a conformal isodose configuration and a steep fall-off into other surrounding structures in order to provide long-term tumour control with a low morbidity profile.

Several machines have been developed or implemented to deliver stereotactic treatments and are currently in use: Gamma Knife, linear accelerators, Cyberknife, and dedicated proton equipments are the most used and have been compared in several plan-comparison studies. At the same time, in the treatment of SB tumours, many studies have shown the effectiveness of SRS and HSRT with photons and, though less frequently, with protons. Considering the continuous advancement of technology in delivering SRS and HSRT with photons and the increased use of protons, we deemed it useful to review this topic by evaluating differences with photons and possible advantages of the use of protons. An analysis of the fundamental principles and differences underlying photon- and proton-based SRS/HSRT as well as clinical outcomes in SB tumours is provided and discussed.

2. Radiobiological background

Experimental and clinical data suggest that the radiobiological principles may differ when irradiation is delivered with different fractionation regimens (fractionated versus large single doses) [3] or when a different type of radiation, such as protons, is employed [4].

This section provides a brief overview on the radiobiological principles underlying radiation therapy and their applications to single or (hypo)fractionated radiotherapy. For a comprehensive analysis of the topic, the reader is referred to specific textbooks and articles [4-6].

The first principle points out that hypoxic cells are highly resistant to the radiation-related killing [7] when radiations with low linear energy transfer are employed.

Secondly, the dose-response relationship differs according to the type of tissues. Those containing mainly non-cycling cells (classified as "late reacting tissues" [8]), are more sensitive to large doses per fraction than tissues containing mainly cycling cells (classified as "early reacting tissues" [8]).

Finally, experimental data show that cells have different radiation sensitivities in different parts of the cell cycle [9].

Taking into account such knowledge, the employment of a fractionated regimen allows hypoxic cells to reestablish their oxygenation state [6] so that they will be more sensitive to a second, and subsequent, dose fraction. Dose fractionation also spares late reacting (healthy) tissues more than early reacting (malignant tumor) tissues [5]. Finally, it allows part of the cells to leave the resistant phase while entering in a more sensitive phase. As an overall result, a more effective cell killing takes place.

Conversely, SRS exploits a different pattern of dose distribution, rather than radiobiological differences between normal and tumour tissue, to achieve effective tumour destruction. Theoretically, the use of large single dose does not allow reoxygenation [4] and may be more damaging if the target is in close proximity of or embedded within late responding organs at risk [10]. Provided that SRS dose falloff is steep enough to spare surrounding structures, the delivery of high single dose should translate into a greater rate of local tumour control, while still offering a low rate of complications. Moreover, the delivery of a single large dose does not allow redistribution of cells into a more radiosensitive phase of the cell cycle. However, the argument for the use of SRS is the relevant radiobiological effect of single-session radiation cell kill or cell division capability arrest, regardless of the mitotic phase [10].

Protons and photons differ in terms of physical properties and interaction with matter, which ultimately translate into different dose distribution as well as biological effectiveness [2]. To date, such a difference has been quantified in a 1.1 relative biological effectiveness (RBE) of protons over photons [11]. Despite the fact that this generic RBE may not be true, its variations do not show sufficient degree to be clinically relevant [11]. As a consequence, all of the above stated radiobiological principles as well as the corresponding clinical applications keep their validity regardless the employed type of radiation so that there is no difference between photon- and proton-based stereotactic irradiation.

However, experimental data [11] have shown that proton RBE values increase over the last few millimeters of the range, ultimately leading to an increased linear energy transfer. The corresponding effect may be equivalent to the expansion of 2 mm or more of the distal penumbra [11], which may be clinically relevant for the surrounding healthy structures. From the radiobiological standpoint, this issue probably represents the most relevant difference between photon- and proton-based stereotactic radiotherapy. Therefore, it is wise to take into account the biological effects of this high-RBE component during the planning.

3. Dosimetrical features

The stereotactic delivering modalities and techniques have been compared in several plan comparison studies [12-15]. The corresponding efficacy has been investigated also on the basis of the normal tissue complication probability (NTCP) and tumour control probability (TCP) models in the attempt to set the results also on a biological basis [14,16].

In general, the differences among photon-based techniques (GK, multi- non-coplanar arcs or shaped beams linac treatment) are negligible [12-15]. Conversely, the modality (photons or protons) can be what is more important. Target features such as size, shape and location within the brain can influence the choice for the best stereotactic modality. In fact, all modalities are equally good if the target is small and regular [14,15].

Based on the normal brain dose, the dosimetrical advantage of charged particles relative to photons is evident in all types of targets [12,14,15]. Such a difference is more relevant under the 60% dose level regardless of the target features [14]. Moreover, the larger the target volume the greater the difference [12,14,15], which peaks for regular shaped targets larger than 24-26 cc, even though it can be relevant even for smaller and irregular targets (about 6 cc) [14,15].

All of the above-stated considerations also apply with respect to the lesion's shape and location: charged particles perform better than photon techniques.

All of the above-mentioned quantitative differences have been confirmed when the analysis was approached on a biological basis, being the NTCP different according to the treatment modality, size, shape and location of the target [14,16]. Again, protons demonstrated the lowest NTCP for medium-large regular and irregular shaped lesions [14,16]. In this scenario, charged particles scored NTCP values 4-6% smaller than photon techniques.

In this context, it is noteworthy that radiation-induced tumours have been reported after photon SRS [17,18]. It is well-known that protons feature a low integral dose to healthy structures providing the potential to reduce this risk. However, the tissue volume that can benefit from this feature may be very small in SRS and the corresponding clinical gain may be difficult to detect.

In conclusion, in the attempt to customize the treatment according to the clinical scenario it is possible to state that small to medium regularly-shaped lesions can be effectively managed by all photon-based techniques although at the expense of some target dose inhomogeneity. The charged particle capability to simultaneously provide high-target conformity and dose homogeneity maximizes for regularly and irregularly-shaped, medium to large lesions.

Finally, it is noteworthy that despite such comparisons included several planning and treatment strategies, further improvements, such as intensity-modulated photon and proton RT, have been introduced. These certainly deserve further investigation.

4. Clinical results of photon and proton SRS/HSRT for skull base tumours

4.1. Search strategy and selection criteria

Data for this review were obtained searching MEDLINE databases for publications dated between January 1980 and December 2011.

The search terms were: "skull base" and "stereotactic radiosurgery". Further research was conducted by adding the definitions of different SB tumours ("meningioma", "schwannoma / acoustic neuroma", "pituitary adenoma", "chordoma", "chondrosarcoma", "craniopharyngioma", "olfactory neuroblastoma / esthesioneuroblastoma", "glomus jugulare / chemodectoma", "proton") to the previously-searched keywords.

This search was limited to articles written in English. Editorials, case reports, letters of opinion, and congress abstracts were excluded, even if they added valuable information. In case of repeated publications by the same institution, only the most updated was used for the analysis. Papers were reviewed and prioritized according to content relevancy. Reference lists from these sources were searched for additional publications. A systematic review was beyond the aim of the paper; the following results are reported in the form of a narrative summary.

4.2. Clinical outcomes

Photon-based SRS and HSRT have been increasingly employed as primary or post-operative treatments with more than 10.000 patients reported in published studies over the last two decades. Less data are available on the treatment with proton-based SRS and HSRT even though several types of tumour in benign and malignant settings, and also non-tumoural lesions as arteriovenous malformations, have been treated since its early use showing that it as a viable option for larger volumes.

To date, no randomized or non-randomized study has compared photon SRS/HSRT with proton SRS/HSRT, and almost all the studies available in literature are retrospective. Clinical outcomes are presented in the following, according to histopathological classification.

A brief summary is provided in Table 1.

Tumor type	Delivery technique	Doses	Five-year tumor control
Benign meningioma	SRS	12 – 18 Gy	> 92%
	HSRT	14 – 25 Gy / two-five fractions	93.5%
Pituitary adenoma	SRS	15 – 22 Gy (non functioning) 18 – 26 Gy (secreting)	94%
	HSRT	17 – 25 Gy / three-five fractions	98% (three-years)

Tumor type	Delivery technique	Doses	Five-year tumor control
Acoustic neuroma	SRS	12 – 13 Gy	92%-100%
	HSRT	30 – 36 Gy /six fractions 20 – 25 Gy /five fractions	94%-100%
Craniopharyngioma	SRS	3 – 25 Gy	36%-91.6%
	HSRT	NA	NA
Chordoma and chondrosarcoma	SRS	15 – 20 Gy	Chordoma: 32-72% Chondrosarcoma: 63-100%
	HSRT	20 – 43.6 Gy / two-five fractions	Chordoma: 100% (two-years)

Table 1. Main clinical outcomes regarding the most frequent tumours of the skull base treated with stereotactic radiosurgery (SRS) and hypofractionated stereotactic radiotherapy (HSRT).

- Meningioma

Meningiomas represent approximately 25% of all intracranial tumours, the majority of which are benign (grade I according to the World Health Organization classification).

These lesions can be observed or treated with surgery or RT. Surgical resection is the preferred treatment for accessible tumours that can be safely removed. RT is used when surgery is not possible for the location of the lesion or when the patient is not a suitable surgical candidate. Other indications are the risk of progression after partial excision or the salvage after a relapse. Atypical or malignant meningioma are usually irradiated adjuvantly after complete surgical excision [19]. Recently-published multicenter series [20] and review [21] on benign lesions show a 5-year control rate ≥ 92%. Radiosurgical doses between 12 and 18 Gy have been used in the control of skull base meningiomas. A similar 5-year actuarial tumour control rate in the range of 90-95% has been observed with doses of 15-16 Gy or 12-14 Gy. Large meningiomas are associated with worse long-term local control [22,23].

Radiation-induced toxicity has been shown in up to 40% after SRS, being represented by either transient or permanent neurological complications; however, the reported rate of significant complications at doses of 12-15 Gy, as currently used in most centres, is relatively low. Reference [22] reported permanent neurological deficits of 6.3% for cavernous sinus meningiomas treated with GK SRS. Reference [24] showed late transient or permanent complications in 4.5% of patients, and similar complication rates have been reported in the majority of published series [21]. Other complications, such as epilepsy, internal carotid occlusion, and hypopituitarism have been rarely reported (less than 1-2%).

Only few studies report on the use of HSRT for skull base meningiomas [25-27]. In a series of 157 patients treated with Cyberknife [27], 5-year control was 93.5%. Interestingly, local control in tumours bigger than 8 ml and/or situated close to critical structures and treated with two to five daily fractions was similar to that obtained in smaller meningiomas treated with single fraction SRS.

http://dx.doi.org/10.5772/55692

Protons have been used in this context usually with conventional fractionation and in association with photons for benign [28-32] or atypical lesions [33,34], but also with HSRT or single session SRS [35-37]. In reference [35], 23 patients were treated, 18 with three fractions HSRT, and five with HSRT in 16 or more fractions: the mean reference dose was 20.3 Cobalt Gray equivalent (CGyE). In the HSRT group, clinical control was 89% (16/18) and radiological local control was 88%. Two patients (11%) developed transient new cranial nerve neuropathy after radiosurgery, which gradually recovered. Two more patients (11%) developed late side effects. The results of 51 cases of benign meningioma treated, between 1996 and 2007, with proton SRS as primary treatment (n = 32) or for residual tumour following surgery (n = 8), or recurrent tumour following surgery (n = 10) were recently published [37]. The median dose delivered was 13 CGyE (range, 10 -15.5 CGyE) prescribed to the 90% isodose line. After a median follow-up of 32 months (range, 6-133 months), MRI revealed 33 meningiomas with stable, 13 with decreased, and five with increased size. The 3-year actuarial tumour control rate was 94%. Symptoms were improved in 47% (16/34) of patients. Potentially permanent adverse effects after SRS were recorded in 3/51 (5.9%) patients. The main limitation of these studies is that longer follow-up is needed to assess the durability of tumour control.

- Pituitary adenoma

There are two general categories of pituitary tumours: non-secreting and secreting lesions. Functioning tumours cause an excess secretion of one or more pituitary hormones. Although pituitary adenomas are histologically benign, successful management of these tumours can be challenging. Treatment options include microresection, medical therapy, fractionated RT, and SRS. The role of RT in pituitary adenomas is well-established [38], particularly when medical and surgical options have been exhausted. Therapeutic goals when performing RT for pituitary tumours are: stopping the tumour growth by preventing problems from mass effect, and normalization of excessive hormone secretion.

All main published results on the long-term effectiveness of SRS in patients with non-functioning and secreting pituitary adenomas have been recently reviewed [39,40]. In 15 studies reporting 684 patients with non-functioning adenomas treated with SRS at doses of 15-22 Gy, the reported 5-year actuarial tumour control rate was 94%. A similar local control was observed in patients with secreting pituitary adenomas, although higher doses in the range of 18-26 Gy are usually employed with the aim to achieve normalization of hormone hypersecretion. SRS data for 1215 patients with acromegaly have been reported in 29 studies [39]. At a median follow-up of 50 months, the 5-year and 10-year biochemical remission rates were 44% (range, 15-60%) and 74% (range, 46-86%), respectively. Time to response ranged from 12 to 66 months. Results of SRS were reported for 280 patients with Cushing's disease in 12 studies [40]. At a corrected median follow-up of 45 months, 48% of patients had biochemical remission of disease, with a reported time to hormonal response ranging from 3 months to 3 years. SRS is rarely used in the treatment of prolactinomas since medical treatment with dopamine agonists can achieve tumour shrinkage and normalize prolactin (PRL) levels in more than 80% of patients. When employed in patients who fail surgery and medical therapy, at a median follow-up of 29 months normalization of elevated PRL levels has been observed in 33% of 353 patients included in 18 studies, with a reported time to hormonal response ranging from 5 to 40 months [40]. The reported overall rate of serious complications after SRS is low. The main complication is hypopituitarism, which is reported in up to 47% of patients, with higher rates in those series with a longer median follow-up.

HSRT has been employed in patients with tumours involving the optic apparatus and patients who are not considered suitable for SRS. Initial experiences with Cyberknife in treating patients with pituitary adenomas are promising [25,41,42]. Reference [25] reported high rates of tumour control and preservation of visual function in a small group of patients with pituitary adenomas within two mm of the optic apparatus treated to doses of 18-24 Gy delivered in two to five sessions. Although hypofractionated treatment schedules may offer a reduced risk of radiation-related adverse effects as compared to single fraction SRS, its efficacy needs to be evaluated in large prospective studies.

Data on proton treatment in pituitary adenomas are available both with the option of conventional fractionation [43] or with SRS [44-47]. In a small series of 22 patients treated with proton SRS for persistent acromegaly at a median follow-up of 6.3 years, the biochemical remission of disease was observed in 13 patients (59%) [44]. Time to response was 42 (range, 6-62) months. In a retrospective series of 33 patients with Cushing's disease at a median follow-up of 62 months, normalization of plasma and urinary free cortisol was achieved in 17 (52%) patients, with a time to remission of 18 (range, 5-49) months [45]. In both series, the only reported toxicity was represented by new pituitary deficits, which occurred in up to 52% of patients, whereas no visual complications, seizures, or secondary tumours were noted. The small number of cases treated and limited follow-up precludes drawing firm conclusions, even though it supports the hypothesis that proton SRS may offer better dosimetric coverage of the pituitary gland than photon-based treatments.

- Acoustic neuroma/vestibular schwannoma

Acoustic neuroma is a benign primary intracranial tumor of the vestibulocochlear nerve that can be treated with surgery or with several stereotactic irradiation techniques. Studies in the literature are poorly comparable because of the lack of uniform-reporting evaluation criteria [48].

SRS as an effective treatment for acoustic neuroma has evolved over the last decades, leading to an improvement of local control and reduction of long-term toxicity. At doses of 12-13 Gy, as used in most recent studies, SRS results in an actuarial 5-year tumour control between 92 and 100% with a low incidence of radiation-induced complications [49]. The reported local control is similar to that reported with higher doses in the range of 15-18 Gy as used in early experiences of SRS, however with a lower incidence of radiation-induced complications. A recent review of more than 2000 patients included in 23 studies has shown an overall facial nerve preservation rate of 96% after GK, with a significant better facial nerve preservation rate in patients receiving ≤ 13 Gy of radiation at the marginal dose and with a tumor volume ≤ 1.5 cm^3 [50]. Using similar doses, an overall hearing preservation, as defined by the maintenance of Gardner-Robertson Grade I or II after SRS, has been reported in 51% (range, 32-71%) of 4234 patients included in 45 publications [51]. Equivalent tumor control and hearing preservation rates have been reported for larger acoustic neuromas compressing the brainstem, with a reported balance improvement or stabilization in more than 85% of patients who had imbalance at presentation [52]. Neurological toxicity, including facial and trigeminal neuropathies, and balance disturbances may occur in 0-3% of patients. Hydrocephalus has been observed in 1-2% of patients, whereas radiation-induced tumors or malignant transformation of acoustic neuroma have been reported rarely [49].

There are only few reports regarding the use of HSRT in patients with vestibular schwannomas [53,54]. The reference [53] employed a regimen of 30 or 36 Gy in six fractions. At a median follow-up of 4.5 years, absolute tumor control, as well as hearing, facial and trigeminal preservation were 100%.

In reference [54], 20 or 25 Gy were delivered in five fractions. Five-year tumor control, trigeminal, facial, and hearing preservation were 94%, 98%, 97%, and 61%, respectively. It is noteworthy that in the latter reference HSRT provided equivalent tumor control, facial and hearing preservation with respect to SRS. Conversely, trigeminal preservation was significantly improved in patients treated with HSRT.

Also in this site, proton beam has been used with conventional fractionation [55] or with SRS with a satisfactory level of hearing, facial nerve, trigeminal nerve preservation, and with tumor-control rates of 84-100% [56-58]. Reference [56] reported on 88 patients with vestibular schwannomas treated at the Massachusetts General Hospital between 1992 and 2000 with proton SRS. At a median follow-up period of 38.7 months (range, 12-102), the actuarial 2- and 5-year tumor control was 95.3% and 93.6%, respectively. Hearing was preserved in 33% of 21 (24% of the total) patients with functional hearing before treatment. Actuarial 5-year normal facial and trigeminal nerve function preservation rates were 91% and 89%, respectively. Three patients (3.4%) underwent shunting for hydrocephalus.

Figure 1 shows a representative case of vestibular schwannoma treated with proton SRS.

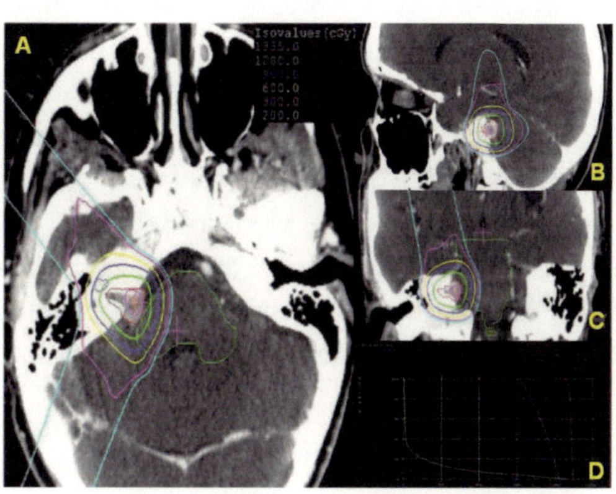

Courtesy of Francis H. Burr Proton Therapy Center – Massachusetts General Hospital, Boston (USA).

Figure 1. Dose distribution in axial (A), sagittal (B), and coronal (C) views of a right vestibular schwannoma treated by proton radiosurgery. Tumor volume (in red) was 1 cubic centimeter. A dose of 12 Cobalt Gray Equivalent was prescribed to 90% isodose. Three equally weighted passive scattering beams were employed. The dose-volume histogram graph (D) shows the doses to organs at risk (right cochlea in blue and brainstem in green) and tumor volume (in red).

Reference [58] reported on 51 patients treated with proton HSRT with a dose of 26 CGyE in three fractions. At a median follow-up of 72 months, the 5-year local control was 98%. Hearing, facial nerve, and trigeminal nerve preservation rates were 42%, 90.5% and 93% at 5 years, respectively.

- Craniopharyngioma

Craniopharyngioma is a rare and mostly benign epithelial paediatric brain tumour of the sellar and suprasellar region. The treatment is based on a surgical approach with transcranial approaches or endoscopic endonasal surgery followed by RT, mainly in form of fractionated regimens with a local control of 80-90% at 5-10 years [59]. The proximity of craniopharyngiomas to the optic pathways provides a major limitation to the use of SRS, although in selected series of relatively small residual tumours, a local control of 34-88% has been reported [60-62]. Tumor control was achieved with a median dose of 22-24 Gy (marginal dose 11-12 Gy), whereas the use of lower radiation results in an unsatisfactory tumor control [63]. The reported late toxicity after SRS ranges from 0 to 38%, mainly represented by visual and endocrinological deficits [59].

To date, there are no data dealing with the delivery of HSRT in patients with craniopharyngioma.

Protons have been recently used for the treatment of this tumour but only with conventional fractionated regimens [64-66], and to date no experience with proton SRS has been reported.

- Chordoma and chondrosarcoma

Chordomas and chondrosarcomas of the SB are rare bone tumours with locally aggressive behaviour. Safe, maximal resection is the mainstay of treatment, usually followed by adjuvant RT. Protons are used with conventional fractionation schemes utilizing doses of 70 Gy in chondrosarcoma and, 74-78 in chordoma with valuable results [67,68]. The improvements in surgical techniques allow more radical tumour resection, while frequently providing small residual lesions suitable also for SRS or HSRT. Few clinical data was published on this issue, showing, however, promising preliminary results. Both for chordomas and chondrosarcomas, SRS has been employed to treat small tumour volumes: with few exceptions, corresponding median or mean values were less than 20 cm^3. Median delivered dose was 15-20 Gy in most series, depending on the proximity with organs at risk. Such dose levels translated into actuarial local control rates of 32-72% at 5 years for chordomas [67] and 63-100% for chondrosarcomas [68]. It is noteworthy that most series have mean or median follow-up of less than 5 years.

Concerning the delivery of HSRT, literature shows very limited data [69-71]. None of them reports outcomes regarding chondrosarcomas. Total dose was 20-43.6 Gy delivered in 2 to 5 fractions. When reported, tumour volumes were again limited in size (less than 20 cm^3). Only one series reports specific outcomes for patients treated with HSRT: at a median follow-up of just 24 months, absolute local control was 100% [70].

Both for SRS and HSRT severe radiation-related side effects were rare [67].

Even though such data need to be confirmed at a longer follow-up, it seems that SRS and HSRT could represent viable treatment options for small sized chordomas and chondrosarcomas residual after surgery or relapsing.

No data are available at this moment concerning the use of proton SRS or HSRT.

- Chemodectoma/glomus jugulare tumours

Radiation has been found to be helpful in controlling glomus jugulare tumour growth by inducing fibrosis around the supplying vessels. A recent comprehensive review identified 109 studies for a total of 869 patients described outcomes for patients with glomus jugulare tumours [72]. Patients undergoing SRS had the lowest rates of recurrence and the most favourable rates of tumour control. In particular, those treated with subtotal resection plus SRS had a control rate of 71% at 96 months of follow-up. At a median follow-up of 71 months, patients undergoing SRS alone had a tumour control rate of 95%. A recent meta-analysis [73] found 19 eligible studies. SRS marginal dose ranged between 12 and 20.4 Gy. Ninety-seven percent of patients achieved tumour control, and 95% of patients achieved clinical control suggesting the useful utilization of SRS for the primary management of glomus jugulare tumours in particular for patients with preserved glossopharyngeal and vagus nerve function, after surgical recurrence, in the elderly, and in patients with serious pre-existing medical conditions [74].

So far, data dealing with the use of HSRT in patients with chemodectoma or tumors of glomus jugulare are very limited. In reference [75], part of the patient sample received a slight hypofractionated regimen: 2.67 Gy per fraction (median dose 45 Gy). Overall, the 10-year tumour control rate was 92%. In reference [76] 49 patients received a median dose of 45 Gy in 15 or 16 fractions. At both 5 and 10 years, 92% of cases were recurrence-free. More recently, 18 patients were treated with a median dose of 20 Gy in 3 fractions [77]. At a median follow-up of 22 months, local control was 100%.

No data are available for the use of protons in this field.

- Olfactory neuroblastoma/Esthesioneuroblastoma

Olfactory neuroblastoma or esthesioneuroblastoma is a rare tumour of the frontal SB. It is characterized by high rates of tumour recurrence and mortality. A recent meta-analysis [78] demonstrated that the most effective management of these lesions is usually based on surgery followed by post-operative irradiation. For early stage tumours, where the risk of cervical nodes involvement is very low, the combination of SRS (15-34 Gy marginal dose) with endoscopic sinus surgery seems a promising treatment option [79,80].

To date, there are no data dealing with the delivery of HSRT in patients with olfactory neuroblastoma or esthesioneuroblastoma.

In the only report concerning the use of protons in this field, 14 patients received irradiation as definitive treatment [81]. Total dose was 65 CGyE, with 2.5 CGyE per fraction. Actuarial 5-year local progression-free survival rate was 84%.

5. Conclusions

Stereotactic irradiation is highly effective in the management of SB benign tumours and long-term data clearly indicate a tumour control in more than 90% of cases after 5 and 10 years, with an acceptable incidence of complications. In most series, radiosurgical dose has been delivered using GK, although outcome is similar for patients with SB tumours treated with Linac SRS.

Even though protons are increasingly used in the clinical community, only few studies have been performed to assess the efficacy and toxicity of proton SRS and HSRT in skull base tumors. The number of Institutions that are currently using protons is small, particularly those performing proton-based stereotactic techniques. Proton beam, while utilizing a different type of radiation, also represents a similar highly focused and targeted radiation tool. The physical properties of protons offer superior conformality in dose distribution with respect to photons. This advantage becomes more apparent as the lesion volume increases. However, current results do not clearly indicate that proton SRS/HSRT is superior to photon SRS/HSRT. Clinical results are probably confounded by a bias toward reserving proton beams for the treatment of larger and more complex lesions; but conclusions about the presumed superiority of protons in comparison to other photons-based techniques are difficult to draw.

With respect to the small number of treated patients and short follow-up, toxicity was similar with the use of the different techniques; however, the evaluation of complications is often completely subjective and unsatisfactory. Proton SRS may represent a treatment alternative to photon SRS especially for larger and/or irregularly shaped tumors close to sensitive structures. The difference between techniques may be small and large numbers of patients followed for long periods would be required to demonstrate any clinically significant advantage. The more widespread use of protons could allow comparative multi-institutional trials to select the appropriate modality for each tumour type.

Acknowledgements

We thank Valentina Piffer (ATreP, Trento – Italy) for her language editing of the manuscript.

Author details

Dante Amelio[1], Marco Cianchetti[1], Barbara Rombi[1], Sabina Vennarini[1], Francesco Dionisi[1], Maurizio Amichetti[1] and Giuseppe Minniti[2]

1 ATreP – Provincial Agency for Proton Therapy, Trento, Italy

2 Department of Radiation Oncology, University La Sapienza, S. Andrea Hospital, Rome, Italy

The authors have no conflicts of interest. All authors have contributed to the review.

References

[1] Balagamwala EH. Principles of Radiobiology of Stereotactic Radiosurgery and Clinical Applications in the Central Nervous System. Technol Cancer Res Treat 2012;11(1) 3-13.

[2] Suit H. Proton beams to replace photon beams in radical dose treatments. Acta Oncol 2003; 42(8) 800-808.

[3] Kirkpatrick JP. The linear-quadratic model is inappropriate to model high dose per fraction effects in radiosurgery. Semin Radiat Oncol 2008;18(4) 240–243.

[4] Breuer H, Smit BJ. Proton therapy and radiosurgery. Heidelberg: Springer-Verlag; 2010.

[5] Chin LS, Regine WF. Principles and practice of stereotactic radiosurgery. New York: Springer; 2008.

[6] Hall EJ. The radiobiology of radiosurgery: rationale for different treatment regimens for AVMs and malignancies. Int J Radiat Oncol Biol Phys 1993;25(2) 381-385.

[7] Overgaard J. Modification of hypoxia-induced radioresistance in tumors by the use of oxygen and sensitizers. Semin Radiat Oncol 1996;6(1) 10-21.

[8] Whiters HR, Thames HD, Peters LJ. Progress in radio-oncology, vol 2. New York: Raven Press; 1982.

[9] Whiters HR. Cell cycle redistribution as factor in multifractionation irradiation. Radiology 1975;114(1) 199-202.

[10] Larson DA. Radiobiology of radiosurgery. Int J Radiat Oncol Biol Phys 1993;25(3) 557-561.

[11] Paganetti H. Relative biological effectiveness (RBE) values for proton beam therapy. Int J Radiat Oncol Biol Phys 2002;53(2) 407-421.

[12] Phillips MH. Comparison of different radiation types and irradiation geometries in stereotactic radiosurgery. Int J Radiat Oncol Biol Phys 1990;18(1) 211-220.

[13] Luxton G. Stereotactic radiosurgery: principles and comparison of treatment methods. Neurosurgery 1993;32(2) 241-259.

[14] Serago CF. Comparison of proton and x-ray conformal dose distributions for radiosurgery applications. Med Phys 1995;22(12) 2111-2116.

[15] Verhey LJ. Comparison of radiosurgery treatment modalities based on physical dose distributions. Int J Radiat Oncol Biol Phys 1998;40(2) 497-505.

[16] Smith V. Comparison of radiosurgery treatment modalities based on complication and control probabilities. Int J Radiat Oncol Biol Phys 1998;40(2):507-513.

[17] Yu JS. Glioblastoma induction after radiosurgery for meningioma. Lancet 2000;356(9241) 1576-1577.

[18] Loeffler JS. Second tumors after radiosurgery: tip of the iceberg or a bump in the road? Neurosurgery 2003;52(6) 1436-40; discussion 1440-1442.

[19] Hanft S. A review of malignant meningiomas: diagnosis, characteristics, and treatment. J Neurooncol 2010;99(3) 433-443.

[20] Santacroce A. Long term tumor control of benign intracranial meningiomas after radiosurgery in a series of 4565 patients. Neurosurgery 2012;70(1) 32-39.

[21] Minniti G. Radiotherapy and radiosurgery for benign skull base meningiomas. Radiat Oncol 2009;4 42.

[22] Kondziolka D. Radiosurgery as definitive management of intracranial meningiomas. Neurosurgery 2008;62(1) 53-58.

[23] DiBiase SJ. Factors predicting local tumor control after gamma knife stereotactic radiosurgery for benign intracranial meningiomas. Int J Radiat Oncol Biol Phys 2004;60(5) 1515–1519.

[24] Nicolato A. The role of Gamma Knife radiosurgery in the management of cavernous sinus meningiomas. Int J Radiat Oncol Biol Phys 2002;53(4) 992-1000.

[25] Adler JR Jr. Visual field preservation after multisession cyberknife radiosurgery for perioptic lesions. Neurosurgery 2008;62(Suppl 2) 733-743.

[26] Tuniz F. Multisession cyberknife stereotactic radiosurgery of large, benign cranial base tumors: preliminary study. Neurosurgery 2009;65(5) 898-907.

[27] Colombo F. Cyberknife radiosurgery for benign meningiomas: short term results in 199 patients. Neurosurgery 2009;64(Suppl 2) A7-13.

[28] Noël G. Highly conformal therapy using proton component in the management of meningiomas. Preliminary experience of the Centre de Protonthérapie d'Orsay. Strahlenther Onkol 2002;178(9) 480-485.

[29] Wenkel E. Benign meningioma: Partially resected, biopsied, and recurrent intracranial tumors treated with combined proton and photon radiotherapy. Int J Radiat Oncol Biol Phys 2000;48(5) 1363–1370.

[30] Weber DC. Spot Scanning-based Proton Therapy for Intracranial Meningioma: Long-term Results from the Paul Scherrer Institute. Int J Radiat Oncol Biol Phys 2012;83(3) 865-871.

[31] Noël G. Functional outcome of patients with benign meningioma treated by 3D conformal irradiation with a combination of photons and protons. Int J Radiat Oncol Biol Phys 2005;62(5) 1412-1422.

[32] Arvold ND. Visual outcome and tumor control after conformal radiotherapy for patients with optic nerve sheath meningioma. Int J Radiat Oncol Biol Phys 2009;75(4) 1166-1172.

[33] Boskos C. Combined proton and photon conformal radiotherapy for intracranial atypical and malignant meningioma. Int J Radiat Oncol Biol Phys 2009;75(2) 399-406.

[34] Hug EB. Management of atypical and malignant meningiomas: role of high-dose, 3D-conformal radiation therapy. J Neurooncol 2000;48(2) 151-160.

[35] Vernimmen FJ. Stereotactic proton beam therapy of skull base meningiomas. Int J Radiat Oncol Biol Phys 2001;49(1) 99-105.

[36] Gudjonsson O. Stereotactic irradiation of skull base meningiomas with high energy protons. Acta Neurochir 1999;141(9) 933–940.

[37] Halasz LM. Proton stereotactic radiosurgery for the treatment of benign meningiomas. Int J Radiat Oncol Biol Phys 2011;81(5) 1428-1435.

[38] Loeffler JS. Radiation therapy in the management of pituitary adenomas. J Clin Endocrinol Metab 2011;96(7) 1992-2003.

[39] Minniti G. Radiation techniques for acromegaly. Radiat Oncol 2011;6 167.

[40] Minniti G. Modern techniques for pituitary radiotherapy. Rev Endocr Metab Disord 2009;10(2) 135-144.

[41] Iwata H. Hypofractionated stereotactic radiotherapy with CyberKnife for nonfunctioning pituitary adenoma: high local control with low toxicity. Neuro Oncol 2011;13(8) 916-922.

[42] Killory BD. Hypofractionated CyberKnife radiosurgery for perichiasmatic pituitary adenomas: early results. Neurosurgery 2009;64(Suppl 2) A19-25.

[43] Ronson BB. Fractionated proton beam irradiation of pituitary adenomas. Int J Radiat Oncol Biol Phys 2006;64(2) 425-434.

[44] Petit JH. Proton stereotactic radiosurgery in management of persistent acromegaly. Endocr Pract 2007;13(7) 726-734.

[45] Petit JH. Proton stereotactic radiotherapy for persistent adrenocorticotropin-producing adenomas. J Clin Endocrinol Metab 2008;93(2) 393-399.

[46] Yock TI. Stereotactic Proton Beam Radiosurgery for ACTH Producing Adenomas in the MRI/CT Era. Int J Radiat Oncol Biol Phys 2001;51(Supplement 1)162.

[47] Aghi MK. Management of Recurrent and Refractory Cushing's Disease with Reoperation and/or Proton Beam Radiosurgery. Clin Neurosurg 2008;55 141-144.

[48] Bassim MK. Radiation therapy for the treatment of vestibular schwannoma: a critical evaluation of the state of the literature. Otol Neurotol 2010;31(4) 567-573.

[49] Murphy ES. Radiotherapy for vestibular schwannomas: a critical review. Int J Radiat Oncol Biol Phys 2011;79(4) 985-997.

[50] Yang I. A comprehensive analysis of hearing preservation after radiosurgery for vestibular schwannoma. J Neurosurg 2010;112(4) 851-859.

[51] Sughrue ME. Preservation of facial nerve function after resection of vestibular schwannoma. Br J Neurosurg 2010;24(6) 666-671.

[52] Nakaya K. Gamma knife radiosurgery for benign tumors with symptoms from brainstem compression. Int J Radiat Oncol Biol Phys 2010;77(4) 988-995.

[53] Kalapurakal JA. Improved trigeminal and facial nerve tolerance following fractionated stereotactic radiotherapy for large acoustic neuromas. Br J Radial 1999;72(864) 1202-1207.

[54] Meijer OW. Single-fraction vs. fractionated LINAC-based stereotactic radiosurgery for vestibular schwannoma: a single institution study. Int J Radiat Oncol Biol Phys 2003;56(5) 1390-1396.

[55] Bush DA. Fractionated proton beam radiotherapy for acoustic neuroma. Neurosurgery 2002;50(2) 270-273.

[56] Weber DC. Proton beam radiosurgery for vestibular schwannoma: tumor control and cranial nerve toxicity. Neurosurgery 2003;53(3) 577-586.

[57] Harsh GR. Proton beam stereotactic radiosurgery of vestibular schwannomas. Int J Radiat Oncol Biol Phys 2002;54(1) 35-44.

[58] Vernimmen FJ. Long-term results of stereotactic proton beam radiotherapy for acoustic neuromas. Radiother Oncol 2009;90(2) 208-212.

[59] Minniti G. The role of fractionated radiotherapy and radiosurgery in the management of patients with craniopharyngioma. Neurosurg Rev 2009;32(2) 125-132.

[60] Kobayashi T. Long-term results of gamma knife surgery for the treatment of craniopharyngioma in 98 consecutive cases. J Neurosurg 2005;103(Suppl 6) 482–488.

[61] Mokry M. Craniopharyngiomas: a six year experience with Gamma Knife radiosurgery. Stereotact Funct Neurosurg 1999;72(Suppl 1) 140–149.

[62] Niranjan A. Radiosurgery for craniopharyngioma. Int J Radiat Oncol Biol Phys 2010;78(1) 64-71.

[63] Ulfarsson E. Gamma knife radiosurgery for craniopharyngiomas: long-term results in the first Swedish patients. J Neurosurg 2002; 97(Suppl 5) 613–622.

[64] Beltran C. On the Benefits and Risks of Proton Therapy in Pediatric Craniopharyngioma. Int J Radiat Oncol Biol Phys 2012;82(2) e281-287.

[65] Luu QT. Fractionated proton radiation treatment for pediatric craniopharyngioma: preliminary report. Cancer J 2006;12(2) 155-159.

[66] Fitzek MM. Combined proton and photon irradiation for craniopharyngioma: long-term results of the early cohort of patients treated at Harvard Cyclotron Laboratory and Massachusetts General Hospital. Int J Radiat Oncol Biol Phys 2006;64(5) 1348-1354.

[67] Amichetti M. Proton therapy in chordoma of the base of the skull: a systematic review. Neurosurg Rev 2009;32(4) 403-416.

[68] Amichetti M. A systematic review of proton therapy in the treatment of chondrosarcoma of the skull base. Neurosurg Rev 2010;33(2) 155-165.

[69] Chang SD. Stereotactic radiosurgery and hypofractionated stereotactic radiotherapy for residual or recurrent cranial base and cervical chordomas. Neurosurg Focus 2001;10(3) E5.

[70] Gwak HS. Hypofractionated stereotactic radiation therapy for skull base and upper cervical chordoma and chondrosarcoma: preliminary results. Stereotact Funct Neurosurg 2005;83(5-6) 233-243.

[71] Henderson FC. Treatment of chordomas with CyberKnife: Georgetown University experience and treatment recommendations. Neurosurgery 2009;64(Suppl 2) A44-53.

[72] Ivan ME. A meta-analysis of tumor control rates and treatment-related morbidity for patients with glomus jugulare tumors. J Neurosurg 2011;114(5) 1299-1305.

[73] Guss ZD. Radiosurgery of glomus jugulare tumors: a meta-analysis. Int J Radiat Oncol Biol Phys 2011;81(4) e497-502.

[74] Hafez RF. The safety and efficacy of gamma knife surgery in management of glomus jugulare tumor. World J Surg Oncol 2010;8 76.

[75] Krych AJ. Long-term results of irradiation for paraganglioma. Int J Radiat Oncol Biol Phys 2006;65(4) 1063-1066.

[76] Pemberton LS. Radical radiotherapy alone for glomus jugulare and tympanicum tumours. Oncol Rep 2005;14(6) 1631-1633.

[77] Wegner RE. Linac-based stereotactic body radiation therapy for treatment of glomus jugulare tumors. Radiother Oncol 2010;97(3) 395-398.

[78] Dulguerov P. Esthesioneuroblastoma: a meta-analysis and review. Lancet Oncol 2001;2(11) 683–690.

[79] Walch C. The minimally invasive approach to olfactory neuroblastoma: combined endoscopic and stereotactic treatment. Laryngoscope 2000;110(4) 635-640.

[80] Unger F. Combined endoscopic surgery and radiosurgery as treatment modality for olfactory neuroblastoma (esthesioneuroblastoma). Acta Neurochir (Wien) 2005;147(6) 595-601.

[81] Nishimura H. Proton-beam therapy for olfactory neuroblastoma. Int J Radiat Oncol Biol Phys 2007;68(3) 758-762.

Chapter 12

Hyperthermia: Cancer Treatment and Beyond

Ahmed Bettaieb, Paulina K. Wrzal and
Diana A. Averill-Bates

Additional information is available at the end of the chapter

http://dx.doi.org/10.5772/55795

1. Introduction

The three mainstays for cancer treatment include surgical removal of tumors, radiation therapy and chemotherapy, which have led to improved patient survival for certain types of cancer, but there is still much room for improvement. Cancer is one of the leading causes of death worldwide and accounted for 7.6 million deaths (13% of all deaths) in 2008 (World Health Organization, 2012). The 2012 Report to the Nation on the Status of Cancer indicated that there was a decrease in overall cancer mortality and incidence in the U.S.A. from 1999 to 2008, particularly for the four major cancer sites: lung, colorectum, breast and prostate [1]. However, there were increases in the incidence of other types of cancer, including those of the pancreas, kidney, thyroid and liver, as well as melanoma and adenocarcinoma of the esophagus, from 1999 to 2008.

Over the past decades, the struggle against cancer has led to the discovery of new strategies to fight this disease and to bring hope to patients. These new strategies include hyperthermia (also commonly known as thermal therapy or thermotherapy), biological therapies (e.g. immunotherapy), photodynamic therapy, laser treatment, gene therapy, and inhibitors of angiogenesis. Most of these strategies still need optimization, and in some cases (e.g. hyperthermia, photodynamic therapy), improved equipment is required. Moreover, a better understanding of the biological mechanisms involved in their anticancer action would certainly be beneficial. Hyperthermia is one of the few strategies to be adopted as a promising therapy among the alternative methods to treat cancer.

Hyperthermia is defined as moderate elevation in temperature. Hyperthermia can either have a pathological origin, resulting from the fever response of the organism to viral or bacterial infections, or may occur during exposure to high temperatures as during heat stroke. It is relatively recent as a clinical procedure, in which body tissues are exposed to elevated temperatures in the range of 39°C to 45°C. These high temperatures can damage and kill cancer cells with minimal injury to normal tissues [2]. During the last two decades, hyperthermia has been used as an efficient complement to standard cancer treatments such as radiation therapy and chemotherapy [2,3] (Figure 1). A further advantage is that hyperthermia can eliminate drug-resistant and radio-resistant tumour cells. Another form of hyperthermia involves very high temperatures (> 60°C), which can destroy or «cook» tumours by a technique known as thermal ablation (see review, [4]). The present review will address the therapeutic potential of moderate hyperthermia (39°C to 45°C).

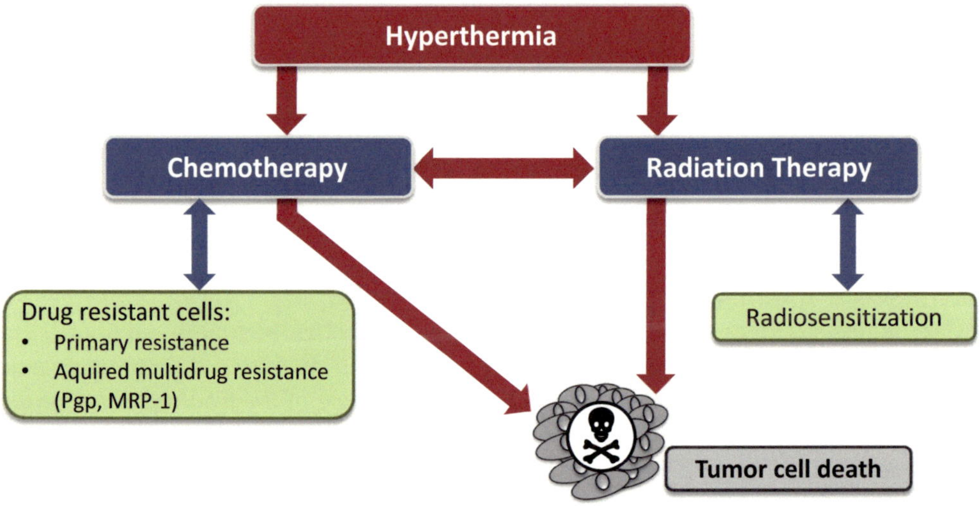

Figure 1. Hyperthermia complements standard cancer treatments such as chemotherapy and radiation therapy in destroying tumour cells.

2. Hyperthermia

2.1. Scientific history

The use of heat to treat disease, including cancer, is a concept that dates back to early Egyptian times, over 5000 years ago (see review, [5]). Indeed, the Egyptian medical papyrus recounts an attempt to treat breast cancer with a "heated stick" [6]. Likewise, many Greek doctors, among them Hippocrates, suggested cauterizing superficial tumours by using heated metal. Many ancient cultures, including the Roman, Chinese, Indian and Japanese cultures have used this concept for the treatment of a variety of diseases. During the late 1800s, there were numerous observations by astute clinicians of spontaneous remissions of cancer in patients suffering from a variety of infections [7]. Dr. William B. Coley found 47 case reports in which simultaneous infection seemed to have caused the remission of an incurable neoplastic malignancy (see review, [8]). In the late 1800s, he used "Coley's Mixed Toxins" (bacterial pyrogenic toxins) as a deliberate fever-inducing treatment to control tumor growth [9]. Despite promising observations during several decades, these cancer treatments were difficult to administer in a controlled manner, and responses were unpredictable [10]. Using a different approach, Westermark reported the use of localized, non-fever producing heat treatments (42-44°C) by means of water-circulating cisterns that resulted in the long-term remission of inoperable cancer of the cervix [11]. As different techniques were developed, such as surgery, radiation therapy and chemotherapy, further development of hyperthermia for cancer treatment was put on the back burner. There was a resurgence of interest in the use of hyperthermia in cancer treatment based on scientific studies initiated in the 1960s and 1970s. A turning point was a study conducted in transplanted mouse tumors that illustrated novel biological phenomena: cytotoxicity of hyperthermia was dependent on time and temperature; increased sensitivity of large versus small tumors to hyperthermia (later attributed to vascular events); heat-induced thermotolerance of normal and tumor tissue; and hyperthermia-induced sensitization to radiation [12]. These promising observations led to quantitative experimental studies and a rapid increase in our understanding of the biological effects of hyperthermia. Furthermore, they frame the rationale for the clinical use of hyperthermia, and the development of more effective technologies for the precise application of heat to tumors and for the measurement of heat distribution in tumors by thermometry.

2.2. Cellular changes

Temperatures in the range of moderate hyperthermia can be non-lethal (39 to 42°C) or lethal (>42°C). Temperatures above 42°C were shown to kill cancer cells in a time- and temperature-dependent manner that was measured by the clonogenic cell survival assay [13]. However, despite numerous studies during at least three decades, which have improved our understanding of hyperthermia biology, the mechanisms involved in heat-induced cytotoxicity are still ill-defined [14]. Hyperthermia causes many changes in cells and leads to a loss of cellular homeostasis [15-17]. A key event appears to be protein denaturation and aggregation, which results in cell cycle arrest, inactivation of protein synthesis, and inhibition of DNA repair processes [18]. Other cellular effects of hyperthermia include: (1) the inhibition of DNA synthesis, transcription, RNA processing and translation; (2) increased degradation of aggregated/misfolded proteins through the proteasomal and lysosomal pathways; (3) disruption of the membrane cytoskeleton; (4) metabolic changes (e.g. uncoupling of oxidative phosphorylation) that lead to decreased levels of ATP; and (5) alterations in membrane permeability that cause increases in intracellular levels of Na^+, H^+ and Ca^{2+} (see reviews, [19,20].

Hyperthermia can cause changes in lipids but these appear to be reversible [21]. The viscosity of the plasma membrane decreases with increasing temperature [22], and this may be associated with altered transport functions of the membrane. Changes in membrane viscosity were linked to an elevation in the activity of the ATP-dependent sodium-potassium pump [22], which maintains Na^+ and K^+ levels across the plasma membrane against a concentration gradient. During hyperthermia, membrane permeability towards several compounds is altered, including polyamines, glucose, and anticancer drugs [23-25].

Despite the large number of documented cellular changes, the nature of the critical lesions that lead to cell death following heat treatment remains unknown. Proteins appear to be the first target of hyperthermia in the clinically-relevant temperature range of 39 to 45°C (Figure 2). The alteration of cellular homeostasis after exposure to hyperthermia entails a certain number of post-translational modifications such as glycosylation, acylation, phosphorylation, farnelysation and ubiquitination [18,26]. Several studies reported that hyperthermia can cause DNA fragmentation and the formation of double strand breaks (DBSs) [27,28], which could arise from the inhibition of DNA repair mechanisms [21]. However, it appears that nuclear protein damage may be the key factor rather than direct DNA damage itself. Nuclear proteins, in particular, appear to be very sensitive to hyperthermia and undergo aggregation [21]. Nuclear protein aggregation has been linked to the inhibition of transcription and DNA replication.

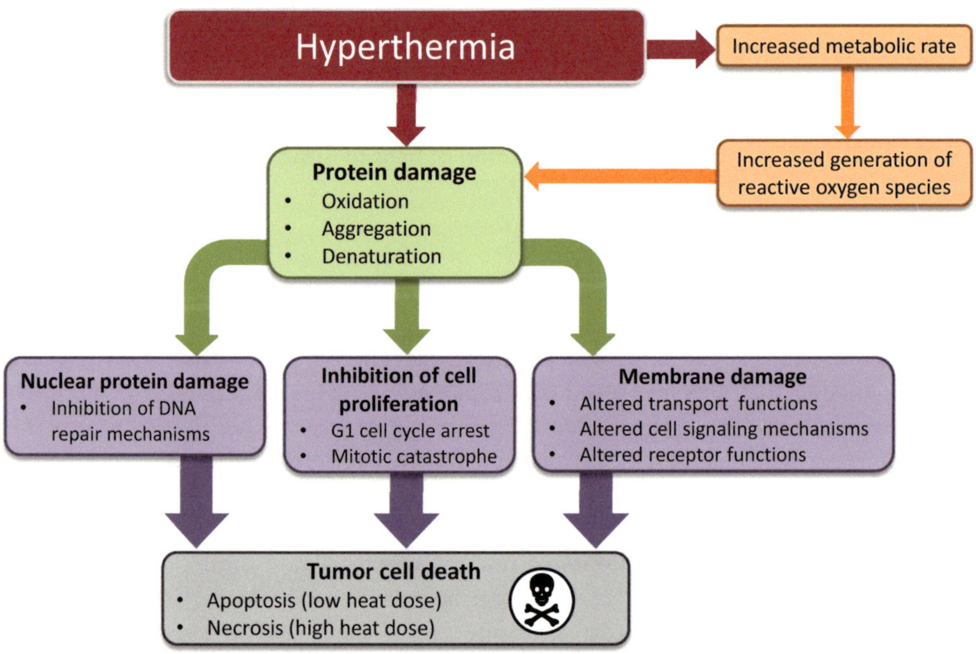

Figure 2. Hyperthermia-induced cellular changes that could lead to tumour cell death.

Elevated temperatures can increase the rates of biochemical reactions and this would increase cell metabolism, which should cause increased oxidative stress (Figure 2). Levels of reactive oxygen species (ROS) were shown to increase after exposure to both lethal (≥42°C) [29-31] and non-lethal (40°C) temperatures [32,33]. This would arise principally from the increased generation of ROS such as superoxide and hydrogen peroxide (H_2O_2), likely as a result of dysfunction of the mitochondrial respiratory chain. Other potential sources of increased ROS generation would be increased activity of superoxide-producing enzymes such as NADPH oxidase and xanthine oxidase at elevated temperatures. Hyperthermia could also increase the reactivity of these ROS; indeed, the cytotoxicity of hydrogen peroxide was increased at elevated temperatures (41 to 43°C) compared to the physiological temperature (37°C) [34]. Hyperthermia also inactivated cellular antioxidant defenses against H_2O_2 such as the pentose phosphate pathway [35], which maintains the intracellular antioxidant glutathione in its reduced form, GSH [36]. An increase in the generation of ROS can cause oxidative damage to proteins, lipids and nucleic acids. A hyperthermia-induced decrease in tumor growth was accompanied by an increase in lipid peroxidation in rabbits [37]. Another consequence of increased ROS generation by hyperthermia is that molecules such as H_2O_2 can perturb mitochondrial membrane potential [38]. A temperature-induced increase in cell metabolism could also cause acidosis of the tumor tissue [39,40].

2.3. Cytotoxicity of hyperthermia

As a consequence of different cellular changes, hyperthermia causes mitotic catastrophe, permanent G1 arrest and a loss of clonogenic or reproductive cell capacity [21] (Figure 2). Cells can die by processes such as apoptosis and/or necrosis, which are dependent on the cell type as well as the temperature and duration of heat exposure [32,41]. Another consequence is that cells can become sensitized to other cytotoxic modalities such as radiation [16]. Hyperthermia was reported to cause centrosomal dysfunction and mitotic catastrophe [42], which have been implicated in thermal radio-sensitization [43]. Hyperthermia (42 to 44°C) has been reported to cause chromatin condensation and apoptotic DNA fragmentation (formation of DNA ladders) leading to apoptosis in many different cell types including HeLa cells [44], T lymphocytes [45,46], HL-60 leukemic cells [47], and mice embryonic fibroblasts [48]. In rats treated with whole body hyperthermia (41.5°C for 2 h), both the extent and kinetics of hyperthermia-induced apoptosis differed between two different tumor types (fibrosarcoma and colon carcinoma) [49]. Additionally, the same study revealed another important advantage; the induction of apoptosis was higher in tumor tissues in comparison to normal tissues. Most of the studies that have investigated the mechanisms of heat shock-induced cytotoxicity concluded that apoptosis is the main form of cell death and proposed the pro-apoptotic effects of hyperthermia as the potential desired outcome of hyperthermia in cancer therapy.

2.4. Hyperthermia and physiological changes

Several physiological factors including oxygenation, pH and blood flow were shown to play a role in the sensitivity of cells/tissues to moderate hyperthermia. The intrinsic sensitivity to heat varies significantly among different cell types. Several studies indicate that cancer cells are more susceptible to heat injury than normal cells [21,50]. This could be caused, at least in part, by the differential expression of heat shock proteins (Hsps) and other proteins involved in the cellular defense system against different stressors, including heat shock. However, there is no consistency in findings about heat sensitivity between tumor and normal cells [21]. The sensitivity of cells to heat also varies with phase of the cell cycle, where cells in S phase and mitosis were reported to be most sensitive [51].

Another reason for the use of hyperthermia in cancer treatment is the fact that tumor tissues are poorly vascularized in comparison to normal tissues. This may lead to a differential heating, with higher temperatures being achieved in tumors compared with normal tissue, where heat may be dissipated by circulating blood. Hyperthermia also appears to be complementary to other forms of treatment by being able to destroy tumor cells that are relatively resistant to radiation therapy or chemotherapy. Tumor cells located in the hypoxic centers of tumors are relatively resistant to chemotherapy due to poor drug delivery. Several chemotherapeutic drugs also require oxygen to generate free radicals in order to cause tumor cytotoxicity. Further, most chemotherapeutic drugs are more effective against proliferating cells. However, hypoxia has been shown to cause decreased proliferation, which may partially explain the reason for resistance of tumor cells to chemotherapy [52-54]. Cells located in hypoxic areas of tumors are also resistant to radiation therapy.

Heating of human tumours is heterogeneous. Some areas of the tumour reach cytotoxic temperatures such as 43 to 45°C, whereas other areas only reach 39 to 42°C. It is more difficult to heat larger or deep-seated tumours to cytotoxic temperatures that are adequate to cause cell death or vascular damage.

Tumors are unable to adapt their blood circulation to the effects of high temperatures (≥42°C), which enables hyperthermia to cut off the supply of nutrients and oxygen, leading to lower interstitial pH and a collapse in tumor vasculature [55]. These conditions render cells more susceptible to heat treatment. Indeed, cells at lower (acidic) pH and decreased oxygen tension, as in the center of tumors, are more sensitive to heat treatment [56,57]. Cells in a nutrient-deprived environment are also more sensitive to elevated temperatures. This effect appears to correlate with changes in cellular ATP levels [58]. Cells that were deprived of glucose exhibited increased sensitivity to the cytotoxicity of hyperthermia [35]. This effect could be linked to a decrease in antioxidant defenses involving the glutathione redox cycle, since glucose metabolism, through the pentose phosphate pathway, is required for maintaining intracellular levels of GSH. On the other hand, heating at milder temperatures (e.g. 39° to 42°C) can increase tumor blood flow, which leads to improved tumor oxygenation [59,60]. This could render tumors more sensitive to radiation and certain anticancer drugs.

Hyperthermia (≥42°C) has been shown to cause vascular damage in rodent tumours, which leads to decreased oxygenation and necrosis [61]. Although, the vasculature of human tumours appears to be more resistant to hyperthermia than that of rodent tissues, hyperthermia has been shown to cause disturbances in the microcirculation of cancer tissue in human osteosarcoma [62].

Milder temperatures in the range of 40 to 41°C appear to be able to stimulate various elements of the immune system, thus increasing immune surveillance and protecting against tumor growth (see reviews, [63-65]). The exposure of immune effector cells (e.g. macrophages, T cells, and natural killer (NK) cells) to mild temperatures has been shown to: (1) enhance the migration of immune cells to target sites, which could allow better control of infection and tumor burden; (2) increase the expression of cell surface molecules (e.g. involved in antigen presentation); (3) increase the release of soluble factors involved in immune effector cell activity (e.g. pro-inflammatory cytokines including tumor necrosis factor-alpha (TNF-α), interleukin-1 (IL-1), IL-6, IL-10, and IL-12; (4) regulate immune cell proliferation; and (5) increase the cytotoxicity of immune cells against target (tumor) cells.

2.5. Thermotolerance: The other side of hyperthermia

The exposure of cells to lethal temperatures such as 43 to 45°C during short periods of time, ranging from 10 to 30 minutes, allows the development of tolerance towards subsequent exposure to multiple stresses; this phenomenon is termed "thermotolerance" [66,67]. Thermotolerance is an adaptive survival response induced by heat preconditioning whereby cells become resistant to a subsequent lethal insult such as that triggered by heat shock, reactive oxygen species (ROS), and environmental stressors including heavy metals [68,69]. If the level of stress is very low, cells attempt to survive by activating stress responses that protect essential biochemical processes such as DNA repair, protein folding, and the elimination of damaged proteins [70]. Once the stress stimulus is removed, cells can recover their normal cellular function. If the stress continues or is too severe, then the cell will likely die by apoptosis or necrosis.

The acquisition of thermotolerance is characterized by numerous biochemical and molecular changes. Thermotolerance is generally associated with the accumulation of Hsps [19,63,68,71-73]. Hsp expression is regulated by a stress-responsive transcription factor known as heat shock factor 1 (HSF-1), through its interaction with the heat shock element (HSE) [74]. In addition, changes in the expression of about 50 to 200 other genes, not traditionally considered Hsps, have been found during or after heat stress (see review, [20]). These include genes for transcription factors, protein degradation, DNA repair enzymes, metabolic enzymes, cell cycle arrest, transport and detoxification, and signal transduction. The reason for the induction of these other cell-protective pathways by heat shock is probably to protect nascent chain synthesis and folding, prevent protein misfolding and aggregation, and to promote recovery from stress-induced damage [75]. Proteomic analyses showed a change in the phosphorylation of 93 proteins between control RIF-1 and their thermotolerant derivatives, TR-RIF-1 cells [76]. These phosphorylated proteins are responsible for a range of cellular functions, which include chaperones, ion channels, signal transduction, transcription and translation, biosynthesis of amino acids, oxidoreduction, energy metabolism, and cell motility or structure.

The heat shock response is highly conserved in all organisms from yeast to humans, which suggests that it is important for survival in a stressful environment [74]. In addition to heat, the heat shock response can be induced by other insults such as oxidative stress, heavy metals, ethanol, toxins and bacterial infections.

The major classes of Hsps induced by the heat shock response are Hsp90, Hsp70, Hsp60, and Hsp27. Hsps appear to play an important role in thermotolerance. Many studies suggest a correlation between the accumulation of Hsp70 and the acquisition of a thermotolerant state in mammals, amphibians, insects [77-79] and fish [80]. Under conditions of stress, Hsp70s can prevent the formation of protein aggregates and assist the refolding of aggregated proteins into their native structures [19]. Other studies have shown that the state of thermotolerance correlated with an increase in the expression of Hsp110 [81]. Hsp110 is as effective as Hsp70 in preventing protein aggregation, and contributes, along with Hsp70 and Hsp40, to the refolding of denatured proteins. In addition to their protective role against a subsequent lethal heat shock, Hsps are known to protect cells against other forms of stress, such as oxidative stress and radiation [82].

Hsps play an important and yet complex role in the regulation of apoptosis. The specific roles of different Hsps such as Hsp27, Hsp60, Hsp70 and Hsp90 in the regulation of the mitochondrial and death receptor pathways of apoptosis have been reviewed [82-85]. The induction of apoptosis through the Fas death receptor can be regulated by Hsp70 and Hsp27 [86,87]. Hsp27 and Hsp70 can regulate the death receptor pathway of apoptosis by preventing t-Bid translocation to mitochondria, which in turn inhibits cytochrome c release [88, 89]. Hsp90 was shown to be a negative regulator of caspase-2 activation [90]. Hsp27, Hsp70, and Hsp90 can attenuate apoptosis upstream of mitochondria [91], as well as interfering with apoptosome formation, post-mitochondrial events, and caspase activation [92]. Furthermore, Hsp70 and phosphorylated Hsp27 can protect cells against oxidative stress, a potent activator of apoptosis [93,94].

The development of thermotolerance by lethal hyperthermia has been the subject of intensive studies during the past three decades, whereas thermotolerance induced at mild, fever-range temperatures has received relatively little attention. Thermotolerance can be developed following exposure for shorter times (e.g. 30 min) to lethal temperatures (42 to 45°C) [68,71], or during continuous heating (e.g. 3 to 24 h) at non-lethal temperatures (39 to 41.5°C) [95,96]. The development of thermotolerance by exposure of cells to mild hyperthermia (40°C) for 3 to 24 h led to the accumulation of Hsps 27, 32, 60, 70, 90 and 110 [32,95]. This phenomenon is of notable importance for fundamental research given that it is a physiological fever-range temperature and suggests that thermotolerance could protect healthy tissue against stressors during clinical therapies. The treatment of BALB/c mice *in vivo* with fever-range whole body hyperthermia (39.5 to 40°C) for 6h led to increased expression of Hsp70 and Hsp110 in several mouse tissues [97].

Mild thermotolerance developed at 40°C created an apoptosis-resistant phenotype. The activation of the mitochondrial pathway of apoptosis by moderate hyperthermia (42 to 43°C) was attenuated in these thermotolerant cells [44]. Similarly, activation of the death receptor signaling pathway through the Fas receptor by lethal heat shock (42 to 43°C) was inhibited in thermotolerant cells [32]. Furthermore, thermotolerance developed at 40°C protected cells against the induction of apoptosis by oxidative stress (H_2O_2), mediated through the mitochondrial and death receptor pathways [33,38]. This apoptosis-resistant phenotype could be conferred by increased levels of both Hsps (Hsps 27, 32, 60, 70, 90, and 110 kDa) and antioxidants (catalase, manganese superoxide dismutase, glutathione) [32,33]. Mild thermotolerance also inhibited hyperthermia-induced ROS generation [32], and this could be explained by the ROS-inhibitory effect of Hsps such as Hsp27 and Hsp70 [93,94].

Hsps play overlapping roles in tumour development and growth by promoting cell proliferation and by inhibiting cell death pathways [98]. Hsp70 is a survival protein that is overexpressed in various malignant tumors and its expression correlates with increased cell proliferation, poor differentiation and poor therapeutic outcome in human breast cancer [99]. The increased expression of Hsp70 in tumors can prevent the activation of caspases and proteases, and thus abolish apoptotic cell death [98]. Moreover, the increased expression of Hsps appears to be involved in the acquisition of drug-resistant phenotypes. Several studies have reported that Hsp27 may be involved in the development of resistance to chemotherapeutic agents such as doxorubicin and cisplatin [100-104].

2.6. Hyperthermia in cancer therapy

The biological rational for the use of hyperthermia in cancer treatment is very strong. Temperatures of 42.5°C and above are able to kill cancer cells. Findings from *in vitro* studies generally indicate that there is no intrinsic difference in heat sensitivity between normal and tumour cells [105]. However, a tumour selective effect of hyperthermia could occur at higher temperatures *in vivo*. In solid tumours, the vascular system is chaotic, which results in regions with hypoxia and low pH levels, compared to normal tissues. These conditions render cells more sensitive to the cytotoxic effects of hyperthermia. Therefore, hyperthermia can be beneficial by causing direct cytotoxicity to tumour cells, in addition to selective destruction of tumour cells in hypoxic and low pH environments within solid tumours. A further benefit is that mild hyperthermia can activate certain responses of the immune system, which could also provide protection against tumour growth [64,106]. In the clinic, hyperthermia has been shown to be most beneficial when used in combination with radiation therapy and/or chemotherapy.

2.6.1. Hyperthermia in combination with radiotherapy

One of the most promising aspects of hyperthermia in cancer treatment is the ability to eliminate radiation-resistant tumour cells [see review, 5]. Indeed, this renders hyperthermia as one of the most effective radiation sensitizers known. The basis for this effect is that hyperthermia has the ability to kill cells that are under conditions of hypoxia, low pH and that are in the S-phase of cell division, which are all conditions that render cells resistant to radiation. The mechanisms responsible for heat-induced radio-sensitization are not entirely understood, particularly for milder temperatures [21]. For temperatures of 43°C and above, nuclear protein damage is considered to be a critical event [107]. It was suggested that hyperthermia interferes with the repair of radiation-induced DNA damage. In support of this idea, hyperthermia increased the amount of radiation-induced chromosomal aberrations [13, 108]. It was suggested that heat-induced enhancement of chromosomal aberrations could arise from the inhibition of repair of radiation-induced DNA damage. Hyperthermia could exert its major effect on radio-sensitization by specifically inhibiting base excision repair of DNA damage [109,110].

2.6.2. Hyperthermia in combination with chemotherapy

The combined use of regional hyperthermia with systemic chemotherapy has considerable potential in cancer treatment mainly because localized heat delivery could enhance cytotoxic activity of anticancer drugs within a defined target region. This may lead to an improved therapeutic ratio by allowing targeting of chemotherapy, as can be achieved with radiation therapy. At present, targeted treatment with anticancer drugs can only be accomplished when they are administered either topically or intra-arterially. There is also evidence to suggest that the cytotoxic effects of hyperthermia and anticancer drugs may prove to be complementary. Tumour cells that are located in less well-vascularized regions of a tumour, such as the tumour center, may be relatively resistant to systemic chemotherapy because they are exposed to lower concentrations of drug. The benefit of hyperthermia is that it kills cells most efficiently in the low pH and hypoxic environment of the tumour core. Furthermore, the temperature achieved in poorly vascularized regions of the tumour may be higher because of less efficient cooling by circulating blood. Another potential benefit is that regional hyperthermia at 40–43°C causes an increase in tumour blood supply [111]. Blood flow and vascular permeability, which are increased by hyperthermia, are critical factors for drug uptake [112].

Laboratory and *in vivo* studies have shown that the combined use of hyperthermia and chemotherapy leads to increased cytotoxic effects of several anticancer drugs such as cisplatin, anthracyclines, cyclophosphamide, ifosfamide, nitrosoureas, bleomycin, mitomycin, and nitrogen mustards such as melphalan [16,25,105,113-118]. Optimal heat enhancement of drug cytotoxicity generally occurs between 40.5°C and 43°C. For drugs such as cisplatin, alkylating agents, and nitrosoureas, interactions between heat and drug are more than additive (or synergistic), whereas in other cases, interactions are simply additive [119]. For bleomycin and Adriamycin, there is a threshold temperature of about 42.5°C to 43°C for enhancement of drug cytotoxicity. The antimetabolites (e.g. 5-fluorodeoxyuridin and methotrexate) and Vinca alkaloids or taxanes have independent interactions with hyperthermia. In general, the most effective heat-drug sequence is drug treatment immediately before heat delivery. The mechanisms of heat-induced enhancement of drug cytotoxicity are not well understood. Possible mechanisms include improved drug delivery to the tumour due to increased blood perfusion, increased intracellular uptake of drugs, and increased rates of reaction of drugs with cellular targets (e.g. increased drug alkylation, increased DNA damage).

2.6.2.1. Resistance to chemotherapeutic agents

One of the major limitations to the successful use of chemotherapy in cancer treatment is the development of resistance to multiple anticancer drugs. Cross-resistance occurs between different anticancer agents that have distinct structures and mechanisms of cytotoxicity. Multidrug resistance (MDR) is characterized by cross-resistance to four classes of commonly used anticancer drugs such as Vinca alkaloids, anthracyclines, taxanes, and epipodophyllotoxins. Classical MDR was discovered about 35 years ago and was initially related to the overexpression of the cellular 170-kDa protein P-glycoprotein (Pgp) [120], a member of the ATP-binding cassette (ABC) transporters. Pgp acts as an ATP-dependent transmembrane pump. Once anticancer drugs enter cells, they are immediately expulsed out of cells by Pgp. This results in decreased levels of drugs inside cells, rendering the drugs less effective against the tumour cells. In addition to Pgp, several other transporter proteins have been implicated in MDR in human cancer: multidrug resistance-associated protein 1 (MRP1), lung resistance protein (LRP) and breast cancer resistance protein (BCRP) [121]. MRP1 is a 190-kDa member of the ABC transporter family of proteins [122]. MRP1-mediated transport requires GSH, as well as ATP binding and hydrolysis. The overexpression of the protein MRP1 can cause cellular resistance to several anticancer drugs, including Adriamycin (doxorubicin), epipodophyllotoxins, and Vinca alkaloids such as vincristine, [123]. The substrate spectrum of MRP proteins also comprises amphiphilic anion conjugates of lipophilic compounds with glutathione (GSH), glucuronate, or sulfate [124], as well as cysteinyl leukotriene (LTC4), prostaglandins, and the anticancer drug methotrexate [125].

Eventually, other distinct mechanisms were also implicated in the MDR phenotype [126]. These mechanisms engage other proteins involved in cellular defenses such as glutathione S-transferase (GST), an enzyme involved in the cellular detoxification of xenobiotics, which include certain anticancer drugs, toxins and environmental pollutants that undergo conjugation with the antioxidant GSH [127]. Other cellular defenses utilized by the MDR phenotype include metallothionein, thioredoxin, thymidylate synthase, dihydrofolate reductase, Hsps and topoisomerase II [126].

Clinical drug resistance appears to be a very complex and multifactorial problem [128] with multiple mechanisms involved. There is often overlapping substrate specificity between different drug transporters, and they are commonly co-expressed in many normal tissues and tumours. Overcoming MDR in cancer treatment presents a formidable challenge [129].

To date, three generations of inhibitors have been used to increase the efficacy of chemotherapy by inhibiting transporter-mediated drug efflux. However, the development of clinical inhibitors of ABC transporters as targets for clinical intervention in oncology has been difficult and new approaches are clearly needed. Clinical drug resistance is a major barrier which, if overcome, should lead to a significant improvement in patient survival.

2.6.2.2. Hyperthermia and reversal of resistance to chemotherapeutic agents

A beneficial effect of hyperthermia is its ability to reverse resistance to certain chemotherapeutic drugs [130]. Hyperthermia increased the cytotoxicity of anticancer drugs such as methotrexate [131], cisplatin [132], and mitomycin c [133] in cells exhibiting primary drug resistance. In addition, hyperthermia enhanced the cytotoxicity of melphalan in MDR Chinese hamster ovary CH^RC5 cells that overexpress Pgp [117]. CH^RC5 cells are resistant to anticancer drugs such as colchicine, Vinca alkaloids, Adriamycin, and melphalan [134].

Among the earlier strategies to overcome MDR, Pgp-modulating agents such as cyclosporin A and verapamil were developed. These chemosensitizers appear to act by decreasing Pgp-mediated efflux of anticancer drugs from cells, which allows increased accumulation of drugs to more cytotoxic levels inside cells. However, clinical studies showed that these chemosensitizers were effective only at toxic doses [128]. Therefore, chemosensitizers with improved MDR-reversing ability and lower toxicity need to be developed, as well as novel approaches. Hyperthermia (42 to 43°C) showed beneficial effects by reversing MDR involving Pgp when melphalan or Adriamycin was combined with Pgp modulators such as cyclosporin A [135,136]) or verapamil [137,138]. When combined with hyperthermia (43°C), the Pgp modulator PSC 833 reduced resistance to vinblastine in MDR K562 leukaemia cells and MESSA leiomyosarcoma cells [139]. Moreover, ultrasound-induced hyperthermia (USHT) increased Adriamycin cytotoxicity in the MDR human lung adenocarcinoma cell line MV522 [140]. The alkylating agent melphalan is mainly detoxified through conjugation with GSH, which can be catalyzed by GST [141]. In addition to overexpression of Pgp, CH^RC5 cells also overexpress the alpha and pi forms of GST, compared to the drug-sensitive AuxB1 cells [142]. Hyperthermia was beneficial by enhancing melphalan cytotoxicity in MDR cells when GST was inhibited using ethacrynic acid [142].

2.6.2.3. Sensitivity of multidrug resistant cells to hyperthermia

Another important advantage for the clinical use of hyperthermia is that MDR cells overexpressing Pgp or MRP1 do not display cross-resistance to heat [25,143]. Indeed, these MDR cells exhibit equivalent sensitivity to the cytotoxic and apoptosis-inducing effects of hyperthermia (41-45°C) as their drug-sensitive counterparts. Moreover, drug-resistant sub-clones of human T-lineage acute lymphoblastic leukaemia (ALL) and acute myeloblastic leukaemia (AML) cells were as sensitive to hyperthermia as were the drug-sensitive sub-clones [144]. Results from these studies indicate that, in addition to enhancing drug cytotoxicity in resistant cells, hyperthermia alone can successfully eliminate MDR cells. Together, these findings clearly show that hyperthermia could be useful by destroying subpopulations of drug-resistant tumour cells, which have survived chemotherapy treatments, where the overexpression of Pgp and MRP1 is involved.

Apoptosis is considered to be a physiological mechanism for the elimination of damaged and abnormal cells, such as tumour cells. One of the hallmark characteristics of tumour cells is their ability to evade destruction by apoptosis [145]. The up-regulation of different anti-apoptotic proteins, to provide a survival advantage, has been a frequent explanation for the resistance of cancer cells to elimination by apoptosis [146]. The induction of death receptor and mitochondria-mediated signaling pathways of apoptosis by hyperthermia (41 to 43°C) in MDR $CH^{R}C5$ cells was compared to drug-sensitive CHO cells [147]. Differences were found between MDR and drug-sensitive cells in terms of induction of apoptosis by hyperthermia. For death receptor-mediated apoptosis, MDR cells contained higher levels of the anti-apoptosis protein c-FLIP and they had a lower level of activation of initiator caspase-8 and caspase-10 in response to hyperthermia. In the mitochondria-mediated pathway of heat-induced apoptosis, MDR cells showed higher mitochondrial levels of the pro-apoptosis proteins Bax and tBid, more pronounced mitochondrial membrane depolarization, and increased levels of the apoptosome protein Apaf-1 (apoptosis protease activating factor 1). The MDR cells appeared to show some resistance to death receptor-mediated apoptosis [147], in agreement with other studies in leukaemia cells [148, 149], but this resistance appeared to be compensated for by the pro-apoptosis changes in mitochondrial apoptosis. For the execution stage of apoptosis, the MDR and drug-sensitive cells showed similar levels of hyperthermia-induced caspase-3 activation, as well cleavage of caspase-3 substrates poly (ADP-ribose) polymerase (PARP) and inhibitor of caspase-activated DNase (ICAD) [147]. Similar levels of nuclear chromatin condensation were induced by hyperthermia, showing that overall, MDR cells are not resistant to hyperthermia-induced apoptosis compared to the drug-sensitive cells. In summary, MDR and drug-sensitive cells showed similar responses to heat in terms of clonogenic cell survival and apoptosis, which indicates that hyperthermia could be a promising strategy for eradicating MDR tumour cells in the cancer clinic.

2.7. Hyperthermia in the cancer clinic

2.7.1. Techniques to increase tumour temperatures

In the cancer clinic, hyperthermia is administered by exposing tumour tissues to conductive heat sources, or non-ionizing radiation (e.g. electromagnetic or ultrasonic fields). Hyperthermia can be applied by either invasive or noninvasive techniques, using externally applied power. To increase tumour temperatures, hyperthermia can be applied by several different techniques: local hyperthermia by external or internal energy sources, perfusion hyperthermia of organs, limbs, or body cavities, and whole body hyperthermia [150].

2.7.1.1. Local hyperthermia

Local hyperthermia entails elevating the temperature of superficial or deep-seated subcutaneous tumours while sparing the surrounding normal tissue, using external, intraluminal or interstitial heating modalities. The area can be heated externally with high-frequency waves (e.g. electromagnetic or ultrasound energy) aimed at the tumour from a device outside the body. To achieve internal heating, one of several types of sterile probes may be used, including thin heated wires, hollow tubes filled with warm water, implanted microwave antennae, radiofrequency electrodes and ultrasound. Local hyperthermia has allowed the use of hyperthermia in conjunction with other modalities of antineoplastic therapy. Local hyperthermia is more appropriate for the treatment of solid tumours, rather than blood diseases such as leukaemia. Despite advances in the technology of heating, the non-homogeneous character of the treatment region (i.e. tissue characteristics and blood flow) can often affect the uniformity of the heat dispersion in the treated area. This means that it can be difficult to obtain a uniform regional rise in the temperature that is reproducible [151-155]. Deep regional hyperthermia combined with chemotherapy, also known as hyperthermic intraperitoneal chemotherapy, is one of the promising methods for the treatment of prostate carcinoma [156,157] and bladder cancer [158].

2.7.1.2. Perfusion hyperthermia

This technique involves regional heating through the perfusion of a limb, organ (liver, pelvis, stomach), or body cavity using heated fluids [159-161]. In perfusion, the patient's blood can be removed, heated, and then pumped into the region that is to be heated internally. Perfusion hyperthermia can be applied with or without a cytotoxic drug. When applied to limbs without a cytotoxic agent, a temperature of about 43°C can be used for about two hours. Lower temperatures are used when perfusion is performed in combination with cytotoxic agents, to avoid drug toxicity.

2.7.1.3. Whole body hyperthermia

Externally-induced whole body hyperthermia can be used to treat metastatic cancers that have spread throughout the body. Whole body hyperthermia can be applied using different methods and involves heating the patient to a maximum temperature of 41.8 to 42°C. A newer approach is to increase the temperature to about 40°C for a longer duration, and use a combination of mild hyperthermia with cytokines and/or cytotoxic drugs [118].

Many studies are focusing on improving the heating techniques. This is one of the main challenges that currently limit the clinical use of hyperthermia. Furthermore, improvements are required to heat effectively the deep-seated tumours that are localized in internal organs. The use of nanoparticles and the induction heating of magnetic materials that are implanted into tumors are among the new approaches that are currently being investigated for the improved application of hyperthermia.

2.7.2. Progress in the cancer clinic

In the cancer clinic, hyperthermia (40 to 44°C) is mainly used as an adjuvant to radiation and chemotherapy [2,5,16,150]. The major limitations of these conventional cancer treatments are lack of specificity and normal tissue toxicity. An important advantage of hyperthermia is that the cytotoxicity of radiotherapy and chemotherapy can be targeted to the tumour volume, thereby decreasing toxic side effects. The effectiveness of hyperthermia depends on the temperature rise and the duration of treatment at the elevated temperature. At least 19 randomized studies using a combination of hyperthermia with radiotherapy, chemotherapy or both, have shown significant improvement in clinical outcome in oncology patients, without a significant increase in side effects [150]. In all of these studies, the differences were very large. The combination of hyperthermia with radiation resulted in higher (complete) response rates, accompanied by improved local tumour control rates, better palliative effects, and/or better overall survival rates in many Phase II clinical trials [162-171]. These studies focused on many types of cancer including tumors of the head and neck, cervix, rectum, breast, brain, bladder, lung, esophagus, liver, appendix, prostate, peritoneal lining (mesothelioma), soft-tissue sarcoma and melanoma [2,3,105]. Based on results from a randomized study [171], radiation combined with hyperthermia was included in the 2007 Breast Cancer Guidelines for recurrent breast cancer and other localized cancer recurrences by the National Comprehensive Cancer Network (NCCN, U.S.A.).

Despite positive phase III trials, the clinical application of hyperthermia remains limited. This could be partly due to inadequate monitoring of tumour temperatures or thermal dose, during heat treatments. The temperature distribution throughout a tumour during clinical treatment is not homogeneous due to variable tissue properties and changes in blood flow [172] To ensure high quality of treatments, precise tumour temperature measurements and rigorous thermal dosimetric data are essential. Most hyperthermia centers obtain a sparse number of temperature measurements within intraluminal or interstitial catheters [173]. Thermal dose parameters are dependent on the number of measurement sites and on characteristics such as blood flow and tumor size [174]. It is eventually hoped that temperature measurements during hyperthermia treatment can be improved by measuring 3D thermal distribution in tumours by magnetic resonance imaging (MRI) techniques.

In general, hyperthermia treatments are well tolerated by patients. Hyperthermia can cause some toxicity, including skin burns, but this is usually of limited clinical relevance [166]. Normal tissue damage and toxicity do not generally occur during 1 hour of treatment with temperatures that are below 44°C [175]. Nervous and gastrointestinal tissues appear to be most sensitive.

http://dx.doi.org/10.5772/55795

3. Conclusion

Throughout the past two decades, hyperthermia has been used as a particularly efficient complement to standard cancer treatments such as radiation therapy and chemotherapy. Furthermore, considerable progress has been made in our understanding of the biology, physics and bioengineering involved in hyperthermia. Significant improvement in clinical outcome has been demonstrated for many different types of tumours, including head and neck, breast, brain, bladder, cervix, rectum, lung, esophagus, liver, prostate, melanoma and sarcoma [150]. In Europe, hyperthermia is a standard for the treatment of cervical cancer and some sarcomas. It is a successful alternative for the treatment of other types of cancer such as brain, bladder, rectal and esophageal cancer. Moreover, transurethral microwave thermotherapy (TUMT) has been found to be safe and effective as an alternative to surgery and drug treatment for chronic urogenital pathologies such as benign prostatic hyperplasia [176]. TUMT is a minimally invasive therapy that aims to maintain a good quality of life.

In spite of good clinical results, hyperthermia has received little attention [150]. Several problems associated with the acceptance of this promising treatment modality concern the limited availability of equipment for heating tumours, the lack of awareness concerning clinical results, and the lack of financial resources. Hyperthermia is currently under study in many clinical trials, particularly in Europe, Japan and the US, to improve and better understand this promising technique. Future areas of challenge and opportunity for hyperthermia include: improved understanding of thermal biology; improved technologies for delivery and monitoring of heat treatments in patients; successful high-quality clinical trials; and combination of hyperthermia with emerging cancer therapies [170].

Acknowledgements

Financial support is gratefully acknowledged from the Natural Sciences and Engineering Research Council of Canada (NSERC) (DAB).

Author details

Ahmed Bettaieb[1], Paulina K. Wrzal[2] and Diana A. Averill-Bates[3]

1 Department of Nutrition, University of California, Davis, California, USA

2 Department of Pharmacology and Therapeutics, McGill University, Montréal, Québec, Canada

3 Département des sciences biologiques, Université du Québec à Montréal, Succursale Centre-Ville, Montréal, Québec, Canada

References

[1] Eheman C. et al. Annual Report to the Nation on the status of cancer, 1975-2008, featuring cancers associated with excess weight and lack of sufficient physical activity. Cancer, 2012. 118(9): 2338-66.

[2] van der Zee J. Heating the patient: a promising approach? Ann Oncol, 2002. 13(8): p. 1173-84.

[3] Van der Zee J and MC Erasmus. Hyperthermia in addition to radiotherapy. Clin Oncol (R Coll Radiol), 2007. 19(3 Suppl): S18.

[4] Ahmed M and SN Goldberg. Basic science research in thermal ablation. Surg Oncol Clin N Am, 2011. 20(2): 237-58.

[5] Horsman MR and J Overgaard. Hyperthermia: a potent enhancer of radiotherapy. Clin Oncol (R Coll Radiol), 2007. 19(6): 418-26.

[6] Bryan CP. Ancient Egyptian medicine: the Papyrus Ebers Chicago: Ares Publishers. 1974.

[7] Storm FK. Background, principles, and practice. In: Storm, F.K. (ed.) Hyperthermia in cancer therapy. Boston: G.K. Hall; 1983. p. 1-8.

[8] Decker WK and A Safdar. Bioimmunoadjuvants for the treatment of neoplastic and infectious disease: Coley's legacy revisited. Cytokine Growth Factor Rev, 2009. 20(4): 271-81.

[9] Nauts HC, GA Fowler and FH Bogatko. A review of the influence of bacterial infection and of bacterial products (Coley's toxins) on malignant tumors in man; a critical analysis of 30 inoperable cases treated by Coley's mixed toxins, in which diagnosis was confirmed by microscopic examination selected for special study. Acta Med Scand Suppl, 1953. 276: 1-103.

[10] Stewart JR. Prospects for hyperthermia in cancer treatment. In: Urano M. and Douple E. (eds.) Hyperthermia and Oncology. Vol. 1. Utrecht: VSP; 1988. p. 1-12.

[11] Westermark F. Uber die behandlung des ulceration cervix-carcinoma mittels konstanter warme. Zentralbl Gynaekol 1998. 22: 1335.

[12] Crile G Jr. The effects of heat and radiation on cancers implanted on the feet of mice. Cancer Res, 1963. 23: 372-80.

[13] Dewey WC et al. Cellular responses to combinations of hyperthermia and radiation. Radiology, 1977. 123(2): 463-74.

[14] Milleron RS and SB Bratton. 'Heated' Debates in Apoptosis. Cell Mol Life Sci, 2007. 64(18): 2329-33.

[15] Lindquist S. The heat-shock response. Annu Rev Biochem, 1986. 55: 1151-91.

[16] Hildebrandt B et al. The cellular and molecular basis of hyperthermia. Crit Rev Oncol Hematol, 2002. 43(1): 33-56.

[17] Roti Roti JL. Cellular responses to hyperthermia (40-46 degrees C): cell killing and molecular events. Int J Hyperthermia, 2008. 24(1): 3-15.

[18] Lepock JR. How do cells respond to their thermal environment? Int J Hyperthermia, 2005. 21(8): 681-7.

[19] Richter K, M Haslbeck and J Buchner. The heat shock response: life on the verge of death. Mol Cell, 2010. 40(2): 253-66.

[20] Sonna LA et al. Invited review: Effects of heat and cold stress on mammalian gene expression. J Appl Physiol, 2002. 92(4): 1725-42.

[21] Sugahara T et al. Kadota Fund International Forum 2004. Application of thermal stress for the improvement of health, 15-18 June 2004, Awaji Yumebutai International Conference Center, Awaji Island, Hyogo, Japan. Final report. Int J Hyperthermia, 2008. 24(2): 123-40.

[22] Bates DA et al. Effects of thermal adaptation at 40 degrees C on membrane viscosity and the sodium-potassium pump in Chinese hamster ovary cells. Cancer Res, 1985. 45(10): 4895-9.

[23] Gerner EW et al. Factors regulating membrane permeability alter thermal resistance. Ann N Y Acad Sci, 1980. 335: 215-33.

[24] Lecavalier D and WJ Mackillop. The effect of hyperthermia on glucose transport in normal and thermal-tolerant Chinese hamster ovary cells. Cancer Lett, 1985. 29(2): 223-31.

[25] Bates DA and WJ Mackillop. Hyperthermia, adriamycin transport, and cytotoxicity in drug-sensitive and -resistant Chinese hamster ovary cells. Cancer Res, 1986. 46(11): 5477-81.

[26] Bensaude O et al. Heat-shock induced protein modifications and modulation of enzyme activities. EXS, 1996. 77: 199-219.

[27] Kuhl NM, J Kunz and L Rensing. Heat shock-induced arrests in different cell cycle phases of rat C6-glioma cells are attenuated in heat shock-primed thermotolerant cells. Cell Prolif, 2000. 33(3): 147-66.

[28] Lui JC and SK Kong. Heat shock protein 70 inhibits the nuclear import of apoptosis-inducing factor to avoid DNA fragmentation in TF-1 cells during erythropoiesis. FEBS Lett, 2007. 581(1): 109-17.

[29] Flanagan SW, PL Moseley and GR Buettner. Increased flux of free radicals in cells subjected to hyperthermia: detection by electron paramagnetic resonance spin trapping. FEBS Lett, 1998. 431(2): 285-6.

[30] Moriyama-Gonda N et al. Heat-induced cellular damage and tolerance in combination with adriamycin for the PC-3 prostate cancer cell line: relationships with cytotoxicity, reactive oxygen species and heat shock protein 70 expression. Eur Urol, 2000. 38(2): 235-40.

[31] Katschinski DM et al. Role of tumor necrosis factor alpha in hyperthermia-induced apoptosis of human leukemia cells. Cancer Res, 1999. 59(14): 3404-10.

[32] Bettaieb A and DA Averill-Bates. Thermotolerance induced at a fever temperature of 40 degrees C protects cells against hyperthermia-induced apoptosis mediated by death receptor signalling. Biochem Cell Biol, 2008. 86(6): 521-38.

[33] Pallepati P and DA Averill-Bates. Mild thermotolerance induced at 40 degrees C protects HeLa cells against activation of death receptor-mediated apoptosis by hydrogen peroxide. Free Radic Biol Med, 2011. 50(6): 667-79.

[34] Lord-Fontaine S and DA Averill. Enhancement of cytotoxicity of hydrogen peroxide by hyperthermia in chinese hamster ovary cells: role of antioxidant defenses. Arch Biochem Biophys, 1999. 363(2): 283-95.

[35] Lord-Fontaine S and DA Averill-Bates. Heat shock inactivates cellular antioxidant defenses against hydrogen peroxide: protection by glucose. Free Radic Biol Med, 2002. 32(8): 752-65.

[36] Przybytkowski E and DA Averill-Bates. Correlation between glutathione and stimulation of the pentose phosphate cycle in situ in Chinese hamster ovary cells exposed to hydrogen peroxide. Arch Biochem Biophys, 1996. 325(1): 91-8.

[37] Yoshikawa T et al. The role of active oxygen species and lipid peroxidation in the antitumor effect of hyperthermia. Cancer Res, 1993. 53(10 Suppl): 2326-9.

[38] Pallepati P and D Averill-Bates. Mild thermotolerance induced at 40 degrees C increases antioxidants and protects HeLa cells against mitochondrial apoptosis induced by hydrogen peroxide: Role of p53. Arch Biochem Biophys, 2010. 495(2): 97-111.

[39] Vujaskovic Z et al. Temperature-dependent changes in physiologic parameters of spontaneous canine soft tissue sarcomas after combined radiotherapy and hyperthermia treatment. Int J Radiat Oncol Biol Phys, 2000. 46(1): 179-85.

[40] Bicher HI. The physiological effects of hyperthermia. Radiology, 1980. 137(2): 511-3.

[41] Samali A et al. Thermotolerance and cell death are distinct cellular responses to stress: dependence on heat shock proteins. FEBS Lett, 1999. 461(3): 306-10.

[42] Nakahata K et al. Heat shock induces centrosomal dysfunction, and causes non-apoptotic mitotic catastrophe in human tumour cells. Int J Hyperthermia, 2002. 18(4): 332-43.

[43] Mackey MA and F Ianzini. Enhancement of radiation-induced mitotic catastrophe by moderate hyperthermia. Int J Radiat Biol, 2000. 76(2): 273-80.

[44] Bettaieb A and DA Averill-Bates. Thermotolerance induced at a mild temperature of 40 degrees C protects cells against heat shock-induced apoptosis. J Cell Physiol, 2005. 205(1): 47-57.

[45] Boreham DR et al. Heat-induced thermal tolerance and radiation resistance to apoptosis in human lymphocytes. Biochem Cell Biol, 1997. 75(4): 393-7.

[46] Mosser DD and LH Martin. Induced thermotolerance to apoptosis in a human T lymphocyte cell line. J Cell Physiol, 1992. 151(3): 561-70.

[47] Poe BS and KL O'Neill. Inhibition of protein synthesis sensitizes thermotolerant cells to heat shock induced apoptosis. Apoptosis, 1997. 2(6): 510-7.

[48] Buzzard KA et al. Heat shock protein 72 modulates pathways of stress-induced apoptosis. J Biol Chem, 1998. 273(27): 17147-53.

[49] Sakaguchi Y et al. Apoptosis in tumors and normal tissues induced by whole body hyperthermia in rats. Cancer Res, 1995. 55(22): 5459-64.

[50] Babbs CF and DP DeWitt. Physical principles of local heat therapy for cancer. Med Instrum, 1981. 15(6): 367-73.

[51] Yuguchi T et al. Combined use of hyperthermia and irradiation cause antiproliferative activity and cell death to human esophageal cell carcinoma cells-mainly cell cycle examination. Hum Cell, 2002. 15(1): p. 33-42.

[52] Fokas E, WG McKenna and RJ Muschel. The impact of tumor microenvironment on cancer treatment and its modulation by direct and indirect antivascular strategies. Cancer Metastasis Rev, 2012. 31(3-4):823-42.

[53] Cosse JP and C Michiels. Tumour hypoxia affects the responsiveness of cancer cells to chemotherapy and promotes cancer progression. Anticancer Agents Med Chem, 2008. 8(7): 790-7.

[54] Zhou J et al. Tumor hypoxia and cancer progression. Cancer Lett, 2006. 237: 10-21.

[55] Song CW. Physiological factors in hyperthermia. Natl Cancer Inst Monogr, 1982. 61: 169-76.

[56] Song SK et al. Increased intracellular Ca2+: a critical link in the pathophysiology of sepsis? Proc Natl Acad Sci U S A, 1993. 90(9): 3933-7.

[57] Wike-Hooley JL et al. Human tumour pH changes following hyperthermia and radiation therapy. Eur J Cancer Clin Oncol, 1984. 20(5): 619-23.

[58] Oleson JR et al. Biological and clinical aspects of hyperthermia in cancer therapy. Am J Clin Oncol, 1988. 11(3): 368-80.

[59] Song CW, H Park and RJ Griffin. Improvement of tumor oxygenation by mild hyperthermia. Radiat Res, 2001. 155(4): 515-28.

[60] Iwata K et al. Tumour pO2 can be increased markedly by mild hyperthermia. Br J Cancer Suppl, 1996. 27: S217-21.

[61] Song CW. Effect of local hyperthermia on blood flow and microenvironment: a review. Cancer Res, 1984. 44(10 Suppl): 4721s-4730s.

[62] Bogovic J et al. Posttreatment histology and microcirculation status of osteogenic sarcoma after a neoadjuvant chemo- and radiotherapy in combination with local electromagnetic hyperthermia. Onkologie, 2001. 24(1): 55-8.

[63] Calderwood SK, SS Mambula and PJ Gray Jr. Extracellular heat shock proteins in cell signaling and immunity. Ann N Y Acad Sci, 2007. 1113: 28-39.

[64] Peer AJ et al. Diverse immune mechanisms may contribute to the survival benefit seen in cancer patients receiving hyperthermia. Immunol Res, 2010. 46(1-3): 137-54.

[65] Wang XY et al. Current ideas about applications of heat shock proteins in vaccine design and immunotherapy. Int J Hyperthermia, 2005. 21(8): 717-22.

[66] Subjeck JR, JJ Sciandra and RJ Johnson, Heat shock proteins and thermotolerance; a comparison of induction kinetics. Br J Radiol, 1982. 55(656): 579-84.

[67] Samali A and TG Cotter. Heat shock proteins increase resistance to apoptosis. Exp Cell Res, 1996. 223(1): 163-70.

[68] Landry J et al. Synthesis and degradation of heat shock proteins during development and decay of thermotolerance. Cancer Res, 1982. 42(6): 2457-61.

[69] Martindale JL and NJ Holbrook. Cellular response to oxidative stress: signaling for suicide and survival. J Cell Physiol, 2002. 192(1): 1-15.

[70] Morimoto T et al. Hyperthermia enhances spectrin breakdown in transient focal cerebral ischemia. Brain Res, 1997. 746(1-2): 43-51.

[71] Landry J et al. Thermotolerance and heat shock proteins induced by hyperthermia in rat liver cells. Int J Radiat Oncol Biol Phys, 1982. 8(1): 59-62.

[72] Hayashi M et al. Reversal of P-glycoprotein associated multidrug resistance by new isoprenoid derivatives. Anticancer Drug Des, 2001. 16(4-5): 255-60.

[73] Kregel KC. Heat shock proteins: modifying factors in physiological stress responses and acquired thermotolerance. J Appl Physiol, 2002. 92(5): 2177-86.

[74] Akerfelt M, RI Morimoto and L Sistonen. Heat shock factors: integrators of cell stress, development and lifespan. Nat Rev Mol Cell Biol, 2010. 11(8): 545-55.

[75] Morimoto RI. The heat shock response: systems biology of proteotoxic stress in aging and disease. Cold Spring Harb Symp Quant Biol, 2011. 76: 91-9.

[76] Kim HJ, EJ Song and KJ Lee. Proteomic analysis of protein phosphorylations in heat shock response and thermotolerance. J Biol Chem, 2002. 277(26): 23193-207.

[77] Parsell DA and S Lindquist. The function of heat-shock proteins in stress tolerance: degradation and reactivation of damaged proteins. Annu Rev Genet, 1993. 27: 437-96.

[78] Favatier F et al. Variation in hsp gene expression and Hsp polymorphism: do they contribute to differential disease susceptibility and stress tolerance? Cell Stress Chaperones, 1997. 2(3): 141-55.

[79] Krebs RA and ME Feder. Deleterious consequences of Hsp70 overexpression in Drosophila melanogaster larvae. Cell Stress Chaperones, 1997. 2(1): 60-71.

[80] Podrabsky JE and GN Somero. An inducible 70 kDa-class heat shock protein is constitutively expressed during early development and diapause in the annual killifish Austrofundulus limnaeus. Cell Stress Chaperones, 2007. 12(3): 199-204.

[81] Easton DP, Y Kaneko and JR Subjeck. The hsp110 and Grp1 70 stress proteins: newly recognized relatives of the Hsp70s. Cell Stress Chaperones, 2000. 5(4): 276-90.

[82] Sreedhar AS and P Csermely. Heat shock proteins in the regulation of apoptosis: new strategies in tumor therapy: a comprehensive review. Pharmacol Ther, 2004. 101(3): 227-57.

[83] Beere HM. "The stress of dying": the role of heat shock proteins in the regulation of apoptosis. J Cell Sci, 2004. 117(Pt 13): 641-51.

[84] Beere HM and DR Green. Stress management - heat shock protein-70 and the regulation of apoptosis. Trends Cell Biol, 2001. 11(1): 6-10.

[85] Lanneau D et al. Heat shock proteins: essential proteins for apoptosis regulation. J Cell Mol Med, 2008. 12(3): 743-61.

[86] Schett G et al. Activation of Fas inhibits heat-induced activation of HSF1 and up-regulation of hsp70. Faseb J, 1999. 13(8): 833-42.

[87] Mehlen P, K Schulze-Osthoff and AP Arrigo. Small stress proteins as novel regulators of apoptosis. Heat shock protein 27 blocks Fas/APO-1- and staurosporine-induced cell death. J Biol Chem, 1996. 271(28): 16510-4.

[88] Paul C et al. Hsp27 as a negative regulator of cytochrome C release. Mol Cell Biol, 2002. 22(3): 816-34.

[89] Gabai VL et al. Hsp72 and stress kinase c-jun N-terminal kinase regulate the bid-dependent pathway in tumor necrosis factor-induced apoptosis. Mol Cell Biol, 2002. 22(10): 3415-24.

[90] Bouchier-Hayes L et al. Characterization of cytoplasmic caspase-2 activation by induced proximity. Mol Cell, 2009. 35(6): 830-40.

[91] Steel, R., et al., Hsp72 inhibits apoptosis upstream of the mitochondria and not through interactions with Apaf-1. J Biol Chem, 2004. 279(49): 51490-9.

[92] Beere, H.M., Stressed to death: regulation of apoptotic signaling pathways by the heat shock proteins. Sci STKE, 2001. 2001(93): re1.

[93] Musch MW et al. Induction of heat shock protein 70 protects intestinal epithelial IEC-18 cells from oxidant and thermal injury. Am J Physiol, 1996. 270(2 Pt 1): C429-36.

[94] Huot J et al. HSP27 phosphorylation-mediated resistance against actin fragmentation and cell death induced by oxidative stress. Cancer Res, 1996. 56(2): 273-9.

[95] Przybytkowski E et al. Thermal adaptation in CHO cells at 40 degrees C: the influence of growth conditions and the role of heat shock proteins. Radiat Res, 1986. 107(3): 317-31.

[96] Field SB and RL Anderson. Thermotolerance: a review of observations and possible mechanisms. Natl Cancer Inst Monogr, 1982. 61: 193-201.

[97] Ostberg JR, KC Kaplan and EA Repasky. Induction of stress proteins in a panel of mouse tissues by fever-range whole body hyperthermia. Int J Hyperthermia, 2002. 18(6): 552-62.

[98] Calderwood SK and DR Ciocca. Heat shock proteins: stress proteins with Janus-like properties in cancer. Int J Hyperthermia, 2008. 24(1): 31-9.

[99] Barnes JA et al. Expression of inducible Hsp70 enhances the proliferation of MCF-7 breast cancer cells and protects against the cytotoxic effects of hyperthermia. Cell Stress Chaperones, 2001. 6(4): 316-25.

[100] Huot J et al. Increased survival after treatments with anticancer agents of Chinese hamster cells expressing the human Mr 27,000 heat shock protein. Cancer Res, 1991. 51(19): 5245-52.

[101] Oesterreich S et al. Basal regulatory promoter elements of the hsp27 gene in human breast cancer cells. Biochem Biophys Res Commun, 1996. 222(1): 155-63.

[102] Oesterreich S et al. The small heat shock protein hsp27 is correlated with growth and drug resistance in human breast cancer cell lines. Cancer Res, 1993. 53(19): 4443-8.

[103] Garrido C. et al. HSP27 as a mediator of confluence-dependent resistance to cell death induced by anticancer drugs. Cancer Res, 1997. 57(13): 2661-7.

[104] Ciocca DR et al. Biological and clinical implications of heat shock protein 27,000 (Hsp27): a review. J Natl Cancer Inst, 1993. 85(19): 1558-70.

[105] Issels RD. Hyperthermia adds to chemotherapy. Eur J Cancer, 2008. 44(17): 2546-54.

[106] Skitzki JJ, EA Repasky and SS Evans. Hyperthermia as an immunotherapy strategy for cancer. Curr Opin Investig Drugs, 2009. 10(6): 550-8.

[107] Lepock JR. Role of nuclear protein denaturation and aggregation in thermal radiosensitization. Int J Hyperthermia, 2004. 20(2): 115-30.

[108] Dewey WC, SA Sapareto and DA Betten. Hyperthermic radiosensitization of synchronous Chinese hamster cells: relationship between lethality and chromosomal aberrations. Radiat Res, 1978. 76(1): 48-59.

[109] Kampinga HH and E Dikomey. Hyperthermic radiosensitization: mode of action and clinical relevance. Int J Radiat Biol, 2001. 77(4): 399-408.

[110] Kampinga HH et al. Resistance to heat radiosensitization and protein damage in thermotolerant and thermoresistant cells. Int J Radiat Biol, 1997. 71(3): 315-26.

[111] Song CW et al. Implications of increased tumor blood flow and oxygenation caused by mild temperature hyperthermia in tumor treatment. Int J Hyperthermia, 2005. 21(8): 761-7.

[112] Jain RK. Normalization of tumor vasculature: an emerging concept in antiangiogenic therapy. Science, 2005. 307(5706): 58-62.

[113] Hahn GM. Potential for therapy of drugs and hyperthermia. Cancer Res, 1979. 39(6 Pt 2): 2264-8.

[114] Marmor JB. Interactions of hyperthermia and chemotherapy in animals. Cancer Res, 1979. 39(6 Pt 2): 2269-76.

[115] Engelhardt R. Rationale for clinical application of hyperthermia and drugs. Strahlenther Onkol, 1987. 163(7): 428-9.

[116] Dahl O. Interaction of hyperthermia and chemotherapy. Recent Results Cancer Res, 1988. 107: 157-69.

[117] Bates DA and WJ Mackillop. The effect of hyperthermia on the uptake and cytotoxicity of melphalan in Chinese hamster ovary cells. Int J Radiat Oncol Biol Phys, 1989. 16(1): 187-91.

[118] Bull JM. An update on the anticancer effects of a combination of chemotherapy and hyperthermia. Cancer Res, 1984. 44(10 Suppl): 4853s-4856s.

[119] Kampinga HH. Cell biological effects of hyperthermia alone or combined with radiation or drugs: a short introduction to newcomers in the field. Int J Hyperthermia, 2006. 22(3): 191-6.

[120] Ling V. Multidrug resistance: molecular mechanisms and clinical relevance. Cancer Chemother Pharmacol, 1997. 40 Suppl: S3-8.

[121] Kuo MT. Redox regulation of multidrug resistance in cancer chemotherapy: molecular mechanisms and therapeutic opportunities. Antioxid Redox Signal, 2009. 11(1): 99-133.

[122] Cole SP et al. Overexpression of a transporter gene in a multidrug-resistant human lung cancer cell line. Science, 1992. 258(5088): 1650-4.

[123] Hipfner DR, R.G Deeley and SP Cole. Structural, mechanistic and clinical aspects of MRP1. Biochim Biophys Acta, 1999. 1461(2): 359-76.

[124] Jedlitschky G et al. Transport of glutathione, glucuronate, and sulfate conjugates by the MRP gene-encoded conjugate export pump. Cancer Res, 1996. 56(5): 988-94.

[125] Slot AJ, SV Molinski and SP Cole. Mammalian multidrug-resistance proteins (MRPs). Essays Biochem, 2011. 50(1): 179-207.

[126] Volm M. Multidrug resistance and its reversal. Anticancer Res, 1998. 18(4C): 2905-17.

[127] Mannervik B. The isoenzymes of glutathione transferase. Adv Enzymol Relat Areas Mol Biol, 1985. 57: 357-417.

[128] Baird RD and SB Kaye. Drug resistance reversal-are we getting closer? Eur J Cancer, 2003. 39(17): 2450-61.

[129] Tamaki A et al. The controversial role of ABC transporters in clinical oncology. Essays Biochem, 2011. 50(1): 209-32.

[130] Towle LR. Hyperthermia and drug resistance., In: Urano M. and Douple E. (eds.) Hyperthermia and Oncology, Vol. 4. Utrecht: VSP; 1994. p. 91-113.

[131] Herman TS et al. Reversal of resistance to methotrexate by hyperthermia in Chinese hamster ovary cells. Cancer Res, 1981. 41(10): 3840-3.

[132] Raaphorst GP, et al. A comparison of hyperthermia cisplatin sensitization in human ovarian carcinoma and glioma cell lines sensitive and resistant to cisplatin treatment. Cancer Chemother Pharmacol, 1996. 37(6): 574-80.

[133] Wallner KE, M Banda and GC Li. Hyperthermic enhancement of cell killing by mitomycin C in mitomycin C-resistant Chinese hamster ovary cells. Cancer Res, 1987. 47(5): 1308-12.

[134] Ling V and LH Thompson. Reduced permeability in CHO cells as a mechanism of resistance to colchicine. J Cell Physiol, 1974. 83(1): 103-16.

[135] Larrivee B and DA Averill. Melphalan resistance and photoaffinity labelling of P-glycoprotein in multidrug-resistant Chinese hamster ovary cells: reversal of resistance by cyclosporin A and hyperthermia. Biochem Pharmacol, 1999. 58(2): 291-302.

[136] Larrivee B and DA Averill. Modulation of adriamycin cytotoxicity and transport in drug-sensitive and multidrug-resistant Chinese hamster ovary cells by hyperthermia and cyclosporin A. Cancer Chemother Pharmacol, 2000. 45(3): 219-30.

[137] Averill DA and C Su. Sensitization to the cytotoxicity of adriamycin by verapamil and heat in multidrug-resistant Chinese hamster ovary cells. Radiat Res, 1999. 151(6): 694-702.

[138] Averill-Bates DA and B Courtemanche. The effect of hyperthermia and verapamil on melphalan cytotoxicity and transport in multidrug-resistant Chinese hamster ovary cells. Radiat Res, 1995. 143(1): 17-25.

[139] Dumontet C, F Bodin and Y Michal. Potential interactions between antitubulin agents and temperature: implications for modulation of multidrug resistance. Clin Cancer Res, 1998. 4(6): 1563-6.

[140] Liu Z, R Bendayan and XY Wu. Triton-X-100-modified polymer and microspheres for reversal of multidrug resistance. J Pharm Pharmacol, 2001. 53(6): 779-87.

[141] Awasthi S et al. Interactions of melphalan with glutathione and the role of glutathione S-transferase. Drug Metab Dispos, 1996. 24(3): 371-4.

[142] Turcotte S and DA Averill-Bates. Sensitization to the cytotoxicity of melphalan by ethacrynic acid and hyperthermia in drug-sensitive and multidrug-resistant Chinese hamster ovary cells. Radiat Res, 2001. 156(3): 272-82.

[143] Souslova T and DA Averill-Bates. Multidrug-resistant hela cells overexpressing MRP1 exhibit sensitivity to cell killing by hyperthermia: interactions with etoposide. Int J Radiat Oncol Biol Phys, 2004. 60(5): 1538-51.

[144] Uckun FM et al. Radiation and heat sensitivity of human T-lineage acute lymphoblastic leukemia (ALL) and acute myeloblastic leukemia (AML) clones displaying multiple drug resistance (MDR). Int J Radiat Oncol Biol Phys, 1992. 23(1): 115-25.

[145] Indran IR et al. Recent advances in apoptosis, mitochondria and drug resistance in cancer cells. Biochim Biophys Acta, 2011. 1807(6): 735-45.

[146] Reed JC. Dysregulation of apoptosis in cancer. J Clin Oncol, 1999. 17(9): 2941-53.

[147] Wrzal PK, A Bettaieb and DA Averill-Bates. Molecular mechanisms of apoptosis activation by heat shock in multidrug-resistant Chinese hamster cells. Radiat Res, 2008. 170(4): 498-511.

[148] Friesen C et al. Involvement of the CD95 (APO-1/FAS) receptor/ligand system in drug-induced apoptosis in leukemia cells. Nat Med, 1996. 2(5): 574-7.

[149] Ruefli AA et al. P-glycoprotein inhibits caspase-8 activation but not formation of the death inducing signal complex (disc) following Fas ligation. Cell Death Differ, 2002. 9(11): 1266-72.

[150] van der Zee J et al. The Kadota Fund International Forum 2004--clinical group consensus. Int J Hyperthermia, 2008. 24(2): 111-22.

[151] Fiorentini G and A Szasz. Hyperthermia today: electric energy, a new opportunity in cancer treatment. J Cancer Res Ther, 2006. 2(2): 41-6.

[152] Kamisawa T et al. [Thermo-chemo-radiotherapy for advanced biliary carcinoma]. Nippon Rinsho, 2006. 64 Suppl 1: 543-6.

[153] Eveno C et al. [Treatment of peritoneal carcinomatosis with surgery and hyperthermic peroperative intraperitoneal chemotherapy (HIPEC): new aspects and validated indications]. Bull Cancer, 2008. 95(1): 141-5.

[154] Kawai N et al. Effect of heat therapy using magnetic nanoparticles conjugated with cationic liposomes on prostate tumor in bone. Prostate, 2008. 68(7): 84-92.

[155] Kikumori T et al. Anti-cancer effect of hyperthermia on breast cancer by magnetite nanoparticle-loaded anti-HER2 immunoliposomes. Breast Cancer Res Treat, 2009. 113(3): 435-41.

[156] Kuylenstierna J and K Lantorp. [Dangerous drugs in health food store]. Lakartidningen, 1976. 73(33): 691.

[157] Tilly W et al. Regional hyperthermia in conjunction with definitive radiotherapy against recurrent or locally advanced prostate cancer T3 pN0 M0. Strahlenther Onkol, 2005. 181(1): 35-41.

[158] Rampersaud EN, Z Vujaskovic and BA Inman. Hyperthermia as a treatment for bladder cancer. Oncology (Williston Park), 2010. 24(12): 1149-55.

[159] Ginzburg GS, OV Galibin and AI Krasheniuk. [Polarographic study of the rate of dissociation of oxyhemoglobin]. Biofizika, 1972. 17(3): 446-52.

[160] Petrovich Z et al. Deep regional hyperthermia of the liver. A clinical study of 49 patients. Am J Clin Oncol, 1989. 12(5): 378-83.

[161] Petrovich Z et al. Regional hyperthermia of the liver. Strahlenther Onkol, 1989. 165(10): 721-3.

[162] Vernon CC et al. Radiotherapy with or without hyperthermia in the treatment of superficial localized breast cancer: results from five randomized controlled trials. International Collaborative Hyperthermia Group. Int J Radiat Oncol Biol Phys, 1996. 35(4): 731-44.

[163] Overgaard J et al. Randomised trial of hyperthermia as adjuvant to radiotherapy for recurrent or metastatic malignant melanoma. European Society for Hyperthermic Oncology. Lancet, 1995. 345(8949): 540-3.

[164] Valdagni R and M Amichetti. Report of long-term follow-up in a randomized trial comparing radiation therapy and radiation therapy plus hyperthermia to metastatic lymph nodes in stage IV head and neck patients. Int J Radiat Oncol Biol Phys, 1994. 28(1): 163-9.

[165] Datta NR et al. Head and neck cancers: results of thermoradiotherapy versus radiotherapy. Int J Hyperthermia, 1990. 6(3): 479-86.

[166] van der Zee J et al. Point-counterpoint: what is the optimal trial design to test hyperthermia for carcinoma of the cervix? Point: addition of hyperthermia or cisplatin to

radiotherapy for patients with cervical cancer; two promising combinations--no definite conclusions. Int J Hyperthermia, 2002. 18(1): 19-24.

[167] Sharma S et al. Side-effects of local hyperthermia: results of a prospectively randomized clinical study. Int J Hyperthermia, 1990. 6(2): 279-85.

[168] Harima Y et al. A randomized clinical trial of radiation therapy versus thermoradiotherapy in stage IIIB cervical carcinoma. Int J Hyperthermia, 2001. 17(2): 97-105.

[169] Sneed PK et al. Survival benefit of hyperthermia in a prospective randomized trial of brachytherapy boost +/- hyperthermia for glioblastoma multiforme. Int J Radiat Oncol Biol Phys, 1998. 40(2): 287-95.

[170] Hurwitz MD et al. Hyperthermia combined with radiation for the treatment of locally advanced prostate cancer: long-term results from Dana-Farber Cancer Institute study 94-153. Cancer, 2011. 117(3): 510-6.

[171] Jones EL et al. Randomized trial of hyperthermia and radiation for superficial tumors. J Clin Oncol, 2005. 23(13): 3079-85.

[172] Feldmann, H.J., et al., Changes in oxygenation patterns of locally advanced recurrent tumors under thermoradiotherapy. Adv Exp Med Biol, 1994. 345: 479-83.

[173] Paulides, M.M., et al., The clinical feasibility of deep hyperthermia treatment in the head and neck: new challenges for positioning and temperature measurement. Phys Med Biol, 2010. 55(9): 2465-80.

[174] de Bruijne, M., et al., Evaluation of CEM43 degrees CT90 thermal dose in superficial hyperthermia: a retrospective analysis. Strahlenther Onkol, 2010. 186(8): 436-43.

[175] Fajardo, J.E., et al., Chronic meningitis, polyarthritis, lymphadenitis, and pulmonary hemosiderosis. The Journal of pediatrics, 1982. 101(5): 738-40.

[176] Walmsley, K. and S.A. Kaplan, Transurethral microwave thermotherapy for benign prostate hyperplasia: separating truth from marketing hype. J Urol, 2004. 172(4 Pt 1): 1249-55.

Chapter 13

Glioblastomas, Astrocytomas: Survival Amelioration Adding Hyperthermia to Conformal Radiotherapy and Temozolomide — Use of Pegylated Doxorubicin and Hyperthermia in the Treatment of a Recurrent Case

Gianfranco Baronzio, Gurdev Parmar,
Michela De Santis and Alberto Gramaglia

Additional information is available at the end of the chapter

http://dx.doi.org/10.5772/55966

1. Introduction

Fifty per cent of primary brain tumours are Glioblastoma (GBM), the rest is constituted by astrocytomas and less aggressive tumours [1,2]. GBM is biologically an aggressive tumor quickly developing genetic hetereoneity and therapeutic resistance [2,3]. No specific markers exist for GBM at the moment as reported by Kesari [4], but new imaging techniques including diffusion weighted imaging (DWI), perfusion weighted imaging (PWI or MR), are aiding in better defining disease development and progression. According to the World Health Organization (WHO), astrocytomas are classified into four prognostic grades [4,5]. Grade I and two are classified as low grade gliomas whereas grade III and IV are classified as high grade gliomas, despite the fact that these grades indicate tumor aggressiveness they have not been reliable in predicting the response to therapy. Kesari has outlined that other factors such as overexpression of some growth factors and their receptors have prognostic relevance [4]. Overexpression of Platelet derived growth factor (PDGF) and its receptors indicates a tumor is less aggressive and has a better prognosis compared to GBM expressing the Epidermal Growth Factor (EGFR) [4,6].

Almost 45% of GBM have molecular alterations of the enzyme 06-methylguanine-DNA methyltransferase(MGMT) and mutations of isocitrate dehydrogenase 1 (IDH1) [7]. MGMT, affects signalling pathways and has an important role with alkylating cytostatic drugs such as Temozolomide (TMZ). Methylation of MGMT is associated to a better prognosis and response to TMZ [8]. More recently, a specific and target therapy has been suggested by authors such as Reardon and Wen [3] who have provided a complete list of these inhibitors for this disease including: Gefitinib (Iressa®), Ernolitib (Tarceva®),Thalidomide (Thalidomid®), Bezacizumab (Avastin®), and proteasome inhibitors (bortezomid).

Another approach at the moment not completely in use is immunotherapy [9, 10]. EGFR is expressed in near the 50% of patients with GBM [11]. Inhibitors of EGFR, like Iressa and Tarceva have been used with limited success [12]. A phase II study with Gefitinib has been conducted by Rich et al. in which fifty-seven patients have been treated orally once daily with 500 mg of oral Iressa®. No objective responses were seen, possibly because only 21% of patients had measurable disease at treatment initiation. Iressa® was well tolerated and a dose increase was thus suggested [13]. Studies with Tarceva® has given similar results with a minimum benefit not superior to standard treatment of care with radiotherapy and TMZ [14]. Another modest response has been obtained inhibiting the PDGF receptors using imatinib (Gleevec®) [10, 16].

Lasty, as angiogenesis due tumor hypoxia is a common processes in GBM [17,18], the inhibitor of Vascular Endothelial Growth Factor (VEGF) bevacizumab (Avastin) has been studied extensively in treating resistant GBM [17, 19]. Avastin has recently been used as single agent or in combination with several drugs, such as carboplatin [20], Ectoposide [21], Lomustine and TMZ [17]. Avastin, is a recombinant monoclonal immunoglobulin able to inhibit VEGF and to normalize tumor vasculature [21,22], but, the promises on GBM have not been confirmed and 98.8% of patients experienced adverse effects such as fatigue, headache, hypertension, thromboembolism, cerebral haemorrhage, convulsion and infarction [22]. Another antiangiogenetic factor Thalidomide has been used in GBL [23]. Thalidomide exert its anti tumoral activity through several mechanisms, such as: inhibition of angiogenesis, cytokine-mediated pathways and adhesion molecules modulation, inhibition of cyclooxygenase-2 and stimulation of immuno response [24]. Another approach is immunotherapy. As known GBL is an immunogenic tumor exerting an immunosuppressive effects on cell mediated immunity partially by regulatory T cells [25,26,27]. This kind of therapy is however experimental and dependent on laboratory skilled personal.

However, none of these association are really superior to TMZ + radiotherapy, regarding survival, and are also becoming cost - prohibitive [28]. Understanding this issue we have started to add hyperthermia (HT) to TMZ and Conformal Radiotherapy (CRT). The basis for adding HT together radiotherapy have been described since 2006 [29]. Hypoxia, the increased apoptosis induced by heat and the additive response to CRT are the most important reasons for adding HT in the treatment of GBM [29]. Animal and human studies have also indicated that there are significant chemosensitizing effects of adding HT to chemotherapy such as nitrosureas derivates [29, 30]. Previous studies not yet published by our group have shown that HT with TMZ is additive. We have thus be (TMZ) (5F,11 M median age 44.64 ± 9.95 yr), and were eligible to be compared with 15 patients with (GBM) treated with CFRT plus TMZ (see table 2)(15 GBM, 7F,8M; 52.13±16.17 yr). Four of them (Astrocytoma IV) were previous treated with CCNU, with disease progression (see. Table. 1). All patients had a histological proven malignant GBM or anaplastic astrocytomas. Since 2001, we have begun to use capacitive HT in association to TMZ and conformal radiotherapy. Follow up of patients was collected at a mean interval of 65 days, with a large range [40-90] days for those patients with a disease stabilization.

PTS	Year	Gender	Histology	TMZ	CCNU	ECOG	Gy	RTV	Ner HT Cycle	A/D	Survival Ms
1	36	F	GBM	X			45	65.6	2	D	25
2	52	M	GBM	X			42	101	1	D	12
3	54	F	GBM	X			60		1	A	75
4	57	M	GBM	X			14	42	3	A	51
5	51	M	GBM	X			20	57	2	A	20
6	45	F	GBM	X			65	43.4	1	A	20
7	70	M	GBM	X			28	28.4	5	A	96
8	31	M	GBM	X			14	64	1	D	7
9	41	F	GBM			3	41	64	1	D	12
10	33	M	GBM				28	28.4	2	A	83
11	60	F	GBM			1	65	64	1	D	12
12	40	F	Astro IV	X	X	10	25	72.5	1	D	9
13	43	M	Astro IV	X	X	2	47.6	33.6	2	D	7
14	59	M	Astro IV	X	X	4	45	32.9	1	A	19
15	37	M	Astro IV		X	1	42	101	1	D	12
16	45	F	Astro IV			1	44	113	1	A	98
17	44	M	Astro IV			10	39.6		3	A	82
18	44	M	AstroII			10	45	65.6	4	A	111
19	34	M	AstroII	X			39.6	44	1	D	23
20	44	F	AstroII			10	43	112	6	D	17
21	34	M	AstroII				45		1	A	76
22	40	F	Astro II	X					4	D	12
23	30	M	Astro II	X					6	A	60
24	46	M	Astro II	X					6	A	30
25	46	M	Astro II	X					9	A	17
25>		9F- 16M	11GBM, 6 Astro IV, 8 Astro II				39.9±14. 39	62.91±27. 95		13A-12D	39.44±34.2 5

Pts: Patients; GBM: Glioblastomas, Astro: Astrocytomas; RTV: radiotherapeutic volume; Gy: Gray; D: dead, A: Alive; Ms: months

Table 1. Characteristics of patients with GBM – ASTRO- II- IV treated with CFRT+ HT

1.1. Conformal radiotherapy

Computer tomographic (CT) scans using a spiral CT scanner and magnetic resonance scanner (MR) were performed on each patients. These scans are elaborated for determining the cancer size and shape in 3 dimensions (3D). In this way precisely focused, high dose, radiation beams can be delivered to cancer mass in multiple treatment sessions. Before radiation, patients are fitted with a head frame, meantime CT and MR scans are performed to determine treatment planning. After the acquisition of these informations, patients are positioned on treatment couch and the linear accelerator directs arcs of radioactive photon beams to tumor. The pattern of the arc is computer - matched to the tumor shape using specific multileaf collimators. The CT/MR data of patients are sent to a computerized treatment platform. Through, this platform CT/MR images are fused using an image fusion software and the CTV is defined and contoured manually by clinicians and physicists. In our department, an integration of images with metabolic information such as single photon emission computed tomography (SPECT) has also been used. This permits sometimes to obtain a more accurate tumor visualization. The fusion of images is obtained by a commercial software package (Ergo- 3Dline®). Obtained the CTV, normally, a margin over these countered borders must be defined to take into account the possible microscopic extension of the tumour not evidenced on the CT/MR scans. These margins are generally countered 10-30 mm around the CTV obtaining the planned target volume (PTV). After PTV determination a new contour is done ensuring PTV coverage by 95% isodose line with the aim for obtaining a uniform dose homogeneity. Treatment is performed using a Varian Clinac 2100, 6mv. The median dose used for GBM and anaplastic astrocytomas treated with HT were of 36.87±17.75 Gy versus 39.2 ± 15.57 Gy for patients treated with CFRT+TMZ alone. The radiotherapeutic volume were 54.04 ± 22.53 mm3 versus 85.12 ± 50.37 mm^3 respectively.

1.2. Capacitive hyperthermia

For treating our patients we used a device (Synchrotherm) developed by Duer ®, Vigevano, Italy. This device consists of the following components: 1) a Radiofrequency generator (13.56 Mhz) 2) a pair of mobile plates or electrodes with independent superficial cooling system, 3) a heat exchanger, 4) a computerized control console. The thermal profiles to obtain a probable deposition of the energy were obtained by heating patterns produced in a static phantoms. A cylindrical phantom made of 4% agar gel plus 02% NaCl was made and the various isotherms were monitored and reconstructed through computerizations of images obtained by a special film sensible to temperature. A flexible vinyl sheet, forming a space filled with 0.4% NaCl solution, covered the surfaces of the electrodes. The saline solution circulated between the electrode and the heat exchangers. Differently to other cooling system, the two electrodes were independently controlled and were simply adaptable to the contour of the brain patients, thanks to their flexibility These plates are coupled to opposite side of the patient 's brain and kept in place thanks to a girdle permitting a better contact over the irregularity of the skull contour. Capacitive hyperthermia treatment were given to the patients 30 ' after the CFRT; during the HT session 500cc of mannitol at 19%, plus 4-8 mg of desamethazone were infused. HT treatments lasted for all patients 1 hour, and for five days consecutively. Some of these patients received more than one HT treatment/month (median 3 maximum 5 HT treatments).

2. TMZ administration

TMZ was administered orally 200mg/m2 /day on day one to five, after written informed consent. A full blood examination was performed before each new cycle. The treatment cycles were repeated every 28 days. The patients fasted 4 hours before TMZ use, and were submitted to conformal radiotherapy (CFRT), following our standards supplementation with omega-3 fatty acids and silymarin for preventing radionecrosis.

3. Rationale for using liposomal doxorubicin

Temozolomide is an imido-tetrazine readily absorbed orally and able to cross the Blood brain barrier. TMZ has demonstrated activity against Glioblastoma, astrocytoma of various degree and brain metastases [3, 15]. Although TMZ has become the drug of choice in association with radiotherapy for Glioblastoma, many Glioblastoma develop resistance to the drug and become incurable. The reasons for this resistance is at the moment not completely understood and seems linked to the presence of certain subpopulations of cancer- stem cells inside the tumor mass [32]. This possible resistance has forced our group to look for other drugs active on GBM. We have chosed liposomal doxorubicin for various reasons that we will be describe here.

Liposomal doxorubicin (Caelyx®), is a formulation of hydrochloride doxorubicin wrapped by a film composed by phospholipids and polymers of methoxypolyethylene (mPEG) embedded in the lipid surface [33]. This association determines favorable pharmacokinetic profile characterised by an extended circulation time, a reduced volume of distribution, thereby promoting an increased tumour uptake [34, 35]. Tumor abnormal microcirculation and permeability is responsible for the increased uptake and retention of liposomal drugs, see Maeda [36]. This phenomenon is greatly increased by Hyperthermia, as demonstrated by Ponce and Dvorak [37, 38]. Dvorak was one of the first to use the combination of Caelyx® and hyperthermia on hepatocarcinoma and after his study reported that the combination of hyperthermia and doxorubicin itself may be supra-additive, resulting in enhanced antitumor efficacy in the heated region and in decrease of toxicity [38]. Caelyx® has been investigated by Koukoukaris in glioblastoma and in metastatic brain tumours [39]. These authors in agreement with Chua and Lesniak group concluded that liposomal doxorubicin selectively overcome the blood brain barrier and accumulate 13-19 times higher in the Glioblastoma [40, 41]. Furthermore, Chua [40] has demonstated the possibility of using Caelyx® in association with temozolomide in recurrent Glioblastoma. Liposomal doxorubicin was associated with disease stabilization and a modest haematologic toxicity. These studies have convinced our group to use pegylated doxorubicin in a recurrent case of GBM. The case is here briefly described.

4. Case of patient treated with Caelyx

The patient (right handed man) was first surgically treated (Dec 2005) for left posterior parietal Glioblastoma then the patient underwent RT (45 Gy CFRT in 18 fractions followed by a boost CFRT to reduced target of 20 Gy in 4 fractions) and started and continued Temodar (10 cycles) until progression (Jan 07) followed by ACNU (2 Cycles) until progression (March 2007) and then we started LD and Radiofrequency Hyperthermia (HT).

During the first period the cycles were done at 45 days interval then, after a initial good response and stabilization, the treatment was done at larger interval up to 9 CT+HT (the last treatment was done in Nov 2007).

The treatment was as follows: 12 mgm^2 IV + steroids in glucose solution and assumption of 200 mg of Quercetin in day 1 and one hour of HT at least four hour later. From day 2 to 5 the patient underwent 4 further consecutive days of HT and quercetin (100 mg before and after the completion of treatment).

HT was delivered by means of a 13.56 MHz radiofrequency capacitive device (Synchrotherm Duer) via two opposite plates at the maximum tolerated power for at least one hour for five consecutive days.

4.1. Statistical analysis

Survival curves were calculated according to Kaplan-Meier method, Starting on the first day of HT. Survival was compared using the log-rank test and the K-test. Significance was posed as $p \leq 0.05$ [11].

4.2. Results

As it is possible to see comparing table 1 and table 2 there is no statistical difference between the two groups regarding age, gy administered and volume of tumour treated. The difference on survival curves (see Fig. 1) using the log-rank test and the K-test are important and more than the 50% of patients treated with CFRT+HT+TMZ are alive at 26 months. We can object than the comparison of the two groups is not completely homogeneous. In fact, the group in table 2 treated with TMZ + CFRT are only GBM, on the contrary in table 1 there is the presence of Astrocytoma of II degree. At a second look at table 1, an important observation emerges however, the GBM group has a long survival that is sometimes 3 times that of table 2, see pts 1, 3 table 2 and pts 3,7,10 of table1. It seems clear that HT adds something regarding survival and no side effects have been reported by patients. The patient treated with Caelyx® after surgery Dec 2005, had progression of the disease. He received CFRT in February 2006 and 10 cycles of Temodal. The patient on March 2009 shows progression and possible resistance to Temodal, we decided to treat the patient with 11 cycles of Caelyx + HT. The patient situation is illustrated in Fig 1(progression of disease after 10 cycle of Temodal, 2006) and Fig 2 after 11 cycles of Caelyx + HT (2009). The decrease of volume is evident. The patient is still alive and in treatment with a dose of 80 mg of Talidomide taken orally at evening, as a single dose.

Pts	Gender	Age	RTV(cm³)	Gy	D / A	Ms Survival
1	F	30	31.6	36.4	D	30
2	M	52	65.4	20	D	13
3	F	64	108	40.5	D	37
4	M	22	56.8	25	D	9
5	M	69	76.9	45.6	D	15
6	M	57	64.1	70	D	1
7	F	61	175	18	D	2
8	F	65	64.5	35	D	10
9	F	47	19.8	54	D	25
10	M	66	136.9	45.5	D	4
11	M	50	226	42	D	13
12	F	45	19.9	54	D	19
13	M	67	67.9	20.4	D	26
14	M	65	119	20	D	14
15	F	22	45	45	D	5
15	7F- 8M	52.13±16.177	85.12±50.37	39.2±15.57	15 D	14.87±10.7

Pts: Patients; RTV: radiotherapeutic volume; Gy: Gray; D: dead, A: Alive; Ms: months

Table 2. Characteristics of Patients with GBM treated with CFRT + TMZ

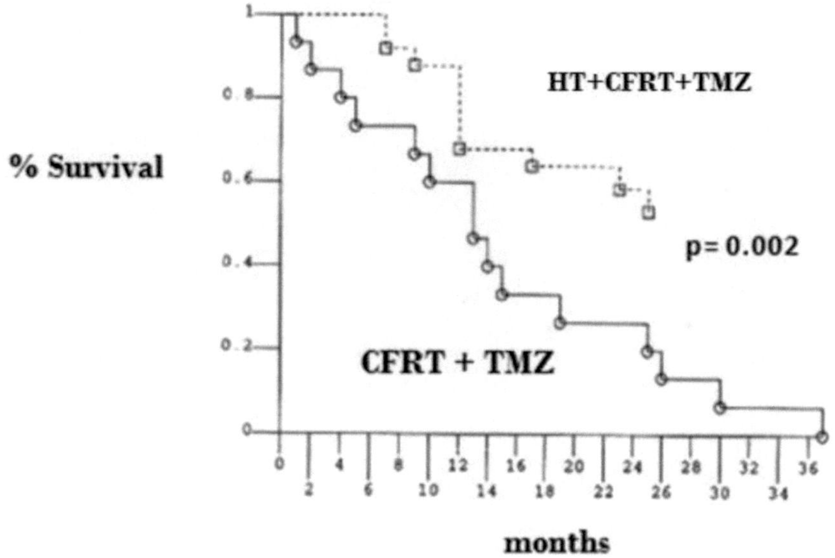

Figure 1. Survival curve of patients treated with HT + CFRT + Temodal, compared with CFRT + Temodal

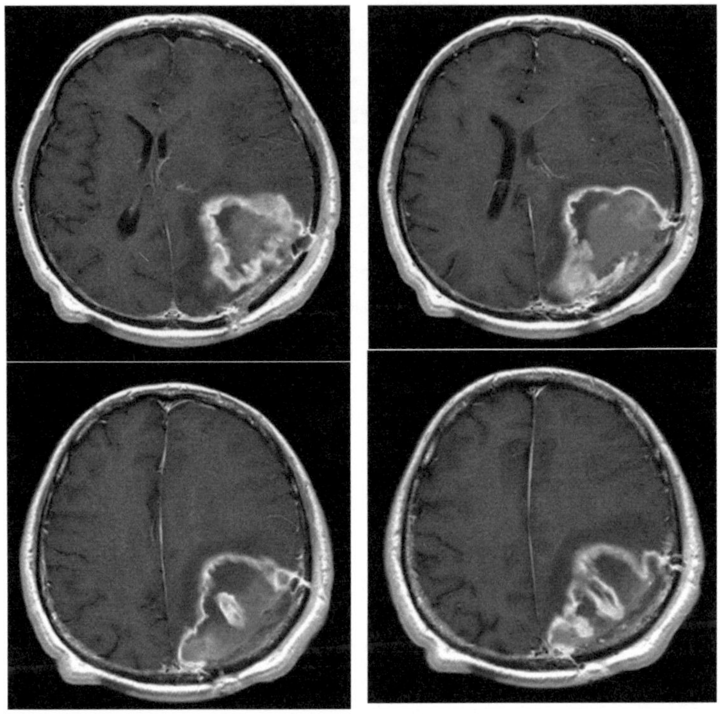

(a)

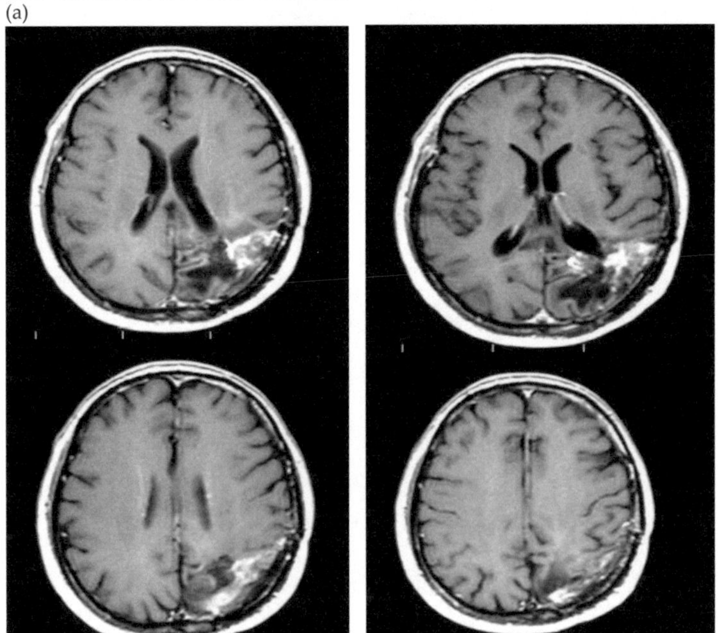

(b)

Figure 2. a. Patient with recurrent and drug resistance before Hyperthermia and Caelyx treatmen. b. Decrease of GBM volume after Hyperthermia and Caelyx treatment

5. Conclusions

Our study, is in agreement with the previous studies on HT [29], and show that the association with themozolomide is feasible and that this triple treatment (Chemotherapy, Conformal Radiotherapy and hyperthermia) represents a promising new approach to the treatment of glioblastomas. In this initial work we have not analyzed patients treated with hyperthermia without TMZ, so we cannot understand if the increase in life survival must be ascribed simply to HT or to the combination with temozolamide. The quantity of patients is limited but we are encouraged to use external capacitive HT in association with the standard therapy of our institution. In a near future, we hope to be able to distinguish the effects of the two therapies. We hope also to analyze the compliance of the patients to hyperthermia and to be able to study the side effects of HT on brain. We want to point out that most of works done on brain and hyperthermia regards studies with interstitial HT [29]. Interstitial HT represents to our opinion a limit to a larger use of this technique in association with CFRT and chemotherapy, whereas capacitive HT show a simpler use and seems to be well tolerated by patients.

Author details

Gianfranco Baronzio[1*], Gurdev Parmar[2], Michela De Santis[3] and Alberto Gramaglia[3]

*Address all correspondence to: barongf@intercom.it

1 Centro Medico Kines, Castano primo, (Mi), Italy

2 Integrated Health Clinic, Fort Langley, B.C., Canada

3 Radiotherapy and Hyperthermia Department, Policlinico di Monza, Monza, Italy

References

[1] Parkin, D. M. Global cancer statistics in the year 2000. Lancet Oncol. (2001). Sep;, 2(9), 533-43.

[2] Lino, M, & Merlo, A. Translating biology into clinic: the case of Glioblastoma. Curr Opin Cell Biol. (2009). Apr;, 21(2), 311-6.

[3] Reardon, D. A, & Wen, P. Y. Therapeutic advances in the treatment of Glioblastoma: rationale and potential role of targeted agents. Oncologist. (2006). Feb;, 11(2), 152-64.

[4] Kesari, S. Understanding glioblastoma tumor biology: the potential to improve current diagnosis and treatments. Semin Oncol. (2011). Dec;38 Suppl 4:S, 2-10.

[5] Schneider, T, Mawrin, C, Scherlach, C, Skalej, M, & Firsching, R. Gliomas in adults. Dtsch Arztebl Int. (2010). Nov;, 107(45), 799-807.

[6] Ekstrand, A. J, Sugawa, N, James, C. D, & Collins, V. P. Amplified and rearranged epidermal growth factor receptor genes in human glioblastomas reveal deletions of sequences encoding portions of the N- and/or C-terminal tails. Proc Natl Acad Sci U S A. (1992). May 15;, 89(10), 4309-13.

[7] Bleeker, F. E, Molenaar, R. J, & Leenstra, S. Recent advances in the molecular understanding of glioblastoma. J Neurooncol. (2012). May;, 108(1), 11-27.

[8] MartinezRamon; Schackert, Gabriele; Yaya-Tur, Ricard; Rojas-Marcos, Iñigo; Herman, James G.; Esteller, Manel ((2006). Frequent hypermethylation of the DNA repair gene MGMT in long-term survivors of glioblastoma multiforme". *Journal of Neuro-Oncology* , 83(1), 91-3.

[9] Daga, A, Bottino, C, Castriconi, R, Gangemi, R, & Ferrini, S. New perspectives in glioma immunotherapy. Curr Pharm Des. (2011). , 17(23), 2439-67.

[10] Polivka J JrPolivka J, Rohan V, Topolcan O, Ferda J. New molecularly targeted therapies for glioblastoma multiforme. Anticancer Res. (2012). Jul;, 32(7), 2935-46.

[11] Rao, S. K, Edwards, J, Joshi, A. D, Siu, I. M, & Riggins, G. J. A survey of glioblastoma genomic amplifications and deletions. J Neurooncol. (2010). Jan;, 96(2), 169-79.

[12] Lassman, A. B, Rossi, M. R, Raizer, J. J, Abrey, L. E, Lieberman, F. S, Grefe, C. N, Lamborn, K, Pao, W, Shih, A. H, Kuhn, J. G, Wilson, R, Nowak, N. J, Cowell, J. K, Deangelis, L. M, Wen, P, Gilbert, M. R, Chang, S, Yung, W. A, Prados, M, & Holland, E. C. Molecular study of malignant gliomas treated with epidermal growth factor receptor inhibitors: tissue analysis from North American Brain Tumor Consortium Trials 01-03 and 00-01. Clin Cancer Res. (2005). Nov 1;, 11(21), 7841-50.

[13] Rich, J. N, Reardon, D. A, Peery, T, Dowell, J. M, Quinn, J. A, Penne, K. L, Wikstrand, C. J, Van Duyn, L. B, Dancey, J. E, Mclendon, R. E, Kao, J. C, & Stenzel, T. T. Ahmed Rasheed BK,Tourt-Uhlig SE, Herndon JE 2nd, Vredenburgh JJ, Sampson JH, Friedman AH, Bigner DD, Friedman HS. Phase II trial of gefitinib in recurrent glioblastoma. J Clin Oncol. (2004). Jan 1;, 22(1), 133-42.

[14] Raizer, J. J, Abrey, L. E, Lassman, A. B, Chang, S. M, Lamborn, K. R, Kuhn, J. G, Yung, W. K, Gilbert, M. R, Aldape, K. A, Wen, P. Y, Fine, H. A, Mehta, M, Deangelis, L. M, Lieberman, F, Cloughesy, T. F, Robins, H. I, & Dancey, J. Prados MD; North American Brain TumorConsortium. A phase II trial of erlotinib in patients with recurrent malignant gliomas and nonprogressive glioblastoma multiforme postradiation therapy. Neuro Oncol. (2010). Jan;, 12(1), 95-103.

[15] Addeo, R, & Caraglia, M. Combining temozolomide with other antitumor drugs and target-based agents in the treatment of brain metastases: an unending quest or chasing a chimera? Expert Opin Investig Drugs. (2011). Jul;, 20(7), 881-95.

[16] Raymond, E, Brandes, A. A, Dittrich, C, Fumoleau, P, Coudert, B, Clement, P. M, Frenay, M, Rampling, R, Stupp, R, Kros, J. M, Heinrich, M. C, Gorlia, T, & Lacombe, D. van den Bent MJ; European Organisation for Research and Treatment of Cancer Brain Tumor Group Study. Phase II study of imatinib in patients with recurrent gliomas of various histologies: a European Organisation for Research and Treatment of Cancer Brain Tumor Group Study. J Clin Oncol. (2008). Oct 1;, 26(28), 4659-65.

[17] Plate, K. H, Scholz, A, & Dumont, D. J. Tumor angiogenesis and anti-angiogenic therapy in malignant gliomas revisited. Acta Neuropathol. (2012). Dec;, 124(6), 763-75.

[18] Yang, L, Lin, C, Wang, L, Guo, H, & Wang, X. Hypoxia and hypoxia-inducible factors in glioblastoma multiforme progression and therapeutic implications. Exp Cell Res. (2012). Nov 15;, 318(19), 2417-26.

[19] Haar, C. P, Hebbar, P, & Wallace, G. C. th, Das A, Vandergrift WA 3rd, Smith JA, Giglio P, Patel SJ, Ray SK, Banik NL. Drug resistance in glioblastoma: a mini review.Neurochem Res. (2012). Jun;, 37(6), 1192-200.

[20] Mrugala, M. M, Crew, L. K, Fink, J. R, & Spence, A. M. Carboplatin and bevacizumab for recurrent malignant glioma. Oncol Lett. (2012). Nov;, 4(5), 1082-1086.

[21] Sweet, J. A, Feinberg, M. L, & Sherman, J. H. The role of avastin in the management of recurrent glioblastoma. Neurosurg Clin N Am. (2012). Apr;, 23(2), 331-41.

[22] Goel, S, Duda, D. G, Xu, L, Munn, L. L, Boucher, Y, Fukumura, D, & Jain, R. K. Normalization of the vasculature for treatment of cancer and other diseases. Physiol Rev. (2011). Jul;, 91(3), 1071-121.

[23] De Boüard, S, & Guillamo, J. S. Angiogenesis and anti-angiogenic strategies for glioblastoma]. Bull Cancer. (2005). Apr;, 92(4), 360-72.

[24] Fanelli, M, Sarmiento, R, Gattuso, D, Carillio, G, Capaccetti, B, Vacca, A, Roccaro, M, & Gasparini, G. Thalidomide: a new anticancer drug? Expert Opin Investig Drugs. (2003). Jul;, 12(7), 1211-25.

[25] Daga, A, Bottino, C, Castriconi, R, Gangemi, R, & Ferrini, S. New perspectives in glioma immunotherapy. Curr Pharm Des. (2011). , 17(23), 2439-67.

[26] Lowther, D. E, & Hafler, D. A. Regulatory T cells in the central nervous system.Immunol Rev. (2012). Jul;, 248(1), 156-69.

[27] Wainwright, D. A, Sengupta, S, Han, Y, & Lesniak, M. S. Thymus-derived rather than tumor-induced regulatory T cells predominate in brain tumors. Neuro Oncol. (2011). Dec;, 13(12), 1308-23.

[28] Holdhoff, M, & Grossman, S. A. Controversies in the adjuvant therapy of high-grade gliomas. Oncologist. (2011). , 16(3), 351-8.

[29] Baronzio, G. F, Cerretta, V, Baronzio, A, Freitas, I, & Mapelli, M. Gramaglia A: Thermochemotherapy association: Biologic rationale, preliminary observations on its use

on malignat Brain tumors. In Hyperthermia in Cancer treatment. A primer. Baronzio GF and Hager D editors (2006). Springer Busines Ed. New York., 128-155.

[30] Schem, B. C, & Dahl, O. Thermal enhancement of ACNU and potentiation of thermochemotherapy with ACNU by hypertonic glucose in the BT4An rat glioma. J Neurooncol. (1991). Jun;, 10(3), 247-52.

[31] Beal, K, Abrey, L. E, & Gutin, P. H. Antiangiogenic agents in the treatment of recurrent or newly diagnosed glioblastoma: analysis of single-agent and combined modality approaches. Radiat Oncol. (2011). Jan 7;6:2.

[32] Johannessen, T. C, & Bjerkvig, R. Molecular mechanisms of temozolomide resistance in glioblastoma multiforme. Expert Rev Anticancer Ther. (2012). May;, 12(5), 635-42.

[33] Green, A. E, & Rose, P. G. Pegylated liposomal doxorubicin in ovarian cancer. Int J Nanomedicine.(2006). , 1(3), 229-39.

[34] Gabizon, A, Shmeeda, H, & Grenader, T. Pharmacological basis of pegylated liposomal doxorubicin: impact on cancer therapy. Eur J Pharm Sci. (2012). Mar 12;, 45(4), 388-98.

[35] Holloway, R. W, Grendys, E. C, Lefebvre, P, Vekeman, F, & Mcmeekin, S. Tolerability,efficacy, and safety of pegylated liposomal Doxorubicin in combination with Carboplatin versus gemcitabine-Carboplatin for the treatment of platinum-sensitive recurrent ovarian cancer: a systematic review. Oncologist.(2010). , 15(10), 1073-82.

[36] Maeda, H. Macromolecular therapeutics in cancer treatment: The EPR effect and beyond. J Control Release. (2012).

[37] Ponce, A. M, Vujaskovic, Z, Yuan, F, Needham, D, & Dewhirst, M. W. Hyperthermia mediated liposomal drug delivery. Int J Hyperthermia. (2006). May;, 22(3), 205-13.

[38] Dvorak, J, Zoul, Z, Melichar, B, Petera, J, Vesely, P, Vosmik, M, & Dolezel, M. Liposomal doxorubicin combined with regional hyperthermia: reducing systemic toxicity and improving locoregional efficacy in the treatment of solid tumors. J Chemother. (2004). Nov;16 Suppl , 5, 34-6.

[39] Koukourakis, M. I, Koukouraki, S, Fezoulidis, I, Kelekis, N, Kyrias, G, Archimandritis, S, & Karkavitsas, N. High intratumoural accumulation of stealth liposomal doxorubicin (Caelyx) in glioblastomas and in metastatic brain tumours. Br J Cancer. (2000). Nov;, 83(10), 1281-6.

[40] Chua, S. L, Rosenthal, M. A, Wong, S. S, Ashley, D. M, Woods, A. M, Dowling, A, & Cher, L. M. Phase 2 study of temozolomide and Caelyx in patients with recurrent Glioblastoma multiforme. Neuro Oncol. (2004). Jan;, 6(1), 38-43.

[41] Lesniak, M. S, Upadhyay, U, Goodwin, R, Tyler, B, & Brem, H. Local delivery of doxorubicin for the treatment of malignant brain tumors in rats. Anticancer Res. (2005). Nov-Dec;25(6B):, 3825-31.

Section 3

The Immunotherapy of Cancer

Chapter 14

Targeted Cancer Therapy by Dendritic Cell Vaccine

Hiroyuki Abe, Touko Shimamoto,
Shinichiro Akiyama and Minako Abe

Additional information is available at the end of the chapter

http://dx.doi.org/10.5772/55450

1. Introduction

The unpredictability of efficacy and toxicity of treatment are limitations of current standard cancer treatments. The clinical results obtained by standard therapies suggest a need for a paradigm change in cancer treatment. In recent years, immune cell therapy has been in the spotlight with the expectation of opening the door to a new area of cancer therapy. Targeted cancer therapy, which selectively takes action against targets expressed in the tumor surface, seems to be promising.

The immune system can control various types of tumors. Antigen-non-specific innate immunity and antigen-specific adaptive immunity can reject tumors.

The identification of tumor antigens recognized by T cells has facilitated the development of immune cell therapy in clinical oncology. The dendritic cell based cancer vaccine aims to induce tumor specific effector T cells (cytotoxic T lymphocyte, CTL) that can reduce tumor mass as well as tumor specific memory T cells that can control tumor relapse.

In this text, immune cell target therapy in clinical oncology will be discussed and hopefully this will be helpful in daily clinical practice.

2. Role of natural killer cells

Natural killer (NK) cells are present in the peripheral blood and number approximately 10-15% in the lymphocyte fraction. NK cells are the most important innate immune cell because of their ability to directly kill target cells as well as produce immunoregulatory cytokines. NK cells are defined by the surface expression of CD56, a neural cell adhesion molecule and lacks the T cell antigen CD3 [1]. The function of NK cells are direct cytotoxic activity against virus-infected cells and tumor cells [2]. There are two distinct subsets of human NK cells based on the density of surface CD56 expression [3]. Approximately 90% of human NK cells are CD 56^{dim} and have high density expression of CD16, others are CD56^{bright} and CD16$^{dim/neg}$. The CD56^{bright} and CD56^{dim} NK cell subsets show an important difference in cytotoxic potential, capacity for cytokine production and response to cytokine activation (Table 1) [4].

	CD56^{bright}	CD56^{dim}
NK receptors		
FcγRIII (CD16)	-/+	+++
KIR	-/+	+++
CD94/NKG2	+	-/+
Cytokine receptors		
IL-2Rαβγ	++	-
IL-2Rβγ	++	++
CCR7	++	-
Adhesion molecules	++	-/+
Effector functions		
ADCC	-/+	+++
Natural cytotoxicity	-/+	+++
Cytokine production	+++	-/+

*KIR indicated killer immunoglobulin-like receptor; IL, interleukin; ADCC, antibody-dependent cellular cytotoxicity.

Table 1. Functional Differences in Natural Killer (NK) cell Subsets* [2]

NK cells can mediate antibody-dependent cellular cytotoxicity (ADCC) through membrane FcγRIII (CD16) expressed on the majority of NK cells. CD56^{dim} NK cells are more cytotoxic against NK-sensitive targets than CD56^{bright} NK cells and respond to IL-2 with increased cytotoxicity. It is of clinical importance to know that CD56^{bright} cells, after activation with IL-2, can exhibit similar or enhanced cytotoxicity against NK targets compared with CD56^{dim} cells [5-7]. In addition, more than 95% of all CD56^{dim} NK cells express CD16 (FcγRIII) and are capable of ADCC. On the other hand, 50% to 70% of CD56^{bright} NK cells lack expression of CD16 or have only low-density expression of CD16 and therefore function minimally in ADCC.

It is well known that major histocompatibility complex (MHC) class I molecules are critical for the inhibition of NK cell-mediated lysis of normal autologous cells [8, 9]. NK cells selectively lyse autologous cell that have lost MHC class I self-expression [10].

In humans, two families of paired inhibitory and activating NK receptors have been identified, killer immunoglobulin (Ig)-like receptor (KIR) family and the heterodimeric CD94/NKG2 C-type lectin family. In this text, these receptors are not discussed in order to simplify the clinical application of NK cell therapy. Although the activating KIR and CD95/NKG2 receptors are important in mediating NK cytotoxicity, Natural Cytotoxicity Receptors (NCR) and the homodimeric NKG 2D receptors may be important in mediating cytotoxicity against abnormal, MHC class I-deficient, or class I-negative targets. This biological information will result in the clinical application of NK cell-based therapies for cancer. Table 2 shows the incidence of MHC class I deficient or negative cancer cells.

Tumor cell		Incidence (%)
Uterine cervical cancer		90
Osteosarcoma		
	Primary	52
	Metastatic	88
Breast cancer		81
Pancreatic cancer		76
Prostate cancer		74
Colon cancer		
	Primary	32
	Metastatic	72
Sarcoma		62
Melanoma		
	Primary	16
	Metastatic	58
Head and neck cancer		49
Hepatoma		42
Renal cell carcinoma		38
Lung cancer		38
Ovarian cancer		37
Pharyngeal cancer		56
Urinary bladder cancer		25

Table 2. Incidence of MHC class I deficient or negative cancer cells [11]

It is presumed that the difference of MHC class I expression may be the difference in the clinical efficacy of NK cell based immune therapy. Because of the variety of cancer cells, it is not enough to kill all cancer cells by NK cell-based therapy. It is necessary to target a cancer specific antigen by cytotoxic T cells, which are activated by a Dendritic Cell (DC)-based cancer vaccine (Figure 1).

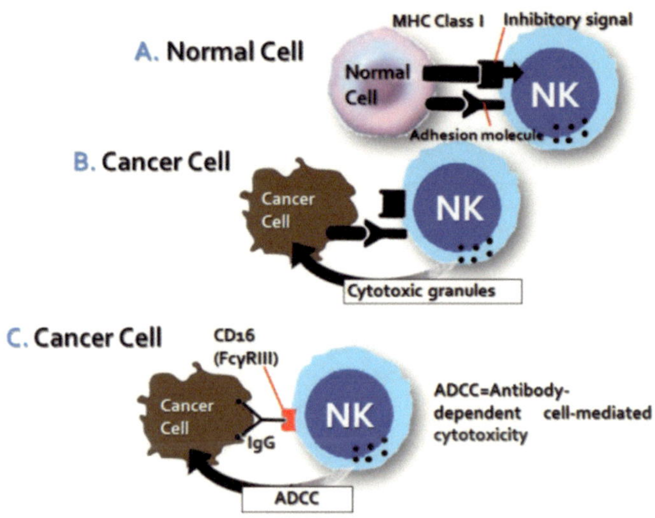

Figure 1. Cytotoxicity of NK cells [11]

3. Strategies using dendritic cell vaccine

Dendritic cells (DCs) are key regulators of both T- and B-cell immunity, because of their superior ability to take up, process and present antigens compared with other antigen presenting cells (APCs) [12]. DCs can also activate NK cells and natural killer T (NKT) cells [13]. Because of these functions, DCs can conduct all of the elements of the immune orchestra and they are therefore a fundamental target and tool for vaccines [14]. Cancer related antigens are a key factor implicated in the design of DC vaccine strategies. If a patient's own cancer cells are available for lysate, this will be used for the production of an individual DC-based vaccine, which is utilized for the optimally matched tumor surface antigen. In most instances, however, if a patient's own cancer cells are not available, then artificial cancer antigens are utilized for the production of a DC-based cancer vaccine.

A pilot project by the National Cancer Institute reported on the prioritization of cancer antigens to develop a well-vetted, priority-ranked list of cancer vaccine target antigens based on predefined and preweighted objective criteria [15]. Antigen prioritization involves developing a list of ideal cancer antigen criteria (Figure 2).

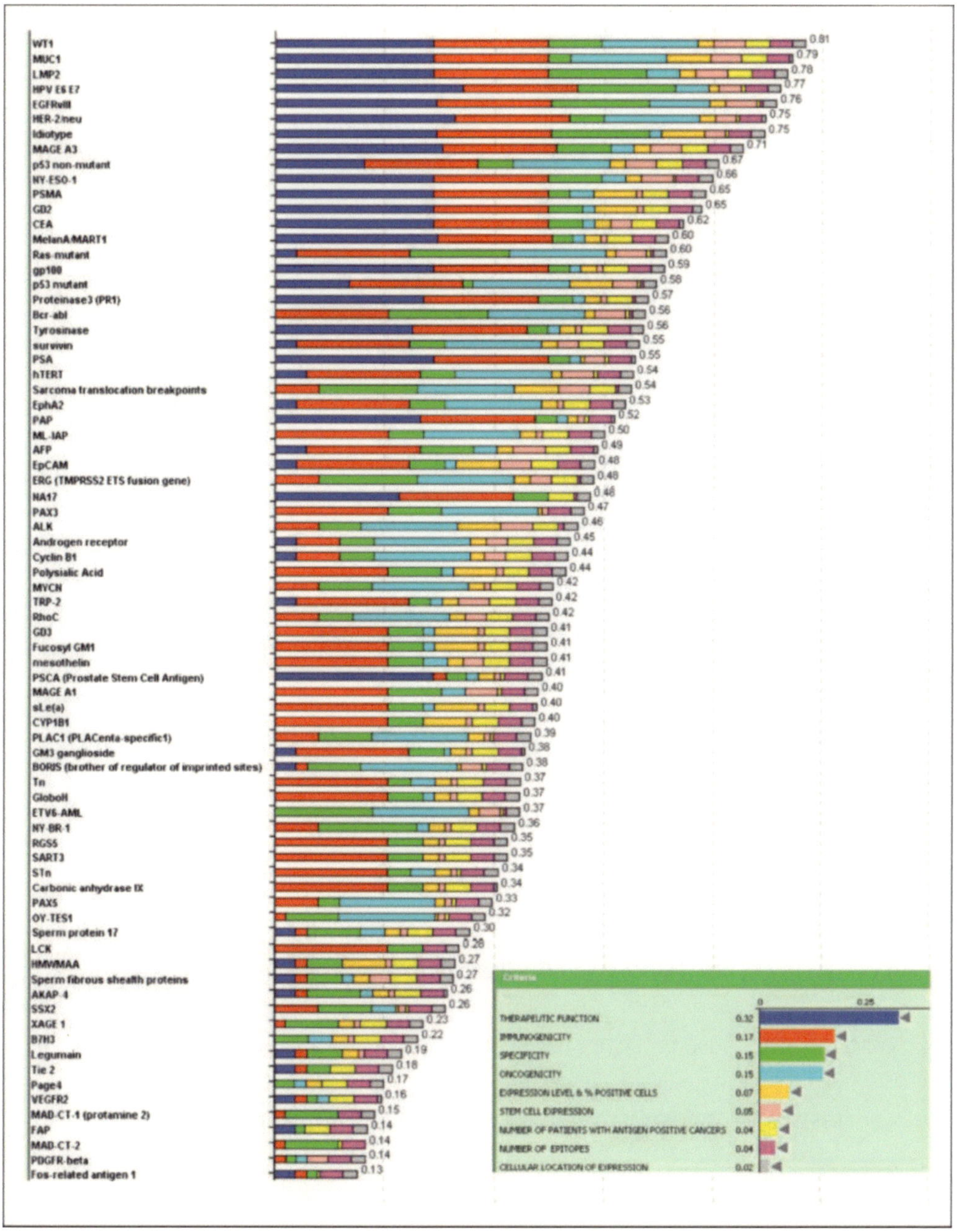

Figure 2. Cancer antigen pilot prioritization: representation of ranking based on predefined and preweighted criteria and subcriteria. Inset, the color used to designate each criterion and its relative weight. Number at the end of each bar, relative rank of that antigen. [15]

Among these, frequently used artificial tumor antigens are listed below. Some of these are restricted by HLA-A1 or HLA-A24, so that an HLA study is needed to select and match the tumor antigens to the DCs (Table 3). Certain artificial tumor antigens cannot apply depending on HLA types on DCs and tumor cells.

HLA-A2 or HLA-A24 restricted	Non-restricted
WT1	MUC1
CEA	CA125
MAGE-1, MAGE-3	PSA
HER 2	NY-ESO-2
gp100	
NY-ESO-1	
PSMA	
SART-1, SART-3	
MART-1	
Melan-A	
HPV16-E7	

Table 3. Typical artificial tumor antigens.

WT1 peptide is a part of long chain of WT1 protein (Figure 3).

10	20	30	40	50
MGSDVRDLNA	LLPAVPSLGG	GGGCALPVSG	AAQWAPVLDF	APPGASAYGS
60	70	80	90	100
LGGPAPPPAP	PPPPPPPPHS	FIKQEPSWGG	AEPHEEQCLS	AFTVHFSGQF
110	120	130	140	150
TGTAGACRYG	PFGPPPPSQA	SSGQARMFPN	APYLPSCLES	QPAIRNQGYS
160	170	180	190	200
TVTFDGTPSY	GHTPSHHAAQ	FPNHSFKHED	PMGQQGSLGE	QQYSVPPPVY
210	220	230	240	250
GCHTPTDSCT	GSQALLLRTP	YSSDNLYQMT	SQLECYTWNQ	MNLGATLKGV
260	270	280	290	
AAGSSSSVKW	TEGQSNHSTG	YESDNHTTPI	LCGAQYRIHT	HGVFRGIQDV
310	320	330	340	350
RRVPGVAPTL	VRSASETSEK	RPFMCAYPGC	NKRYFKLSHL	QMHSRKHTGE
360	370	380	390	400
KPYQCDFKDC	ERRFSRSDQL	KRHQRRHTGV	KPFQCKTCQR	KFSRSDHLKT
410	420	430	440	449
HTRTHTGKTS	EKPFSCRWPS	CQKKFARSDE	LVRHHNMHQR	NMTKLQLAL

Figure 3. Amino acid sequence of WT1 protein (Total length 449, mass (Da) 49,188)

Wild sequence: RMFPNAPYL (126-135), HLA-A2 restricted

Modified sequence: CYTWNOMNL (235-243), HLA-A24 restricted

The sequence RMFPNAPYL is called wild type and is HLA-A2 restricted. Another sequence CYTWNQMNL is a modified type and is HLA-A24 restricted. WT1 is expressed on the cell surface of carcinomas such as esophageal, gastric, colorectal, pancreas, biliary tract, liver, breast, uterus, brain, lung (non-small cell), malignant melanoma, sarcoma, acute myeloid and lymphoid leukemia, salivary gland and prostate, etc.

Another important tumor antigen to be targeted is MUC1 which is the cell membrane associated protein. The sequence of this peptide is TRPAPGSTAPPAHGVTSAPDTRPAPGSTAP and is HLA-non restricted (Figure 4). MUC1 is presented over the surface of cancer cells of the esophagus, stomach, colorectal, pancreas, biliary tract, breast, uterus, ovary, salivary gland, lung (adenocarcinoma), prostate and so on.

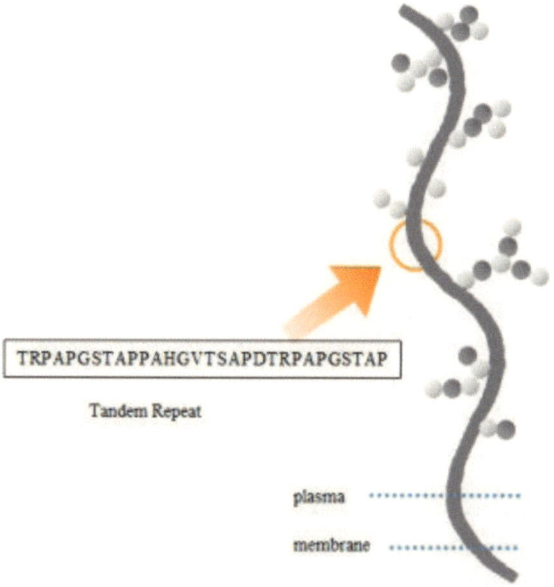

Figure 4. Sequence of MUC1 peptide.

Recently, new therapy strategies that focus on tumor associated antigens (TAAs) have been suggested as additional options to currently available treatments, due to their fewer adverse events and better tolerability. The establishment and maintenance of immune cell therapy for cancer relies on special TAAs, such as WT1 and MUC1 which have become primary targets for cancer vaccines [16, 17].

The high risk of metastatic recurrence suggests that cancer cell dissemination may occur early in most carcinomas, and therefore it seems that active immunotherapy may have a place among treatment modalities [18]. Among TAAs, above mentioned WT1 and MUC1 have received particular attention as potential targets for vaccine-based immunotherapy, because with the exception of very few tissues such as the splenic capsule and stroma, they are not expressed in normal human tissues and become activated in a number of cancers [19-21]. Therefore vaccination is an effective medical procedure in clinical oncology, based on the induction of a long-lasting immunologic memory and characterized by mechanisms endowed with high destructive potential and specificity. These functions will elicit a persistent immune memory that can eliminate residual cancer cells and protect against relapses.

On this basis, vaccination strategies employing DCs have been regarded as a promising therapeutic approach, even for advanced cancer. DCs internalize the cancer antigen, process their protein and then displays them, as short peptides on their extra cellular surface in conjunction with major histocompatibility complex (MHC) class I and II molecules. DCs then migrate into corresponding lymph nodes, where they mature and present the antigen to naïve T lymphocytes. Helper T cells ($CD4^+$) recognize their cognate antigens (MHC class II molecules) on DCs, where $CD8^+$ cytotoxic T lymphocytes (CTLs) recognize foreign or cancer cells that display the complementary peptide-MHC class I molecule on their cell surface. Adapting single peptides for the development of vaccines is not an optimal approach. It has been shown that after a complete objective response to the NY-ESO-1 peptide vaccine, a NY-SEO-1 negative tumor later recurred, showing that single-target immunization approaches can result in the development of immune escape tumor variants [22]. Since MHC expression levels vary with tumor types and stages, it is difficult to eradicate cancer by administration of NK cells alone. So, it is rational to use NK cell together with cancer vaccine, which we call hybrid immune therapy. CTLs activated by DC-based vaccine target MHC expressing cancer cells, where NK cells attack cancers that do not express MHC. We have proposed WT1, MUC1, CEA, CA125 and HER2/neu as potential cancer antigens for DC-based cancer vaccine, according to the patient's primary lesions and the tumor markers [23-26]. It has been reported that WT1 and MUC1 are antigens with high immunogenicity and their targeted immunotherapy has confirmed their safety and clinical efficiency. However, there are few studies regarding cancer vaccines that simultaneously use WT1 and MUC1 as antigens [27].

Preparations of DCs are as follows; PBMC-rich fraction is obtained usually by leukapheresis using COM. TEC (Fresenius Kabi, Hamburg, Germany). PBMCs were isolated from the heparinized leukapheresis products by Fi-coll-Hypaque gradient density centrifugation [28]. These PBMCs are placed into 100mm plastic tissue culture plates (Becton Dickinson Labware, Franklin Lakes, NJ) in AIM-V medium (Gibco, Gaithersburg, MD). Following 30 min incubation at 37deg C, non-adherent cells are removed and adherent cells were cultured in AIM-V medium containing granulocyte-macrophage colony stimulating factor (GM-CSF, 500ng/ml, Primmune Inc., Kobe, Japan) and IL-4 (250ng/ml, R&D Systems Inc., Minneapolis, MN), to generate immature DCs [29]. The population of adherent cells remaining in the wells is composed of 95.6 +/- 3.3% $CD14^+$ cells. After 5 days of cultures, the immature DCs are stimulated with OK-432 (10μ/mL) and prostaglandin E2 (50ng/mL, Daiichi Fine Chemical Co., Ltd., Toyama, Japan) for 24 hours to induce differentiation. Then, WT1, MUC1 and other antigens or proteins are pulsed onto the DCs in the same culture media are incubated for 24 hours. The concentrations usually used are shown (Table 4).

WT1	20μg/mL
MUC1, long peptide (30-mer)	20μg/mL
CEA peptides	20μg/mL
CA125 protein	500μg/mL
HER2	20μg/mL
Autologous tumor lysates	50μg/mL

Table 4. Concentrations of peptide using DC vaccine

To prepare the autologous tumor lysates, tumor masses were obtained by surgical resection exclusion and are homogenized. Aliquots of isolated tumor cells were then lysed by 10 cycles of repeated freeze in liquid nitrogen and thaw in a 37deg C water bath. The lysed cells were centrifuged at 14,000G for 5 min, and supernatants are passed through a 0.22μm filter (Millipore Corporation, Bedford, MA). Protein concentrations in the resultant cell-free lysates are determined using DC protein assay kits (Bio-Rad Laboratories, Hercules, CA). Aliquots (500μg/tube) are then cryopreserved at -135deg C until use [30]. Surface molecules are determined using flow cytometry. The cells defined as mature DCs are $CD14^-$, $HLA\text{-}DR^+$, $HLA\text{-}ABC^+$, $CD83^+$, $CD86^+$, $CD40^+$ and $CCR7^+$. Vaccine quality control and FACS analysis are as follow; All vaccines are subjected to quality control evaluation, which involves assessing the total number of live DCs, monocyte-derived DC characteristics and percentage of viable cells. For vaccine to be deemed "adequate" $4x10^7$ viable DCs are required. The frozen DC cells are allowed to thaw quickly in a 37deg C water bath and are retrieved from the cryopreservation tube by rinsing with 0.02% albumin-containing FACS buffer cell Wash™ (Bioscience, San Hose, CA). The FACS analysis is performed for cell surface antigen detection. FITC-labeled anti-human CD14, CD40, CD80, HLA-A, B, C, PE-labeled anti-human CD11C, CD83, CD197 ($CCR7^+$), HLA-DR and the FACS Calibur flow cytometer were used from DC Biosciences (Franklin Lakes, NJ).

4. Role of hyperthermia in DC vaccine therapy

Hyperthermia is widely used to enhance the efficiency of chemotherapy or radiation in patients with inoperable cancer [31]. It has been given much attention for the cellular response to heat stress with respect to the immune system in cancer. The anti-tumor immune response can be markedly enhanced by treatment with hyperthermia particularly in the fever range [32]. Immunological effects of mild hyperthermia are twofold. One is the effect on dendritic and other immune cells [33]. The other is the effect is on tumor cells. Protein or peptides derived from cancer which are chaperoned by heat-shock protein (HSP) are possible sources of antigens, transferred to antigen presenting cells for priming $CD8^+$ T cell responses [34]. Human tumor-derived HSP70 peptide complexes (HSP70-PC) have the immunogenic potential to instruct DCs and cross-present endogenously expressed, nonmutated, tumor antigenic peptides. The cross-presentation of a shared human tumor Ag together with its exquisite efficacy is an important new aspect for HSP70-based immunotherapy in clinical anticancer vaccination strategies, and suggest a potential extension of HSP70-based vaccination protocols from a patient-individual treatment modality to its use in an allogeneic setting [35]. The other studies support various clinical use of hyperthermia as part of an immunotherapeutic strategy in treating cancer [32, 36].

The mechanisms by which a tumor cell can escape CTL is critical for the design and modification of effective vaccine strategies against cancer. These mechanisms fall into four broad categories: (i) inadequate antigen presentation by tumor cells resulting in their poor sensitivity to lysis by CTL; (ii) inhibitory signals provided by the tumor microenvironment; (iii) inability of TAA-specific CTL to localize at a tumor site; and (iv) inability of the tumor microenvironment to sustain T cell function in vivo [37]. Therefore, adequate antigen expression by tumor cells is of crucial importance. Many research papers show the possible augmentation of MHC class I antigen presentation via heat shock protein expression by hyperthermia. It has been demonstrated that the cell surface presentation of MHC class I antigen is increased in tandem with increased heat shock protein 70 (HSP 70) [38]. It is clear that mild hyperthermia enhances both the expression of TAA on the surface of tumors and also increased presentation of TAA chaperoned by HSP on the dendritic cell. These findings are encouraging for usage of hyperthermia at the time of DC vaccination.

5. Clinical results in miscellaneous cancers

Indications for the DC-based cancer vaccine is summarized as follows:

1. Patients with advanced cancer refractory to standard treatments.
2. Cancer patients treated with standard treatments without satisfactory results.
3. Efficiency of current standard therapy is not expected, but there are some possibilities to improve quality of life and prolong survival time by use of DC-based vaccine.

Prevention of relapse or metastasis after surgery or other standard treatments.

In this communication, the results of the retrospective study of the DC-based vaccine are presented in cancers common in Japan. Most of these patients are called "cancer refugees" who are told that no further effective treatments are available. Patient evaluations included a medical history and physical examination which include measurement of performance status (PS), total protein, albumin, hemoglobin, WBC count, platelet count, blood urea nitrogen (BUN), creatinine, alkaline phosphatase, LDH, AST, ALT, bilirubin, HbA1c, tumor marker level and HLA. As an image marker, computed tomography (CT) scans or magnetic resonance image (MRI) as well as ultrasound studies were included. To be eligible, patients were required to have an ECOG PS of <3. They were also required to have adequate hematologic and hepatorenal functions as determined by the flowing parameters:

WBC counts of≧2,500/μL, platelet counts of≥80,000/μL, hemoglobin value of≧9.0g/dL, BUN<50mg/dL, serum bilirubin level <5.0mg/dL and AST level<50DIU/L.

Autologous DCs (1x10^7 cells) were administered intradermally at 14-day intervals, for a total of 6-8 times. Tolerable 1 to 5 KE doses of OK-432 (Chugai Pharmaceutical Co., Ltd., Tokyo, a streptococcus immunological adjuvant) was administered together with the DC vaccine. NK cells were simultaneously injected intravenously in some patients at 14-day intervals. Clinical response was evaluated according to the Response Evaluation Criteria in Solid Tumors (RECIST) version 1.0 as follows: complete remission (CR), partial remission (PR), stable disease (SD) and progressive disease (PD). Adverse events were evaluated by grading the toxicity according to the National Cancer Institute (NCI) Common Terminology Criteria for Adverse Events (CTCAE) version 4.0. The most common advanced cancers that were refractory to standard treatments that were treated by our DC-based cancer vaccine were as follows: breast cancer, lung cancer, pancreatic cancer, and colorectal cancer (Figures 5-8). The most important factor for prolonged survival was good PS before entry into DC vaccine treatment. Patients in the better PS group had a significantly longer survival time compared to those in the poorer group. The overall survival (OS) based on our risk score was significantly better for patients with clinical response of CR, PR and SD compared to those with a response of PD group. Therapy was well tolerated during treatment and for 3 months after the final treatment. None of the patients experienced adverse events of grade 3 or higher during the treatment period. Grade 1 to 2 fevers and grade 1 injection site reactions, consisting of erythema, induration and tenderness lasting 1-5 days after injection occurred in most patients and did not result in any dosage modifications or delayed treatments. No signs of autoimmune disease (arthritis, rash, colitis, etc.) were observed either during or after therapy.

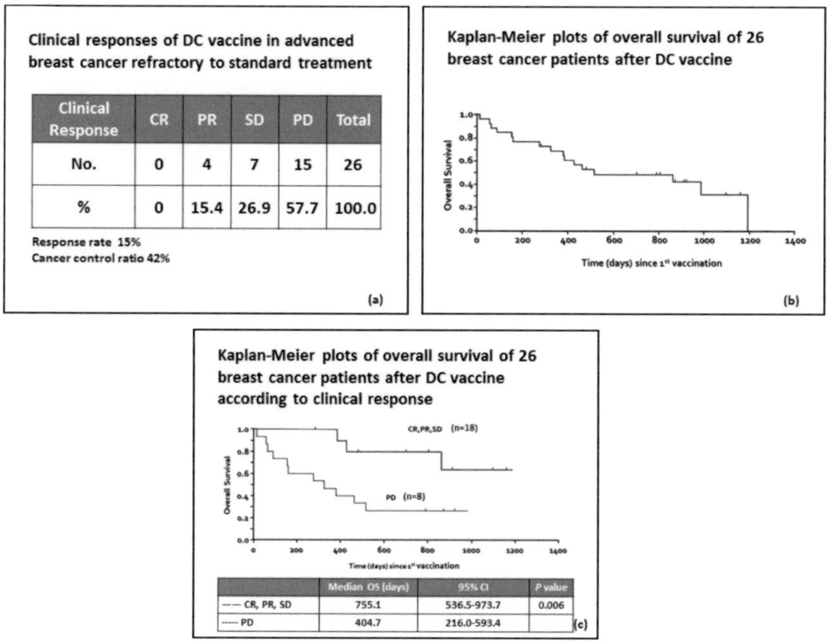

Figure 5. Clinical response of DC vaccine in advanced breast cancer refractory to standard treatment.

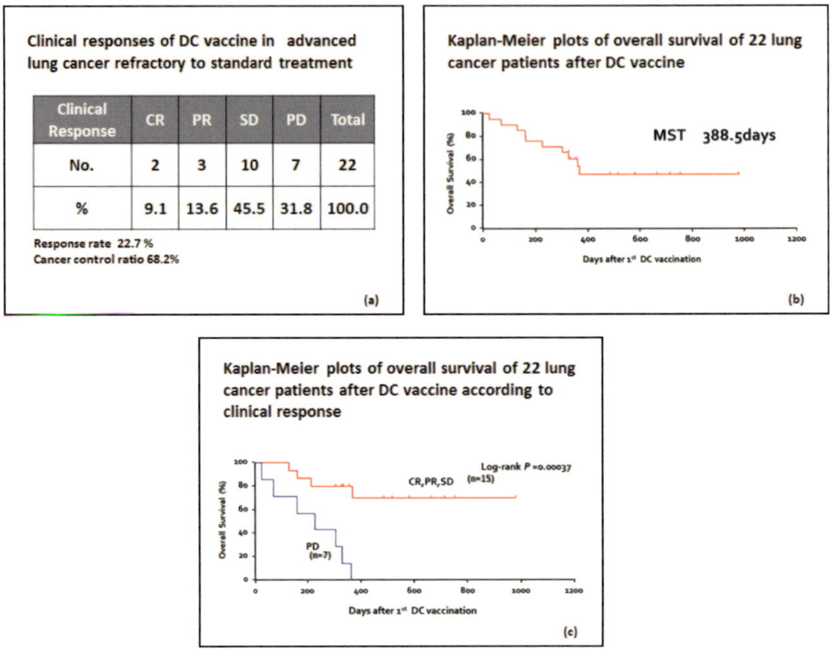

Clinical Response	CR	PR	SD	PD	Total
No.	2	3	10	7	22
%	9.1	13.6	45.5	31.8	100.0

Figure 6. Clinical response of DC vaccine in advanced lung cancer refractory to standard treatment.

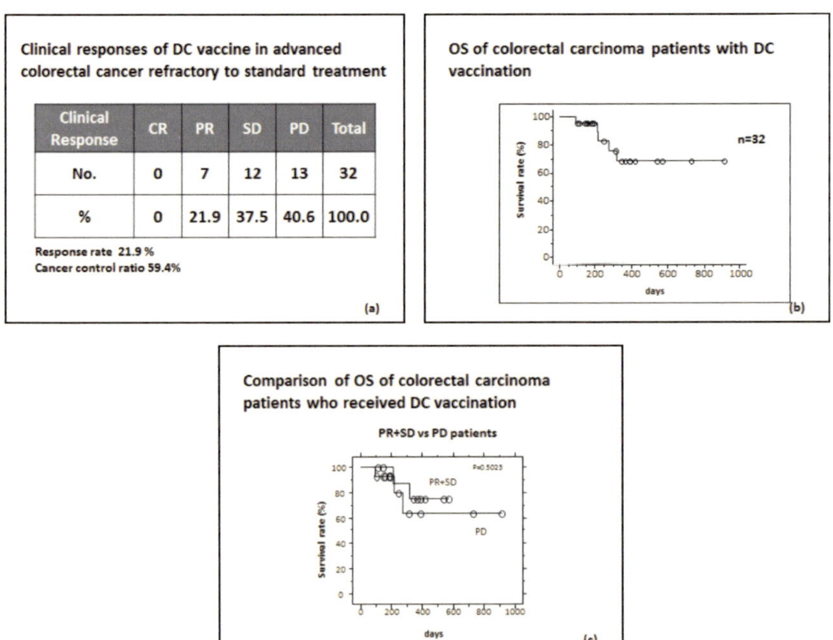

Clinical Response	CR	PR	SD	PD	Total
No.	0	7	12	13	32
%	0	21.9	37.5	40.6	100.0

Figure 7. Clinical response of DC vaccine in advanced colorectal cancer refractory to standard treatment.

http://dx.doi.org/10.5772/55450

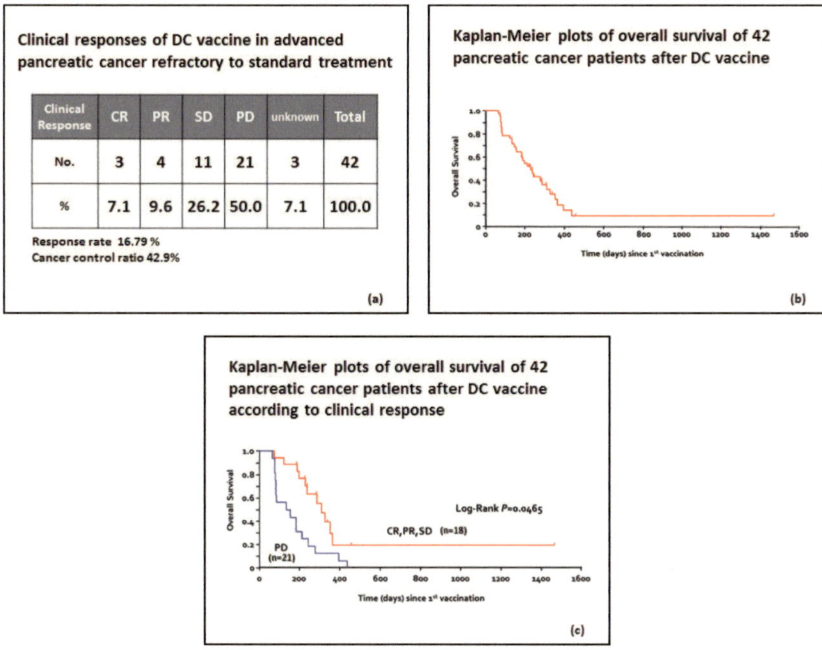

Clinical Response	CR	PR	SD	PD	unknown	Total
No.	3	4	11	21	3	42
%	7.1	9.6	26.2	50.0	7.1	100.0

Figure 8. Clinical response of DC vaccine in advanced pancreatic cancer refractory to standard treatment.

The current results show that the DC-based vaccine is clinically applicable to any patient with a good PS at the initiation of DC-based therapy and can clinically benefit from continuing therapy beyond disease progression. Of the professional APCs, DCs are the most potent stimulators of T cell responses and play a crucial role in the initiation of primary immune responses [12]. Despite several immunotherapeutic approaches tested in colon cancer patients, only one has reported clinical results in a prospective randomized trial [39]. Preclinical data suggest that DC-based vaccines exert cytotoxic actions and that prolonged vaccine exposure is necessary for continued cancer suppression [40]. However, precisely when the full efficacy of antitumor vaccines will be realized, and when this approach will become routine therapy is difficult to predict. To date, most of peptide-based vaccines have targeted HLA class I-restricted peptides. However, there is increasing evidence that tumor-specific $CD4^+$ T cells may also be important in inducing effective antitumor immunity. An ideal TAA is a protein that is essential for sustaining the malignant phenotype but which is not removed or down-regulated by the immune reaction. TAAs have been categorized according to their characteristics, such as therapeutic function, immunogenicity, oncogenicity, specificity, expression level, number of positive cells, and cancer stem cell expression.

It is important to understand the immunological mechanisms underlying the significant increase in cancer control ratios. Our results indicate that WT1 and /or MUC1-pulsed DC-based vaccination can have significant clinical benefits, even for advanced cancer patients that are refractory to standard therapies. These encouraging preliminary results suggest that WT1- and/or MUC1-pulsed DC-based vaccination strategies warrant further study as novel therapeutic approaches to patients with advanced carcinomas. The combination of cytotoxic therapy with immune stimulation against cancer has been studied preclinically for a variety of common tumor types and could be directly translated to clinical use [41-43]. The current result clearly supports the idea that quality specifications are of the highest priority and must be important considerations in any future vaccine-based study.

Moreover, the induction of memory T and B cells underlies immunological memory induced by vaccination [44]. The ability of memory T cells to confer protective immunity depends on the number and quality of the cells produced [45, 46]. In the current study patients with an outcome of SD lived for a relatively long time, which is unusual for other therapeutic modalities. This tendency may due to CTL proliferation and differentiation into effector memory CD8 cells.

Given the wide interest for vaccine intervention in treating miscellaneous cancers, our findings may help in guiding and designing future trials. Additional studies are necessary to identify appropriate targets for vaccine development in this new era of molecular-targeted agents for cancer treatment.

6. Discussion and conclusion

A better understanding of cancer molecular biology would enhance the design of novel therapies for cancer. Currently the scope of cancer immunotherapy is limited because most targeted antigens are restricted to a subset of patients. Molecular target DC vaccines evoke the power of each patient's immune system to help prevent recurrence and increase the long-term survival rate. If the patient's resected tumor is available, lysate is used as molecular antigens. Using this lysate, the vaccine induces an immune response against cancerous cells and creates immunologic memory. Because it is derived from the individual patient's tumor cells, this vaccine is a true targeted and personalized cancer therapy. When patient's own tumor cells are not available, integrating several candidates of peptides such as WT1, MUC1, CEA, CA125, Her2, PSA etc. can be used for the design of an anti-tumor vaccine which are restricted to the patient's HLA typing. Among these antigens, it is known that WT1 and MUC1 are the most important antigens expressed in cancer stem cells. Cancer stem cells form new tumors and may not be eliminated by chemotherapy or radiation. This has changed the perspective with regard to new approaches for treating cancer. Cancer stem cells are slow-dividing and inherently chemotherapy resistant. Eradication of these cancer stem cells may be necessary for the long-term success in cancer treatment. Using this strategy, a DC vaccine pulsed with WT1 and MUC1 and other tumor specific antigens would be used to eliminate cancer stem cells in individual patients. Hyperthermia is often used to activate immune system. There is evidence that when DCs take up HSPs together with the peptide they chaperone, the accompanying peptides are delivered into the antigen-processing pathways, leading to peptide presentation by MHC molecules. When DCs travel to the lymph nodes, T cells recognize the antigenic peptides and are specifically activated against cancer cells bearing these peptides [47]. Finally, the clinical results of molecular target cell therapy for cancers involving different organs, using the DC vaccine and or combination with natural killer cells are discussed. The response rate and cancer control rate of advanced breast cancer, lung cancer, colorectal cancer and pancreatic cancer are 12% and 38%, 22.7% and 68.2%, 21.9% and 59.4%, 16.9% and 42.9%, respectively. Overall survival rates were more than that of expected in advanced cancer refractory to standard therapy. These findings of DC based vaccines suggest the usefulness for treating cancer patients. Given the wide interest for targeted vaccine intervention in treating miscellaneous cancers, our findings may help in guiding and designing future trials and the development of novel cancer treatment strategies.

Author details

Hiroyuki Abe*, Touko Shimamoto, Shinichiro Akiyama and Minako Abe

*Address all correspondence to: drabeqqq@yahoo.co.jp

Abe Cancer Clinic, Japan

References

[1] Melder RJ, Whiteside TL, Vujanovic NL, Hiserodt JC, Herberman RB. A new approach to generating antitumor effectors for adoptive immunotherapy using human adherent lymphokine-activated killer cells. Cancer Res. 1988 Jun 15;48(12):3461-3469.

[2] Farag SS, VanDeusen JB, Fehniger TA, Caligiuri MA. Biology and clinical impact of human natural killer cells. Int J Hematol. 2003 Jul;78(1):7-17.

[3] Nagler A, Lanier LL, Cwirla S, Phillips JH. Comparative studies of human FcRIII-positive and negative natural killer cells. J Immunol. 1989;143(10):3183-3191.

[4] Miller JS, Oelkers S, Verfaillie C, McGlave P. Role of monocytes in the expansion of human activated natural killer cells. Blood. 1992;80(9):2221-2229.

[5] Baume DM, Caligiuri MA, Manley TJ, Daley JF, Ritz J. Differential expression of CD8a and CD8b associated with MHC-restricted and non-MHC-restricted cytolytic effector cells. Cell Immunol. 1990;131: 352-365.

[6] Rabinowich H, Pricop L, Herberman RB. Whiteside T.L. Expression and function of CD7 molecule on human natural killer cells. J Immunol. 1994;152(2):517-526.

[7] Lee DM, Patel DD, Pendergast AM, Haynes BF. Functional association of CD7 with phosphatidylinositol 3-kinase: interaction via a YEDM motif. Int Immunol. 1996;8(8): 1195-1203.

[8] Keever CA, Pekle K, Gazzola MV, Collins NH, Gillio A. NK and LAK activities from human marrow progenitors. I. The effects of interleukin-2 and interleukin-1. Cell Immunol. 1990;126(1):211-226.

[9] Trinchieri G, Matsumoto-Kobayashi M, Clark SC, Seehra J, London L, Perussia B. Response of resting human peripheral blood natural killer cells to interleukin 2. J Exp Med. 1984;160(4):1147-1169.

[10] Baume DM, Robertson MJ, Levine H, Manley TJ, Schow PW, Ritz J. Differential responses to interleukin 2 define functionally distinct subsets of human natural killer cells. Eur J Immunol. 1992;22(1):1-6.

[11] Abe H, Akiyama S, Okamoto M. Clinical Cancer Immunotherapy: Molecular Targeting Immunotherapy. J Integ Med. 2008;1(1):38-46.

[12] Banchereau J, Steinman RM. Dendritic cells and the control of immunity. Nature. 1998 Mar 19;392(6673):245-252.

[13] Kadowaki N, Antonenko S, Ho S, Rissoan MC, Soumelis V, Porcelli SA, et al. Distinct cytokine profiles of neonatal natural killer T cells after expansion with subsets of dendritic cells. J Exp Med. 2001 May 21;193(10):1221-1226.

[14] Banchereau J, Palucka AK. Dendritic cells as therapeutic vaccines against cancer. Nat Rev Immunol. 2005 Apr;5(4):296-306.

[15] Martin A. Cheever, James P. Allison, Andrea S. Ferris, et al. The Prioritization of Cancer Antigens: A National Cancer Institute Pilot Project for the Acceleration of Translational Research. Clin Cancer Res 2009;15:5323-5337.

[16] Akiyama S, Hamaya K, Ito Y, et al. Retrospective analysis of clinical responses in patients with gastroenterological cancer treated with dendritic cell vaccination. Int J Integ Med. 2011;3:12-24.

[17] Akiyama S, Abe H. Successful treatment by hybrid immune therapy and high dose vitamin C therapy against hepatocellular carcinoma. Int J Integ Med. 2011;3:147-151.

[18] Mittendorf EA, Peoples GE, Singletary SE. Breast cancer vaccines: promise for the future of pipe dream? Cancer. 2007;15:1677-1686.

[19] Brieger J, Weidmann E, Fenchel K, et al. The expression of the Wilms' tumor gene in acute myelocytic leukemia as a possible maker for leukemic blast cells. Leukemia. 1994;8:2138-2143.

[20] Menssen HD, Renkl HJ, Rodeck U, Maurer J, Notter M, Schwartz S, et al. Presence of Wilms' tumor gene (wt1) transcripts and the WT1 nuclear protein in the majority of human acute leukemias. Leukemia. 1995;9(6):1060-1067.

[21] Ogawa H, Tamaki H, Ikegame K, Soma T, Kawakami M, Tsuboi A, et al. The usefulness of monitoring WT1 gene transcripts for the prediction and management of re-

lapse following allogeneic stem cell transplantation in acute type leukemia. Blood. 2003 1;101(5):1698-1704.

[22] Odunsi K, Qian F, Matsuzaki J, Mhawech-Fauceglia P, Andrews C, Hoffman EW, et al. Vaccination with an NY-ESO-1 peptide of HLA class I/II specificities induces integrated humoral and T cell responses in ovarian cancer. Proc Natl Acad Sci U S A. 2007 31;104(31):12837-12842.

[23] Sugiyama H. Cancer immunotherapy targeting Wilms' tumor gene WT1 product. Expert Rev Vaccines. 2005;4(4):503-512.

[24] Mukherjee P, Ginardi AR, Madsen CS, Sterner CJ, Adriance MC, Tevethia MJ, et al. Mice with spontaneous pancreatic cancer naturally develop MUC-1-specific CTLs that eradicate tumors when adoptively transferred. J Immunol. 2000;165(6): 3451-3460.

[25] Nair SK, Hull S, Coleman D, Gilboa E, Lyerly HK, Morse MA. Induction of carcinoembryonic antigen (CEA)-specific cytotoxic T-lymphocyte responses in vitro using autologous dendritic cells loaded with CEA peptide or CEA RNA in patients with metastatic malignancies expressing CEA. Int J Cancer. 1999;82(1):121-124.

[26] Larbouret C, Robert B, Navarro-Teulon I, Thèzenas S, Ladjemi MZ, Morisseau S, at al. In vivo therapeutic synergism of anti-epidermal growth factor receptor and anti-HER2 monoclonal antibodies against pancreatic carcinomas. Clin Cancer Res. 2007 Jun 1;13(11):3356-3362.

[27] Ramanathan RK, Lee KM, McKolanis J, Hitbold E, Schraut W, Moser AJ, at al. Phase I study of a MUC1 vaccine composed of different doses of MUC1 peptide with SB-AS2 adjuvant in resected and locally advanced pancreatic cancer. Cancer Immunol Immunother. 2005 Mar;54(3):254-264.

[28] Böyum A. Isolation of mononuclear cells and granulocytes from human blood. Isolation of monuclear cells by one centrifugation, and of granulocytes by combining centrifugation and sedimentation at 1 g. Scand J Clin Lab Invest Suppl. 1968;97:77-89.

[29] Okamoto M, Furuichi S, Nishioka Y, Oshikawa T, Tano T, Ahmed SU, at al. Expression of toll-like receptor 4 on dendritic cells is significant for anticancer effect of dendritic cell-based immunotherapy in combination with an active component of OK-432, a streptococcal preparation. Cancer Res. 2004 Aug 1;64(15):5461-5470.

[30] Nagayama H, Sato K, Morishita M, Uchimaru K, Oyaizu N, Inazawa T, et al. Results of a phase I clinical study using autologous tumour lysate-pulsed monocyte-derived mature dendritic cell vaccinations for stage IV malignant melanoma patients combined with low dose interleukin-2. Melanoma Res. 2003 Oct;13(5):521-530.

[31] Feyerabend T, Wiedemann GJ, Jäger B, Vesely H, Mahlmann B, Richter E. Local hyperthermia, radiation, and chemotherapy in recurrent breast cancer is feasible and ef-

fective except for inflammatory disease. Int J Radiat Oncol Biol Phys. 2001 Apr 1;49(5):1317-1325.

[32] Calderwood SK, Theriault JR, Gong J. How is the immune response affected by hyperthermia and heat shock proteins? Int J Hyperthermia. 2005 Dec;21(8):713-716.

[33] Srivastava P. Interaction of heat shock proteins with peptides and antigen presenting cells: chaperoning of the innate and adaptive immune responses. Annu Rev Immunol. 2002;20:395-425.

[34] Binder RJ, Srivastava PK. Peptides chaperoned by heat-shock proteins are a necessary and sufficient source of antigen in the cross-priming of CD8+ T cells. Nat Immunol. 2005 Jun;6(6):593-599.

[35] Noessner E, Gastpar R, Milani V, Brandl A, Hutzler PJ, Kuppner MC, at al. Tumor-derived heat shock protein 70 peptide complexes are cross-presented by human dendritic cells. J Immunol. 2002 Nov 15;169(10):5424-5432.

[36] Ostberg JR, Repasky EA. Emerging evidence indicates that physiologically relevant thermal stress regulates dendritic cell function. Cancer Immunol Immunother. 2006 Mar;55(3):292-298.

[37] Marincola FM, Jaffee EM, Hicklin DJ, Ferrone S. Escape of human solid tumors from T-cell recognition: molecular mechanisms and functional significance. Adv Immunol. 2000;74:181-273.

[38] Ito A, Shinkai M, Honda H, Wakabayashi T, Yoshida J, Kobayashi T. Augmentation of MHC class I antigen presentation via heat shock protein expression by hyperthermia. Cancer Immunol Immunother. 2001 Dec;50(10):515-522.

[39] Vermorken JB, Claessen AM, van Tinteren H, et al. Active specific immunotherapy for stage II and stage III human colon cancer: a randomised trial. Lancet. 1999;353:345-350.

[40] Sadanaga N, Nagashima H, Mashino K, Tahara K, Yamaguchi H, Ohta M, et al. Dendritic cell vaccination with MAGE peptide is a novel therapeutic approach for gastrointestinal carcinomas. Clin Cancer Res. 2001 Aug;7(8):2277-2784.

[41] Meng Y, Carpentier AF, Chen L, Boisserie G, Simon JM, Mazeron JJ, et al. Successful combination of local CpG-ODN and radiotherapy in malignant glioma. Int J Cancer. 2005 Oct 10;116(6):992-927.

[42] Najar HM, Dutz JP. Topical CpG enhances the response of murine malignant melanoma to dacarbazine. J Invest Dermatol. 2008 Sep;128(9):2204-2210.

[43] VanOosten RL, Griffith TS. Activation of tumor-specific CD8+ T Cells after intratumoral Ad5-TRAIL/CpG oligodeoxynucleotide combination therapy. Cancer Res. 2007 Dec 15;67(24):11980-11990.

[44] Pulendran B, Ahmed R. Immunological mechanisms of vaccination. Nat Immunol. 2011;12:509-517.

[45] Gourley TS, Wherry EJ, Masopust D, Ahmed R. Generation and maintenance of immunological memory. Semin Immunol. 2004 Oct;16(5):323-333.

[46] Hand TW, Kaech SM. Intrinsic and extrinsic control of effector T cell survival and memory T cell development. Immunol Res. 2009;45(1):46-61.

[47] Li Z, Qiao Y, Liu B et al. Combination of imatinib mesylate with autologous leukocyte-derived heat shock protein and chronic myelogenous leukemia . Clin Cancer Res. 2005 11:4460-4468.

Chapter 15

Immunotherapy of Urinary Bladder Carcinoma: BCG and Beyond

Yi Luo, Eric J. Askeland, Mark R. Newton,
Jonathan R. Henning and Michael A. O'Donnell

Additional information is available at the end of the chapter

http://dx.doi.org/10.5772/55283

1. Introduction

Urothelial carcinoma of the bladder is the second most common urologic neoplasm after prostate carcinoma in the United States, with an estimated 70,510 new cases and 14,880 deaths in 2012 [1]. Global prevalence of bladder cancer is estimated at >1 million and is steadily increasing. This disease places enormous economic burden on the U.S. health care system due to its requirements of surgical resection, repeated intravesical therapies, and lifelong medical follow-up. Urothelial carcinoma accounts for 90% of bladder tumors. At the time of diagnosis, 20-25% of cases are muscle invasive (stage T2 or higher) and are typically treated with surgical resection (radical cystectomy) [2]. The remainders are confined to layers above the muscularis propria – so-called nonmuscle invasive bladder cancer (NMIBC). These cancers (also termed "superficial bladder cancer") include tumors confined to the urothelium (Ta), tumors invading the lamina propria (T1), and carcinoma *in situ* (Tis, a flat erythematous lesion), occurring in 70%, 20% and 10% of NMIBC cases, respectively [2]. Transurethral resection of bladder tumor (TURBT) is the standard primary treatment for Ta and T1 lesions; however, recurrence rates for TURBT alone can be as high as 70% with up to 30% progressing to muscle invasive disease requiring cystectomy [3]. The high rates of recurrence and significant risk of progression in higher grade tumors mandate additional therapy with intravesical agents. While limiting the systemic exposure, intravesical therapy allows the destruction of residual microscopic tumor and circulating tumor cells after TURBT by exposure to therapeutic agents, thereby preventing reimplantation. To date, intravesical therapy has been used as an adjuvant treatment after TURBT to prevent recurrence and progression of the disese and is also the treatment of choice for Tis that is not feasible for TURBT.

Chemotherapeutic agents such as mitomycin C, doxorubicin and epirubicin have long been used as intravesical therapies for NMIBC [3,4]. Recently, intravesical use of gemcitabine, valrubicin, and apaziquone have also been evaluated [5-7]. With respect to immunotherapy, BCG, a live attenuated strain of *Mycobacterium bovis* widely used as a vaccine against tuberculosis, was first introduced as an intravesical therapy for bladder cancer in 1976 by Morales and associates [8]. Since then, BCG has been extensively evaluated and demonstrated to be superior to any other single chemotherapeutic agent for reducing recurrence and preventing progression of the disease [3,9]. To date, BCG has become the mainstay of therapy for NMIBC and remains the most effective treatment [3,9]. However, despite its favorable effects, a significant proportion of patients do not respond to BCG or tolerate treatment. In addition, recurrence and side effects are common. Therefore, research has been pursued and efforts made to improve BCG therapy. During the past decades, cytokine-based therapies have been developed. To date, multiple cytokines with Th1 stimulating properties, such as IFN-α, IL-2 and IL-12, have been evaluated, alone or in combination with BCG for the treatment of bladder cancer. In addition, pre-clinical research continues, aiming to identify new BCG therapeutic modalities. This chapter reviews the progress of bladder cancer immunotherapy, focusing on the clinical use of BCG and cytokines. In addition, we describe our own experience with BCG and cytokine therapies as well as research on BCG combination therapy and genetic engineering of BCG to secrete Th1 cytokines. Finally, we describe the future directions for research with regard to BCG immunotherapy.

2. BCG immunotherapy of bladder cancer

2.1. Clinical use of BCG in bladder cancer treatment

Intravesical administration of BCG is currently the most common therapy employed for NMIBC. Since its advent in 1976, BCG has been extensively used to reduce recurrence and progression of NMIBC in an attempt to preserve the bladder. Although various BCG strains (e.g. Pasteur, Tice, Connaught, Frappier, RIVM and Tokyo) have been used, there is no evidence of a difference in efficacy or toxicity profile among these strains [9]. Many prospective randomized studies and meta-analyses have demonstrated the effectiveness of intravesical BCG therapy. Typical complete response rates are 55-65% for papillary tumors and 70-75% for Tis, which inversely indicates that 30-45% of patients will fail BCG treatment [3,9-12]. Adjuvant intravesical therapy was noted by the 2007 American Urological Association (AUA) panel to reduce recurrences by 24% and treatment with BCG was recommended by the panel [10]. Unfortunately, of complete responders, up to 50% will develop recurrent tumors within the first 5 years [13]. Furthermore, up to 90% of patients experience side effects ranging from cystitis and irritative voiding symptoms to much more uncommon life-threatening BCG sepsis. Up to 20% of patients are BCG intolerant due to these side effects [14].

The optimum dosing, schedule and duration for BCG treatment of NMIBC are unknown. Both induction and maintenance courses are largely empirical. According to the AUA's 2007 clinical practice guidelines [10], BCG therapy should be initiated 2-3 weeks following TURBT to allow healing of the urothelium and reduce the risk of side effects. The induction course consists of six weekly intravesical instillations. The recommended dose varies in weight from strain to strain, but each provides approximately 1-5 X 10^8 colony-forming units (CFU) of viable mycobacteria. Lyophilized powder BCG is reconstituted in 50 ml of saline and administered via urethral catheter into an empty bladder with a dwell time of 2 hours. Maintenance is given as three weekly intravesical instillations at 3 and 6 months and then every 6 months for up to 3 years. Maintenance BCG is more effective in decreasing recurrence as compared to induction therapy alone. Multiple meta-analyses support BCG maintenance and it is now firmly established in clinical practice. The European Association of Urology (EAU) and the AUA recommend at least one year of maintenance for high risk patients [10,15]. The optimum schedule and duration of therapy have yet to be determined; however, most who use maintenance follow some permutation of the Southwest Oncology Group (SWOG) program, a 3-week "mini" series given at intervals of 3, 6, 12, 18, 24, 30 and 36 months for a total of 27 instillations over 3 years [3,9,16]. Other schedules, such as single maintenance instillations of BCG at 3, 6, 9 and 12 months after induction therapy, have also produced promising results [17]. Recently, the EAU updated its guidelines on NMIBC and recommended a minimum of one year of intravesical BCG therapy for intermediate or high risk disease [18]. The International Bladder Cancer Group (IBCG) also reviewed the current guidelines and recommended the use of intravesical BCG with maintenance for intermediate or high risk disease [19]. Intravesical BCG is contraindicated under the following situations: TURBT within the past 2 weeks, traumatic catheterization, macroscopic hematuria, urethral stenosis, active tuberculosis, prior BCG sepsis, immunosuppression, and urinary tract infection.

At our own institution, a BCG induction course is typically initiated at 2-3 weeks post-TURBT with six weekly installations and a 1-2 hour dwell time. For patients with Tis, severe dysplasia, Grade 3/high grade or poorly differentiated pathology, and/or stage T1 disease, formal restaging under anesthesia is performed 6 weeks later and includes bilateral upper tract cytology, retrograde pyelograms, 4-5 random bladder biopsies, and prostatic urethral biopsies. If this pathology and restaging is negative, maintenance cycles may be initiated in 6 weeks. We classify three maintenance cycles A, B and C. Maintenance A consists of 3 weekly instillations followed by cystoscopy 6 weeks later. Cytology and fluorescence *in situ* hybridization (FISH) in urine specimens may be obtained at this time. If cystoscopy/cytology is negative, maintenance B may be initiated 6 months after the conclusion of cycle A, again for three weekly treatments. Maintenance C is initiated 6 months after the conclusion of cycle B. Following cycle C, cystoscopy/cytology is repeated every 3 months for 2 years from the original diagnosis at which time it is extended to every 6 months for 2 years, and then annually.

2.2. Mechanism of BCG action

Understanding of the mechanisms of BCG action is critical to improving the efficacy of BCG therapy. Although the exact mechanisms of BCG action currently remain elusive, many details have been discovered during the past decades. It has become clear that a functional host immune system is a necessary prerequisite for successful BCG therapy. It has also been known that the effects of intravesical BCG depend on the induction of a complex inflammatory cascade event in the bladder mucosa reflecting activation of multiple types of immune cells and bladder tissue cells [20,21] (Figure 1). The initial step after BCG instillation is binding of BCG to fibronectin expressed on the urothelial lining through fibronectin attachment protein (FAP) [22]. Attached BCG is then internalized and processed by both normal and malignant cells, resulting in secretion of an array of proinflammatory cytokines and chemokines such as IL-1, IL-6, IL-8, tumor necrosis factor (TNF)-α, and granulocyte-macrophage colony stimulating factor (GM-CSF) [23,24]. Following urothelial cell activation, an influx of various leukocyte types into the bladder wall occurs including neutrophils, monocytes/macrophages, lymphocytes, natural killer (NK) cells, and dendritic cells (DC) [25-27]. These infiltrating leukocytes are activated and produce a variety of additional proinflammatory cytokines and chemokines and also form BCG-induced granuloma structures in the bladder wall [25,27]. Subsequently, a large number of leukocyte types such as neutrophils, T cells and macrophages are expelled into the bladder lumen and appear in patients' voided urine [28-31]. In addition, transient massive cytokines and chemokines can be detected in voided urine including IL-1β, IL-2, IL-6, IL-10, IL-12, IL-18, IFN-γ, TNF-α, GM-CSF, macrophage colony-stimulating factor (M-CSF), macrophage-derived chemokine (MDC), monocyte chemoattractant protein (MCP)-1, macrophage inflammatory protein (MIP)-1α, interferon-inducible protein (IP)-10, monokine induced by γ-interferon (MIG), and eosinophil chemoattractant activity (Eotaxin) [30,32-37]. The urine of animals treated with intravesical BCG also showed increased levels of numerous cytokines and chemokines [27]. It has been noted that the development of a predominant Th1 cytokine profile (e.g. IFN-γ, IL-2 and IL-12) is associated with the therapeutic effects of BCG, whereas the presence of a high level of Th2 cytokines (e.g. IL-10) is associated with BCG failure [33,35, 36]. Thus, a shift of the cytokines produced towards a Th1 milieu is necessary for succesful BCG immunotherapy of bladder cancer. To support this, it has been observed that both IFN-γ and IL-12 but not IL-10 are required for local tumor surveillance in an animal model of bladder cancer [38]. Mice deficint in IL-10 genetically (IL-$10^{-/-}$) or functionally via antibody neutralization or receptor blockage can also develop enhanced anti-bladder cancer immunity in response to intravesical BCG [36,39].

Multiple immune cell types participate in the inflammatory response induced by BCG in the bladder. It is well accepted that macrophages, an indispensable cellular component of the innate immune system, serve as the first line of defense in mycobacterial infection. Activation, maturation and cytokine production of macrophages are primarily induced by Toll-like receptor (TLR) 2 ligation [40]. Following BCG instillation, an increased number of macrophages can be observed in bladder cancer infiltrates and the peritumoral bladder wall. Voided urine after BCG instillation also contains an increased number of macrophages and the cytokines and chemokines predominantly produced by macrophages such as TNF-α, IL-6, IL-10, IL-12 and IL-18 [28,30,32,35-37]. In addition to presenting BCG antigens, macrophages are capable of functioning as tumoricidal cells toward bladder cancer cells upon activation by BCG [41-45]. The killing of bladder cancer cells by macrophages relies on direct cell-to-cell contact and release of various soluble effector factors such as cytotoxic cytokines TNF-α and IFN-γ and apoptotic mediators such as nitric oxide (NO) [43-45,46]. Th1 cytokines (e.g. IFN-γ) enhance the induction of macrophage cytotoxicity whereas Th2 cytokines (e.g. IL-10) inhibit the induction of macrophage cytotoxicity [44,45].

http://dx.doi.org/10.5772/55283

Neutrophils also compose the early responding cells to BCG instillation of the bladder and can be observed in the bladder wall and urine shortly after BCG instillation [27,28,30]. Neutrophils are central mediators of the innate immunity in BCG infection and are activated by signalling through TLR2 and TLR4 in conjunction with the adaptor protein myeloid differentiation factor 88 (MyD88) [47]. In addition to secretion of proinflammatory cytokines and chemokines (e.g. IL-1α, IL-1β, IL-8, MIP-1α, MIP-1β, MCP-1, transforming growth factor (TGF)-β, and growth-related oncogene (GRO)-α) that lead to the recruitment of other immune cells [48], recent studies revealed that neutrophils are the primary source of TNF-related apoptosis-inducing ligand (TRAIL) found in the urine after BCG instillation [49,50]. TRAIL is a member of the TNF family that induces apoptosis in malignant cells but not in normal cells. Studies have indicated that the neutrophil TRAIL response is specific to BCG stimulation rather than nonspecific immune activation. Studies have also revealed a positive correlation between urinary TRAIL level and a favorable response to BCG treatment [49]. These observations suggest an important

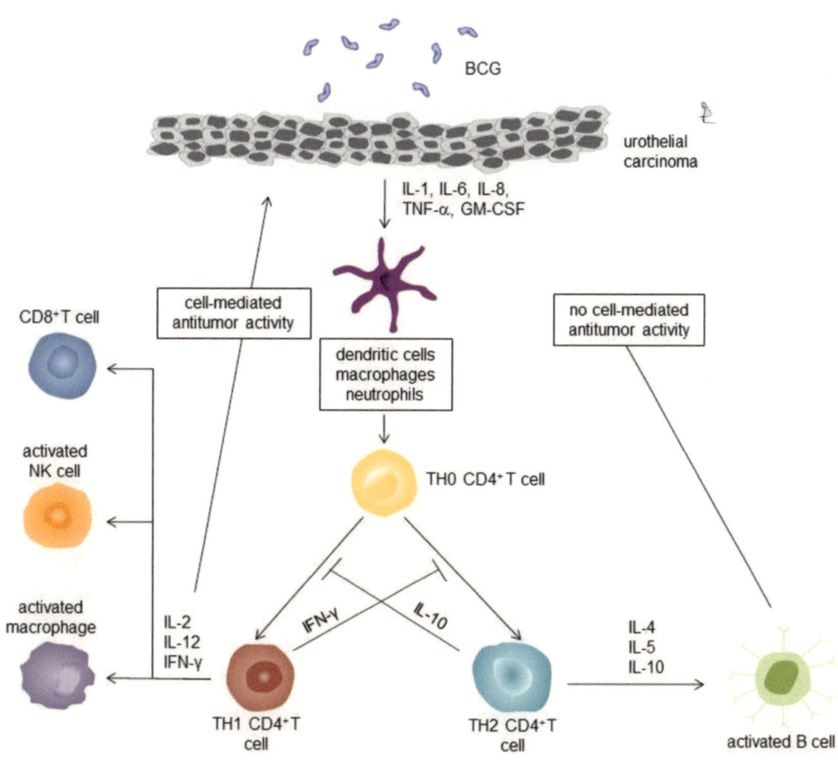

Figure 1. Suggested cascade of immune responses in bladder mucosa induced by intravesical BCG instillation. Attachment of BCG to urothelial cells including carcinoma cells triggers release of cytokines and chemokines from these cells, resulting in recruitment of various types of immune cells into the bladder wall. Activation of phagocytes and the new cytokine environment lead to the differentiation of naïve CD4⁺ T cells into TH1 and/or TH2 cells that direct immune responses toward cellular or humoral immunity, respectively. The therapeutic effect of BCG depends on a proper induction of TH1 immune responses. IL-10 inhibits TH1 immune responses whereas IFN-γ inhibits TH2 immune responses. Blocking IL-10 or inducing IFN-γ can lead to a TH1 dominated immunity that is essential for BCG-mediated bladder cancer destruction.

role of neutrophils in BCG-induced anti-bladder cancer immunity. Indeed, it has been observed that depletion of neutrophils resulted in a reduced BCG-induced anti-bladder cancer response in a mouse model of bladder cancer [48].

Following the activation of macrophages and neutrophils in the bladder wall, driven by chemoattractants, recruitment of other immune cell types including $CD4^+$ T cells, $CD8^+$ T cells, NK cells, and DC takes place [25,26]. As for neutrophils and macrophages, these cell types can be found in the voided urine of patients after BCG instillation [28-30]. These effector cells produce various cytokines and chemokines to further promote BCG-induced anti-bladder cancer immune responses in the local milieu. In addition, DC, together with macrophages, trigger an anti-BCG specific immune response via antigen presentation to T cells that also amplifies the BCG-induced antitumor immunity. Like neutrophils and macrophages, both T cells and NK cells are cytotoxic toward bladder cancer cells upon activation. They kill target cells via the major histocompatibility complex (MHC) restricted (e.g. for cytotoxic T lymphocytes (CTL)) and/or MHC non-restricted pathways (e.g. for NK cells) [41,51,52]. Perforin-mediated lysis and apoptosis-associated killing (e.g. via Fas ligand and TRAIL) have been implicated as the major molecular effector mechanisms underlying the eradication of bladder cancer cells. These effector cell types are crucial for BCG immunotherapy of bladder cancer, as depletion of these cell types failed to develop effective anti-bladder cancer responses *in vivo* and kill bladder cancer cells *in vitro* [53,54].

It has been shown that stimulation of human peripheral blood mononuclear cells (PBMC) by viable BCG *in vitro* leads to the generation of a specialized cell population called BCG-activated killer (BAK) cells [55,56]. BAK cells are a $CD3^-CD8^+CD56^+$ cell population whose cytotoxicity is MHC non-restricted [56,57]. BAK cells kill bladder cancer cells through the perforin-mediated lysis pathway and effectively lyse NK cell-resistant bladder cancer cells [55-57]. Macrophages and $CD4^+$ T cells have been found to be indispensable for the induction of BAK cell killing activity but have no such activity by themselves [56]. Th1 cytokines IFN-γ and IL-2 have been found to be required for the induction of BAK cell cytotoxicity, as neutralizing antibodies specific to these cytokines could inhibit BCG-induced cytotoxicity [56]. BAK cells, together with lymphokine-activated killer (LAK) cells, a diverse population with NK or T cell phenotypes that are generated by IL-2 [58-60], have been suggested to be the major effector cells during intravesical BCG therapy of bladder cancer. Other potential cytotoxic effector cells include CD1 restricted $CD8^+$ T cells [61], $\gamma\delta$ T cells [62-64], and natural killer T (NKT) cells [63-65].

Activation of the innate immune system is a prerequisite for BCG-induced inflammatory responses and the subsequent eradication of bladder cancer by intravesical BCG. In BCG instillation, TLRs participate in neutrophil, macrophage and DC recognition, maturation and activation. Both TLR2 and TLR4 appear to serve important but distinct roles in the induction of host immune responses to BCG or BCG cell-wall skeleton [40]. TLR9 also contributes to DC recognition of BCG [66]. Like other microbes, BCG has surface components called pathogen-associated molecular patterns (PAMPs) that are recognized by cells of the innate immune system through TLRs during infection [67]. It is this interaction between TLRs and PAMPs that activates the cells of the innate immune system, leading to BCG-induced inflammatory responses and subsequent eradication of bladder cancer. It is known that the antitumor effect of intravesical BCG depends on its proper induction of a localized Th1 immune response. However, a systemic immune response appears also to be involved in intravesical BCG therapy. It has been documented that purified protein derivative (PPD) skin test often converts from negative to positive after BCG instillation and the effective treatment is associated with the development of delayed-type hypersensitivity (DTH) reaction to PPD [68]. Animal studies have also demonstrated the importance of DTH in the antitumor activity of intravesical BCG therapy [36]. Moreover, studies have shown increased levels of cytokines and chemokines in the serum (e.g. IL-2, IFN-γ, MCP-1 and RANTES), along with production of these cytokines and chemokines in the urine and/or bladder, during the course of BCG instillation [34,69]. Furthermore, studies have also shown an increase in PBMC cytotoxicity against urothelial carcinoma cells (UCC) after BCG instilation [34].

In addition to the ability of BCG to elicit host immune responses, evidence supports a direct effect of BCG on the biology of UCC. *In vitro* studies have shown that BCG is anti-proliferative and even cytotoxic to UCC [41,70], and induces UCC expression of cytokines and chemokines (e.g. IL-1β, IL-6, IL-8, TNF-α and GM-CSF) [24], antigen-presenting molecules (e.g. MHC class II, CD1 and B7-1) [71], and intercellular adhesion molecules (e.g. ICAM-1) [71]. Analysis of tumor biopsy specimens from bladder cancer patients who underwent intravesical BCG therapy further supported the ability of BCG to induce UCC expression of these molecules *in vivo* [26]. Moreover, the bladder urothelium of animals treated with intravesical BCG shows upregulation of HLA antigens (e.g. MHC class I and II) and changes of many other molecules [72]. Recent studies have revealed that by cross-linking $\alpha5\beta1$ integrin receptors, BCG exerts its direct biological effects on UCC, including activation of the signal transduction pathways involving activator protein (AP) 1, NFkB and CCAAT-enhancer-binding protein (C/EBP) [73], upregulation of gene expressions such as IL-6 and cyclin dependant kinase inhibitor p21 [73,74], and cell cycle arrest at the G1/S transition [75]. Although some studies showed the ability of BCG to induce apoptosis in UCC [76], other studies showed no such an ability or even induction of apoptotic resistance in UCC [77]. Further studies revealed that BCG induced UCC death in a caspase-independent manner [77] and that p21 played an important role in modulating the direct effects of BCG on UCC [78].

3. Recombinant cytokines for bladder cancer treatment

Prompted by the burden of patients either with BCG refractory disease or intolerance to BCG treatment, the search goes on for therapeutic improvements. Given that the effect of BCG depends on a proper induction of Th1 immune responses, decades of research have focused on enhancing the BCG induction of Th1 immune responses. Th1 stimulating cytokines, such as IFN-α, IL-2, IL-12, IFN-γ, TNF-α and GM-CSF, have been used alone or in combination with BCG and demonstrated to be favorable in the treatment of bladder cancer. Particularly, combination therapies potentially allow the use of a lower and safer dose of BCG while preserving or even enhancing BCG efficacy.

3.1. Recombinant IFN-α

IFNs are glycoproteins initially isolated in the 1950s and valued for their anti-viral properties. Three types have been isolated, IFN-α (which is actually a family of interferons), IFN-β, and IFN-γ. IFN-α and IFN-β are grouped as "Type I" interferons whereas IFN-γ is a "Type II" interferon. The Type I interferon receptor has 2 components, IFNAR-1 and IFNAR-2, which subsequently bind and phosphorylate Jak molecules initiating a cascade resulting in gene transcription [79]. The IFN-α family is well known to stimulate NK cells, induce MHC class I response, and increase antibody recognition [80]. They have antineoplastic properties by direct antiproliferative effects and complex immunomodulatory effects [79], both of which could be advantageous for bladder cancer treatment. Clinically available preparations include IFN-α2a (Roferon-A, recombinant, Roche Laboratories, Nutley, NJ) and IFN-α2b (Intron-A, recombinant, Schering Plough, Kenilworth, NJ), though to date most research involves IFN-α2b. There has been interest in IFN-α2b both alone and combination with BCG, where a synergistic response has been described. Conceptually, combining BCG and IFN makes sense. BCG efficacy depends on the induction of a robust Th1 cytokine profile and IFN-α2b has been shown to potentiate the Th1 immune response [81]. However, despite theoretical promise, data after translation to clinical practice has been mixed.

For many years, IFN-α was thought to exert antitumor activity primarily through direct antiproliferative properties [82]. At least part of this effect has been shown to be mediated by directly inducing tumor cell death. IFN-α has been documented to independently induce tumor necrosis factor related apoptosis inducing ligand (TRAIL) expression in UM-UC-12 bladder cancer cells [83], which subsequently triggers apoptosis in cells expressing the appropriate cell death receptor. Cell death occurs ultimately by Fas-associated protein with death domain (FADD) dependent activation of the death inducing signaling complex (DISC) followed by activation of caspase-8. Furthermore, Tecchio and associates have demonstrated that IFN-α can stimulate TRAIL mRNA as well as the release of a bioactive soluble TRAIL protein from neutrophils and monocytes, which induces apoptotic activity on TRAIL sensitive leukemic cell lines [84]. It also appears that IFN-α apoptotic effects may not be limited to TRAIL; rather it may trigger caspase-8 via both cell death receptor dependent and independent pathways [85]. Much like IFN-α, BCG has also been shown to induce TRAIL [49,50], which has correlated with patient response to BCG therapy and has been a source of overlapping research interest. Other direct IFN-α effects include enhancing cytotoxicity of $CD4^+$ T cells, increasing antigen detection by up-regulating MHC class I expression [82,86,87]. Direct suppression of proliferation by induction of tumor suppressor genes or inhibition of tumor oncogenes has also been described [82]. Also contributing to antiproliferative properties, IFN-α has been documented to decrease angiogenesis and basic fibroblast growth factor. Additionally, it down-regulates matrix metalloprotease-9 (MMP-9) mRNA as well as the MMP-9 translational protein in murine bladder tumors [88]. Interestingly, it has also been demonstrated that an optimal biologic dose with higher frequency, rather than maximal tolerated dose, produced the most significant decreases in angiogenesis. Significantly decreased angiogenesis has also been documented in human urothelium during and after IFN-α2b treatment following TURBT [89].

In vivo monotherapy with IFN-α2b for bladder cancer has been explored by multiple groups. In 1990, Glashan published data from a randomized controlled trial evaluating high dose (100 million unit) and low dose (10 million unit) IFN-α2b regimens in patients with Tis [90]. Patients were treated weekly for 12 weeks and monthly thereafter for 1 year. The high and low dose groups had complete response rates of 43% and 5%, respectively. Of the high dose patients achieving a complete response, 90% remained disease-free at a notably short 6 months of follow-up. The primary side effects of treatment were flu-like symptoms (8% low dose, 17% high dose) but without the irritative symptoms seen so often in BCG therapy. When IFN-α2b was investigated alone to treat BCG failures, eight of twelve patients had recurrence at initial three-month evaluation and only one of twelve was disease-free at 24 months [91]. Another trial conducted by Portillo and associates randomized 90 pT1 bladder cancer patients to either intravesical treatment or placebo groups as primary prophylaxis after complete resection [92]. They utilized a similar dosing schedule but used 60 million units IFN-α2b. At 12 months of follow-up, recurrence rates were significantly lower for IFN-α2b group than placebo, 28.2% vs 35.8%, respectively. However, after 43 months rates were similar - 53.8% and 51.2% respectively, indicating that treatment benefit of IFN-α2b alone may not be durable.

Given the described antiproliferative and immunomodulatory effects of IFN-α, combination therapy with BCG has held tantalizing promise. Gan and associates found significantly greater antitumor activity with combination therapy than BCG alone: 14/15 mice receiving BCG/IFN-α2b versus 8/15 mice receiving only BCG became tumor-free after 5 weekly intralesional treatments [93]. In an *in vitro* study comparing BCG plus IFN-α2b to BCG alone, our group demonstrated a 66-fold increase in IFN-γ production in peripheral blood mononuclear cell (PBMC) cultures [81]. Since IFN-γ is a major Th1 restricted cytokine found in patients responding to BCG therapy, it has been used routinely as a surrogate marker for Th1 immune response in studies examining effect of IFN-α [81]. It appears that IFN-α2b by itself generates a negligible Th1 response, as no significant levels of IFN-γ were detected after IFN-α2b was incubated alone with the PBMCs. We have also demonstrated that the augmented IFN-γ production persisted even with reduced doses of BCG. These findings give credence to the idea that adding Th1 stimulating cytokines may allow for a decrease in BCG doses, thereby decreasing side effects thought to be directly related to BCG. Further augmenting Th1 differentiation, IFN-α was found to increase levels of several Th1 cytokines, including IL-12 and TNF-α as well as decreasing known Th1 inhibitory cytokines IL-10 and IL-6 by 80-90% and 20-30%, respectively [94].

Clinical investigations with the combination of IFN-α2b and BCG began initially in BCG refractory patients but were subsequently expanded to BCG naïve patients. Stricker and associates found the combination to be safe, with a similar side effect profile to BCG alone [95]. In 2001, O'Donnell and associates reported on combination therapy administered to 40 patients who had failed at least 1 course of BCG alone [96]. At 24 months, 53% of patients were disease-free. Patients with two or more prior BCG failures faired similarly to patients with only one. Lam and associates in 2003 reported on the treatment of 32 patients, of which 20 (63%) were BCG failures. At 22 months' median follow-up, 12 of the 20 BCG failure patients (60%) remained disease-free [97]. In a smaller trial, Punnen and associates documented a 50%

disease-free rate after combination therapy at 12 months' follow-up in 12 patients with BCG refractory disease [98]. A subsequent large community based phase II clinical trial examined 1106 patients from 125 sites with NMIBC, which were split into BCG naïve and BCG refractory groups [99]. At median 24 months' follow-up, tumor-free rates were 59% and 45%, respectively. In this larger trial, patients who had two or more courses of prior BCG therapy had a worse outcome when compared to patients who had 1 or less, likely indicating more resistant disease. A recent study limited to BCG naïve patients demonstrated similar disease-free rate of 62% but with much longer median follow-up of 55.8 months [100]. Furthermore, after evaluating failure patterns and response rates to BCG plus IFN-α, Gallagher and associates found that patients who recurred more than 12 months after initial BCG treatments had similar tumor-free rates at 24 months when compared to BCG naïve patients [101]. However, patients who recurred within a year of receiving their initial BCG treatments did significantly worse, with disease-free rates of 34-43% at 24 months, indicating that additional immunotherapy may not be appropriate. Overall, while promising, these data are unable to define any treatment benefit of combination therapy over BCG alone in previously BCG untreated patients.

To date, the only randomized trial comparing BCG alone to BCG plus IFN was a multi-center study of 670 BCG naïve patients with Tis, Ta, or T1 urothelial carcinoma [102]. This was a four-arm trial evaluating efficacy of megadose vitamins as well as BCG and IFN. Patients were randomized to 1 of 4 groups: BCG plus recommended daily vitamins, BCG plus megadose daily vitamins, BCG plus IFN-α2b plus recommended daily vitamins, and BCG plus IFN-α2b plus megadose daily vitamins. At 24 month follow up, median recurrence-free survival was similar across all groups, though the two IFN-α2b groups experienced higher incidence of constitutional symptoms and fever ($p<0.05$).

In general, a BCG/IFN-α2b combination thearpy is appropriate for patients with previous BCG failures, those with Tis, and the elderly [103]. Optimal dose and schedule have yet to be defined in controlled trials and debate continues on the subject. At our institution, we use 1/3 the standard dose of BCG plus 50 MU of IFN-α2b. The dose may be lowered for those patients experiencing lower urinary tract symptoms or low grade fever. For maintenance cycle A, we adjust the BCG dose for week 1 consisting of 1/3 the standard dose of BCG plus 50 MU of IFN-α2b. For weeks 2 and 3, the BCG dose is lowered to 1/10 the standard dose plus 50 MU of rIFN-α2b. Maintenance cycles B and C utilize similar dosing.

There are multiple areas where additional research is warranted. A recent evolution in combination therapy has been the development of an IFN-α2b expressing strain of recombinant BCG (rBCG-IFN-α) from the Pasteur strain of BCG. An initial *in vitro* study documented enhanced IFN-γ expression in PBMCs after incubation with rBCG-IFN-α as compared to standard BCG [104]. A subsequent study reported that rBCG-IFN-α increased cytotoxicity up to 2-fold over standard BCG in PBMC cultures. Both $CD56^{+}CD8^{-}$ NK cells and $CD8^{+}$ T cells were identified as primary contributors to the increased cytotoxicity [105]. Combining IFN-α2b with other antiproliferative agents has shown *in vitro* promise. Louie and associates reported that a combination of IFN-α2b and maitake mushroom D-fraction (PDF) could reduce T24 bladder cancer cell proliferation by 75%, accompanied by G_1 cell cycle arrest [106]. A recently reported study indicated that adding grape seed proanthocyanin significantly enhanced antiproliferative effects of IFN-α2b, with >95% growth reduction in T24 bladder cancer cells [107]. Cell cycle analysis also revealed G_1 cell cycle arrest, with Western blots confirming expression of G_1 cell cycle regulators. Lastly, several groups have investigated gene therapy with a recombinant adenovirus delivery system (rAd-IFN/Syn3), which could potentially result in sustained therapeutic IFN-α2b levels for long periods of time. Nagabhushnan and associates were able to demonstrate delivery and expression of IFN in the bladder as well as significant tumor regression in mice. Phase I trials with rAd-IFN/Syn3 were ongoing at the time of their publication in 2007 [108].

3.2. Recombinant IL-2

The discovery and characterization of IL-2 was one of the most important breakthroughs in the field of immunology. Prior to its discovery, lymphocytes were thought to be terminally differentiated and incapable of proliferation [109,110]. In 1975 it was discovered that the supernatant of murine splenic cell cultures could stimulate thymocytes, suggesting a native effector protein was responsible for this mitogenic activity [110,111]. When initially examined independently by different investigators, this "effector protein" was given multiple working names including thymocyte stimulating factor (TSF), thymocyte mitogenic factor (TMF), T cell growth factor (TCGF), co-stimulator, killer cell helper factor (KHF), and secondary cytotoxic T cell-inducing factor (SCIF) [112]. In 1979 it was recognized that these factors likely represented the same entity and the nomenclature was standarized with the term "interleukin" (between leukocytes). Thus, the "effector protein" was named IL-2, differentiating it from the only other interleukin known at that time, IL-1 [112]. Regardless of the nomenclature, this protein was recognized to promote proliferation of primary T cells *in vitro* which revolutionized the experimental armamentarium in the field of immunology [109,111,113].

Since the discovery of IL-2 mediated control of T cell growth in culture, there has been much progress in elucidating its mechanisms. It was discovered relatively early that IL-2 enhances the production of cytotoxic lymphocytes which are capable of lysing tumor cells while leaving normal cells unharmed [113-116]. These IL-2 activated lymphocytes became known as "lymphokine-activated killer" (LAK) cells and were thought to play a large role in antitumor immune function [113-116]. Additionally, it was noted that IL-2 functions to augment the cytotoxic activity of NK cells and monocytes [117,118]. It has even been discovered that IL-2 is important for the activation of B cells [119]. As the $CD4^+$ Th1 and Th2 cell cytokine profiles were defined, it became clear that IL-2 is predominantly a Th1 secreted cytokine [120].

The cytotoxic antitumor capabilities induced in lymphocytes by IL-2 make it a potential cancer immunotherapeutic agent. To date, multiple studies have demonstrated regression of metastatic disease following systemic IL-2 treatment in some cancers [121]. Rosenberg and associates reported on 157 patients with a heterogenous mix of metastatic cancers refractory to other treatments including renal cell, colon cancer, breast cancer and lymphoma. Patients were treated with either IL-2 and LAK cells or IL-2 alone. Between the two groups, 9 complete and 20 partial responses were obtained. Significant morbidity has been reported with systemic IL-2 much of which is secondary to increased capillary permeability [121,122] and includes weight gain, hypotension, oliguria, elevated creatinine and bilirubin. These tend to resolve with cessation of IL-2 therapy [121]; however, Rosenberg reported 4 treatment related deaths among their 157 patients. Despite the reports of morbidity, IL-2 seemed to offer hope to patients with few treatment options.

With regard to bladder cancer, interest was stimulated after multiple investigators identified elevated IL-2 levels (as well as other cytokines) in urine of patients following BCG, suggesting an immunomodulatory effect of BCG [30,32,33,123-129]. Additionally, an elevation in IL-2 receptor expression has been documented on T cells in voided urine after BCG therapy [30,128]. Increased levels of urinary IL-2 have also been found to correlate with BCG response, which supports the concept that a Th1 cytokine profile confers a favorable response to BCG [35]. Furthermore, elevated IL-2 has been reported in the serum of patients following BCG instillation, which suggests both a local and systemic immune response to therapy [34,130]. These findings led to the conclusion that IL-2 may have a therapeutic use in bladder cancer.

One of the first clinical trials reported evidence of bladder tumor regression following intralesional injections of IL-2, with no adverse events recorded [131]. Multiple murine studies have demonstrated that systemic administration of IL-2, with or without BCG, can significantly decrease tumor size, suppress tumor growth and improve mean survival [132-134]. A small clinical study investigating systemic IL-2 administration effects on low stage bladder cancer found a complete and partial response rate in 5 of 12 patients, though 2 patients discontinued therapy due to toxicity [135]. The poor side effect profile of systemic IL-2 administration subsequently prompted a shift to utilize IL-2 as an intravesical therapy. Reports of intravesical use revealed a much improved side effect profile as well as some efficacy alone or when combined with BCG [136-141]. Den Otter and associates administered intravesical IL-2 alone after incomplete transurethral resection of grade 1-2, T1 papillary urothelial carcinoma, and documented "marker lesion" regression in 8 of 10 patients [142]. Additional experiments have focused on developing recombinant-IL-2 secreting strains of BCG [42,143-147]. Animal models using this approach have shown that compared to native BCG, IL-2 secreting BCG strains have increased IFN-γ production, induced a more favorable IFN-γ to IL-4 ratio, improved antigen-specific proliferation, enhanced antitumor cytotoxicity, and mounted a Th1 cytokine profile even in immunosuppressed or IL-4 transgenic mice (two conditions which favor a Th2 response) [42,143-147]. More recent animal and *in vitro* studies have investigated IL-2 transfecting dendritic cells (DCs), immobilized streptavidin-tagged bioactive IL-2 on the biotinylated surface of murine bladder mucosa, and development of a murine IL-2 surface modified bladder cancer vaccine [148-151]. Since IL-2 plays a crucial role in the Th1 response, it will continue to be a source of interest for immunotherapy of bladder cancer.

3.3. Recombinant IL-12

IL-12 has been the focus of significant cancer research among cytokines as well. In 1987, it was discovered through *in vitro* experiments that there existed a factor which synergized with IL-2 in promoting a CTL response [151]. This factor was given the name cytotoxic lymphocyte maturation factor (CLMF) [151]. Shortly thereafter a factor was discovered that induced IFN-γ production, enhanced T cell responses to mitogens, and augmented NK cell cytotoxicity [152]. This factor was provisionally called natural killer cell stimulatory factor (NKSF) [152].

It didn't take long to discover that these factors represented the same entity, thus the nomenclature converged and this protein was termed IL-12 [153-157].

Although initially discovered in a B cell lymphoma, it was subsequently found that IL-12 is primarily involved with the regulation of T cells, causing proliferation of both activated $CD4^+$ and $CD8^+$ T cell subsets while causing minimal proliferation of resting PBMCs [152,154]. This concept is supported by studies demonstrating that the IL-12 receptor is upregulated in activated T and NK cells, but not in activated B cells [157]. IL-12 potentiates a Th1 specific immune response, and it was later discovered that DCs produce IL-12 and thus direct the development of Th1 cells from naïve $CD4^+$ T cells [158,159]. Additionally, IL-12 can, by itself, stimulate the activation of nonspecific LAK cells and facilitate the generation of an allogeneic CTL response [160]. IL-12 has even been found to play a role in the activation of neutrophils [161,162]. Multiple studies have shown that IL-12 strongly inhibits neovascularization, thought to be mediated through its induction of IFN-γ [163,166]. Furthermore, the mechanism by which IL-12 enhances the cytolytic effect of NK cells has been found to be via the perforin pathway [167,168].

Multiple animal studies have shown tumor responsiveness to immunomodulation with IL-12. Using systemic or peri-tumoral injections, IL-12 showed antitumor properties in murine sarcoma, melanoma, renal cell carcinoma, lung cancer, colon cancer, breast cancer, and bladder cancer models [164,169-173]. Increases in serum IFN-γ were observed in mice treated with IL-12 [170]. Antitumor efficacy was lost in $CD8^+$ depleted mice, but not $CD4^+$ depleted mice or NK deficient mice, suggesting that the primary mediators of the antitumor IL-12 effect are $CD8^+$ T cells [169,170]. Some of these studies saw effectiveness even with metastatic disease, including bladder cancer [169,170,173]. Multiple murine studies have also revealed added effectiveness with IL-12 administered in combination with chemotherapeutic agents [171,174-176]. Additionally, IL-12 therapy has shown synergistic activity when combined with radiation therapy in mice [172,177]. Various delivery systems for IL-12 therapy have been tested in mice using viral and retroviral vectors to elicit an IL-12 response [178-182]. These constructs have shown some effectiveness as antitumor therapeutics [178-181]. IL-12 as intravesical therapy for bladder cancer has shown great success in mouse models. BCG was found to be a potent stimulus for IL-12 expression, and neutralization of IL-12 significantly dampened the induction of IFN-γ by BCG [183]. BCG therapy for murine bladder cancer was essentially found to be ineffective in IL-12 knock-out mice, suggesting a crucial role for IL-12 in the BCG response [184]. When IL-12 is used as a therapy with BCG it causes a synergistic induction of IFN-γ [183]. Intravesical IL-12 treatment alone was found to be effective for the treatment of orthotopically placed bladder tumors in mice, and urinary IFN-γ was subsequently found to be significantly elevated [173,185,186]. These observations further support to importance of IFN-γ induction for effective immunotherapy of bladder cancer. More recently, multiple attempts have been made to improve the delivery of intravesical IL-12 to the bladder mucosa to improve efficacy. One method utilized cationic liposome-mediated IL-12 gene therapy which showed improved survival and tumor-specific immunologic memory in mice [187]. Another method utilized chitosan, a mucoadhesive biopolymer, to increase IL-12 delivery to urothelial surfaces [188]. This method showed improved efficacy over IL-12 alone in a mouse model [188].

The great success of IL-12 in treating various murine cancers subsequently led to experiments testing its use on human cancers, though with mixed success. Initial trials focused on systemic IL-12 treatment for metastatic cancer, though progress was initially halted when several patients suffered severe toxic effects from the treatment and two patients died from the therapy [189]. A phase I trial of systemically administered IL-12 in 40 patients with advanced malignancy found a dose-dependent increase in circulating IFN-γ with administration [190]. Experiments on the peripheral blood of these patients showed augmented NK cell cytolytic activity and enhanced T cell proliferation [191]. Unfortunately, of these 40 patients there was only one partial response and one transient complete response [190]. Further studies looking at chronic administration of twice weekly IL-12 in patients with metastatic cancer found that it is well tolerated and induces co-stimulatory cytokines (including IFN-γ) [192]. However, in a cohort of 28 patients there was only one patient with a partial response and two with prolonged disease stabilization, with one of these patients eventually exhibiting tumor regression [192]. Similar low response rates have been seen with systemic IL-12 in other studies of advanced malignancies [193-197]. Various combinations of immunotherapy have been tested with systemic IL-12 in humans. A phase I study examined systemic IL-12 with low dose IL-2 and showed it was well tolerated, and the addition of IL-2 significantly augmented IFN-γ production as well as the NK response [198]. Of 28 patients there was one partial response and two pathologic responses [198]. Another phase I study using systemic IL-12 with IFN-α2b showed acceptable toxicity, but with no response in 41 patients [199]. As discussed previously, intravesical IL-12 showed great promise for the topical treatment of bladder cancer in a mouse model, however this success has not translated clinically. A phase I study of intravesical IL-12 therapy in patients with superficial bladder cancer showed minimal toxicity, but disappointing efficacy [200]. A total of 15 patients were enrolled in this study, of which 12 had no visible pretreatment lesions [200]. Of these 12 patients, 7 remained disease-free and 5 had recurrence within 4 weeks. The remaining 3 patients with pretreatment lesions had persistent disease at follow-up [200]. Perhaps the most disparaging results were that there was negligible IFN-γ induced in the urine and serum of these patients post-treatment, suggesting minimal immunologic effect from intravesical IL-12 therapy [200]. Despite the disappointing results from human studies, IL-12 remains an important target for the treatment of bladder cancer.

3.4. Other recombinant cytokines

In addition to the above-mentioned cytokines, several phase I and II trials have shown that other Th1 stimulating cytokines such as IFN-γ, TNF-α and GM-CSF, when intravesically administrated, are well tolerated and effective in the treatment of bladder cancer. Giannopoulos and associates conducted a study of 123 patients with stage Ta/T1, grade 2 tumors who were followed for a median of 26.5 months. They demonstrated that intravesical IFN-γ therapy prevented tumor recurrence after TURBT and was more effective than intravesical mitomycin C therapy [201]. The effect of IFN-γ was associated with significant increases of leukocytes in the bladder wall including $CD4^+$ T cells, $CD8^+$ T cells, NK cells and B cells, suggesting the involvement of a primary cellular immune response in the mechanism of IFN-γ action. A separate study consisting of 54 patients with stage Ta/T1 tumors also supported the safety and anti-bladder cancer activity of intravesical IFN-γ therapy in preventing tumor recurrence after

TURBT during a mean follow-up time of 12.1 months [202]. Serretta and associates demonstrated in two studies that intravesical TNF-α therapy was well tolerated and resulted in approximately a 24.5% complete response rate in 42 patients with superficial bladder cancer [203,204]. Two separate studies also supported the excellent tolerability and some antitumor effects of intravesical TNF therapy in patients with superficial bladder cancer [205,206]. Studies demonstrated that intravesical administration of GM-CSF for patients with stage Ta/T1 tumors after TURBT induced immunomodulatory effects on macrophage activities [207]. In correlation with regression of marker lesions, migration of macrophages to the surface layer was observed. Macrophages showed an extensive lysosomal system and pseudopodia. In addition, intravesical GM-CSF therapy was also observed to enhance lymphocyte recruitment into the bladder wall and activation in the bladder mucosa [208]. These clinical trials suggest that intravesical use of recombinant cytokines are favorable for the treatment of bladder cancer and further investigations are warranted.

4. Advances in BCG immunotherapy research

4.1. BCG therapy in conjunction with IL-10 blockage

Unlike Th1 stimulating cytokines discussed above, IL-10 is distinct in that its primary effect is to promote a Th2 response and thus dampen the immunotherapeutic effects of BCG for the treatment of bladder cancer [36,45]. As a result, it may have therapeutic value not by its native function, but by abrogation of its native function. IL-10 was first characterized in 1989. It was initially termed cytokine synthesis inhibitory factor (CSIF), a rather fitting name, because it was found to inhibit the production of several cytokines produced by Th1 clones [209]. The most important of these cytokines was IFN-γ, which was recognized as an important player in the Th1 response. As discussed previously, it is a key contributor in the immunotherapeutic effectiveness of BCG [209,210]. Further studies showed that IL-10 prevented DTH response to BCG and the neutralization or abrogation of IL-10 prolonged a response, thus further supporting its role in the Th1/2 response [36,211]. Several human tumors, including melanoma, non-small cell lung carcinoma, renal cell carcinoma and bladder cancer, have been found to have elevated expression of IL-10 [212-216]. It is speculated that production of IL-10 by tumor cells may represent an "escape mechanism" whereby tumor cells avoid Th1 immune mediated tumoricidal effects [212].

There has been significant progress in determining the regulation and mechanism of IL-10 function since its discovery, particularly with regard to its role in tumor immunology. It is secreted by multiple cell types including Th2 cells, B cells and monocytes/macrophages [209,217-219]. Like many other cytokines, IL-10 is known to auto-regulate itself by down-regulating its own mRNA synthesis [219]. It has been shown to block the accumulation of macrophages and DCs at tumor sites, which are important players in the cellular immune response [220,221]. Additionally, it compromises DCs ability to stimulate T cells causing induction of antigen-specific anergy of T cells [222]. Furthermore, it down-regulates the expression of MHC class II and co-stimulatory molecules, thus preventing a cellular immune response to tumor cells [223-225]. During activation of CD4⁺ T cells, the presence of IL-10 can cause them to differentiate into T regulatory cells 1 (Tr1), leading to peripheral tolerance [226]. IL-10 further reduces cellular tumoricidal activity by preventing release of reactive nitrogen/oxygen intermediates by macrophages and NK cells, a key step in their efficacy during cellular immune defense [45,227].

Successful treatment of bladder cancer with BCG, as discussed previously, requires a Th1 cytokine profile. IL-10 antagonizes the production of a Th1 milieu, thus its neutralization has been targeted as a potential means to augment the BCG response. Several murine studies have demonstrated that after IL-10 knock-out mice are inoculated with bladder cancer, they have improved BCG response with amplified local immune response, increased bladder mononuclear infiltrate, enhanced DTH responses, greater antitumor activity, and prolonged survival [36,212]. Although murine IL-10 knock-out studies are conceptually important, studies focused on IL-10 neutralization hold more promise as clinically useful therapeutics. Murine bladder cancer studies utilizing anti-IL-10 neutralizing monoclonal antibody (mAb) have shown similar results, with BCG treatment inducing an enhanced DTH response and increased bladder mononuclear infiltrate [36,211]. More recent efforts have been placed at targeting the IL-10 receptor. The IL-10 receptor is composed of two known subunits (IL-10R1 and IL-10R2) and the IL-10R1 subunit plays the predominant role in signal transduction [228]. In *in vitro* studies we have recently shown that splenocytes incubated with BCG and anti-IL-10R1 mAb produced significantly higher IFN-γ than those incubated with BCG plus anti-IL-10 neutralizing mAb [39], suggesting that interference with IL-10 signal transduction may be more effective than neutralizing IL-10 protein. In *in vivo* studies mice treated with BCG and anti-IL-10R1 mAb showed increased urinary IFN-γ production compared to BCG controls [39]. In a similar murine experiment, there was improved overall and tumor-free state in mice treated with BCG plus anti-IL-10R1 mAb compared to BCG treatment controls, though this difference did not reach statistical significance [39]. Most recently, in an experiment designed to follow murine survival after inoculation with a luciferase-expressing MB49 bladder cancer cells, we discovered that control mice and BCG only treated mice developed histologically confirmed lung metastasis, whereas mice treated with BCG and anti-IL-10R1 mAb developed no metastasis [unpublished data]. This difference was statistically significant and raises questions as to anti-IL-10R1 mAb's role as more than just an augmentation to BCG for local bladder cancer control. Confirmatory experiments and mechanistic studies are necessary, but anti-IL-10R1 mAb shows great potential in not only local bladder cancer control, but also possibly systemic immunomodulation for the prevention of metastatic bladder cancer.

4.2. Development of recombinant BCG strains

BCG in combination with Th1 stimulating cytokines (e.g. IFN-α2b) has demonstrated to improve BCG efficacy in the treatment of bladder cancer. However, these strategies require multiple applications and a large quantity of recombinant cytokines. Genetic manipulation of BCG to secrete Th1 stimulating cytokines provides an opportunity to overcome the drawbacks. To date, numerous recombinant BCG (rBCG) strains capable of secreting cytokines or chemokines, mainly Th1 stimulating cytokines such as IL-2, IL-12, IL-18, IFN-γ and IFN-α, have been developed

[229-250] (Table 1). Most of these rBCG strains have demonstrated to be superior to BCG in the induction of Th1 immune responses and antitumor immunity in pre-clinical settings.

Strain	Cytokine	Species	Immunological Effect	Reference
IL-2 BCG (RBD)	IL-2	m	Th1 cyt prod, Antitumor, Cytotoxicity	[143]
IL-2 BCG (MAO)	IL-2	r	Th1 cyt prod	[143]
BCG-CI	IL-2	h	Anti-BCG	[229]
BCG-CII	IL-2	h	Anti-BCG	[229]
BCG-IL-2	IL-2	m	CI, Th1 & Th2 cyt prod	[144]
BCG-GM-CSF	GM-CSF	m	CI, Th1 & Th2 cyt prod, DC act, Anti-*M.tb*	[144, 230]
BCG-IFN-γ	IFN-γ	m	CI, Th1 & Th2 cyt prod, Anti-BCG	[144, 231]
rBCG/IL-2	IL-2	m	CI, Th1 cyt prod, Anti-BCG	[145, 147, 232]
rBCG-IL-2/GFP	IL-2	m	CI, Th1 cyt prod, Anti-BCG	[146]
rBCG(α-Ag-IL-2)	IL-2	m	Th1 cyt prod, Cytotoxicity	[42]
BCG-IFN-γ	IFN-γ	m	Th1 cyt prod, Anti-BCG	[233]
rBCG-IFN-α	IFN-α2b	h	Th1 cyt prod, Cytotoxicity	[104]
rBCG/IL-18	IL-18	m	no clear effect	[232]
BCG IL-18	IL-18	m	Th1 & Th2 cyt prod	[234, 235]
BCG-hIL2MUC1	IL-2	h	CI, Th1 cyt prod, Antitumor	[236, 237]
rBCG-IFN-γ	IFN-γ	m	CI, Th1 cyt prod, Antitumor	[238]
rBCG-IL-18	IL-18	m	Th1 cyt prod, Anti-BCG, Cytotoxicity	[43]
rBCG-huIL-2-ESAT6	IL-2	h	CI, Th1 cyt prod, Cytotoxicity, HI	[239]
rBCG-IL-2	IL-2	h	Th1 cyt prod	[240]
BCGMCP-3	MCP-3	m	CI, Anti-BCG	[241]
rBCG-AEI	IFN-γ	m	CI, HI, Anti-*M.tb*	[242]
rBCG-Ag85B-IL15	IL-15	m	CI, Th1 cyt prod, Anti-*M.tb*	[243]
rBCG-MVNTR4-CSF	GM-CSF	h	CI, Th1 cyt prod, Antitumor	[244, 245]
rBCG-MVNTR8-CSF	GM-CSF	h	CI, Th1 cyt prod, Antitumor	[244, 245]
rBCG-Ag85B-Esat6-TNF-α	TNF-α	m	CI, HI	[246]
rBCG-IE	IL-12	h	CI, Th1 cyt prod	[247]
rBCG:GE	GM-CSF	h	CI, Th1 cyt prod, HI	[248]
rBCG::Ag85B-CFP10-IL-12	IL-12	h	CI, HI, Anti-*M.tb*	[249]
rBCG-IFN-α–2b	IFN-α2b	h	CI, Cytotoxicity	[250]

Anti-BCG: anti-BCG infection; Anti-*M.tb*: anti-Mycobacterium tuberculosis infection; CI: cellular immunity; DC act: dendritic cell activation; h: human; HI: humoral immunity; m: mouse; r: rat; Th1 cyt prod: T helper type 1 cytokine production; Th2 cyt prod: T helper type 2 cytokine production.

Table 1. Cytokine- and chemokine-expressing rBCG strains

BCG is a potent immunoadjuvant and induces a primary Th1 immune response that is required for effective treatment of most cancer types. Genetic manipulation of BCG to secrete Th1 stimulating cytokines with simultaneous coexpression of tumor-associated antigens may therefore potentiate the induction of specific antitumor immune responses. Early studies demonstrated that IL-2 secreting rBCG was at least equally effective to wild-type BCG when used as an intratumoral injection or a vaccine therapy in conjunction with irradiated tumor cells in a murine melanoma model [251]. However, it was not until recently that the potential of rBCG for treating cancer has gained further appreciation. We and others have developed rBCG strains that deliver the breast cancer-associated antigen mucin-1 (MUC1) in a form of multiple tandem repeats with coexpression of human IL-2 or human GM-CSF [236,237,244,245]. Severe combined immunodeficient (SCID) mice reconstituted with human peripheral blood lymphocytes (PBL) followed by immunization with the rBCG strains developed MUC1-specific cellular immune respnses and enhanced protection against MUC1-positive human breast cancer xenografts, compared to control mice reconstituted with human PBL and immunized with non-cytokine secreting BCG. Studies have also demonstrated that the antitumor effects of the rBCG strains were correlated with the number of MUC1 tandem repeats delivered by BCG [244,245]. These results suggest that these MUC1 rBCG strains coexpressing Th1 stimulating cytokines are promising candidates as breast cancer vaccines and thus warrant further investigation.

It has been known that BCG stimulation of human PBMC leads to the generation of effector cells cytotoxic to bladder cancer cells *in vitro* [55,56]. We recently demonstrated that stimulation of human PBMC with rBCG-IFN-α, a rBCG strain secreting human IFN-α2b [104], *in vitro* for 7 days induced enhanced PBMC cytotoxicity toward human bladder cancer cell lines T24, J82, 5637, TCCSUP and UMUC-3 by up to 2-fold compared to control BCG carrying an empty vector [105]. This induction of enhanced PBMC cytotoxicity was correlated with increased production of IFN-γ and IL-2 by rBCG stimulated PBMC. Studies further revealed that this enhancement in PBMC cytotoxicity was dependent on BCG secreted IFN-α as well as endogenously expressed IFN-γ and IL-2, as blockage of IFN-α, IFN-γ or IL-2 by neutralizing antibodies during BCG stimulation reduced or abolished the induction of this enhanced PBMC cytotoxicity. Studies using NK and $CD8^+$ T cells isolated from human PBMC revealed that both cell types were responsible for the enhanced PBMC cytotoxicity induced by rBCG-IFN-α with the former cell type being more predominant [105]. A similar rBCG strain secreting human IFN-α2b has also been recently demonstrated to stimulate PBMC proliferation and cytotoxicity toward bladder cancer cell lines T24 and 5637 [250].

An early study demonstrated that human peripheral monocytes/macrophages were capable of functioning as tumoricidal cells toward bladder cancer UCRU-BL-17 cells upon activation by BCG *in vitro* [41]. It was observed that the cytotoxic activity of human monocytes/macrophages was significantly enhanced after BCG stimulation, while the naïve cells exhibited only minimum cytotoxicity. Later, more studies including ours further demonstrated that murine macrophages could also function as tumoricidal cells toward bladder cancer cells upon activation by BCG *in vitro* [42-45]. Stimulation of thioglycollate-elicited peritoneal macrophages by BCG for 24 hour resulted in macrophage-mediated killing of bladder cancer MBT-2 (C3H background) and MB49 (C57BL/6 background) cells in a dose-dependent manner [44,45]. Studies also revealed that endogenous Th1 cytokines (e.g. IL-12, IL-18, IFN-γ and TNF-α)

http://dx.doi.org/10.5772/55283

played an important role in BCG-induced macrophage cytotoxicity, as blockage of these cytokines during BCG stimulation led to substantially reduced macrophage cytotoxicity toward bladder cancer cells [44]. In contrast, supplementation of BCG with Th1 cytokines (e.g. IL-2, IL-12 or IL-18) increased macrophage cytotoxicity by approximately 2-fold. Consistent with these observations, rBCG strains secreting murine IL-2 or IL-18 showed enhanced macrophage-mediated killing on bladder cancer MBT-2 cells, which was correlated with increased expression of IFN-γ, TNF-α and IL-6 by rBCG stimulated macrophages [44]. The effect of murine IL-2 secreting rBCG strain on the induction of macrophage cytotoxicity toward bladder cancer MBT-2 cells was also demonstrated by a separate study [42].

Although the *in vitro* studies have suggested the potential usefulness of Th1 cytokine-secreting rBCG strains for the treatment of bladder cancer, unfortunately, the effect of rBCG on treating bladder cancer *in vivo* has not well been studied. Up to date, only an rBCG strain secreting IFN-γ (rBCG-IFN-γ) has been studied in a murine MB49 syngeneic orthotopic tumor model [238]. This study showed that, with a low-dose treatment regimen, intravesical administration of rBCG-IFN-γ significantly prolonged animal survival compared to medium-treated controls, whereas BCG carrying an empty vector only slightly increased survival. In a similar experiment using the MB49 syngeneic orthotopic tumor model in IFN-γ knockout mice, intravesical treatment with rBCG-IFN-γ failed to prolong survival of mice, indicating that rBCG-derived IFN-γ had no measurable antitumor effect in the absence of endogenous IFN-γ. Studies also provided the mechanisms underlying the effect of rBCG-IFN-γ on treating bladder cancer. As demonstrated, this rBCG-IFN-γ strain could specifically upregulate the expression of MHC class I molecules on MB49 cells *in vitro* compared to control BCG, as the MHC class I upregulation could be blocked by an inhibitory antibody to IFN-γ. This rBCG strain also enhanced recruitment of $CD4^+$ T cells into the bladder and further induced the local expression of IL-2 and IL-4 mRNA compared to control BCG. In addition, we have also evaluated the effects of rBCG strains secreting murine IL-2 or IP-10 (a Th1 chemokine) on treating bladder cancer in the MB49 syngeneic orthotopic tumor model and observed survival benefits of these rBCG strains [unpublished data]. All these observations suggest that rBCG strains secreting Th1 cytokines or chemokines possess improved antitumor properties and may offer new opportunities for the treatment of bladder cancer.

Supporting Th1 cytokine-secreting rBCG, *Mycobacterium smegmatis* (*M. smegmatis*), a closely related non-pathogenic mycobacterial organism, has been engineered to secrete murine TNF-α (*M. smegmatis*/TNF-α) and tested in a transplantable MB49 tumor model [252]. Studies demonstrated that lymphocytes from tumor-bearing mice vaccinated with *M. smegmatis*/TNF-α produced elevated and prolonged IFN-γ but no IL-10 in response to mycobacterial antigen or tumor lysate stimulation *in vitro*. Histopathology revealed significantly increased infiltrating $CD3^+$ lymphocytes in the tumor nodules of mice receiving the recombinant vaccine compared to those of mice receiving wild-type bacteria. These observations indicated that *M. smegmatis*/TNF-α induced cell-mediated immunity. Importantly, mice implanted subcutaneously with MB49 tumor and treated at an adjacent site with the recombinant vaccine exhibited significantly reduced tumor growth with a 70% durable tumor-free survival compared to those treated with wild-type bacteria or BCG (a 10-20% long-term survival). Interestingly, treatment with *M. smegmatis*/TNF-α also resulted in similar tumor growth inhibition in T cell-deficient athymic nude mice and reduced but not abolished tumor growth inhibition in NK cell-deficient Beige mice. These observations indicated that NK cells contribute to the antitumor effect of *M. smegmatis*/TNF-α but are not solely responsible for the eradication of tumor. Like immunocompetent mice, Beige mice also developed tumor specific memory after treatment with *M. smegmatis*/TNF-α. A study also demonstrated enhanced immunotherapeutic potential of a human TNF-α secreting recombinant *M. smegmatis* for treating bladder cancer [253]. The ability to deliver immunomodulatory cytokines with no pathogenic effects makes *M. smegmatis* attractive as an alternative intravesical mycobacterial agent for bladder cancer treatment.

5. Conclusion and future perspectives

Intravesical administration of BCG for NMIBC represents one of the most successful immunotherapies for solid malignancy. However, BCG therapy is associated with a considerable side-effect profile and is ineffective in a significant proportion of patients. Therefore, multiple Th1 stimulating cytokines (e.g. IFN-α, IL-2 and IL-12) have been investigated either as adjuncts with BCG or as a solo replacement therapy in both clinical and pre-clinical studies. Combination of BCG with IL-10 blocking mAb and genetic engineering of BCG to secrete Th1 cytokines have also been conducted in pre-clinical studies. These treatment strategies potentially allow the use of a lower and safer dose of BCG while preserving or even enhancing BCG efficacy. Despite a multitude of encouraging *in vitro* and murine studies, no clinical data has yet been reported which is compelling enough to change the current standard of care, yet many practitioners continue to use adjunctive immunotherapy based on basic science data and theoretical benefit. Further studies are needed and should focus on the optimization of combination therapies including dosing, schedule and duration. The mechanisms through which supplemental agents enhance BCG-induced Th1 immune responses and antitumor immunity need to be explored in both effector and memory phases. In addition to classical effector cells, influence of combination therapy on Th17 and regulatory T (Treg) cells should be evaluated, as the importance of these cell types in bladder cancer has emerged. Today, research continues and efforts have been made to increase our understanding of tumor biology, human immunology, and the treatment of urothelial carcinoma. The pace of research must be maintained if we are to improve this gold standard therapy for bladder cancer. BCG combination therapy merits further appraisal as an improved modality for the treatment of bladder cancer.

Author details

Yi Luo, Eric J. Askeland, Mark R. Newton, Jonathan R. Henning and Michael A. O'Donnell

University of Iowa, Department of Urology Iowa City, Iowa, USA

References

[1] Siegel R, Naishadham D, Jemal A. Cancer statistics, 2012. CA Cancer Journal for Clinicians 2012;62(1):10-29.

[2] Ro JY, Staerkel GA, Ayala AG. Cytologic and histologic features of superficial bladder cancer. The Urologic Clinics of North America 1992;19(3):435-453.

[3] Williams SK, Hoenig DM, Ghavamian R, Soloway M. Intravesical therapy for bladder cancer. Expert Opinion on Pharmacotherapy 2010:11(6):947-958.

[4] Weizer AZ, Tallman C, Montgomery JS. Long-term outcomes of intravesical therapy for non-muscle invasive bladder cancer. World Journal of Urology 2011;29(1):59-71.

[5] Shelley MD, Jones G, Cleves A, Wilt TJ, Mason MD, Kynaston HG. Intravesical gemcitabine therapy for non-muscle invasive bladder cancer (NMIBC): a systematic review. British Journal of Urology International 2012;109(4):496-505.

[6] Dinney CP, Greenberg RE, Steinberg GD. Intravesical valrubicin in patients with bladder carcinoma in situ and contraindication to or failure after bacillus Calmette-Guérin. Urologic Oncology 2012;PMID:22575238.

[7] Yutkin V, Chin J. Apaziquone as an intravesical therapeutic agent for urothelial non-muscle-invasive bladder cancer. Expert Opinion on Investigational Drugs 2012;21(2): 251-260.

[8] Morales A, Eidinger D, Bruce AW. Intracavitary Bacillus Calmette-Guerin in the treatment of superficial bladder tumors. The Journal of Urology 1976;116(2):180-3.

[9] Sylvester RJ. Bacillus Calmette-Guérin treatment of non-muscle invasive bladder cancer. International Journal of Urology 2011; 18(2):113-120.

[10] Hall MC, Chang SS, Dalbagni G, Pruthi RS, Seigne JD, Skinner EC, Wolf JS Jr, Schellhammer PF. Guideline for the management of nonmuscle invasive bladder cancer (stages Ta, T1, and Tis): 2007 update. The Journal of Urology 2007;178(6):2314-2330.

[11] Lamm DL, Blumenstein BA, Crawford ED, Montie JE, Scardino P, Grossman HB, Stanisic TH, Smith JA Jr, Sullivan J, Sarosdy MF, et al. A randomized trial of intravesical doxorubicin and immunotherapy with bacille Calmette-Guérin for transitional-cell carcinoma of the bladder. The New England Journal of Medicine 1991;325(17): 1205-1209.

[12] Morales A, Ottenhof P, Emerson L. Treatment of residual, non-infiltrating bladder cancer with bacillus Calmette-Guerin. The Journal of Urology 1981;125(5):649-651.

[13] Malmström PU, Wijkström H, Lundholm C, Wester K, Busch C, Norlén BJ. 5-year followup of a randomized prospective study comparing mitomycin C and bacillus Calmette-Guerin in patients with superficial bladder carcinoma. Swedish-Norwegian Bladder Cancer Study Group. The Journal of Urology 1999;161(4):1124-1127.

[14] van der Meijden AP, Sylvester RJ, Oosterlinck W, Hoeltl W, Bono AV; EORTC Genito-Urinary Tract Cancer Group. Maintenance Bacillus Calmette-Guerin for Ta T1 bladder tumors is not associated with increased toxicity: results from a European Organisation for Research and Treatment of Cancer Genito-Urinary Group Phase III Trial. European Urology 2003;44(4):429-434.

[15] Babjuk M, Oosterlinck W, Sylvester R, Kaasinen E, Böhle A, Palou-Redorta J; European Association of Urology (EAU). EAU guidelines on non-muscle-invasive urothelial carcinoma of the bladder. European Urology 2008;54(2):303-314.

[16] Lamm DL, Blumenstein BA, Crissman JD, Montie JE, Gottesman JE, Lowe BA, Sarosdy MF, Bohl RD, Grossman HB, Beck TM, Leimert JT, Crawford ED. Maintenance bacillus Calmette-Guerin immunotherapy for recurrent TA, T1 and carcinoma in situ transitional cell carcinoma of the bladder: a randomized Southwest Oncology Group Study. The Journal of Urology 2000;163(4)1124-1129.

[17] Koga H, Ozono S, Tsushima T, Tomita K, Horiguchi Y, Usami M, Hirao Y, Akaza H, Naito S; BCG Tokyo Strain Study Group. Maintenance intravesical bacillus Calmette-Guérin instillation for Ta, T1 cancer and carcinoma in situ of the bladder: randomized controlled trial by the BCG Tokyo Strain Study Group. International Journal of Urology 2010;17(9):759-766.

[18] Babjuk M, Oosterlinck W, Sylvester R, Kaasinen E, Böhle A, Palou-Redorta J, Rouprêt M; European Association of Urology (EAU). EAU guidelines on non-muscle-invasive urothelial carcinoma of the bladder, the 2011 update. European Urology 2011;59(6): 997-1008.

[19] Brausi M, Witjes JA, Lamm D, Persad R, Palou J, Colombel M, Buckley R, Soloway M, Akaza H, Böhle A. A review of current guidelines and best practice recommendations for the management of nonmuscle invasive bladder cancer by the International Bladder Cancer Group. The Journal of Urology 2011;186(6):2158-2167.

[20] Brandau S, Suttmann H. Thirty years of BCG immunotherapy for non-muscle invasive bladder cancer: a success story with room for improvement. Biomedicine and Pharmacotherapy 2007;61(6)299-305.

[21] Alexandroff AB, Nicholson S, Patel PM, Jackson AM. Recent advances in bacillus Calmette-Guerin immunotherapy in bladder cancer. Immunotherapy 2010;2(4)551-560.

[22] Kavoussi LR, Brown EJ, Ritchey JK, Ratliff TL. Fibronectin-mediated Calmette-Guerin bacillus attachment to murine bladder mucosa. Requirement for the expression of an antitumor response. Journal of Clinical Investigation 1990;85(1):62-67.

[23] Becich MJ, Carroll S, Ratliff TL. Internalization of bacille Calmette-Guerin by bladder tumor cells. The Journal of Urology 1991;145(6):1316-1324.

[24] Bevers RF, Kurth KH, Schamhart DH. Role of urothelial cells in BCG immunotherapy for superficial bladder cancer. British Journal of Cancer 2004;91(4):607-612.

[25] Böhle A, Gerdes J, Ulmer AJ, Hofstetter AG, Flad HD. Effects of local bacillus Calmette-Guerin therapy in patients with bladder carcinoma on immunocompetent cells of the bladder wall. The Journal of Urology 1990;144(1)53-58.

[26] Prescott S, James K, Hargreave TB, Chisholm GD, Smyth JF. Intravesical Evans strain BCG therapy: quantitative immunohistochemical analysis of the immune response within the bladder wall. The Journal of Urology 1992;147(6)1636-1642.

[27] Saban MR, Simpson C, Davis C, Wallis G, Knowlton N, Frank MB, Centola M, Gallucci RM, Saban R. Discriminators of mouse bladder response to intravesical Bacillus Calmette-Guerin (BCG). BMC Immunology 2007;8:6.

[28] De Boer EC, de Jong WH, van der Meijden AP, Steerenberg PA, Witjes F, Vegt PD, Debruyne FM, Ruitenberg EJ. Leukocytes in the urine after intravesical BCG treatment for superficial bladder cancer. A flow cytofluorometric analysis. Urological Research 1991;19(1):45-50.

[29] De Boer EC, de Jong WH, van der Meijden AP, Steerenberg PA, Witjes JA, Vegt PD, Debruyne FM, Ruitenberg EJ. Presence of activated lymphocytes in the urine of patients with superficial bladder cancer after intravesical immunotherapy with bacillus Calmette-Guérin. Cancer Immunology and Immunotherapy 1991;33(6):411-416.

[30] De Boer EC, de Jong WH, Steerenberg PA, van der Meijden AP, Aarden LA, Debruyne FM, Ruitenberg EJ. Leukocytes and cytokines in the urine of superficial bladder cancer patients after intravesical immunotherapy with bacillus Calmette-Guerin. In Vivo 1991;5(6):671-677.

[31] Simons MP, O'Donnell MA, Griffith TS. Role of neutrophils in BCG immunotherapy for bladder cancer. Urologic Oncology 2008;26(4):341-345.

[32] Böhle A, Nowc C, Ulmer AJ, Musehold J, Gerdes J, Hofstetter AG, Flad HD. Elevations of cytokines interleukin-1, interleukin-2 and tumor necrosis factor in the urine of patients after intravesical bacillus Calmette-Guerin immunotherapy. The Journal of Urology 1990;144(1)59-64.

[33] De Reijke TM, De Boer EC, Kurth KH, Schamhart DH. Urinary cytokines during intravesical bacillus Calmette-Guerin therapy for superficial bladder cancer: processing, stability and prognostic value. The Journal of Urology 1996;155(2):477-482.

[34] Taniguchi K, Koga S, Nishikido M, Yamashita S, Sakuragi T, Kanetake H, Saito Y. Systemic immune response after intravesical instillation of bacille Calmett-Guérin (BCG) for superficial bladder cancer. Clinical and Experimental Immunology 1999;115(1):131-135.

[35] Saint F, Patard JJ, Maille P, Soyeux P, Hoznek A, Salomon L, Abbou CC, Chopin DK. Prognostic value of a T helper 1 urinary cytokine response after intravesical bacillus

Calmette-Guerin treatment for superficial bladder cancer. The Journal of Urology 2002;167(1):364-367.

[36] Nadler R, Luo Y, Zhao W, Ritchey JK, Austin JC, Cohen MB, O'Donnell MA, Ratliff TL. Interleukin 10 induced augmentation of delayed-type hypersensitivity (DTH) enhances Mycobacterium bovis bacillus Calmette-Guérin (BCG) mediated antitumour activity. Clinical and Experimental Immunology 2003;131(2):206-216.

[37] Luo Y, Chen X, O'Donnell MA. Mycobacterium bovis bacillus Calmette-Guérin (BCG) induces human CC- and CXC-chemokines in vitro and in vivo. Clinical and Experimental Immunology 2007;147(2):370-378.

[38] Riemensberger J, Böhle A, Brandau S. IFN-gamma and IL-12 but not IL-10 are required for local tumour surveillance in a syngeneic model of orthotopic bladder cancer. Clinical and Experimental Immunology 2002;127(1):20-26.

[39] Bockholt NA, Knudson MJ, Henning JR, Maymi JL, Weady P, Smith GJ 3rd, Eisenbraun MD, Fraser JD, O'Donnell MA, Luo Y. Anti-IL-10R1 monoclonal antibody enhances bacillus Calmette-Guerin induced T-helper type 1 immune responses and antitumor immunity in a mouse orthotopic model of bladder cancer. The Journal of Urology 2012;187(6):2228-2235.

[40] Heldwein KA, Liang MD, Andresen TK, Thomas KE, Marty AM, Cuesta N, Vogel SN, Fenton MJ. TLR2 and TLR4 serve distinct roles in the host immune response against Mycobacterium bovis BCG. Journal of Leukocyte Biology 2003;74(2):277-286.

[41] Pryor K, Goddard J, Goldstein D, Stricker P, Russell P, Golovsky D, Penny R. Bacillus Calmette-Guerin (BCG) enhances monocyte- and lymphocyte-mediated bladder tumour cell killing. British Journal of Cancer 1995;71(4):801-807.

[42] Yamada H, Matsumoto S, Matsumoto T, Yamada T, Yamashita U. Murine IL-2 secreting recombinant Bacillus Calmette-Guerin augments macrophage-mediated cytotoxicity against murine bladder cancer MBT-2. The Journal of Urology 2000;164(2): 526-531.

[43] Luo Y, Yamada H, Chen X, Ryan AA, Evanoff DP, Triccas JA, O'Donnell MA. Recombinant Mycobacterium bovis bacillus Calmette-Guérin (BCG) expressing mouse IL-18 augments Th1 immunity and macrophage cytotoxicity. Clinical and Experimental Immunology 2004;137(1):24-34.

[44] Luo Y, Yamada H, Evanoff DP, Chen X. Role of Th1-stimulating cytokines in bacillus Calmette-Guérin (BCG)-induced macrophage cytotoxicity against mouse bladder cancer MBT-2 cells. Clinical and Experimental Immunology 2006;146(1):181-188.

[45] Luo Y, Han R, Evanoff DP, Chen X. Interleukin-10 inhibits Mycobacterium bovis bacillus Calmette-Guérin (BCG)-induced macrophage cytotoxicity against bladder cancer cells. Clinical and Experimental Immunology 2010;160(3):359-368.

[46] Jansson OT, Morcos E, Brundin L, Lundberg JO, Adolfsson J, Söderhäll M, Wiklund NP. The role of nitric oxide in bacillus Calmette-Guérin mediated anti-tumour effects in human bladder cancer. British Journal of Cancer 1998;78(5):588-592.

[47] Godaly G, Young DB. Mycobacterium bovis bacille Calmette Guerin infection of human neutrophils induces CXCL8 secretion by MyD88-dependent TLR2 and TLR4 activation. Cellular Microbiology 2005;7(4):591-601.

[48] Suttmann H, Riemensberger J, Bentien G, Schmaltz D, Stöckle M, Jocham D, Böhle A, Brandau S. Neutrophil granulocytes are required for effective Bacillus Calmette-Guérin immunotherapy of bladder cancer and orchestrate local immune responses. Cancer Research 2006;66(16):8250-8257.

[49] Ludwig AT, Moore JM, Luo Y, Chen X, Saltsgaver NA, O'Donnell MA, Griffith TS. Tumor necrosis factor-related apoptosis-inducing ligand: a novel mechanism for Bacillus Calmette-Guérin-induced antitumor activity. Cancer Research 2004;64(10): 3386-3390.

[50] Kemp TJ, Ludwig AT, Earel JK, Moore JM, Vanoosten RL, Moses B, Leidal K, Nauseef WM, Griffith TS. Neutrophil stimulation with Mycobacterium bovis bacillus Calmette-Guerin (BCG) results in the release of functional soluble TRAIL/Apo-2L. Blood 2005;106(10):3474-3482.

[51] Suttmann H, Jacobsen M, Reiss K, Jocham D, Böhle A, Brandau S. Mechanisms of bacillus Calmette-Guerin mediated natural killer cell activation. The Journal of Urology 2004;172(4 Pt 1):1490-1495.

[52] Liu W, O'Donnell MA, Chen X, Han R, Luo Y. Recombinant bacillus Calmette-Guérin (BCG) expressing interferon-alpha 2B enhances human mononuclear cell cytotoxicity against bladder cancer cell lines in vitro. Cancer Immunology and Immunotherapy 2009;58(10):1647-1655.

[53] Ratliff TL, Ritchey JK, Yuan JJ, Andriole GL, Catalona WJ. T-cell subsets required for intravesical BCG immunotherapy for bladder cancer. The Journal of Urology 1993;150(3):1018-1023.

[54] Brandau S, Riemensberger J, Jacobsen M, Kemp D, Zhao W, Zhao X, Jocham D, Ratliff TL, Böhle A. NK cells are essential for effective BCG immunotherapy. International Journal of Cancer 2001;92(5):697-702.

[55] Böhle A, Thanhäuser A, Ulmer AJ, Ernst M, Flad HD, Jocham D. Dissecting the immunobiological effects of Bacillus Calmette-Guérin (BCG) in vitro: evidence of a distinct BCG-activated killer (BAK) cell phenomenon. The Journal of Urology 1993;150(6):1932-1937.

[56] Brandau S, Böhle A, Thanhäuser A, Ernst M, Mattern T, Ulmer AJ, Flad HD. In vitro generation of bacillus Calmette-Guérin-activated killer cells. Clinical Infectious Diseases 2000;31(Suppl 3):S94-S100.

[57] Brandau S, Suttmann H, Riemensberger J, Seitzer U, Arnold J, Durek C, Jocham D, Flad HD, Böhle A. Perforin-mediated lysis of tumor cells by Mycobacterium bovis Bacillus Calmette-Guérin-activated killer cells. Clinical Cancer Research 2000;6(9): 3729-3738.

[58] Wang MH, Flad HD, Bohle A, Chen YQ, Ulmer AJ. Cellular cytotoxicity of human natural killer cells and lymphokine-activated killer cells against bladder carcinoma cell lines. Immunology Letters 1991;27(3):191-197.

[59] Jackson AM, Hawkyard SJ, Prescott S, Ritchie AW, James K, Chisholm GD. An investigation of factors influencing the in vitro induction of LAK activity against a variety of human bladder cancer cell lines. The Journal of Urology 1992;147(1):207-211.

[60] Shemtov MM, Cheng DL, Kong L, Shu WP, Sassaroli M, Droller MJ, Liu BC. LAK cell mediated apoptosis of human bladder cancer cells involves a pH-dependent endonuclease system in the cancer cell: possible mechanism of BCG therapy. The Journal of Urology 1995;154(1):269-274.

[61] Kawashima T, Norose Y, Watanabe Y, Enomoto Y, Narazaki H, Watari E, Tanaka S, Takahashi H, Yano I, Brenner MB, Sugita M. Cutting edge: major CD8 T cell response to live bacillus Calmette-Guérin is mediated by CD1 molecules. Journal of Immunology 2003;170(11):5345-5348.

[62] Wang MH, Chen YQ, Gercken J, Ernst M, Bohle A, Flad HD, Ulmer AJ. Specific activation of human peripheral blood gamma/delta + lymphocytes by sonicated antigens of Mycobacterium tuberculosis: role in vitro in killing human bladder carcinoma cell lines. Scandinavian Journal of Immunology 1993;38(3):239-246.

[63] Naoe M, Ogawa Y, Takeshita K, Morita J, Iwamoto S, Miyazaki A, Yoshida H. Bacillus Calmette-Guerin-pulsed dendritic cells stimulate natural killer T cells and gammadeltaT cells. International Journal of Urology 2007;14(6):532-538.

[64] Higuchi T, Shimizu M, Owaki A, Takahashi M, Shinya E, Nishimura T, Takahashi H. A possible mechanism of intravesical BCG therapy for human bladder carcinoma: involvement of innate effector cells for the inhibition of tumor growth. Cancer Immunology and Immunotherapy 2009;58(8):1245-1255.

[65] Emoto M, Emoto Y, Buchwalow IB, Kaufmann SH. Induction of IFN-gamma-producing CD4+ natural killer T cells by Mycobacterium bovis bacillus Calmette Guérin. European Journal of Immunology 1999;29(2):650-659.

[66] von Meyenn F, Schaefer M, Weighardt H, Bauer S, Kirschning CJ, Wagner H, Sparwasser T. Toll-like receptor 9 contributes to recognition of Mycobacterium bovis Bacillus Calmette-Guerin by Flt3-ligand generated dendritic cells. Immunobiology 2006;211(6-8):557-565.

[67] Aderem A, Ulevitch RJ. Toll-like receptors in the induction of the innate immune response. Nature 2000;406(6797):782-787.

[68] Bilen CY, Inci K, Erkan I, Ozen H. The predictive value of purified protein derivative results on complications and prognosis in patients with bladder cancer treated with bacillus Calmette-Guerin. The Journal of Urology 2003;169(5):1702-1705.

[69] Reale M, Intorno R, Tenaglia R, Feliciani C, Barbacane RC, Santoni A, Conti P. Production of MCP-1 and RANTES in bladder cancer patients after bacillus Calmette-Guerin immunotherapy. Cancer Immunology and Immunotherapy 2002;51(2):91-98.

[70] Pook SH, Rahmat JN, Esuvaranathan K, Mahendran R. Internalization of Mycobacterium bovis, Bacillus Calmette Guerin, by bladder cancer cells is cytotoxic. Oncology Reports 2007;18(5):1315-1320.

[71] Ikeda N, Toida I, Iwasaki A, Kawai K, Akaza H. Surface antigen expression on bladder tumor cells induced by bacillus Calmette-Guérin (BCG): A role of BCG internalization into tumor cells. International Journal of Urology 2002;9(1):29-35.

[72] Saban MR, Hellmich HL, Simpson C, Davis CA, Lang ML, Ihnat MA, O'Donnell MA, Wu XR, Saban R. Repeated BCG treatment of mouse bladder selectively stimulates small GTPases and HLA antigens and inhibits single-spanning uroplakins. BMC Cancer 2007;7:204.

[73] Chen FH, Crist SA, Zhang GJ, Iwamoto Y, See WA. Interleukin-6 production by human bladder tumor cell lines is up-regulated by bacillus Calmette-Guérin through nuclear factor-kappaB and Ap-1 via an immediate early pathway. The Journal of Urology 2002;168(2):786-797.

[74] Zhang G, Chen F, Cao Y, See WA. Bacillus Calmette-Guérin induces p21 expression in human transitional carcinoma cell lines via an immediate early, p53 independent pathway. Urologic Oncology 2007;25(3):221-227.

[75] Chen F, Zhang G, Iwamoto Y, See WA. BCG directly induces cell cycle arrest in human transitional carcinoma cell lines as a consequence of integrin cross-linking. BMC Urology 2005;5:8.

[76] Ping SY, Wu CL, Yu DS. Sunitinib can enhance BCG mediated cytotoxicity to transitional cell carcinoma through apoptosis pathway. Urologic Oncology 2010;PMID: 20884251.

[77] See WA, Zhang G, Chen F, Cao Y, Langenstroer P, Sandlow J. Bacille-Calmette Guèrin induces caspase-independent cell death in urothelial carcinoma cells together with release of the necrosis-associated chemokine high molecular group box protein 1. British Journal of Urology International 2009;103(12):1714-1720.

[78] See WA, Zhang G, Chen F, Cao Y. p21 Expression by human urothelial carcinoma cells modulates the phenotypic response to BCG. Urologic Oncology 2010;28(5): 526-533.

[79] Jonasch E, Haluska FG. Interferon in oncological practice: Review of Interferon Biology, Clinical Applications, and Toxicities. The Oncologist 2001;6(1):34-55.

[80] Kamat AM, Lamm DL. Immunotherapy for bladder cancer. Current Urology Reports 2001;2(1):62-69.

[81] Luo Y, Chen X, O'Donnell MA. Role of Th1 and Th2 cytokines in BCG-induced IFN-gamma production: cytokine promotion and simulation of BCG effect. Cytokine 2003;21(1):17-26.

[82] Belardelli F, Ferrantini M, Proietti E, Kirkwood JM. Interferon-alpha in tumor immunity and immunotherapy. Cytokine and Growth Factor Reviews 2002;13(2): 119-134.

[83] Papageorgiou A, Lashinger L, Millikan R, Grossman HB, Benedict W, Dinney CP, McConkey DJ. Role of tumor necrosis factor-related apoptosis-inducing ligand in interferon-induced apoptosis in human bladder cancer cells. Cancer Research 2004;64(24):8973-8979.

[84] Tecchio C, Huber V, Scapini P, Calzetti F, Margotto D, Todeschini G, Pilla L, Martinelli G, Pizzolo G, Rivoltini L, Cassatella MA. IFNalpha-stimulated neutrophils and monocytes release a soluble form of TNF-related apoptosis-inducing ligand (TRAIL/ Apo-2 ligand) displaying apoptotic activity on leukemic cells. Blood 2004;103(10): 3837-3844.

[85] Papageorgiou A, Dinney CP, McConkey DJ. Interferon-alpha induces TRAIL expression and cell death via an IRF-1-dependent mechanism in human bladder cancer cells. Cancer Biology and Therapeutics 2007;6(6):872-879.

[86] Droller MJ, Gomolka D. Enhancement of natural cytotoxicity in lymphocytes from animals with carcinogen-induced bladder cancer. The Journal of Urology 1983;129(3): 625-629.

[87] Parronchi P, De Carli M, Manetti R, Simonelli C, Sampognaro S, Piccinni MP, Macchia D, Maggi E, Del Prete G, Romagnani S. IL-4 and IFN (alpha and gamma) exert opposite regulatory effects on the development of cytolytic potential by Th1 or Th2 human T cell clones. Journal of Immunology 1992;149(9):2977-2983.

[88] Slaton JW, Perrotte P, Inoue K, Dinney CP, Fidler IJ. Interferon-alpha-mediated down-regulation of angiogenesis-related genes and therapy of bladder cancer are dependent on optimization of biological dose and schedule. Clinical Cancer Research 1999;5(10):2726-2734.

[89] Giannopoulos A, Adamakis I, Evangelou K, Giannopoulou M, Zacharatos P, Zsantoulis P, Perunovic B, Athanasiou A, Retalis G, Constandinidis C, Gorgoulis VG. Interferon-a2b reduces neo-microvascular density in the 'normal' urothelium adjacent to the tumor after transurethral resection of superficial bladder carcinoma. Onkologie 2003;26(2):147-152.

[90] Glashan RW. A randomized controlled study of intravesical alpha-2b-interferon in carcinoma in situ of the bladder. The Journal of Urology 1990;144(3):658-661.

[91] Hudson MA, Ratliff TL. Failure of intravesical interferon-alfa-2b for the treatment of patients with superficial bladder cancer previously failing intravesical BCG Therapy. Urologic Oncology 1995;1(3):115-118.

[92] Martin B, Hernandez R, Correas M, Gutierrez J, Del Valle J, Roca A, Vega A, Villanueva A, Gutierrez R. Results at 43 months' follow-up of a double-blind, randomized, prospective clinical trial using intravesical interferon alpha-2b in the prophylaxis of stage pT1 transitional cell carcinoma of the bladder. Urology 1997;49(2):187-190.

[93] Gan YH, Zhang Y, Khoo HE, Esuvaranathan K. Antitumour immunity of Bacillus Calmette-Guerin and interferon alpha in murine bladder cancer. European Journal of Cancer 1999;35(7):1123-1129.

[94] Luo Y, Chen X, Downs TM, DeWolf WC, O'Donnell MA. IFN-alpha 2B enhances Th1 cytokine responses in bladder cancer patients receiving Mycobacterium bovis bacillus Calmette-Guérin immunotherapy. Journal of Immunology 1999;162(4):2399-2405.

[95] Stricker P, Pryor K, Nicholson T, Goldstein D, Golovsky D, Ferguson R, Nash P, Ehsman S, Rumma J, Mammen G, Penny R. Bacillus Calmette-Guérin plus intravesical interferon alpha-2b in patients with superficial bladder cancer. Urology 1996;48(6): 957-961.

[96] O'Donnell MA, Krohn J, DeWolf WC. Salvage intravesical therapy with interferon-alpha 2b plus low dose bacillus Calmette-Guerin is effective in patients with superficial bladder cancer in whom bacillus Calmette-Guerin alone previously failed. The Journal of Urology 2001;166(4):1300-1304.

[97] Lam JS, Benson MC, O'Donnell MA, Sawczuk A, Gavazzi A, Wechsler MH, Sawczuk IS. Bacillus Calmete-Guérin plus interferon-alpha2B intravesical therapy maintains an extended treatment plan for superficial bladder cancer with minimal toxicity. Urologic Oncology 2003;21(5):354-360.

[98] Punnen SP, Chin JL, Jewett MA. Management of bacillus Calmette-Guerin (BCG) refractory superficial bladder cancer: results with intravesical BCG and Interferon combination therapy. The Canadian Journal of Urology 2003;10(2):1790-1795.

[99] Smith BJ, O'Donnell MA; National BCG-Interferon Phase 2 Investigator Group. Final results from a national multicenter phase II trial of combination bacillus Calmette-Guérin plus interferon alpha-2B for reducing recurrence of superficial bladder cancer. Urologic Oncology 2006;24(4):344-348.

[100] Bazarbashi S, Soudy H, Abdelsalam M, Al-Jubran A, Akhtar S, Memon M, Aslam M, Kattan S, Shoukri M. Co-administration of intravesical bacillus Calmette-Guérin and interferon α-2B as first line in treating superficial transitional cell carcinoma of the urinary bladder. British Journal of Urology International 2011;108(7):1115-1118.

[101] Gallagher BL, Joudi FN, Maymí JL, O'Donnell MA. mpact of previous bacille Calmette-Guérin failure pattern on subsequent response to bacille Calmette-Guérin plus interferon intravesical therapy. Urology 2008;71(2):297-301.

[102] Nepple KG, Lightfoot AJ, Rosevear HM, O'Donnell MA, Lamm DL; Bladder Cancer Genitourinary Oncology Study Group. Bacillus Calmette-Guérin with or without interferon α-2b and megadose versus recommended daily allowance vitamins during induction and maintenance intravesical treatment of nonmuscle invasive bladder cancer. The Journal of Urology 2010;184(5):1915-1919.

[103] Joudi FN, Smith BJ, O'Donnell MA; National BCG-Interferon Phase 2 Investigator Group. Final results from a national multicenter phase II trial of combination bacillus Calmette-Guérin plus interferon alpha-2B for reducing recurrence of superficial bladder cancer. Urologic Oncology 2006;24(4):344-348.

[104] Luo Y, Chen X, Han R, O'Donnell MA. Recombinant bacille Calmette-Guérin (BCG) expressing human interferon-alpha 2B demonstrates enhanced immunogenicity. Clinical and Experimental Immunology 2001;123(2):264-270.

[105] Liu W, O'Donnell MA, Chen X, Han R, Luo Y. Recombinant bacillus Calmette-Guérin (BCG) expressing interferon-alpha 2B enhances human mononuclear cell cytotoxicity against bladder cancer cell lines in vitro. Cancer Immunology and Immunotherapy 2009;58(10):1647-1655.

[106] Louie B, Rajamahanty S, Won J, Choudhury M, Konno S. Synergistic potentiation of interferon activity with maitake mushroom d-fraction on bladder cancer cells. British Journal of Urology International 2010;105(7):1011-1015.

[107] Fishman AI, Johnson B, Alexander B, Won J, Choudhury M, Konno S. Additively enhanced antiproliferative effect of interferon combined with proanthocyanidin on bladder cancer cells. Journal of Cancer 2012;3:107-112.

[108] Nagabhushan TL, Maneval DC, Benedict WF, Wen SF, Ihnat PM, Engler H, Connor RJ. Enhancement of intravesical delivery with Syn3 potentiates interferon-alpha2b gene therapy for superficial bladder cancer. Cytokine and Growth Factor Reviews 2007;18(5-6):389-394.

[109] Gillis S, Smith KA. Long term culture of tumour-specific cytotoxic T cells. Nature 1977;268(5616):154-156.

[110] Di Sabato G, Chen DM, Erickson JW. Production by murine spleen cells of an activity stimulating the PHA-responsiveness of thymus lymphocytes. Cell Immunology 1975;17(2):495-504.

[111] Chen DM, Di Sabato G. Further studies on the thymocyte stimulating factor. Cellular Immunology 1976;22(2):211-224.

[112] Mizel SB, Farrar JJ. Revised nomenclature for antigen-nonspecific T-cell proliferation and helper factors. Cellular Immunology 1979;48(2):433-436.

[113] Shaw J, Monticone V, Mills G, Paetkau V. Effects of costimulator on immune responses in vitro. Journal of Immunology 1978;120(6):1974-1980.

[114] Yron I, Wood TA Jr, Spiess PJ, Rosenberg SA. In vitro growth of murine T cells. V. The isolation and growth of lymphoid cells infiltrating syngeneic solid tumors. Journal of Immunology 1980;125(1):238-245.

[115] Lotze MT, Grimm EA, Mazumder A, Strausser JL, Rosenberg SA. Lysis of fresh and cultured autologous tumor by human lymphocytes cultured in T-cell growth factor. Cancer Research 1981;41(11 Pt 1):4420-4425.

[116] Rayner AA, Grimm EA, Lotze MT, Chu EW, Rosenberg SA. Lymphokine-activated killer (LAK) cells. Analysis of factors relevant to the immunotherapy of human cancer. Cancer 1985;55(6):1327-1333.

[117] Henney CS, Kuribayashi K, Kern DE, Gillis S. Interleukin-2 augments natural killer cell activity. Nature 1981;291(5813):335-338.

[118] Malkovský M, Loveland B, North M, Asherson GL, Gao L, Ward P, Fiers W. Recombinant interleukin-2 directly augments the cytotoxicity of human monocytes. Nature 1987;325(6101):262-265.

[119] Waldmann TA, Goldman CK, Robb RJ, Depper JM, Leonard WJ, Sharrow SO, Bongiovanni KF, Korsmeyer SJ, Greene WC. Expression of interleukin 2 receptors on activated human B cells. Journal of Experimental Medicine 1984;160(5):1450-1466.

[120] Mosmann TR, Cherwinski H, Bond MW, Giedlin MA, Coffman RL. Two types of murine helper T cell clone. I. Definition according to profiles of lymphokine activities and secreted proteins. Journal of Immunology 1986;136(7):2348-2357.

[121] Rosenberg SA, Lotze MT, Muul LM, Chang AE, Avis FP, Leitman S, Linehan WM, Robertson CN, Lee RE, Rubin JT, et al. A progress report on the treatment of 157 patients with advanced cancer using lymphokine-activated killer cells and interleukin-2 or high-dose interleukin-2 alone. The New England Journal of Medicine 1987;316(15): 889-897.

[122] Webb DE, Austin HA 3rd, Belldegrun A, Vaughan E, Linehan WM, Rosenberg SA. Metabolic and renal effects of interleukin-2 immunotherapy for metastatic cancer. Clinical Nephrology 1988;30(3):141-145.

[123] Ratliff TL, Haaff EO, Catalona WJ. Interleukin-2 production during intravesical bacille Calmette-Guerin therapy for bladder cancer. Clinical Immunology and Immunopatholgy 1986;40(2):375-379.

[124] Haaff EO, Catalona WJ, Ratliff TL. Detection of interleukin 2 in the urine of patients with superficial bladder tumors after treatment with intravesical BCG. The Journal of Urology 1986;136(4):970-974.

[125] De Jong WH, De Boer EC, Van der Meijden AP, Vegt P, Steerenberg PA, Debruyne FM, Ruitenberg EJ. Presence of interleukin-2 in urine of superficial bladder cancer

patients after intravesical treatment with bacillus Calmette-Guérin. Cancer Immunology and Immunotherapy 1990;31(3):182-186.

[126] Böhle A, Nowc C, Ulmer AJ, Musehold J, Gerdes J, Hofstetter AG, Flad HD. Detection of urinary TNF, IL 1, and IL 2 after local BCG immunotherapy for bladder carcinoma. Cytokine 1990;2(3):175-181.

[127] De Boer EC, De Jong WH, Steerenberg PA, Aarden LA, Tetteroo E, De Groot ER, Van der Meijden AP, Vegt PD, Debruyne FM, Ruitenberg EJ. Induction of urinary interleukin-1 (IL-1), IL-2, IL-6, and tumour necrosis factor during intravesical immunotherapy with bacillus Calmette-Guérin in superficial bladder cancer. Cancer Immunology and Immunotherapy 1992;34(5):306-312.

[128] Balbay D, Ozen H, Ozkardes H, Barut A, Bakkaloglu M, Tasar C, Remzi D. Detection of urinary interleukin-2, interleukin-2 receptor, and tumor necrosis factor levels in patients with superficial bladder tumors after intravesical BCG immunotherapy. Urology 1994;43(2):187-190.

[129] de Reijke TM, De Boer EC, Kurth KH, Schamhart DH. Urinary interleukin-2 monitoring during prolonged bacillus Calmette-Guerin treatment: can it predict the optimal number of instillations? The Journal of Urology 1999;161(1):67-71.

[130] Magno C, Melloni D, Galì A, Mucciardi G, Nicocia G, Morandi B, Melioli G, Ferlazzo G. The anti-tumor activity of bacillus Calmette-Guerin in bladder cancer is associated with an increase in the circulating level of interleukin-2. Immunology Letters 2002;81(3):235-238.

[131] Pizza G, Severini G, Menniti D, De Vinci C, Corrado F. Tumour regression after intralesional injection of interleukin 2 (IL-2) in bladder cancer. Preliminary report. International Journal of Cancer 1984;34(3):359-367.

[132] Lee KE, Weiss GH, O'Donnell RW, Cockett AT. Reduction of bladder cancer growth in mice treated with intravesical Bacillus Calmette Guerin and systemic interleukin 2. The Journal of Urology 1987;137(6):1270-1273.

[133] Ikemoto S, Kamizuru M, Wada S, Nishio S, Kishimoto T, Maekawa M. Combined effect of interleukin 2 and bacillus Calmette-Guérin in the therapy of mice with transitional cell carcinoma. Urologia Internationalis 1991;47(4):250-254.

[134] Riggs DR, Tarry WF, DeHaven JI, Sosnowski J, Lamm DL. Immunotherapy of murine transitional cell carcinoma of the bladder using alpha and gamma interferon in combination with other forms of immunotherapy. The Journal of Urology 1992;147(1):212-214.

[135] Tubaro A, Velotti F, Stoppacciaro A, Santoni A, Vicentini C, Bossola PC, Galassi P, Pettinato A, Morrone S, Napolitano T, et al. Continuous intra-arterial administration of recombinant interleukin-2 in low-stage bladder cancer. A phase IB study. Cancer 1991;68(1):56-61.

[136] Merguerian PA, Donahue L, Cockett AT. Intraluminal interleukin 2 and bacillus Calmette-Guerin for treatment of bladder cancer: a preliminary report. The Journal of Urology 1987;137(2):216-219.

[137] Huland E, Huland H. Local continuous high dose interleukin 2: a new therapeutic model for the treatment of advanced bladder carcinoma. Cancer Research 1989;49(19):5469-5474.

[138] Cockett AT, Davis RS, Cos LR, Wheeless LL Jr. Bacillus Calmette-Guerin and interleukin-2 for treatment of superficial bladder cancer. The Journal of Urology 1991;146(3):766-769.

[139] Gomella LG, McGinnis DE, Lattime EC, Butler K, Baltish M, Thompson I, Marshall ME. Treatment of transitional cell carcinoma of the bladder with intravesical interleukin-2: a pilot study. Cancer Biotherapy 1993;8(3):223-227.

[140] Nouri AM, Hyde R, Oliver RT. Clinical and immunological effect of intravesical interleukin-2 on superficial bladder cancer. Cancer Immunology and Immunotherapy 1994;39(1):68–70.

[141] Ferlazzo G, Magno C, Iemmo R, Rizzo M, Lupo G, Semino C, et al. Treatment of superficial bladder cancer with intravesical perfusion of rIL-2: a follow-up study. Anticancer Research 1996;16(2):979–980.

[142] Den Otter W, Dobrowolski Z, Bugajski A, Papla B, Van Der Meijden AP, Koten JW, Boon TA, Siedlar M, Zembala M. Intravesical interleukin-2 in T1 papillary bladder carcinoma: regression of marker lesion in 8 of 10 patients. The Journal of Urology 1998;159(4):1183-1186.

[143] O'Donnell MA, Aldovini A, Duda RB, Yang H, Szilvasi A, Young RA, DeWolf WC. Recombinant Mycobacterium bovis BCG secreting functional interleukin-2 enhances gamma interferon production by splenocytes. Infection and Immunity 1994;62(6): 2508-2514.

[144] Murray PJ, Aldovini A, Young RA. Manipulation and potentiation of antimycobacterial immunity using recombinant bacille Calmette-Guérin strains that secrete cytokines. Proceedings of the National Academy of Sciences of the United States of America 1996;93(2):934-939.

[145] Slobbe L, Lockhart E, O'Donnell MA, MacKintosh C, De Lisle G, Buchan G. An in vivo comparison of bacillus Calmette-Guérin (BCG) and cytokine-secreting BCG vaccines. Immunology 1999;96(4):517-523.

[146] Luo Y, Chen X, Szilvasi A, O'Donnell MA. Co-expression of interleukin-2 and green fluorescent protein reporter in mycobacteria: in vivo application for monitoring antimycobacterial immunity. Molecular Immunology 2000;37(9):527-536.

[147] Young SL, O'Donnell MA, Buchan GS. IL-2-secreting recombinant bacillus Calmette Guerin can overcome a Type 2 immune response and corticosteroid-induced immu-

nosuppression to elicit a Type 1 immune response. International Immunology 2002;14(7):793-800.

[148] Li YG, Wang ZP, Tian JQ, Tian BQ, Rodrigues R, Shang PF, Zhang T. Dendritic cell transfected with secondary lymphoid-tissue chemokine and/or interleukin-2 gene-enhanced cytotoxicity of T-lymphocyte in human bladder tumor cell S in vitro. Cancer Investigation 2009;27(9):909-917.

[149] Huang X, Yu HS, Chen Z, Li JL, Hu ZM, Gao JM. A novel immunotherapy for superficial bladder cancer by the immobilization of streptavidin-tagged bioactive IL-2 on the biotinylated mucosal surface of the bladder wall. Chinese Journal of Cancer 2010;29(6):611-616.

[150] Zhang X, Shi X, Li J, Hu Z, Guo F, Huang X, Zhang Z, Sun P, Jing Y, Gao J, Tan W. Novel immunotherapy for metastatic bladder cancer using vaccine of human interleukin-2 surface-modified MB49 cells. Urology 2011;78(3):722.e1-722.e6.

[151] Wong HL, Wilson DE, Jenson JC, Familletti PC, Stremlo DL, Gately MK. Characterization of a factor(s) which synergizes with recombinant interleukin 2 in promoting allogeneic human cytolytic T-lymphocyte responses in vitro. Cellular Immunology 1988;111(1):39-54.

[152] Kobayashi M, Fitz L, Ryan M, Hewick RM, Clark SC, Chan S, Loudon R, Sherman F, Perussia B, Trinchieri G. Identification and purification of natural killer cell stimulatory factor (NKSF), a cytokine with multiple biologic effects on human lymphocytes. Journal of Experimental Medicine 1989;170(3):827-845.

[153] Stern AS, Podlaski FJ, Hulmes JD, Pan YC, Quinn PM, Wolitzky AG, Familletti PC, Stremlo DL, Truitt T, Chizzonite R, et al. Purification to homogeneity and partial characterization of cytotoxic lymphocyte maturation factor from human B-lymphoblastoid cells. Proceedings of the National Academy of Sciences of the United States of America 1990;87(17):6808-6812.

[154] Gately MK, Desai BB, Wolitzky AG, Quinn PM, Dwyer CM, Podlaski FJ, Familletti PC, Sinigaglia F, Chizonnite R, Gubler U, et al. Regulation of human lymphocyte proliferation by a heterodimeric cytokine, IL-12 (cytotoxic lymphocyte maturation factor). Journal of Immunology 1991;147(3):874-882.

[155] Gubler U, Chua AO, Schoenhaut DS, Dwyer CM, McComas W, Motyka R, Nabavi N, Wolitzky AG, Quinn PM, Familletti PC, et al. Coexpression of two distinct genes is required to generate secreted bioactive cytotoxic lymphocyte maturation factor. Proceedings of the National Academy of Sciences of the United States of America 1991;88(10):4143-4147.

[156] Schoenhaut DS, Chua AO, Wolitzky AG, Quinn PM, Dwyer CM, McComas W, Familletti PC, Gately MK, Gubler U. Cloning and expression of murine IL-12. Journal of Immunology 1992;148(11):3433-3440.

[157] Desai BB, Quinn PM, Wolitzky AG, Mongini PK, Chizzonite R, Gately MK. IL-12 receptor. II. Distribution and regulation of receptor expression. Journal of Immunology 1992;148(10):3125-3132.

[158] Manetti R, Parronchi P, Giudizi MG, Piccinni MP, Maggi E, Trinchieri G, Romagnani S. Natural killer cell stimulatory factor (interleukin 12 [IL-12]) induces T helper type 1 (Th1)-specific immune responses and inhibits the development of IL-4-producing Th cells. Journal of Experimental Medicine 1993;177(4):1199-1204.

[159] Macatonia SE, Hosken NA, Litton M, Vieira P, Hsieh CS, Culpepper JA, Wysocka M, Trinchieri G, Murphy KM, O'Garra A. Dendritic cells produce IL-12 and direct the development of Th1 cells from naive CD4+ T cells. Journal of Immunology 1995;154(10):5071-5079.

[160] Gately MK, Wolitzky AG, Quinn PM, Chizzonite R. Regulation of human cytolytic lymphocyte responses by interleukin-12. Cell Immunology 1992;143(1):127-142.

[161] Collison K, Saleh S, Parhar R, Meyer B, Kwaasi A, Al-Hussein K, Al-Sedairy S, Al-Mohanna F. Evidence for IL-12-activated Ca2+ and tyrosine signaling pathways in human neutrophils. Journal of Immunology 1998;161(7):3737-3745.

[162] Yeaman GR, Collins JE, Currie JK, Guyre PM, Wira CR, Fanger MW. IFN-gamma is produced by polymorphonuclear neutrophils in human uterine endometrium and by cultured peripheral blood polymorphonuclear neutrophils. Journal of Immunology 1998;160(10):5145-5153.

[163] Voest EE, Kenyon BM, O'Reilly MS, Truitt G, D'Amato RJ, Folkman J. Inhibition of angiogenesis in vivo by interleukin 12. Journal of the National Cancer Institute 1995;87(8):581-586.

[164] Dias S, Boyd R, Balkwill F. IL-12 regulates VEGF and MMPs in a murine breast cancer model. International Journal of Cancer 1998;78(3):361-365.

[165] Coughlin CM, Salhany KE, Gee MS, LaTemple DC, Kotenko S, Ma X, Gri G, Wysocka M, Kim JE, Liu L, Liao F, Farber JM, Pestka S, Trinchieri G, Lee WM. Tumor cell responses to IFNgamma affect tumorigenicity and response to IL-12 therapy and anti-angiogenesis. Immunity 1998;9(1):25-34.

[166] Coughlin CM, Salhany KE, Wysocka M, Aruga E, Kurzawa H, Chang AE, Hunter CA, Fox JC, Trinchieri G, Lee WM. Interleukin-12 and interleukin-18 synergistically induce murine tumor regression which involves inhibition of angiogenesis. The Journal of Clinical Investigation 1998;101(6):1441-1452.

[167] Hashimoto W, Osaki T, Okamura H, Robbins PD, Kurimoto M, Nagata S, Lotze MT, Tahara H. Differential antitumor effects of administration of recombinant IL-18 or recombinant IL-12 are mediated primarily by Fas-Fas ligand- and perforin-induced tumor apoptosis, respectively. Journal of Immunology 1999;163(2):583-589.

[168] Kawamura T, Takeda K, Mendiratta SK, Kawamura H, Van Kaer L, Yagita H, Abo T, Okumura K. Critical role of NK1+ T cells in IL-12-induced immune responses in vivo. Journal of Immunology 1998;160(1):16-19.

[169] Brunda MJ, Luistro L, Warrier RR, Wright RB, Hubbard BR, Murphy M, Wolf SF, Gately MK. Antitumor and antimetastatic activity of interleukin 12 against murine tumors. Journal of Experimental Medicine 1993;178(4):1223-1230.

[170] Nastala CL, Edington HD, McKinney TG, Tahara H, Nalesnik MA, Brunda MJ, Gately MK, Wolf SF, Schreiber RD, Storkus WJ, et al. Recombinant IL-12 administration induces tumor regression in association with IFN-gamma production. Journal of Immunology 1994;153(4):1697-1706.

[171] Teicher BA, Ara G, Buxton D, Leonard J, Schaub RG. Optimal scheduling of interleukin 12 and chemotherapy in the murine MB-49 bladder carcinoma and B16 melanoma. Clinical Cancer Research 1997;3(9):1661-1667.

[172] Teicher BA, Ara G, Buxton D, Leonard J, Schaub RG. Optimal scheduling of interleukin-12 and fractionated radiation therapy in the murine Lewis lung carcinoma. Radiation Oncology Investigations 1998;6(2):71-80.

[173] O'Donnell MA, Luo Y, Hunter SE, Chen X, Hayes LL, Clinton SK. Interleukin-12 immunotherapy of murine transitional cell carcinoma of the bladder: dose dependent tumor eradication and generation of protective immunity. The Journal of Urology 2004;171(3):1330-1335.

[174] Zagozdzon R, Giermasz A, Gołab J, Stokłosa T, Jalili A, Jakóbisiak M. The potentiated antileukemic effects of doxorubicin and interleukin-12 combination are not dependent on nitric oxide production. Cancer Letters 1999;147(1-2):67-75.

[175] Zagozdzon R, Golab J, Mucha K, Foroncewicz B, Jakobisiak M. Potentiation of antitumor effects of IL-12 in combination with paclitaxel in murine melanoma model in vivo. International Journal of Molecular Medicine 1999;4(6):645-648.

[176] Golab J, Zagozdzon R, Kozar K, Kaminski R, Giermasz A, Stoklosa T, Lasek W, Jakobisiak M. Potentiatied anti-tumor effectiveness of combined therapy with interleukin-12 and mitoxantrone of L1210 leukemia in vivo. Oncology Reports 2000;7(1): 177-181.

[177] Teicher BA, Ara G, Menon K, Schaub RG. In vivo studies with interleukin-12 alone and in combination with monocyte colony-stimulating factor and/or fractionated radiation treatment. International Journal of Cancer 1996;65(1):80-84.

[178] Lieu FH, Hawley TS, Fong AZ, Hawley RG. Transmissibility of murine stem cell virus-based retroviral vectors carrying both interleukin-12 cDNAs and a third gene: implications for immune gene therapy. Cancer Gene Therapy 1997;4(3):167-175.

[179] Bramson JL, Hitt M, Addison CL, Muller WJ, Gauldie J, Graham FL. Direct intratumoral injection of an adenovirus expressing interleukin-12 induces regression and

long-lasting immunity that is associated with highly localized expression of interleukin-12. Human Gene Therapy 1996;7(16):1995-2002.

[180] Addison CL, Bramson JL, Hitt MM, Muller WJ, Gauldie J, Graham FL. Intratumoral coinjection of adenoviral vectors expressing IL-2 and IL-12 results in enhanced frequency of regression of injected and untreated distal tumors. Gene Therapy 1998;5(10):1400-1409.

[181] Meko JB, Yim JH, Tsung K, Norton JA. High cytokine production and effective antitumor activity of a recombinant vaccinia virus encoding murine interleukin 12. Cancer Research 1995;55(21):4765-4770.

[182] Zitvogel L, Tahara H, Cai Q, Storkus WJ, Muller G, Wolf SF, Gately M, Robbins PD, Lotze MT. Construction and characterization of retroviral vectors expressing biologically active human interleukin-12. Human Gene Therapy 1994;5(12):1493-1506.

[183] O'Donnell MA, Luo Y, Chen X, Szilvasi A, Hunter SE, Clinton SK. Role of IL-12 in the induction and potentiation of IFN-gamma in response to bacillus Calmette-Guérin. Journal of Immunology 1999;163(8):4246-4252.

[184] Riemensberger J, Böhle A, Brandau S. IFN-gamma and IL-12 but not IL-10 are required for local tumour surveillance in a syngeneic model of orthotopic bladder cancer. Clinical and Experimental Immunology 2002;127(1):20-26.

[185] O'Donnell MA, Luo Y, Hunter SE, Chen X, Hayes LL, Clinton SK. The essential role of interferon-gamma during interleukin-12 therapy for murine transitional cell carcinoma of the bladder. The Journal of Urology 2004;171(3):1336-1342.

[186] Clinton SK, Canto E, O'Donnell MA. Interleukin-12. Opportunities for the treatment of bladder cancer. The Urologic Clinics of North America 2000;27(1):147–155.

[187] Horinaga M, Harsch KM, Fukuyama R, Heston W, Larchian W. Intravesical interleukin-12 gene therapy in an orthotopic bladder cancer model. Urology 2005;66(2): 461-466.

[188] Zaharoff DA, Hoffman BS, Hooper HB, Benjamin CJ Jr, Khurana KK, Hance KW, Rogers CJ, Pinto PA, Schlom J, Greiner JW. Intravesical immunotherapy of superficial bladder cancer with chitosan/interleukin-12. Cancer Research 2009;69(15): 6192-6199.

[189] Cohen J. IL-12 deaths: explanation and a puzzle. Science 1995;270(5238):908.

[190] Atkins MB, Robertson MJ, Gordon M, Lotze MT, DeCoste M, DuBois JS, Ritz J, Sandler AB, Edington HD, Garzone PD, Mier JW, Canning CM, Battiato L, Tahara H, Sherman ML. Phase I evaluation of intravenous recombinant human interleukin 12 in patients with advanced malignancies. Clinical Cancer Research 1997;3(3):409-417.

[191] Robertson MJ, Cameron C, Atkins MB, Gordon MS, Lotze MT, Sherman ML, Ritz J. Immunological effects of interleukin 12 administered by bolus intravenous injection to patients with cancer. Clinical Cancer Research 1999;5(1):9-16.

[192] Gollob JA, Mier JW, Veenstra K, McDermott DF, Clancy D, Clancy M, Atkins MB. Phase I trial of twice-weekly intravenous interleukin 12 in patients with metastatic renal cell cancer or malignant melanoma: ability to maintain IFN-gamma induction is associated with clinical response. Clinical Cancer Research 2000;6(5):1678-1692.

[193] Hurteau JA, Blessing JA, DeCesare SL, Creasman WT. Evaluation of recombinant human interleukin-12 in patients with recurrent or refractory ovarian cancer: a gynecologic oncology group study. Gynecologic Oncology 2001;82(1):7-10.

[194] Motzer RJ, Rakhit A, Thompson JA, Nemunaitis J, Murphy BA, Ellerhorst J, Schwartz LH, Berg WJ, Bukowski RM. Randomized multicenter phase II trial of subcutaneous recombinant human interleukin-12 versus interferon-alpha 2a for patients with advanced renal cell carcinoma. Journal of Interferon and Cytokine Research 2001;21(4): 257-263.

[195] Lenzi R, Rosenblum M, Verschraegen C, Kudelka AP, Kavanagh JJ, Hicks ME, Lang EA, Nash MA, Levy LB, Garcia ME, Platsoucas CD, Abbruzzese JL, Freedman RS. Phase I study of intraperitoneal recombinant human interleukin 12 in patients with Müllerian carcinoma, gastrointestinal primary malignancies, and mesothelioma. Clinical Cancer Research 2002;8(12):3686-3695.

[196] Lenzi R, Edwards R, June C, Seiden MV, Garcia ME, Rosenblum M, Freedman RS. Phase II study of intraperitoneal recombinant interleukin-12 (rhIL-12) in patients with peritoneal carcinomatosis (residual disease < 1 cm) associated with ovarian cancer or primary peritoneal carcinoma. Journal of Translational Medicine 2007;5:66.

[197] Younes A, Pro B, Robertson MJ, Flinn IW, Romaguera JE, Hagemeister F, Dang NH, Fiumara P, Loyer EM, Cabanillas FF, McLaughlin PW, Rodriguez MA, Samaniego F. Phase II clinical trial of interleukin-12 in patients with relapsed and refractory non-Hodgkin's lymphoma and Hodgkin's disease. Clinical Cancer Research 2004;10(16): 5432-5438.

[198] Gollob JA, Veenstra KG, Parker RA, Mier JW, McDermott DF, Clancy D, Tutin L, Koon H, Atkins MB. Phase I trial of concurrent twice-weekly recombinant human interleukin-12 plus low-dose IL-2 in patients with melanoma or renal cell carcinoma. Journal of Clinical Oncology 2003;21(13):2564-2573.

[199] Eisenbeis CF, Lesinski GB, Anghelina M, Parihar R, Valentino D, Liu J, Nadella P, Sundaram P, Young DC, Sznol M, Walker MJ, Carson WE 3rd. Phase I study of the sequential combination of interleukin-12 and interferon alfa-2b in advanced cancer: evidence for modulation of interferon signaling pathways by interleukin-12. Journal of Clinical Oncology 2005;23(34):8835-8844.

[200] Weiss GR, O'Donnell MA, Loughlin K, Zonno K, Laliberte RJ, Sherman ML. Phase 1 study of the intravesical administration of recombinant human interleukin-12 in pa-

tients with recurrent superficial transitional cell carcinoma of the bladder. Journal of Immunotherapy 2003;26(4):343-348.

[201] Giannopoulos A, Constantinides C, Fokaeas E, Stravodimos C, Giannopoulou M, Kyroudi A, Gounaris A. The immunomodulating effect of interferon-gamma intravesical instillations in preventing bladder cancer recurrence. Clinical Cancer Research 2003;9(15):5550-5558.

[202] Stavropoulos NE, Hastazeris K, Filiadis I, Mihailidis I, Ioachim E, Liamis Z, Kalomiris P. Intravesical instillations of interferon gamma in the prophylaxis of high risk superficial bladder cancer--results of a controlled prospective study. Scandinavian Journal of Urology and Nephrology 2002;36(3):218-222.

[203] Serretta V, Corselli G, Piazza B, Franks CR, Palmer PA, Roest GJ, Pavone-Macaluso M. Intravesical therapy of superficial bladder transitional cell carcinoma with tumor necrosis factor-alpha: preliminary report of a phase I-II study. European Urology 1992;22(2):112–114.

[204] Serretta V, Piazza B, Pavone C, Piazza S, Pavone-Macaluso M. Is there a role for recombinant tumor necrosis facto alpha in the intravesical treatment of superficial bladder tumors?—a phase II study. International Journal of Urology 1995;2(2):100–103.

[205] Glazier DB, Bahnson RR, McLeod DG, von Roemeling RW, Messing EM, Ernstoff MS. Intravesical recombinant tumor necrosis factor in the treatment of superficial bladder cancer: an Eastern Cooperative Oncology Group study. The Journal of Urology 1995;154(1):66–68.

[206] Grampsas SA, Kahn K, Crawford ED. Intravesical RTNF therapy of superficial bladder cancer. A phase I study of recombinant tumor necrosis factor administered intravesically to patients with superficial bladder cancer. The Online Journal of Current Clinical Trials 1994; PMID:8136939.

[207] Stravoravdi P, Toliou T, Kirtsis P, Natsis K, Konstandinidis E, Barich A, Gigis P, Dimitriadis K. A new approach in the management of urothelial tumors using GM-CSF on marker lesions: an ultrastructural and immunohistochemical study on the macrophage population in bladder mucosa. Journal of Interferon Cytokine Research 1999;19(3):221-225.

[208] Theano T, Pelagia S, Konstantinos N, Petros K, Alfred B, Konstantinos D, Panagiotis G. Lymphocyte activation by granulocyte macrophage-colony stimulating factor in human bladder cancer. Journal of Experimental Therapeutics and Oncology 2002;2(3):153-157.

[209] Fiorentino DF, Bond MW, Mosmann TR. Two types of mouse T helper cell. IV. Th2 clones secrete a factor that inhibits cytokine production by Th1 clones. Journal of Experimental Medicine 1989;170(6):2081-2095.

[210] Fiorentino DF, Zlotnik A, Vieira P, Mosmann TR, Howard M, Moore KW, O'Garra A. IL-10 acts on the antigen-presenting cell to inhibit cytokine production by Th1 cells. The Journal of Immunology 1991;146(10):3444-3451.

[211] Ferguson TA, Dube P, Griffith TS. Regulation of contact hypersensitivity by interleukin 10. Journal of Experimental Medicine 1994;179(5):1597-1604.

[212] Halak BK, Maguire HC Jr, Lattime EC. Tumor-induced interleukin-10 inhibits type 1 immune responses directed at a tumor antigen as well as a non-tumor antigen present at the tumor site. Cancer Research 1999;59(4):911-917.

[213] Lattime EC, Mastrangelo MJ, Bagasra O, Li W, Berd D. Expression of cytokine mRNA in human melanoma tissues. Cancer Immunology and Immunotherapy 1995;41(3):151-156.

[214] Krüger-Krasagakes S, Krasagakis K, Garbe C, Schmitt E, Hüls C, Blankenstein T, Diamantstein T. Expression of interleukin 10 in human melanoma. British Journal of Cancer 1994;70(6):1182-1185.

[215] Huang M, Wang J, Lee P, Sharma S, Mao JT, Meissner H, Uyemura K, Modlin R, Wollman J, Dubinett SM. Human non-small cell lung cancer cells express a type 2 cytokine pattern. Cancer Research 1995;55(17):3847-3853.

[216] Nakagomi H, Pisa P, Pisa EK, Yamamoto Y, Halapi E, Backlin K, Juhlin C, Kiessling R. Lack of interleukin-2 (IL-2) expression and selective expression of IL-10 mRNA in human renal cell carcinoma. International Journal of Cancer 1995;63(3):366-371.

[217] Mosmann TR, Schumacher JH, Fiorentino DF, Leverah J, Moore KW, Bond MW. Isolation of monoclonal antibodies specific for IL-4, IL-5, IL-6, and a new Th2-specific cytokine (IL-10), cytokine synthesis inhibitory factor, by using a solid phase radioimmunoadsorbent assay. Journal of Immunology 1990;145(9):2938-2945.

[218] O'Garra A, Stapleton G, Dhar V, Pearce M, Schumacher J, Rugo H, Barbis D, Stall A, Cupp J, Moore K, et al. Production of cytokines by mouse B cells: B lymphomas and normal B cells produce interleukin 10. International Immunology 1990;2(9):821-832.

[219] de Waal Malefyt R, Abrams J, Bennett B, Figdor CG, de Vries JE. Interleukin 10(IL-10) inhibits cytokine synthesis by human monocytes: an autoregulatory role of IL-10 produced by monocytes. Journal of Experimental Medicine 1991;174(5):1209-1220.

[220] Qin Z, Noffz G, Mohaupt M, Blankenstein T. Interleukin-10 prevents dendritic cell accumulation and vaccination with granulocyte-macrophage colony-stimulating factor gene-modified tumor cells. Journal of Immunology 1997;159(2):770-776.

[221] Richter G, Krüger-Krasagakes S, Hein G, Hüls C, Schmitt E, Diamantstein T, Blankenstein T. Interleukin 10 transfected into Chinese hamster ovary cells prevents tumor growth and macrophage infiltration. Cancer Research 1993;53(18):4134-4137.

[222] Steinbrink K, Wölfl M, Jonuleit H, Knop J, Enk AH. Induction of tolerance by IL-10-treated dendritic cells. Journal of Immunology 1997;159(10):4772-4780.

[223] de Waal Malefyt R, Haanen J, Spits H, Roncarolo MG, te Velde A, Figdor C, Johnson K, Kastelein R, Yssel H, de Vries JE. Interleukin 10 (IL-10) and viral IL-10 strongly reduce antigen-specific human T cell proliferation by diminishing the antigen-presenting capacity of monocytes via downregulation of class II major histocompatibility complex expression. Journal of Experimental Medicine 1991;174(4):915-924.

[224] Ding L, Linsley PS, Huang LY, Germain RN, Shevach EM. IL-10 inhibits macrophage costimulatory activity by selectively inhibiting the up-regulation of B7 expression. Journal of Immunology 1993;151(3):1224-1234.

[225] Willems F, Marchant A, Delville JP, Gérard C, Delvaux A, Velu T, de Boer M, Goldman M. Interleukin-10 inhibits B7 and intercellular adhesion molecule-1 expression on human monocytes. European Journal of Immunology 1994;24(4):1007-1009.

[226] Groux H, O'Garra A, Bigler M, Rouleau M, Antonenko S, de Vries JE, Roncarolo MG. A CD4+ T-cell subset inhibits antigen-specific T-cell responses and prevents colitis. Nature 1997;389(6652):737-742.

[227] Cenci E, Romani L, Mencacci A, Spaccapelo R, Schiaffella E, Puccetti P, Bistoni F. Interleukin-4 and interleukin-10 inhibit nitric oxide-dependent macrophage killing of Candida albicans. European Journal of Immunology 1993;23(5):1034-1038.

[228] Moore KW, de Waal Malefyt R, Coffman RL, O'Garra A. Interleukin-10 and the interleukin-10 receptor. Annual Review of Immunology 2001;19:683-765.

[229] Kong D, Kunimoto DY. Secretion of human interleukin 2 by recombinant Mycobacterium bovis BCG. Infection and Immunity 1995;63(3):799-803.

[230] Ryan AA, Wozniak TM, Shklovskaya E, O'Donnell MA, Fazekas de St Groth B, Britton WJ, Triccas JA. Improved protection against disseminated tuberculosis by Mycobacterium bovis bacillus Calmette-Guerin secreting murine GM-CSF is associated with expansion and activation of APCs. Journal of Immunology 2007;179(12): 8418-8424.

[231] Wangoo A, Brown IN, Marshall BG, Cook HT, Young DB, Shaw RJ. Bacille Calmette-Guérin (BCG)-associated inflammation and fibrosis: modulation by recombinant BCG expressing interferon-gamma (IFN-gamma). Clinical and Experimental Immunology 2000;119(1):92-98.

[232] Young S, O'Donnell M, Lockhart E, Buddle B, Slobbe L, Luo Y, De Lisle G, Buchan G. Manipulation of immune responses to Mycobacterium bovis by vaccination with IL-2- and IL-18-secreting recombinant bacillus Calmette Guerin. Immunology and Cell Biology 2002;80(3):209-215.

[233] Moreira AL, Tsenova L, Murray PJ, Freeman S, Bergtold A, Chiriboga L, Kaplan G. Aerosol infection of mice with recombinant BCG secreting murine IFN-gamma parti-

ally reconstitutes local protective immunity. Microbial Pathogenesis 2000;29(3): 175-185.

[234] Biet F, Kremer L, Wolowczuk I, Delacre M, Locht C. Mycobacterium bovis BCG producing interleukin-18 increases antigen-specific gamma interferon production in mice. Infection and Immunity 2002;70(12):6549-6557.

[235] Biet F, Duez C, Kremer L, Marquillies P, Amniai L, Tonnel AB, Locht C, Pestel J. Recombinant Mycobacterium bovis BCG producing IL-18 reduces IL-5 production and bronchoalveolar eosinophilia induced by an allergic reaction. Allergy 2005;60(8): 1065-1072.

[236] He J, Shen D, O'Donnell MA, Chang H. Induction of MUC1-specific cellular immunity by a recombinant BCG expressing human MUC1 and secreting IL2. International Journal of Oncology 2002;20(6):1305-1311.

[237] Chung MA, Luo Y, O'Donnell M, Rodriguez C, Heber W, Sharma S, Chang HR. Development and preclinical evaluation of a Bacillus Calmette-Guérin-MUC1-based novel breast cancer vaccine. Cancer Research 2003;63(6):1280-1287.

[238] Arnold J, de Boer EC, O'Donnell MA, Böhle A, Brandau S. Immunotherapy of experimental bladder cancer with recombinant BCG expressing interferon-gamma. Journal of Immunotherapy 2004;27(2):116-123.

[239] Fan XL, Yu TH, Gao Q, Yao W. Immunological properties of recombinant Mycobacterium bovis bacillus Calmette-Guérin strain expressing fusion protein IL-2-ESAT-6. Acta Biochimica et Biophysica Sinica (Shanghai) 2006;38(10)683-690.

[240] Chen X, O'Donnell MA, Luo Y. Dose-dependent synergy of Th1-stimulating cytokines on bacille Calmette-Guérin-induced interferon-gamma production by human mononuclear cells. Clinical and Experimental Immunology 2007;149(1):178-185.

[241] Ryan AA, Spratt JM, Britton WJ, Triccas JA. Secretion of functional monocyte chemotactic protein 3 by recombinant Mycobacterium bovis BCG attenuates vaccine virulence and maintains protective efficacy against M. tuberculosis infection. Infection and Immunity 2007;75(1):523-526.

[242] Xu Y, Zhu B, Wang Q, Chen J, Qie Y, Wang J, Wang H, Wang B, Wang H. Recombinant BCG coexpressing Ag85B, ESAT-6 and mouse-IFN-gamma confers effective protection against Mycobacterium tuberculosis in C57BL/6 mice. FEMS Immunology and Medcal Microbiology 2007;51(3):480-487.

[243] Tang C, Yamada H, Shibata K, Maeda N, Yoshida S, Wajjwalku W, Ohara N, Yamada T, Kinoshita T, Yoshikai Y. Efficacy of recombinant bacille Calmette-Guérin vaccine secreting interleukin-15/antigen 85B fusion protein in providing protection against Mycobacterium tuberculosis. Journal of Infectious Diseases 2008;197(9):1263-1274.

[244] Yuan S, Shi C, Han W, Ling R, Li N, Wang T. Effective anti-tumor responses induced by recombinant bacillus Calmette-Guérin vaccines based on different tandem repeats of MUC1 and GM-CSF. European Journal of Cancer Prevention 2009;18(5):416-423.

[245] Yuan S, Shi C, Ling R, Wang T, Wang H, Han W. Immunization with two recombinant Bacillus Calmette-Guérin vaccines that combine the expression of multiple tandem repeats of mucin-1 and colony stimulating-factor suppress breast tumor growth in mice. Journal of Cancer Research and Clinical Oncology 2010;136,(9):1359-1367.

[246] Shen H, Wang C, Yang E, Xu Y, Liu W, Yan J, Wang F, Wang H. Novel recombinant BCG coexpressing Ag85B, ESAT-6 and mouse TNF-alpha induces significantly enhanced cellular immune and antibody responses in C57BL/6 mice. Microbiolgy and Immunology 2010;54(8):435-441.

[247] Deng Y, Bao L, Yang X. Evaluation of immunogenicity and protective efficacy against Mycobacterium tuberculosis infection elicited by recombinant Mycobacterium bovis BCG expressing human Interleukin-12p70 and Early Secretory Antigen Target-6 fusion protein. Microbiology and Immunology 2011;55(11):798-808.

[248] Yang X, Bao L, Deng Y. A novel recombinant Mycobacterium bovis bacillus Calmette-Guerin strain expressing human granulocyte macrophage colony-stimulating factor and Mycobacterium tuberculosis early secretory antigenic target 6 complex augments Th1 immunity. Acta Biochimica et Biophysica Sinica (Shanghai) 2011;43(7): 511-518.

[249] Lin CW, Su IJ, Chang JR, Chen YY, Lu JJ, Dou HY. Recombinant BCG coexpressing Ag85B, CFP10, and interleukin-12 induces multifunctional Th1 and memory T cells in mice. Acta Pathologica, Microbiologica et Immunologica Scandinavica 2012;120(1): 72-82.

[250] Ding GQ, Yu YL, Shen ZJ, Zhou XL, Chen SW, Liao GD, Zhang Y. Antitumor effects of human interferon-alpha 2b secreted by recombinant bacillus Calmette-Guérin vaccine on bladder cancer cells. Journal of Zhejiang University-Science B. 2012;13(5): 335-341.

[251] Duda RB, Yang H, Dooley DD, Abu-Jawdeh G. Recombinant BCG therapy suppresses melanoma tumor growth. Annals of Surgical Oncology 1995;3(6):542-549.

[252] Young SL, Murphy M, Zhu XW, Harnden P, O'Donnell MA, James K, Patel PM, Selby PJ, Jackson AM. Cytokine-modified Mycobacterium smegmatis as a novel anticancer immunotherapy. International Journal of Cancer 2004;112(4):653-660.

[253] Haley JL, Young DG, Alexandroff A, James K, Jackson AM. Enhancing the immunotherapeutic potential of mycobacteria by transfection with tumour necrosis factor-alpha. Immunology 1999;96(1):114-121.

Chapter 16

Anti-Angiogenic Active Immunotherapy for Cancers: Dawn of a New Era?

Jianping Pan and Lihuang Zhang

Additional information is available at the end of the chapter

http://dx.doi.org/10.5772/55323

1. Introduction

1.1. Angiogenesis in health and disease

The formation of blood vessels occurs by two mechanisms [1]: vasculogenesis and angiogenesis. Vasculogenesis is the process during which blood vessels are formed *de novo* by *in situ* differentiation of the primitive progenitor (i.e. angioblasts) into mature endothelial cells, which was thought to take place only during embryonic development. However, angiogenesis occurs both during embryonic development and postnatal life. Angiogenesis is defined as a process which gives rise to new blood vessels by proliferation and migration of preexisting differentiated endothelial cells. In embryonic life, angiogenesis is a critical process that leads to formation of stable vasculature comprised of endothelial cells, mural cells (pericytes) and basement membrane in the adult [2]. Vasculature in healthy adult is very stable with the exception of rare events such as cyclical growth of vessels in the ovarian corpus luteum or during pregnancy, angiogenesis activities are rare in adult individuals [2]. In addition to normal development, angiogenesis is known to be an important event in pathological conditions such as tissue repair during wound healing and in the growth of tumors [3].

Tumor angiogenesis, the formation of new blood vessels supplying the tumor mass, plays a critical role in tumor growth, progression, persistence and metastasis, because the proliferation and metastasis of malignant tumors are dependent on the sufficient nutrition supplied by the new vessels [4-6]. Many molecules have been demonstrated as positive regulators of angiogenesis, including vascular endothelial growth factor (VEGF), acidic or basic fibroblast growth factor (aFGF, bFGF), epidermal growth factor (EGF), transforming growth factor-α/β (TGF-α, TGF-β), placental growth factor (PlGF), angiopoietin, angiogenin, endoglin (CD105), prostate-specific membrane antigen (PSMA), the anthrax-toxin-receptor (ATR, TEM8), connective tissue growth factor (CTGF, CCN2), urokinase plasminogen activator (uPA), and several others [7-10]. However, VEGF-mediated signaling through its receptor VEGFR-2 is the key rate-limiting step in tumor angiogenesis, and plays the most important role in neovascularization, development, and progression of various tumors including hematopoietic malignancies [11, 12], breast cancer [13], bladder cancer [14], and renal cell cancer [15]. Importantly, it has been found that tumor growth can be attenuated *via* the suppression of angiogenesis [7].

1.2. Anti-angiogenic strategies for cancer treatment

Given the role of angiogenesis in tumor growth and progression, therapeutic strategies targeting tumor vascular endothelia rather than tumor cells have several merits in comparison to conventional anti-tumor therapies [16, 17]: (a) Vascular endothelial cells have genetically stable MHC expression on the surface, which will not be down-regulated, in contrast to the surface of tumor cells [18]; (b) Effector cells or antibodies can reach targeted endothelial cells more readily than they can reach tumor cells [17]; (c) Treatment by targeting endothelial cells is not restricted to specific tumor entities [16, 17, 19]; (d) As each tumor vessel supplies hundreds of tumor cells, the inhibition or diminishment of a large amount of tumor cells could be achieved merely by the comparatively limited impairment of neovascularized endothelial cells; as a consequence, the efficiency of targeting tumor blood vessel endothelium should be higher than that of targeting tumor cells themselves [15]. (e) Several specific anti-angiogenic agents, such as IFN-γ, have very low toxicity in some cases of drug combination-therapy regimens in both patients and animal models [16]. In recent years, the field of anti-angiogenic therapy for cancers has attracted much attention. In general, anti-angiogenic strategies can be divided into the following five categories:

1. Passive immunotherapy: The use of antibody to neutralize angiogenesis positive regulators such as VEGF. In 2003, the Food & Drug Administration (FDA) of the United States approved Bevacizumab (Avastin®; Genentech Inc.), a humanized variant of VEGF neutralizing monoclonal antibody, as the first anti-angiogenic agent for combinatorial treatment with standard of care in metastatic colorectal cancer [20] and subsequently for treatment of patients with non-small-cell lung cancer [21] or metastatic breast cancer [22]. The combinatorial treatment of Bevacizumab with conventional chemotherapy showed increased therapeutic efficacy, for example in patients with metastatic colorectal cancer, the median survival time was extended by 4.7 months [20]. Besides combining with conventional chemotherapy, bevacizumab could combine with radiation therapy safely and effectively [23].

2. Therapy with VEGF inhibitors: Since the approval of Bevacizumab in the clinical use by FDA, several VEGF inhibitors including small molecules targeting VEGF or its receptors came into different stages of clinical development. For example VEGF-Trap$_{R1-R2}$ (Aflibercept; Regeneron Inc.), a chimeric soluble receptor containing structural elements from VEGFR1 and VEGFR2, has the ability to bind to and neutralize the circulating VEGF [24]. VEGF-Trap$_{R1-R2}$ has shown potent anti-tumor activity in preclinical animal models and is currently in clinical trials [24]. In addition to VEGF inhibitors, several small molecule receptor tyrosine kinase inhibitors (RTKIs) target-

ing VEGF and other signaling pathways have been developed. Some of the most clinically relevant RTKIs are summarized in Table 1.

Compound	Company	Targets	Indications
Sunitinib (SU11248)	Pfizer	VEGFRs, PDGFRB, CSF1R, c-Kit	RCC, GIST
Pazopanib (Votrient)	GSK	VEGFRs, PDGFRs and c-kit	RCC
Sorafenib (Bay 43- 9006; Nexavar®)	Bayer	VEGFR-2 and -3, PDGFR-b, Flt-3, c-kit, Raf kinases	RCC, Inoperable HCC
Vendatanib (Caprelsa)	AstraZeneca	VEGFRs and EGFRs, RET- tyrosine kinases	Late-stage Medullary Thyroid Cancer
Cabozantinib (XL184)	Exelixis	VEGFRs Met	Prostate Cancer
Tivozanib (AV-951, KRN-951)	AVEO Pharmaceutical	VEGFRs	RCC
Axitinib (AG-013736)	Pfizer	VEGFRs	mRCC
Linifanib (ABT-869)	Abbott	VEGFRs, PDGFRB, CSF1R	RCC, NSCLC

Table 1. VEGF RTKIs and their indications in caner patients (adopted from [2])

3. Therapy with angiogenesis negative regulators: Many negative regulators, such as angiostatin, endostatin, interferon-γ etc., are involved in the angiogenesis [25]. Therefore the use of these agents to negatively regulate angiogenesis is another strategy for cancer treatment. For example, recombinant human endostatin has been approved in September 2005 by the State Food and Drug Administration (SFDA), P. R. China. The phase III clinical trial of endostatin in China showed promising effects. Combination of endostatin and NP regimen (vinorelbine and cisplatin) significantly improved the therapeutic efficacy in patients with advanced nonsmall-cell lung cancer and safely extended the median time of tumor progression [26].

4. Therapy with vascular disrupting agents: A strategy directly induce vascular collapse. ASA404, a flavonoid compound, is one of the vascular disrupting agents that induce apoptosis of tumor associated endothelial cells, resulting in the inhibition of blood flow, causing hypoxia and necrosis in tumor mass. ASA404 is currently in advanced stage of clinical trial in combination with standard of care in non-small-cell lung cancer [27].

5. Active immunotherapy: Active immunotherapy targeting tumor angiogenesis is a novel modality for treatment of cancers which is based on several assumptions: a) Tumor-derived endothelial cells (ECs) possess characteristics distinct from those of normal tissue [18]. b) Specific immune responses against self-antigen can be elicited. c) Tumor growth can be attenuated via suppression of angiogenesis [7]. The main aim of the active immunotherapy targeting tumor vessels is to break self immunological tolerance to the positive regulators of angiogenesis, hereby inhibiting tumor angiogenesis and thus leading to the inhibition of tumor growth and metastasis. Anti-angiogenic active immunotherapies can

be divided into two categories: one is based on the immunological cross-reactions mediated by vaccination with xenogeneic homologous molecules associated with angiogenesis, and the other targets non-xenogeneic homologous molecules. Therapeutic targets, vaccines and tumor models used in anti-angiogenic active immunotherapy for cancers are summarized in Table 2.

Strategies	Therapeutic targets	Vaccines	Tumor models	References
Vaccination based on xenogeneic homologous molecules	Murine vascular endothelial cells	Human umbilical vein endothelial cells, human dermal microvascular endothelial cells, and bovine glomerular endothelial cells	Meth A, H22, MA782/5S, FM3A, and Lewis Lung carcinoma	29
	Murine VEGF	Recombinant plasmid encoding VEGF of xenopus laevis	Meth A, H22 and MA782/5S	32
		pMAE5△5 vectors harboring human VEGF 121 gene and mutated human VEGF 121 gene	EL-4, B16, and TC-1	33
	Canine VEGF	Liposome-DNA adjuvant	Soft tissue sarcoma	34
	Murine VEGFR-2	Plasmid DNA encoding quail VEGFR-2	Meth A, EL-4 and MOPC-315,	36
		Plasmid DNA encoding the C terminal 37 amino acids of hCGβ, 5 different CTL epitopes from human surviving and the 3rd and 4th extracellular domains of VEGFR-2	LL/2 lung carcinoma	37
		Bifidobacterium infantis expressing human sKDR	Lewis lung cancer	38
	Murine FGFR-1	cDNA encoding Xenopus FGFR-1	Meth A, H22, and MA782/5S	41
	Murine αvβ3	Plasmid DNA encoding the ligand-binding domain of chicken integrin β3	Meth A, H22, and MA782/5S	43
	Murine MMP-2	Plasmid DNA encoding chicken MMP-2	LL/2, Meth A, H22	48
	Murine RHAMM	Plasmid encoding *Xenopus* RHAMM	B16	49
	Murine DLL4	Plasmid encoding human DLL4	D2F2/E2	55
	Murine Angiomotin	Plasmid encoding human angiomotin	TUBO breast cancer	57, 61

Strategies	Therapeutic targets	Vaccines	Tumor models	References
Vaccination based on non-xenogeneic homologous molecules	Murine VEGFR-2	flk-1 protein pulsed DC	B16, 3LL	62
		flk1 mRNA-transfected DC	B16, MBT-2	64
		Murine sVEGFR-2 and IFN-γ fusion gene-transfected DC	B16, 3LL	68
		Recombinant plasmid encoding flk-1	B16, MC38, D121	63
		H-2D^{b}-restricted KDR2 or KDR3 peptide	MC38	69
		L. monocytogene-based Flk-1	4T1-Luc	71, 72
		pSG.SS.Flk-1$_{ECD}$.C3d3	BTT739	73
	VEGFR-2 in transgenic mice expressing HLA-A*0201	HLA-A*0201-restricted VEGFR-2 epitope peptide	MC38, B16	70
	Human VEGFR-2	HLA-A*2402-restricted VEGFR2-169	Patients with advanced pancreatic cancer	74
	Murine FGF-2	FGF-2 heparin-binding structural domain peptide	B16BL6, LLC-LM	39
	Murine EGFR	Recombinant mouse EGFR ectodomain pulsed DC	Lewis lung carcinoma and mammary cancer	80
	Legumain	Minigene plasmid DNA encoding murine MHC class I antigen epitopes of Legumain	D2F2	85
	Endoglin	Plasmid DNA encoding murine endoglin	D2F2	86
		Listeria-based vaccines encoding murine endoglin	4T1-Luc and NT-2 breast cancer	87
	Endothelium	Endothelium lysates pulsed DC	Colon-26 colon cancer	89
		Glutaraldehyde-fixed HUVECs	Patients with recurrent malignant brain tumour or metastatic colorectal cancer	90

Notes: B16: B16 melanoma; B16BL6: B16BL6 tumor cells; D121: D121 lung carcinoma; D2F2: breast carcinoma cells; D2F2/E2: mammary tumor cells derived from BALB/c mouse and were transfected with the cDNA encoding ERBB2; EL-4: EL-4 lymphoma; FM3A: mammary cancer; H22: H22 hepatoma; LL/2: LL/2 Lewis lung carcinoma; LLC-LM: LLC-LM tumor cells; MA782/5S: MA782/5S mammary cancer; Meth A: Meth A fibrosarcoma; MBT-2: MBT-2 bladder tumor; MC38: MC38 murine colon cancer; MOPC-315: MOPC-315 plasmacytoma; TC-1: TC-1 carcinoma; 3LL: 3LL Lewis lung carcinoma; HUVECs: human umbilical vein endothelial cells.

Table 2. Anti-angiogenic active immunotherapy for cancers

2. Anti-angiogenic active immunotherapy

2.1. Anti-angiogenic active immunotherapy based on xenogeneic homologous molecules

Homologous molecules in different species are formed as the result of evolution. Molecules with essential functions keep the stability of their molecular sequences, although some moderate degree of evolution is essential for adaptation to different environments and physiological requirements in different species. Many genes in the human and mouse genome are similar (but not identical) to the corresponding genome sequences of the fruit fly Drosophila melanogaster and other non-vertebrates such as *Xenopus laevis* [28]. In consequence, effective immune response to self antigens associated with angiogenesis can thus be induced by vaccination with xenogeneic homologous molecules.

2.1.1. Cell vaccine

Neovascular endothelial cells in tumor tissues express proteins not present or not detectable in normal vascular endothelial cells, such as $\alpha v\beta 3$ integrin and receptors for certain angiogenic growth factors [18]. These proteins in murine vascular endothelial cells share homology to varying degree with counterparts of other species including human [18]. Vaccination of mice with paraformaldehyde-fixed xenogeneic human and bovine proliferative vascular endothelial cells, such as human umbilical vein endothelial cells, human dermal microvascular endothelial cells, and bovine glomerular endothelial cells, resulted in successful breaking of the immunological tolerance to autogeneic vascular endothelial cells in several murine tumor models, such as Meth A fibrosarcoma, MA782/5S and FM3A mammary cancer, H22 hepatoma, and Lewis lung carcinoma, generating a protective and therapeutic anti-tumor immunological reaction [29]. Antibodies against the receptors associated with tumor angiogenesis generated in mice immunized with the xenogeneic homologous proliferative vascular endothelial cell vaccines might inhibit the proliferation of endothelial cells in vivo, leading to the regression of established tumor, and the prolonged survival of tumor-bearing mice [29]. Tumor angiogenesis could be suppressed by the adoptive transfer of autoreactive immunoglobulins purified from the immunized mouse, resulting in inhibition of tumor growth in mice [29]. Autoantibody sediments were detected on ECs within tumor tissues in the immunized mice by immunohistochemical analysis [29]. Furthermore, Western blot analysis showed that reactions between the extract from murine ECs and the serum from the immunized mice resulted in several positive bands, at least two of which, with the molecular weight of 220 kDa and 130 kDa, had similar molecular sizes to those of ligand-binding sites of known VEGFR2 and αv integrin, respectively [29], although the authors did not provide direct evidence to demonstrate that the two positive bands aforementioned contained VEGFR2 and αv integrin respectively. Immune cell subset depletion experiments showed that the production of autoantibodies against tumor vascular ECs and the anti-tumor effect were dependent on $CD4^+$ T lymphocytes [29].

In 2006, early-outgrowth progenitor endothelial cells (EO-EPCs) have been characterized on the basis of their dendritic-like phenotypes (such as expression of HLA-DR, CD40, CD54, CD80, and CD86), phagocytotic and antigen-presenting functions, and endothelial markers (such as VEGER2, von Willebrand factor, CD105) [30]. EO-EPCs also incorporated DiLDL and bound UEA-I, which are endothelial features, and additionally, they formed vascular-like structures on Matrigel [30]. Thus, it might be a promising strategy toward anti-angiogenic cancer treatment to use EO-EPCs as cell vaccine to inhibit tumor angiogenesis, since such cells might function both as dendritic-like cells to augment anti-tumor immunity and as xenogeneic proliferative endothelial cells to break self-tolerance, thereby inducing profound anti-angiogenic effects *in vivo*.

2.1.2. Non-cell vaccines

2.1.2.1. VEGF/VEGFR2

VEGF is a potent and crucial vasculogenic and angiogenic factor, which can induce endothelial cell proliferation, promote cell migration, and inhibit endothelial cell apoptosis [5, 6]. In most types of cancers, VEGF is often present at elevated levels, and strategies aimed at blocking its activity usually lead to suppression of tumor angiogenesis and consequently tumor growth inhibition [31]. The amino acid sequence of VEGF in *Xenopus laevis* shares 75 % and 73 % homology with that of VEGF164 in mice and that of VEGF165 in humans, respectively [32]. Recombinant eukaryotic expression plasmids harboring VEGF-encoding gene of mice and *Xenopus laevis*, respectively, designated as MVEGF-P and XVEGF-P, have been constructed. Immunization of mice with XVEGF-P provoked protective and therapeutic anti-tumor immunological effects in mouse tumor models with Meth A fibrosarcoma, MA782/5S mammary cancer and H22 hepatoma [32]. Anti-VEGF specific autoantibody was detected in serum of mice vaccinated with XVEGF-P by Western blot and ELISA [32]. The VEGF levels in the tumor-bearing mice immunized with XVEGF-P was lower than that in the control groups [32]. Furthermore, the frequency of anti-VEGF antibody-producing B cells in the spleen of mice immunized with XVEGF-P was remarkably higher than that in the spleen of control groups where such B cells were undetectable [32]. VEGF-mediated proliferation of ECs could be inhibited *in vitro* by purified immunoglobulins from XVEGF-P-immunized mice. Adoptive transfer of the purified immunoglobulins into non-immunized tumor-bearing mice could also inhibit tumor angiogenesis *in vivo* and generate anti-tumor effects [32]. Anti-$CD4^+$ monoclonal antibody could obstruct the escalation of concentration of immunoglobulin IgG1 and IgG2 in serum and also block the anti-tumor effects of XVEGF-P DNA vaccines, indicating that $CD4^+$ T lymphocytes were responsible for XVEGF-P-induced anti-tumor effects [32]. The possibility that the anti-tumor activity may result from nonspecifically augmented immune response could be ruled out by the findings that no increase in NK activity of spleen cells or in the level of cytokines such as IFN-α, IFN-β, TNF-α, or β-chemokine in sera was found in immunized mice [32]. Recently, it was reported that when immunized with human VEGF isoform 121 gene (hVEGF121) inserted into pMAE5Δ5 vector (pM-VEGF) and later challenged with melanoma or lung carcinoma tumor cells, a reduction of tumor growth and an increased survival of tumor-bearing C57BL/6 mice were observed because the hVEGF121 gene is highly homologous to its murine counterpart [33]. A decrease in tumor cell density around vessels and in mitotic figures, as well as an increase in apoptotic tumor cells were manifested by histopathological analyses of tumors from C57BL/6 mice immunized with hVEGF121 [33]. Spleen cells from mice immunized with pM-VEGF showed a significant enhanced cytotoxic activity against VEGF-secreting tumor cells, including EL-4 lymphoma, B16-F10 melanoma, and TC-1 carcinoma, as compared with those obtained from the mice immunized with the pMAE5Δ5 "empty" vector [33]. IFN-γ ELISPOT assay revealed a significant increase in the number of spots in spleen cells from mice immunized with pM-VEGF [33]. Vaccination with a mutated hVEGF121 gene inserted into the pMAE5Δ5 vector (pM-VEGFmut) produced similar *in vitro* and *in vivo* results, and remarkably reduced the number of spontaneous metastases in a murine model with Lewis lung carcinoma [33]. Serum VEGF levels decreased 8-fold in mice vaccinated with pM-VEGF or pM-VEGFmut as compared with those in pMAE5Δ5 treated mice [33]. A significant correlation was also found between the elevation of serum VEGF level and the increase of the tumor dimensions [33]. However, antibody responses against the GSThVEGF121 fusion protein or GST alone used as capture antigens in ELISA were undetectable in animals vaccinated with pM-VEGF or pM-VEGFmut [33]. These findings indicate that human VEGF-harboring DNA vaccine can be employed for anti-angiogenic active immunotherapy for cancers in mice and direct cell cytotoxicity contributes to the overall anti-tumor effects observed in immunized mice [33].

Previous studies in rodent tumor models have indicated that immunization against xenogeneic growth factors is more likely to induce effective anti-tumor responses than immunization against the syngeneic growth factor [34]. In 2007, an investigation was conducted to assess the safety and anti-tumor and anti-angiogenic effects of a xenogeneic VEGF vaccine in pet dogs with spontaneous cancer. Nine dogs with soft tissue sarcoma were immunized with a recombinant human VEGF vaccine over a 16-week period [34]. The xenogeneic VEGF vaccine was well-tolerated by all dogs and resulted in induction of humoral responses against both human and canine VEGF in animals that remained in the study long enough to receive multiple immunizations [34]. Three of five multiply immunized dogs also experienced sustained decreases in circulating plasma VEGF concentrations and two dogs had a significant decrease in tumor microvessel density [34]. The overall tumor response (>50% decrease in tumor volume) rate was 30% for all treated dogs in the study. Thus, it was concluded that a xenogeneic VEGF vaccine may be a safe and effective alternative means of controlling tumor growth and angiogenesis [34].

VEGF receptor-2 (VEGFR-2, also known as fetal liver kinse-1 (flk-1) in mouse and kinase-containing domain receptor (KDR) in human) is the main receptor responsible for the VEGF-mediated angiogenic activity [6]. The impairment of vasculogenesis and death of embryo at day 8.5 were observed as the result of the targeted inactivation of flk-1 gene in mice [35]. Overexpression of KDR was found on activated endothelial cells of newly formed vessels [6]. It was discovered that the primary sequence of quail VEGFR-2 (qVEGFR-2) was 67% and 70% identical at the amino acid level with mouse and human homologues (flk-1 and KDR), respectively [36]. Immunotherapy with a vaccine based on quail homologous VEGFR-2 elicited protective and therapeutic anti-tumor immunity in both solid and hematopoietic tumor models in mice, such as LL/2 Lewis lung carcinoma, CT26 colon carcinoma, Meth A fibrosarcoma, MOPC-315 plasmacytoma, and EL-4 lymphoma [36]. Autoantibodies against flk-1 in the immunized mice were identified. Sera from qVEGFR-2-

immunized mice recognized not only recombinant qVEGFR-2, but also recombinant mouse VEGFR-2 (mVEGFR) in Western blot analysis [36]. In contrast, the sera isolated from controls showed negative staining [36]. Sera from mice immunized with qVEGFR-2 recognized a single band in flk-1-positive mouse SVEC4-10 endothelial cells and KDR-positive human umbilical vein endothelial cells, with the same size as recognized by commercially available flk-1 or KDR antibodies [36]. Sera from qVEGFR-2-immunized mice also recognized recombinant protein qVEGFR-2 and mVEGFR-2 in ELISA [36]. Detectable IgG1 and IgG2b with significantly elevated concentration in sera were found to be responsible for the immunoglobulin response to VEGFR-2 [36]. Anti-VEGFR-2 specific antibody-producing B cells were detected by ELISPOT. The number of anti-VEGFR-2 antibody-producing B cells was elevated in the spleens of mice immunized with qVEGFR-2, compared with that in controls [36]. Deposition of immunoglobulins on endothelial cells was found within tumors from qVEGFR-2-immunized mice, but not from controls [36]. Adoptive transfer of the purified immunoglobulins from qVEGFR-2-immunized mice resulted in inhibition of VEGF-mediated endothelial cell proliferation and effective protection against tumor growth [36]. Angiogenesis was markedly suppressed within the tumors, and the vascularization of alginate beads was also diminished [36]. Depletion of $CD4^+$ T lymphocyte could abrogate the anti-tumor activity and the production of autoantibodies against flk-1 [36].

Very recently, a DNA vaccine designed by synergizing different tumor antigens with VEGFR2 was constructed. A DNA fragment (HSV) encoding the C terminal 37 amino acids of human chorionic gonadotropin β chain (hCGβ), 5 different HLA-restricted cytotoxic T lymphocyte epitopes from human survivin and the third and fourth extracellular domains of VEGFR2 was inserted into the sequence between the luminal and transmembrane domain of human lysosome-associated membrane protein-1 cDNA for the construction of a novel DNA vaccine (p-L/HSV) [37]. Vaccination of the mice with p-L/HSV elicited potent and long-lasting cellular and humoral immune responses to the specific antigens and showed a prominent anti-tumor effect on the LL/2 lung carcinoma model in syngeneic C57BL/6 mice. In addition, the tumor vasculature was abrogated as observed by immunohistochemistry in p-L/HSV immunized mice [37]. These data indicates that the strategies of combining anti-tumor with anti-angiogenesis cooperate well. Such a study may shed new light on the designing of vaccine for cancer in the future.

Again in 2012, a *Bifidobacterium infantis*-based vaccine that express human extracellular domain of VEGFR2 (sKDR) was established [38]. Immunization of the mice with the *Bifidobacterium infantis*-based vaccine through caudal vein could significantly suppress the tumor growth and prolong the survival of the tumor-bearing mice. On the other hand, this immunization strategy could significantly increase the tumor necrosis, and obviously decrease microvessel density and the blood flow signals in tumor [38].

2.1.2.2. FGFR-1

Fibroblast growth factor receptor-1 (FGFR-1) is expressed on endothelial cells and many types of tumors [39, 40]. The Xenopus homologue of FGFR-1 is 80% and 74% identical at the amino acid level with mouse FGFR-1 and human FGFR-1, respectively [41]. Therefore, FGFR-1 may be used as another ideal target for anti-angiogenesis therapy. Vaccination with Xenopus FGFR-1 (pxFR1) provoked protective and therapeutic effects in three murine tumor models, including Meth A fibrosarcoma cells, H22 hepatoma cells, and MA782/5S mammary carcinoma [41]. FGFR-1-specific autoantibodies were detected in sera of pxFR1-immunized mice by Western blot analysis, and the purified immunoglobulins effectively inhibited endothelial cell proliferation *in vitro* [41]. However, the immunoglobulins had no direct inhibitory effect on the proliferation of above three tumor cell lines [41]. Adoptive transfer of sera or purified immunoglobulin isolated from pxFR1-immunized mice into unimmunized mice provided effective protection against tumor growth, while adsorption of sera or immunoglobulin with FGFR-1-positive endothelial cells before adoptive transfer could abrogate its anti-tumor activity [41]. Autoantibodies deposited on the endothelial cells within tumor tissues and significantly suppressed intratumoral angiogenesis were found in pxFR1-immunized mice by histological examination [41]. Furthermore, this anti-tumor activity and production of FGFR-1-specific autoantibodies were abrogated by depletion of $CD4^+$ T lymphocytes, again pointing to their essential helper function for antibody production [41].

2.1.2.3. Integrins

Integrins are heterodimeric transmembrane proteins consisting of α and β subunits with large extracellular domain and short cytoplasmic tail. They play very crucial roles in angiogenesis as the migration of endothelial cells is dependent on their adhesion to extracellular matrix proteins such as vitronectin [42]. $\alpha v\beta 3$ is not generally found on blood vessels in normal tissues, but its expression is enhanced on newly developing blood vessels in human wound tissue, tumors, diabetic retinopathy, macular degeneration and rheumatoid arthritis, which implies that this integrin may play an important role in angiogenesis and development of neovascularization [42]. This distributive characteristic also makes $\alpha v\beta 3$ an attractive target for tumor therapy [42]. A plasmid DNA encoding the ligand-binding domain of chicken integrin $\beta 3$ was constructed to test this assumption. Immunization with chicken homologous integrin $\beta 3$-based vaccine could elicit both protective and therapeutic anti-tumor immunity in murine tumor models with Meth A fibrosarcoma, H22 hepatoma, or MA782/5S mammary carcinoma [43]. Autoantibodies against integrin $\beta 3$ in sera of the immunized mice were found by Western blot analysis and ELISA [43]. The purified immunoglobulins could effectively inhibit endothelial cell proliferation *in vitro*, and adoptive transfer of the purified immunoglobulins into non-immunized mice could provide effective protection against tumor growth and markedly inhibit tumor angiogenesis [43]. The anti-tumor activity and the production of integrin $\beta 3$-specific autoantibodies were $CD4^+$ T lymphocyte-dependent [43].

2.1.2.4. MMP

Angiogenesis is an invasive process, requiring proteolysis of the extracellular matrix [44]. Inappropriate destruction of extracellular matrix components is involved in certain pathological conditions, including arteriosclerosis, rheumatoid arthritis, and tumor aggression and metastasis [44]. The matrix metalloproteinases (MMPs), a family of extracellular endopeptidases, can selectively degrade components of the extracellular matrix [44]. *In vivo*, elevated stromal MMP-2 and MMP-9 activity is highly correlated with increased metastatic potential in most malignant tumors [45]. Increased activity of MMPs appears to permit the tumor to remodel its surrounding microenvironment, to grow in a permissive space, and to promote the development of supporting stroma, including angiogenesis [46]. Moreover, numerous pathological and clinical studies demonstrated that the MMPs were frequently overexpressed in various solid tumor cells and peritumoral stromal cells [46]. It was reported that the abrogation of MMP-2 alone resulted in the inhibition of the transition from the prevascular to the vascular stage during tumor development and then of tumor growth [47]. Furthermore, the suppression of tumor-induced angiogenesis and of invasion and metastasis of tumor cells could be observed in MMP-2-deficient mice [47]. These findings indicated that MMP-2 alone played an important role in angiogenesis and tumor growth. Sequence comparison analysis showed that the primary sequence of mouse MMP-2 at the amino acid level was 82% and 91% identical with chicken and human homologues, respectively [48]. It was reported that the plasmid DNA vaccination with chicken homologous MMP-2 (c-MMP-2)-based model antigen could induce both protective and therapeutic anti-tumor immunity in murine tumor models with LL/2 Lewis lung carcinoma, Meth A fibrosarcoma, and H22 hepatoma [48]. The elevation of MMP-2 in the sera of tumor-bearing mice was abrogated with the vaccination of c-MMP-2 [48]. The autoimmune response against MMP-2 may be provoked in a cross-reaction by the immunization with c-MMP-2, and the autoantibody targeting to MMP-2 was elevated and probably responsible for the anti-tumor activity [48]. Moreover, gelatinase activity of MMP-2, including both latent MMP-2 and active MMP-2, derived from the above mentioned three murine tumor models was apparently inhibited by the vaccination with c-MMP-2 [48]. However, the vaccination did not inhibit the gelatinase activity of MMP-9 [48]. These findings indicate that the activity of MMP-2 is impaired by immunization with c-MMP-2 in mice. Angiogenesis was apparently inhibited within tumors in immunized mice. The anti-tumor activity and production of auto-antibodies against MMP-2 were abrogated by depletion of $CD4^{+}$ T lymphocytes [48].

2.1.2.5. xRHAMM

In 2010, Yang et al. [49] used a cross-reactive serological expression cloning (SEREX) strategy (CR-SEREX) to identify novel xenogenic angiogenesis- and tumor-associated antigens in oocytes of *Xenopus laevis* and found that *Xenopus* receptor for hyaluronic-acid-mediated motility (xRHAMM) was the most frequently clone among 78 CR-SEREX positive clones, suggesting that xRHAMM has the strongest immunogenic potential for xenogenic immunotherapy. It was demonstrated that expression of RHAMM is restricted to the testis, thymus, placenta, vascular endothelial cells, and various cancer cells, and RHAMM functions in vascular endothelial cell migration, angiogenesis, and in hyaluronic-acid-induced cell mobility [50]. In order to examine the anti-angiogenic effects, a DNA vaccine based on xRHAMM (pcDNA3.1-xRHAMM) was constructed [49]. Intramuscular vaccination of the cationic liposome encapsulated pcDNA3.1-xRHAMM DNA effectively induced a protective anti-tumor immunity against local tumor and lung metastasis in B16 melanoma mouse models. Angiogenesis was inhibited and cell apoptosis was increased within tumors. Anti-tumor activity of xRHAMM was mediated by both the antigen-specific cellular and humoral responses against RHAMM, as confirmed by the depletion of immune cell subsets *in vivo*. Furthermore, the anti-angiogenic and anti-tumor effects induced by vaccination of pcDNA3.1-xRHAMM were significantly stronger than that induced by vaccination of the corresponding autologous counterpart pcDNA3.1-mRHAMM [49].

2.1.2.6. DLL4

Notch signaling has recently emerged as a critical regulator of developmental and tumor angiogenesis. Notch signaling in both endothelial and smooth muscle cells appears to provide critical regulatory information to these cells downstream of the initiating signal induced by VEGF [51, 52]. Studies in humans and mice have demonstrated that Notch ligand delta-like 4 (DLL4) is strongly expressed by the tumor vasculature and generally not by the tumor cells themselves. In various mouse models, strong DLL4 expression was observed in the majority of tumor vessels, contrasting with significantly lower vascular expression in adjacent normal tissues [51]. In humans, DLL4 expression was analyzed in tumors from kidney, bladder, colon, brain and breast [53, 54]. Robust DLL4 expression was observed specifically in the tumor vasculature in all of these tumor types, whereas DLL4 expression was low to undetectable in the vasculature of adjacent normal tissue. Furthermore, at least in the case of breast cancer, the degree of DLL4 expression correlated with outcome: tumors with high DLL4 in the vasculature progressed more rapidly [54]. These findings suggest that DLL4 is an attractive new therapeutic anti-angiogenesis target. To generate the DLL4 plasmid vaccine, the cDNA encoding human DLL4 was cloned into the pVAX1 expression vector (DLL4 vaccine), which is specifically designed for the development of DNA vaccines and approved for use in humans. Immunization of Balb/c mice with DLL4 vaccine could bring about a break in tolerance against the self-antigen, DLL4. Readily detectable titers of serum antibodies against DLL4 were induced. Moreover, immunization with DLL4-encoding plasmid DNA severely retarded the growth of orthotopically implanted D2F2/E2 mammary carcinomas in mice by induction of a non-productive angiogenic response. In addition to the promising therapeutic effects, no evidence for a delayed wound healing response, or for toxicity associated with pharmacological blockade of DLL4 signaling, was observed in mice immunized with the DLL4 vaccine [55].

2.1.2.7. Angiomotin

Angiomotin (Amot), one of angiostatin receptors [56], is a membrane-associated protein present on the endothelial cell surface of angiogenic tissues [57] characterized by conserved coiledcoil and carboxy termini-PDZ domains [58]. A shorter Amot isoform (p80) confers a hyper-migratory and invasive phenotype in transfected cells [59] and induces endothelial cell migration during angiogenesis [60]. The longer (p130) isoform localizes to tight junctions, regulates cell shape and appears to play a role in the later phase of angiogenesis [60]. It was demonstrated that increased Amot expression on tumor endothelia concomitant with the progression from pre-neoplastic lesions to full-fledged carcinoma, therefore, plasmid vaccine encoding human p80 Amot (pAmot) was constructed [57]. Immunization of mice with pAmot can overcome immune tolerance and induce a significant antibody response that mimic the effect of angiostatin. These antibodies inhibit endothelial cell migration, block tumor cell- and bFGF-induced angiogenesis in the matrigel plug assay and prevent growth of transplanted tumors without impairing normal stromal or retina vessels [57]. Very recently, Arigoni et al. further showed that the pAmot-induced antibodies alter tumor vessel permeability and structure. These combined effects of vaccine-induced anti-Amot antibodies lead to inhibition of established clinically evident mammary tumors, massive tumor perivascular necrosis, and an effective tumor antigen presentation in a form of epitope spreading that induces an immune response against other oncoantigens overexpressed by tumor cells [61]. Greater tumor vessel permeability also markedly boosts the local accumulation of doxorubicin and enhances the anti-tumor effect of the drugs [61]. These data provide a rationale for the development of fresh anticancer treatments based on anti-Amot vaccination in conjunction with chemotherapy regimens.

Taken together, it is obvious that vaccination with xenogeneic homologous molecules associated with angiogenesis, such as pro-angiogenic factors, integrins, MMP, could induce anti-tumor immunity and thus might be a feasible strategy for cancer therapy with potential clinical applications.

2.2. Anti-angiogenic active immunotherapies based on non-xenogeneic homologous molecules

Given that vaccination with xenogeneic homologous molecules associated with tumor angiogenesis could effectively induce anti-tumor immunity, it can be assumed that vaccines based on non-xenogeneic homologous molecules, such as allogeneic homologues of some pro-angiogenic factors or other important molecules associated with angiogenesis, could also successfully induce specific and potent anti-tumor immunity. To date, several vaccines based on non-xenogeneic homologous molecules were used in anti-angiogenic active immunotherapy for tumors.

2.2.1. VEGFR-2

As has been discussed above, VEGF-mediated signaling pathway through VEGFR-2 is a rate-limiting step during tumor angiogenesis. Thus, VEGF/VEGFR-2 is still an ideal target in the non-xenogeneic homologous molecules-based anti-angiogenic strategy. Immunization of mice with VEGF receptor-2 (flk-1)-pulsed dendritic cells (DC) can break self-tolerance to VEGFR-2, induce CTL and antibody responses to VEGFR-2 [62]. Significant inhibition of tumor growth and metastasis was observed in both melanoma and Lewis lung carcinoma metastasis murine models [62]. Oral administration of mice with DNA vaccines encoding murine VEGFR-2 carried by attenuated *Salmonella typhimurium* could break the immune tolerance to VEGFR-2, induce CTL response to VEGFR-2, inhibit tumor cell-induced neoangiogenesis, and suppress the formation of spontaneous and experimental pulmonary metastases, with slight impact on wounds healing and no influence on hematopoiesis and pregnancy [63]. Immunization of mice with flk1-encoding mRNA-transfected DC could induce specific CTL response to VEGFR-2, partially inhibit the tumor cell-induced neoangiogenesis, and suppress tumor growth and metastasis in murine B16/F10.9 melanoma and MBT-2 bladder tumor models [64]. We studied the regulatory effects of IFN-γ on the differentiation and development of DC and found that IFN-γ is an autocrine mediator for DC maturation [65]. IFN-γ gene transfection could promote differentiation, development, and functional maturation of DC [66]. IFN-γ gene-modified DC had increased capacity to induce Th1 type immune response, and intratumoral injection of IFN-γ gene-modified DC in a murine model with pre-established B16 melanoma resulted in the potentiation of the anti-tumor effect of DC [66]. On the other hand, it was demonstrated that IFN-γ itself is also a negative regulator of neoangiogenesis [67]. In order to combine the anti-angiogenic immunotherapy with the cytokine immunotherapy, we constructed recombinant plasmid expressing murine VEGFR-2 extracellular domain (sVEGFR-2) and IFN-γ fusion protein, pcDNA3.1/sVEGFR-2-IFN-γ, and found that the fusion protein expressed by recombinant plasmid shared biological activities of both sVEGFR-2 and IFN-γ [68]. Immunization of mice with murine sVEGFR-2-IFN-γ fusion gene-transfected DC could significantly augment the CTL response to murine VEGFR-2 and pronouncedly inhibit tumor cell-induced angiogenensis and tumor metastasis in comparison with murine sVEGFR2 gene-transfected DC [68].

In 2006, three CTL epitope candidates, designated as KDR1, KDR2 and KDR3, respectively, from VEGFR-2 with high binding affinity to the H-2D^{b} molecule were predicted by two computer programs: Bimas and SYFPEITH [69]. Two of them, KDR2 and KDR3, were from the extracellular domain; KDR1 was from the intracellular part of the receptor [69]. Immunization of mice with KDR2 or KDR3 peptide in combination with murine GM-CSF and agonist anti-mouse CD40 antibodies as adjuvant could break self-tolerance and induce specific immune responses in C57BL/6 mice [69]. Furthermore, immunization of mice with these two peptide epitopes elicited pronounced specific CTL responses to murine VEGFR-2, effectively inhibited VEGF-induced angiogenesis, and suppressed tumor growth in MC38 murine colon cancer model [69]. Similarly, the epitope peptides of human VEGFR-2 restricted by HLA-A*0201 and HLA-A*2402 were also identified by analyzing the binding affinities to the corresponding HLA molecules [70]. Antigen based on the epitope peptide with high binding affinity to human HLA-A*0201 could successfully induce specific CTL response *in vitro* [70]. Furthermore, transgenic mice expressing HLA-A*0201, A2/Kb, were generated, and the vascular endothelial cells in that mice could not only express human VEGFR-2 (KDR), but also express human MHC class I molecules [70]. After inoculation of A2/Kb with HLA-A*0201 restricted VEGFR-2 epitope peptide, specific IFN-γ-expressed CTL was induced [70]. Immunization of tumor-bearing A2/Kb transgenic mice with VEGFR-2 epitope peptide could markedly inhibit tumor-induced angiogenesis, hereby inhibiting tumor growth in MC38 colon cancer and B16 melanoma models, and prolong survival of the tumor-bearing animals without fatal adverse effects [70]. To further study whether specific CTL response to KDR can be elicited in human or not, KDR epitope peptide vaccines were used to stimulate peripheral blood mononuclear cells derived from 6 cancer patients *in vitro*, and CTLs specific for the peptide epitope were successfully induced in all patients [70].

In comparison with the full-length protein, peptide vaccines like the aforementioned KDR epitope peptides can be easily synthesized in high purity and are less expensive. Moreover, immunization with such vaccines could avoid the potential dangers involving induction of an infection by recombinant viruses or exposure to a latently allergenic exogenous protein.

In 2009, Seavey, et al developed *Listeria monocytogens* based VEGFR-2 vaccines that encode the peptide of VEGFR-2 extracellular domain fused to the first 441 residues of the microbial adjuvant listeriolysin O (*Lm*-LLO-Flk-E1 and *Lm*-LLO-Flk-E2) and the peptide of VEGFR-2 intracellular domain that also fused to LLO (*Lm*-LLO-Flk-I1), respectively [71, 72]. Immunization of the mice with the *Listeria*-based Flk1 vaccines elicited potent antitumor CTL responses. Lm-LLO-Flk-1 was able to eradicate some established Her-2/neu$^+$ breast tumors, reduce microvascular density in the remaining tumors, protect against tumor rechallenge and experimental metastases, and induce epitope spreading to various regions of the tumor-associated antigen Her-2/neu. Tumor eradication was found to be dependent on epitope spreading to Her-2/neu and was not solely due to the reduction of tumor vasculature [71]. In an autochthonous model for Her-2/neu+ breast cancer, theses vaccines could significantly delay tumor onset, while tumors that grew out overtime accumulated mutations in the Her-2/neu molecule near or within CTL epitopes [72]. Moreover, vaccine efficacy did not affect normal wound healing nor have toxic side effects on pregnancy [71]. These data suggest that an anti-angiogenesis vaccine can overcome tolerance to the host vasculature driving epitope spreading to an endogenous tumor protein and drive active tumor regression.

Recently, a DNA vaccine (pSG.SS.Flk-1_{ECD}.C3d3) encoding Flk-1 extracellular domain and the complement fragment C3d fusion protein was constructed [73]. Vaccination of mice with pSG.SS.Flk-1_{ECD}.C3d3 could also elicit Flk-1 specific antibody response, leading to suppression of angiogenesis and tumor growth in bladder translational cell carcinoma mouse model, suggesting that C3d can be used as an adjuvant to enhance the immune response [73].

In 2010, Miyazawa, et al. [74] reported the results of phase I clinical trial combining of epitope peptide for VEGFR-2 (VEGFR2-169) with gemcitabine for patients with advanced pancreatic cancer. 18 HLA-A*2402-positive patients with metastatic and unresectable pancreatic cancer were enrolled in the trial. Gemcitabine was administered at a dose of 1000 mg/m^2 on days 1, 8, and 15 in a 28-day cycle. The VEGFR2-169 peptide was subcutaneously injected weekly in a dose-escalation manner (doses of 0.5, 1, and 2 mg/body, six patients/one cohort). Safety and immunological parameters were assessed. No severe adverse effect of grade 4 or higher was observed. Of the 18 patients who completed at least one course of the treatment, 15 (83%) developed immunological reactions at the injection sites. VEGFR2-169 specific CTLs were induced in 11 (61%) of the 18 patients. The disease control rate was 67%, and the median overall survival time was 8.7 months. This combination therapy for pancreatic cancer patients was tolerable at all doses. Peptide-specific CTL could be induced by the VEGFR2-169 peptide vaccine at a high rate, even in combination with gemcitabine. Therefore, they suggested that the optimal dose for further clinical trials might be 2 mg/body or higher.

2.2.2. *bFGF*

Basic fibroblast growth factor (bFGF/FGF2) is an important proangiogenic factor, which is secreted by tumor cells and macrophages or released by extracelluar matrix, and functions in the autocrine or paracrine manner. FGF2 can upregulate the expression of several dominant pro-angiogenic factors, such as VEGF [75], and activator of plasminogen [76], and inhibit apoptosis of endothelial cells by bcl-2 pathway [77]. bFGF exerts its biological activities through its binding to high affinity receptor, fibroblast growth factor receptor-1 (FGFR1). It was found that both peptide segments of synthetic human FGF2 heparin-binding structural domain and receptor-binding structural domain could inhibit the *in vitro* proliferation of human umbilical vein endothelial cells [39]. Immunization of mice with vaccine based on heparin-binding structural domain peptide could induce production of anti-FGF2 specific antibody, which could hamper the binding of FGF2 to heparin sulphate, and inhibit tumor-induced angiogenesis in a gelatin sponge model and tumor growth in a tumor metastatic model [39]. Surprisingly, despite an immune response toward FGF2, this modality of treatment did not affect wound healing as shown by the fact that the treatment did not alter the mean time of wound healing [78]. It also did not affect fertility, because the vaccinated females were not impaired in their ability to become pregnant, to support the growth and development of their embryos, and to deliver viable offspring when compared with control animals [78]. Furthermore, histological analyses did not reveal any alterations in organogenesis in these offsprings [78]. Therefore, the authors concluded that although vaccination against FGF2 induced a specific FGF2 antibody response and inhibited angiogenesis and tumor development in a pathological setting, it did not adversely alter normal physiological events dependent on FGF2.

2.2.3. EGFR

Epidermal growth factor receptor (EGFR), a membrane surface sensor with tyrosine kinase activity, is widely distributed on the membrane of mammalian cells [79]. In the physiological condition, EGFR exerts, through binding to ligands (epidermal growth factor, EGF), its physiological activities in regulation of cell division, proliferation and differentiation [79]. Results from clinical studies show that high expression level of EGFR is frequently observed in non-small cell lung cancer, and has been implicated in aggressive biological behavior of tumor cells and poor prognosis of tumor patients [79]. Therefore, immunotherapy targeting EGFR should be another attractive approach to the treatment of EGFR-positive tumors. In murine tumor models with Lewis lung carcinoma and mammary cancer, immunization of mice with DC pulsed with recombinant ectodomain of mouse EGFR (DC-edMER) inhibited tumor angiogenesis, reduced tumor growth, and prolonged the survival of tumor-bearing mice [80]. Spleen cells isolated from DC-edMER-immunized mice showed a high frequency of EGFR-specific antibody-producing cells [80]. Anti-EGFR specific antibody was markedly elevated in sera of immunized mice and was shown to be effective against tumor growth by adoptive transfer [80]. Immunization with DC-edMER vaccine also elicited CTL responses [80]. Depletion of $CD4^+$ T lymphocytes could completely abrogate the anti-tumor activity and generation of EGFR-specific antibody responses, whereas depletion of $CD8^+$ T lymphocytes showed partial abrogation of the anti-tumor activity but antibody was still detected [80]. Furthermore, tumor-induced angiogenesis was suppressed in DC-edMER-immunized mice or mice treated with antibody adoptive transfer [80]. These findings indicate that vaccination with DC-edMER can induce both humoral and cellular anti-tumor immunity, and may suggest novel strategies for the treatment of EGFR-positive tumors through the induction of active immunity against EGFR [80].

2.2.4. *Legumain*

Tumor associated macrophages (TAMs) are well known to play a very important role in tumor angiogenesis and metastasis, as the abrogation of TAMs in tumor tissues effectively reduced several pro-tumor growth and angiogenesis factors, such as VEGF, TGF-β, TNF-α and MMP-9 [81]. Thus, the suppression of TAMs in the tumor-microenvironment provides a novel strategy to inhibit tumor growth and dissemination by remodeling the tumor's stroma. Legumain is an asparaginyl endopeptidase and a member of the C13 family of cystine proteases which was found to be highly upregulated in many murine and human tumor tissues and, furthermore, also overexpressed on TAMs in the murine tumor stroma, but absent or present at only very low levels in all normal tissues from which such tumors arose [81-84]. Recently, several oral minigene vaccines against murine MHC class I antigen epitopes of Legumain were constructed based on the binding predictions for these MHC class I molecules by the HLA peptide binding predictions program [85]. Expression vectors encoding these epitopes were designated as pLegu-H-2D^d and pLegu-H-2K^d respectively [85]. Oral administration of those vaccines by transforming them into attenuated Salmonella typhimurium (Dam$^-$, AroA$^-$) resulted in significant suppression of angiogenesis in tumor tissues of D2F2 breast carcinoma in syngeneic BALB/c mice [85]. The possible mechanism of angiogenic inhibition involved the induction of a specific CTL response capable of killing Legumain positive cells, especially TAMs, which is likely to be responsible for anti-tumor angiogenesis [85]. Generally, the anti-angiogenic effect aided in the protection of BALB/c mice from lethal challenges with D2F2 breast tumor cells in a prophylactic setting [85].

2.2.5. *Endoglin (CD105)*

Endoglin, a 95 kDa cell surface protein expressed as a homodimer, functions as an accessory protein for kinase receptor complexes of the TGF-β superfamily and modulates TGF-β signaling [8]. Expression of CD105 is correlated with vascular density and poor prognosis [8]. Endoglin is over-expressed on proliferating endothelial cells in the breast tumor neovasculature and thus offers a target for anti-angiogenic therapy [8]. It was reported that an oral murine endoglin-encoding DNA vaccine carried by double attenuated Salmonella typhimurium (dam$^-$, AroA$^-$) to a secondary lymphoid organ, i.e., Peyer's patches, resulted in activation of antigen-presenting dendritic cells, induction of immune responses mediated by CD8$^+$ T cells against endoglin-positive target cells, and suppression of angiogenesis and dissemination of pulmonary metastases of D2F2 breast carcinoma cells presumably by eliminating proliferating endothelial cells in the tumor vasculature, thus providing an promising strategy to therapies for breast cancer [86]. More recently, Wood et al. [87] developed *Listeria*-based vaccines directed against CD105, Lm-LLO-CD105A and Lm-LLO-CD105B. The region of CD105 in Lm-LLO-CD105A vaccine contains at least three predicted H-2K^d epitopes, while the region of CD105 in Lm-LLO-CD105B contains at least two predicted H-2K^d epitopes. Immunization of the *Listeria*-based vaccines led to therapeutic responses against primary and metastatic tumors in the 4T1-Luc and NT-2 mouse models of breast cancer. In a mouse model for autochthonous Her-2/neu-driven breast cancer, Lm-LLO-CD105A vaccination prevented tumor incidence in 20% of mice by week 58 after birth while all control mice developed tumors by week 40. In comparison with previous *Listeria*-based vaccines (Lm-LLO-HMWMAA-C [88] and Lm-LLO-FLK-I1 and Lm-LLO-FLK-E2 [71]) targeting tumor vasculature, Lm-LLO-CD105A and Lm-LLO-CD105B demonstrated equivalent or superior efficacy against two transplantable mouse models of breast cancer. Mechanism analysis revealed that the anti-tumor therapeutic efficacy of *Listeria*-based CD105 vaccines was mediated by epitope spreading to endogenous tumor antigens and reduction in tumor vascularity [87]. These data suggest that CD105 therapeutic vaccines are highly effective in stimulating anti-angiogenesis and anti-tumor immune responses leading to therapeutic efficacy against primary and metastatic breast cancer.

2.2.6. Endothelial cell lysates-pulsed dendritic cells

Dendritic cells (DCs) are the most potent professional antigen-presenting cells, they play crucial roles in the initiation of an immune response. DCs prepared from BALB/c mouse were pulsed with lysates of autologous or xenogeneic endothelium, and their anti-tumor effects were tested in two syngeneic models of colon cancer [89]. Immunization of endothelium lysates pulsed DCs could induce a break in self tolerance against endothelial cells and mount both the endothelium-specific CTL response and antibody response, leading to significant inhibition of tumor angiogenesis and the growth of subcutaneous tumors as well as pulmonary metastases in mice. Furthermore, the decrease in the mean vascular density of tumors correlates well with the extent of tumor inhibition [89]. Therefore, immunization of endothelium lysates pulsed DCs is also an effective modality of anti-angiogenic active immunotherapy for cancers, and should have important clinical implications for adjuvant cancer therapy.

2.2.7. Endothelial cell vaccine

In 2008, Okaji Y, et al. [90] reported a pilot phase I clinical study in which glutaraldehyde-fixed human umbilical vein endothelial cells (HUVECs) were used as the vaccine. Six patients with recurrent malignant brain tumour and three patients with metastatic colorectal cancer were given intradermal injections of $5x10^7$ HUVECs/dose, first month weekly, and then every 2 weeks (in total 230 vaccinations). ELISA and flow cytometry revealed immunoglobulin response against HUVECs' membrane antigens. ELISPOT and ^{51}Cr-release cytotoxicity assay revealed a specific cellular immune response against HUVECs, which were lysed in an effectors:targets ratio-dependent manner. Gadolinium-contrasted MRI showed partial or complete tumour responses in three malignant brain tumour patients. Except for a DTH-like skin reaction at the injection site, no adverse effect of vaccination was observed. These results suggested that the endothelial vaccine can overcome peripheral tolerance of self-angiogenic antigens in clinical settings, and therefore could be useful for adjuvant immunotherapy of cancer.

3. Concluding remarks

Recent research achievements have disclosed inspiring pragmatic perspectives of anti-angiogenic active immunotherapy for cancers. In comparison with application of angiogenic inhibitors and angiogenic antibodies, anti-angiogenic active immunotherapy has its obvious merits. Provided that a break of immunological tolerance to positive regulators of angiogenesis is successfully induced, the long-lasting immune response to angiogenesis-related molecule will be present in the body, hereby providing long-lasting inhibitory effects on angiogenesis. Therefore, it is expected to be the more cost-effective strategy than angiogenic inhibitor or anti-angiogenic antibody therapy where continuous use of the drugs is needed.

Here we divided anti-angiogenic active immunotherapy into two categories: therapies based on vaccination with xenogeneic homologous molecules and with non-xenogeneic homologous molecules related to angiogenesis. Presently, it is difficult to point out which one is better for clinical application because most of the outcomes reported to date were based on pre-clinical animal experiments. As VEGF-mediated signaling through its receptor VEGFR-2 is the key rate-limiting step in tumor angiogenesis, and plays the most important role in neovascularization, development, and progression of various tumors [6], as well as human VEGFR2-169 peptide vaccination could effectively break peripheral self tolerance against VEGFR-2 in patients with metastatic and unresectable pancreatic cancer [74], anti-angiogenic active immunotherapy targeting VEGF or VEGFR-2 might be the most effective strategy among all these therapies. Moreover, considering the potential clinical application of anti-angiogenic immunotherapy based on the specific antibodies raised against a variety of angiogenesis-associated molecules in different tumor entities like glioma, renal cell cancer, and breast cancer, etc, a promising clinical application of anti-angiogenic active immunotherapy alone or in combination with other anti-tumor strategies could be expected. However, there exist as well *caveats* and deficiencies in this strategy. Firstly, in the early phase of tumor growth when the tumor diameter is less than 2-3 mm, tumor cells simply depend on passive diffusion rather than blood perfusion to acquire enough oxygen and nutrition indispensable for growth. Therefore, anti-angiogenic therapy against tumor in this early stage might be ineffective when applied alone. Secondly, although current anti-angiogenic active immunotherapy is focused on specific targets, potential adverse effects might include impairment of wound healing and menstrual cycle. Furthermore, this approach has also limited application perspectives in children with cancers. Therefore, along with recent developments in molecular biology and immunology, future studies will focus on multiple approaches, such as series analysis of gene expression to analyze the gene expression in normal endothelial cells and in proliferative endothelial cells, phage display technology to search for new endothelial cell receptors, and proteomics to discover peptide segments or proteins regulating endothelial cell growth. These approaches are expected to discover more tumor-specific endothelial cell markers for the purpose of selecting specific targets for anti-angiogenic active immunotherapy. In addition, further studies are also required to optimize protocols how to construct vaccines to effectively break self-tolerance and to induce efficient immune response. With these issues being solved continuously, anti-angiogenic active immunotherapy for cancers will become more applicable and effective.

Acknowledgements

This work was supported by a grant from the Science and Technology Bureau of Hangzhou, Zhejiang Province, P.R. China (No. 20120633B30).

Author details

Jianping Pan* and Lihuang Zhang

*Address all correspondence to: jppan@zucc.edu.cn

Department of Clinical Medicine, Zhejiang University City College School of Medicine, Hangzhou, P.R. China

References

[1] Arbab AS. Activation of alternative pathways of angiogenesis and involvement of stem cells following anti-angiogenesis treatment in glioma. Histol Histopathol 2012; 27: 549-557.

[2] Shojaei F. Anti-angiogenesis therapy in cancer: current challenges and future perspectives. Cancer Lett 2012; 320:130-137.

[3] Hiratsuka S. Vasculogenensis, angiogenesis and special features of tumor blood vessels. Front Biosci 2011; 16:1413-1427.

[4] Blagosklonny MV. Antiangiogenic therapy and tumor progression. Cancer Cell 2004; 5:13-17.

[5] Ferrara N. VEGF and the quest for tumor angiogenesis factors. Nat Rev Cancer 2002; 2:795-803.

[6] Ferrara N, Gerber HP, LeCouter J. The biology of VEGF and its receptors. Nat Med 2003; 6:669-676.

[7] Ferrara N, Kerbel RS. Angiogenesis as a therapeutic target. Nature 2005; 438:967-974.

[8] Hofmeister V, Schrama D, Becker JC, et al. Anti-cancer therapies targeting the tumor stroma. Cancer Immunol Immunother 2008; 57: 1-17.

[9] Shojaei F, Ferrara N. Antiangiogenesis to treat cancer and intraocular neovascular disorders. Lab Invest 2007; 87:227-230.

[10] Veikkola T, Karkkainen M, Claesson-Welsh L, et al. Regulation of angiogenesis via endothelial growth factor receptors. Cancer Rev 2000; 60:203-212.

[11] Caldini R, Barletta E, Del Rosso M, et al. FGF2-mediated upregulation of urokinase-type plasminogen activator expression requires a MAP-kinase dependent activation of poly (ADP-ribose) polymerase. J Cell Physiol 2005; 202: 125-134.

[12] Ferrajoli A, Manshouri T, Estrov Z, et al. High levels of vascular endothelial growth factor receptor-2 correlate with shortened survival in chronic lymphocytic leukemia. Clin Cancer Res 2001; 7:795-799.

[13] Schneider BP, Sledge GW. Drug insight: VEGF as a therapeutic target for breast cancer. Nat Clin Pract Oncol 2007; 4:181-189.

[14] Kanda S, Miyata Y, Kanetake H. Current status and perspective of antiangiogenic therapy for cancer: urinary cancer. Int J Clin Oncol 2006; 11:90-107.

[15] Rini BI, Rathmell WK. Biological aspects and binding strategies of vascular endothelial growth factor in renal cell carcinoma. Clin Cancer Res 2007; 13:741-746.

[16] Kerbel RS, Folkman J. Clinical translation of angiogenesis inhibitors. Nat Rev Cancer 2002; 2:727-739.

[17] Shant K, Li CG. Targeting of vasculature in cancer and other angiogenic diseases. Trends Immunol 20001; 22:129-133.

[18] St Croix B, Rago C, Velculescu V, et al. Genes expressed in human tumor endothelium. Science 2000; 289:1197-1202.

[19] Reisfeld RA, Niethammer AG, Luo Y, et al. DNA vaccines designed to inhibit tumor growth by suppression of angiogenesis. Int Arch Allergy Immunol 2004; 133:295-304.

[20] Hurwitz H, Fehrenbacher L, Novotny W, et al. Bevacizumab plus irinotecan, fluorouracil, and leucovorin for metastatic colorectal cancer. N Engl J Med 2004; 350:2335-2342.

[21] Sandler A, Gray R, Perry MC, et al. Paclitaxel-carboplatin alone or with bevacizumab for non-small-cell lung cancer. N Engl J Med 2006; 355:2542-2550.

[22] Miller K, Wang M, Gralow J, et al. Paclitaxel plus bevacizumab versus paclitaxel alone for metastatic breast cancer. N Engl J Med 2007; 357:2666-2676.

[23] Willett CG, Duda DG, di Tomaso E, et al. Efficacy, safety, and biomarkers of neoadjuvant bevacizumab, radiation therapy, and fluorouracil in rectal cancer: a multidisciplinary phase II study. J Clin Oncol 2009; 27:3020-3026.

[24] Holash J, Davis S, Papadopoulos N, et al. VEGF-Trap: a VEGF blocker with potent antitumor effects. Proc Natl Acad Sci USA 2002; 99:11393-11398.

[25] Kerbel RS. Tumor angiogenesis. N Engl J Med 2008; 358:2039-2049.

[26] Sun Y, Wang J, Liu Y, et al. Results of phase III trial of rh-endostatin (YH-16) in advanced non-small cell lung cancer (NSCLC) patients. J Clin Oncol 2005; 23:654S.

[27] McKeage MJ, Von Pawel J, Reck M, et al. Randomised phase II study of ASA404 combined with carboplatin and paclitaxel in previously untreated advanced non-small cell lung cancer. Br J Cancer 2008; 99:2006-2012.

[28] Kornberg TB, Krasnow MA. The Drosophila genome sequence: implications for biology and medicine. Science 2000; 287: 2218-2220.

[29] Wei YQ, Wang QR, Zhao X, et al. Immunotherapy of tumors with xenogeneic endothelial cells as a vaccine. Nat Med 2000; 6:1160-1166.

[30] Asakage M, Tsuno NH, Kitayama J, et al. Early-outgrowth of endothelial progenitor cells can function as antigen-presenting cells. Cancer Immunol Immunother 2006; 55: 708-716.

[31] Kerbel RS. Tumor angiogenesis: past, present and the near future. Carcinogenesis 2000; 21:505-515.

[32] Wei YQ, Huang MJ, Yang L, et al. Immunogene therapy of tumors with vaccine based on xenopus homologous vascular endothelial growth factors as a model antigen. Pro Natl Acad Sci USA 2001; 98:11545-11550.

[33] Bequet-Romero M, Ayala M, Acevedo BE, et al. Prophylactic naked DNA vaccination with the human vascular endothelial growth factor induces an anti-tumor response in C57Bl/6 mice. Angiogenesis 2007; 10:23-34.

[34] Kamstock D, Elmslie R, Thamm D, et al. Evaluation of a xenogeneic VEGF vaccine in dogs with soft tissue sarcoma. Cancer Immunol Immunother 2007; 56: 1299-1309.

[35] Shalaby F, Rossant J, Yamaguchi TP, et al. Failure of blood-island formation and vasculogenesis in Flk-1-deficient mice. Nature 1995; 376:62-66.

[36] Liu JY, Wei YQ, Yang L, et al. Immunotherapy of tumors with vaccine based on quail homologous vascular endothelial growth factor receptor-2. Blood 2003; 102:1815-1823.

[37] Wei Y, Sun Y, Song C, et al. Enhancement of DNA vaccine efficacy by targeting the xenogeneic human chorionic gonadotropin, survivin and vascular endothelial growth factor receptor 2 combined tumor antigen to the major histocompatibility complex class II pathway. J Gene Med 2012; 14: 353-362.

[38] Li ZJ, Zhu H, Ma BY, et al. Inhibitory effect of Bifidobacterium infantis-mediated sKDR prokaryotic expression system on angiogenesis and growth of Lewis lung cancer in mice. BMC Cancer 2012; 12:155.

[39] Plum SM, Holaday JW, Ruiz A, et al. Administration of a liposomal FGF-2 peptide vaccine leads to abrogation of FGF-2-mediated angiogenesis and tumor development. Vaccine 2000; 19:1294-1303.

[40] Valesky M, Spang AJ, Fisher GW, et al. Noninvasive dynamic fluorescence imaging of human melanomas reveals that targeted inhibition of bFGF or FGFR-1 in melanoma cells blocks tumor growth by apoptosis. Mol Med 2002; 8: 103-112.

[41] He QM, Wei YQ, Tian L, et al. Inhibition of tumor growth with a vaccine based on xenogeneic homologous fibroblast growth factor receptor-1 in mice. J Biol Chem 2003; 278:21831-21836.

[42] Gutheil JC, Campbell TN, Pierce PR, et al. Targeted antiangiogenic therapy for cancer using Vitaxin: a humanized monoclonal antibody to the Integrin αvβ3. Clin Cancer Res 2000; 6:3056-3061.

[43] Lou YY, Wei QY, Yang L, et al. Immunogene therapy of tumors with vaccine based on the ligand binding domain of chick homologous integrin beta3. Immunol Invest 2002; 31:51-69.

[44] William G, Stetler S. Matrix metalloproteinases in angiogenesis: a moving target for therapeutic intervention. J Clin Invest 1999; 103:1237-1241.

[45] Liotta LA, Steeg PS, Stetler-Stevenson WG. Cancer metastasis and angiogenesis: an imbalance of positive and negative regulation. Cell 1991; 64:327-336.

[46] Albini A, Melchiori A, Santi L, et al. Tumor cell invasion inhibited by TIMP-2. J Natl Cancer Inst 1991; 83: 775-779.

[47] Itoh T, Tanioka M, Yoshida H, et al. Reduced angiogenesis and tumor progression in gelatinase A-deficient mice. Cancer Res 1998; 58:1048-1051.

[48] Su JM, Wei YQ, Tian L, et al. Active immunotherapy of cancer with vaccine on the basis of chicken homologous matrix metalloproteinase-2. Cancer Res 2003; 63:600-607.

[49] Yang HS, Zhang DM, Deng HX, et al.Antitumor and anti-angiogenesis immunity induced by CR-SEREX-identified Xenopus RHAMM.Cancer Sci 2010; 101:862-868.

[50] Hardwick C, Hoare K, Owens R, et al. Molecular cloning of a novel hyaluronan receptor that mediates tumor cell motility. J Cell Biol 1992; 117:1343-1350.

[51] Kuhnert F, Kirshner JR, Thurston G. Dll4-Notch signaling as a therapeutic target in tumor angiogenesis.Vasc Cell 2011; 3:20.

[52] Gu JW, Rizzo P, Pannuti A, et al. Notch signals in the endothelium and cancer "stem-like" cells: opportunities for cancer therapy. Vascular Cell 2012; 4: 7.

[53] Ridgway J, Zhang G, Wu Y, et al. Inhibition of Dll4 signalling inhibits tumour growth by deregulating angiogenesis. Nature 2006; 444:1083-1087.

[54] Jubb AM, Soilleux EJ, Turley H, et al. Expression of vascular notch ligand delta-like 4 and inflammatory markers in breast cancer. Am J Pathol 2010; 176:2019-2028.

[55] Haller BK, Bråve A, Wallgard E, et al. Therapeutic efficacy of a DNA vaccine targeting the endothelial tip cell antigen delta-like ligand 4 in mammary carcinoma. Oncogene 2010; 29:4276-4286.

[56] Troyanovsky B, Levchenko T, Månsson G, et al. Angiomotin: an angiostatin binding protein that regulates endothelial cell migration and tube formation. J Cell Biol. 2001; 152: 1247-1254.

[57] Holmgren L, Ambrosino E, Birot O, et al. A DNA vaccine targeting angiomotin inhibits angiogenesis and suppresses tumor growth. Proc Natl Acad Sci USA 2006; 103: 9208-9213.

[58] Bratt A, Wilson WJ, Troyanovsky B, et al. Angiomotin belongs to a novel protein family with conserved coiled-coil and PDZ binding domains. Gene 2002; 298:69-77.

[59] Levchenko T, Bratt A, Arbiser JL, et al. Angiomotin expression promotes hemangioendothelioma invasion. Oncogene 2004; 23:1469-1473.

[60] Ernkvist M, Birot O, Sinha I, et al. Differential roles of p80- and p130-angiomotin in the switch between migration and stabilization of endothelial cells. Biochim Biophys Acta 2008; 1783: 429-437.

[61] Arigoni M, Barutello G, Lanzardo S, et al. A vaccine targeting angiomotin induces an antibody response which alters tumor vessel permeability and hampers the growth of established tumors. Angiogenesis 2012; 15:305-316.

[62] Li Y, Wang MN, Li H, et al. Active immunization against the vascular endothelial growth factor receptor flk1 inhibits tumor angiogenesis and metastasis. J Exp Med 2002; 195: 1575-1584.

[63] Nithammer AG, Xiang R, Becker JC, et al. A DNA vaccine against VEGF receptor 2 prevents effective angiogenesis and inhibits tumor growth. Nat Med 2002; 8:1369-1375.

[64] Nair S, Boczkowski D, Moeller B, et al. Synergy between tumor immunotherapy and antiangiogenic therapy. Blood 2003; 102: 964-971.

[65] Pan J, Zhang M, Wang J, et al. Interferon-gamma is an autocrine mediator for dendritic cell maturation. Immunol Lett 2004; 94:141-151.

[66] Pan J, Zhang M, Wang J, et al. Intratumoral injection of interferon-gamma genemodified dendritic cells elicits potent antitumor effects: effective induction of tumorspecific CD8+ CTL response. J Cancer Res Clin Oncol 2005; 131:468-478.

[67] Qin Z, Blankenstein T. CD4+ T cell-mediated tumor rejection involves inhibition of angiogenesis that is dependent on IFN gamma receptor expression by nonhematopoietic cells. Immunity 2000; 12:677-686.

[68] Pan J, Heiser A, Marget M, et al. Enhanced antimetastatic effect of fetal liver kinase 1 extracellular domain and interferon-gamma fusion gene-modified dendritic cell vaccine. Gene Ther 2005; 12:742-750.

[69] Dong Y, Qian J, Ramy I, et al. Identification of H-2D^b-specific CD8$^+$ T-cell epitopes from mouse VEGFR2 that can inhibit angiogenesis and tumor growth. J Immunother 2006; 29:32-40.

[70] Wada S, Tsunoda T, Baba T, et al. Rationale for antiangiogenic cancer therapy with vaccination using epitope peptides derived from human vascular endothelial growth factor 2. Cancer Res 2005; 65:4939-4946.

[71] Seavey MM, Maciag PC, Al-Rawi N, et al. An anti-vascular endothelial growth factor receptor 2/fetal liver kinase-1 Listeria monocytogenes anti-angiogenesis cancer vaccine for the treatment of primary and metastatic Her-2/neu+ breast tumors in a mouse model. J Immunol 2009; 182(9):5537-5546.

[72] Seavey MM, Paterson Y. Anti-Angiogenesis immunotherapy induces epitope spreading to Her-2/neu resulting in breast tumor immunoediting. Breast Cancer 2009; 1:19-30.

[73] Liang PH, Zhang KQ, Xu GL, et al. Construction of a DNA vaccine encoding Flk-1 extracellular domain and C3d fusion gene and investigation of its suppressing effect on tumor growth. Cancer Immunol Immunother 2010; 59:93-101.

[74] Miyazawa M, Ohsawa R, Tsunoda T, et al. Phase I clinical trial using peptide vaccine for human vascular endothelial growth factor receptor 2 in combination with gemcitabine for patients with advanced pancreatic cancer. Cancer Sci 2008; 101:433-439.

[75] Tokuda H, Kozawa O, Uematsu T, et al. Basic fibroblast growth factor stimulates vascular endothelial growth factor release in osteoblasts: divergent regulation by p44/p42 mitogen-activated protein kinase and p38 mitogen-activated protein kinase. J Bone Miner Res 2000; 15: 2371-2379.

[76] Dias S, Hattori K, Zhu Z, et al. Autocrine stimulation of VEGFR-2 activates human leukemic cell growth and migration. J Clin Invest 2000; 106: 511-521.

[77] Karsan A, Yee E, Poirier GG, et al. Fibroblast growth factor-2 inhibits endothelial cell apoptosis by Bcl-2-dependent and independent mechanisms. Am J Pathol 1997; 151:1775-1784.

[78] Plum SM, Vu HA, Mercer B, et al. Generation of a specific immunological response to FGF-2 does not affect wound healing or reproduction. Immunopharmacol Immunotoxicol 2004; 26:29-41.

[79] Harari PM. Epidermal growth factor receptor inhibition strategies in oncology. Endocr Relat Cancer 2004; 11: 689-708.

[80] Hu B, Wei YQ, Tian L, et al. Active antitumor immunity elicited by vaccine based on recombinant form of epidermal growth factor receptor. J Immunother 2005; 28:236-244.

[81] Luo Y, Zhou H, Krueger J, et al. Targeting tumor-associated macrophages as a novel strategy against breast cancer. J Clin Invest 2006; 116:2132-2141.

[82] Liu C, Sun C, Huang H, et al. Overexpression of legumain in tumors is significant for invasion / metastasis and a candidate enzymatic target for prodrug therapy. Cancer Res 2003; 63:2957-2964.

[83] Murthy RV, Arbman G, Gao J, et al. Legumain expression in relation to clinicopathologic and biological variables in colorectal cancer. Clin Cancer Res 2005; 11:2293-2299.

[84] Oosterling SJ, van der Bij GJ, Meijer GA, et al. Macrophages direct tumor histology and clinical outcome in a colon cancer model. J Pathol 2005; 207:147-155.

[85] Lewen S, Zhou H, Hu HD, et al. A Legumain-based minigene vaccine targets the tumor stroma and suppresses breast cancer growth and angiogenesis. Cancer Immunol Immunother 2008; 57:507-515.

[86] Lee SH, Mizutani N, Mizutani M, et al. Endoglin (CD105) is a target for an oral DNA vaccine against breast cancer. Cancer Immunol Immunother 2006; 55:1565-1574.

[87] Wood LM, Pan ZK, Guirnalda P, et al. Targeting tumor vasculature with novel Listeria-based vaccines directed against CD105. Cancer Immunol Immunother 2011; 60:931-942.

[88] Maciag PC, Seavey MM, Pan ZK, et al. Cancer immunotherapy targeting the high molecular weight melanoma-associated antigen protein results in a broad antitumor response and reduction of pericytes in the tumor vasculature. Cancer Res 2008; 68: 8066-8075.

[89] Yoneyama S, Okaji Y, Tsuno NH, et al. A study of dendritic and endothelial cell interactions in colon cancer in a cell line and small mammal model. Eur J Surg Oncol 2007; 33:1191-1198.

[90] Okaji Y, Tsuno NH, Tanaka M, et al. Pilot study of anti-angiogenic vaccine using fixed whole endothelium in patients with progressive malignancy after failure of conventional therapy. Eur J Cancer 2008; 44:383-390.

Section 4

Multidisciplinarity in Cancer Therapy: Nutrition and Beyond

Chapter 17

Nutrigenomics and Cancer Prevention

Júlio César Nepomuceno

Additional information is available at the end of the chapter

http://dx.doi.org/10.5772/55429

1. Introduction

Cancer is fundamentally a genetic disease. At the beginning of the process is an alteration in the DNA of a single cell. This change in DNA can be caused by several factors, chemical, physical or biological phenomena. The stage of promotion is the second stage of carcinogenesis. The genetically altered cells, ie, "initiated," suffer the effects of carcinogens classified as oncopromotores. The initiated cell is transformed into a malignant cell, a slow and gradual process. For this transformation to occur, you need a long and continuous contact with the carcinogen promoter. The stage of progression is the third and final stage and is characterized by uncontrolled proliferation of cells and irreversibly changed. At this stage cancer is already installed, progressing to the emergence of the first clinical manifestations of the disease [1]. In this sense, the diet plays a key role in various stages of cancer development. The process of carcinogenesis may be affected by nutritional factors through mechanisms that promote or inhibit its development. Some foods can contain not only carcinogens, but also other substances that act to reduce the damage to the cell's genetic material caused by environmental mutagens. The observation of cancer in an individual does not identify the causative agent(s). However, epidemiological data on populations do indicate that a large fraction of human cancers are associated with lifestyle/ diet. Such studies may also help identify the etiologic agents but unless there are good dose-response data for humans and/or animal models, the probability of identifying the agent is not high. Cancers may result from endogenous reactions, such as oxidations or from exogenous agents, such as tobacco smoke (lung cancer), sunlight exposure (skin cancer), aflatoxin (liver cancer), and relatively high doses of ionizing radiations (many types of cancers) [2].

The importance of nutrition in health is not a new idea. More than two thousand years ago, Hippocrates, the father of Western medicine, wrote: "Let food be thy medicine and medicine be thy food." What has changed since the time of Hippocrates is our understanding of the details of how nutrition affects our health. Researchers are getting more knowledge as to what foods or bioactive food compounds and how they can interact with our bodies promoting health. The Human Genome Project was one of the key factors that enable the study of gene-food interactions and promotion of health. Discoveries in genetics make it possible to understand the effects of nutrients in processes at the molecular level in the body and also the variable effects of dietary components on each individual. Research has shown that the nutrients affect gene expression and formation of several proteins that are important in the formation and maintenance of tissues. So, faced with this interaction genomics and nutrition, emerges Nutrigenomics aiming to understand the functions of all genes and their interactions with food, in order to promote health and reduce the risk of developing diseases [3].

Nutrigenomics studies the modulating effect of the chemical compounds in foods and on the stability of DNA synthesis and gene expression. The nutrients are able to affect the genome and its expression through the synthesis of nucleotides, prevention and repair of DNA damage, or through epigenetic mechanisms including methylation of histones, proteins responsible for chromatin structure that play an important role in regulating gene expression. Those methodological approaches are based on nutrition, molecular biology, and genomics. Integration of these disciplines is leading to identification and understanding of individual and population differences and similarities in gene expression, or phenotype, in response to diet. We can consider nutrigenomics as a multidisciplinary science that applies the genomic techniques besides the biochemical and epidemiological aspects, with the aim to understand the etiologic aspects of chronic diseases such as cardiovascular diseases, diabetes, obesity and cancer [4].

An understanding of scientific information about the composition and functions of genomes, has created unprecedented opportunities for increasing our understanding of how nutrients modulate gene and protein expression and ultimately influence cellular and organismal metabolism. On that basis, the purpose of this chapter is to make a broad review study to evaluate the modulation between compounds found in nutrients and their interactions with on the genomic stability and control of gene expression.

2. Nutrition and epigenetics

All the cells in the body have identical genomes. However, each cell has one of many "epigenomes", unique sets of epigenetic instructions for establishing and maintaining lineage-specific expression profiles. The genome is programmed to express appropriate sets of genes, in particular tissues, at specific time points during the individual's life. Epigenetic events create a memory of cell identity, maintaining genomic functions such as the maintenance of cell identity after differentiation, the propagation of essential features of chromosomal architecture and dosage compensation [5]. Epigenetic mechanisms are capable of modulating gene expression through changes in the chromosomes structure. Chromosomes are formed from the condensation of the chromatin, which is formed by a complex of DNA, and unique proteins called histone. Examples of epigenetic mechanisms may be mentioned as DNA methylation and histone acetylation [3].

DNA methylation occurs at the cytosine bases of eukaryotic DNA, which are converted to 5-methylcytosine. The altered cytosine residues are usually immediately adjacent to a guanine nucleotide, resulting in two methylated cytosine residues sitting diagonally to each other on opposing DNA strands [6]. DNA methylation, which modifies a cytosine base at the CpG dinucleotide residues with methyl groups, is catalyzed by DNA methyltransferases (Dnmt) and regulates gene expression patterns by altering chromatin structures. Currently, 5 different Dnmt are known: Dnmt1, Dnmt2, Dnmt 3a, Dnmt3b and DnmtL [7]. The Polycomb group protein EZH2 directly controls DNA methylation (Figure 1). EZH2 serves as a recruitment platform for DNA methyltransferases, thus highlighting a previously unrecognized direct connection between two key epigenetic repression systems [8].

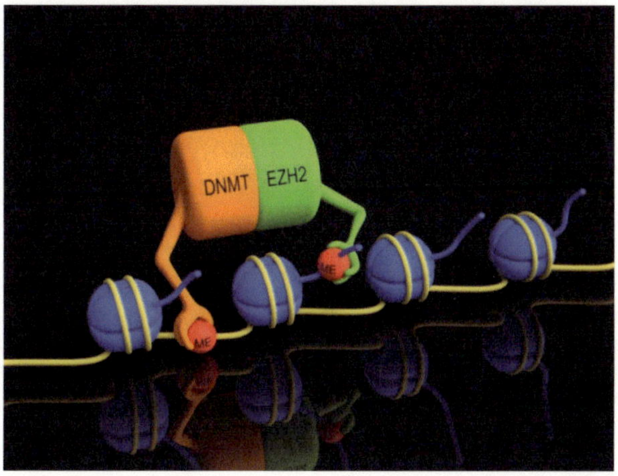

Figure 1. Polycomb Group (PcG) protein EZH2 serves as a recruitment platform for DNA methyltransferases (http://www.ulb.ac.be/medecine/fukslab/research.htm).

DNA methylation is essential for cell differentiation and embryonic development. Moreover, in some cases, methylation has observed to play a role in mediating gene expression. In mammals, methylation is found sparsely but globally, distributed in definite CpG sequences throughout the entire genome, with the exception of CpG islands, or certain stretches (approximately 1 kilobase in length) where high CpG contents are found. The methylation of these sequences can lead to inappropriate gene silencing, such as the silencing of tumor suppressor genes in cancer cells [6]. A large amount of research on DNA methylation and disease has focused on cancer and tumor suppressor genes. Tumor suppressor genes are often silenced in cancer cells due to hypermethylation. In contrast, the genomes of cancer cells have been shown to be hypomethylated overall when compared to normal cells, with the exception of hypermethylation events at genes involved in cell cycle regulation, tumor cell invasion, DNA repair, and other events in which silencing propagates metastasis. In fact, in certain cancers, such as that of the colon, hypermethylation is detectable early and might serve as a biomarker for the disease [6] (See Figure 2).

In the nutritional field, epigenetics is exceptionally important, because nutrients and bioactive food components can modify epigenetic phenomena and alter the expression of genes at the transcriptional level. Nutrients can reverse or change epigenetic phenomena such as DNA

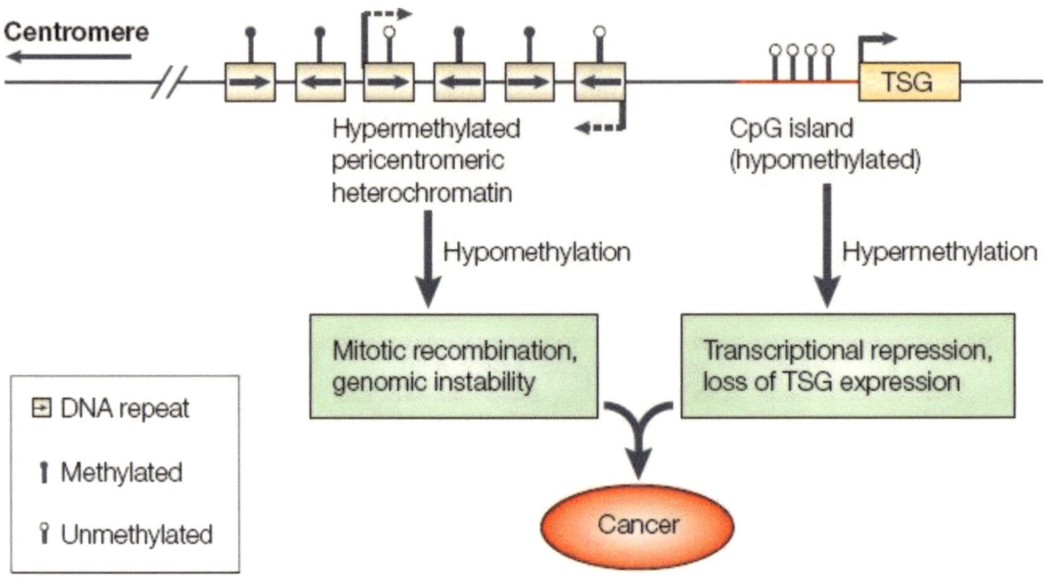

Figure 2. DNA methylation and cancer. This diagram shows a representative region of genomic DNA in a normal cell. The region contains repeat-rich, hypermethylated pericentromeric heterochromatin and an actively transcribed tumor suppressor gene (TSG) associated with a hypomethylated CpG island (indicated in red). In tumor cells, repeat-rich heterochromatin becomes hypomethylated, and this contributes to genomic instability (a hallmark of tumor cells) through increased mitotic recombination events. *De novo* methylation of CpG islands also occurs in cancer cells, and it can result in the transcriptional silencing of growth-regulatory genes. These changes in methylation are early events in tumorigenesis. (See reference [9].)

methylation and histone modifications, thereby modifying the expression of critical genes associated with physiologic and pathologic processes, including embryonic development, aging, and carcinogenesis [7].

The most interesting study linking diet and epigenetics was made by Kucharski et al. [10], about nutritional control of reproductive status in honeybees via DNA methylation. Fertile queens and sterile workers are alternative forms of the adult female honeybee that develop from genetically identical larvae following differential feeding with royal jelly. Royal jelly is a complex, protein-rich substance secreted from glands on the heads of worker bees. A larva destined to become a queen is fed large quantities of royal jelly inside a specially constructed compartment called a queen cup. The authors observed that larvae fed with royal jelly developed functional ovaries and a larger abdomen for egg laying, while worker bees remain sterile. She'll also develop the necessary behaviors to act as queen, such as killing rival queens, making communication sounds known as "piping," and going on "mating flights." The queen is fed royal honey exclusively for the rest of her life. They showed that royal jelly silences a key gene (Dnmt3), which codes for an enzyme involved in genome-wide gene silencing. When Dnmt3 is active in bee larvae, the queen genes are epigenetically silenced and the larvae develop into the default "worker" variety. But when royal jelly turns Dnmt3 off, certain genes jump into action that turn the lucky larvae into queens. The authors suggested that DNA methylation in *Apis* is used for storing epigenetic information, that the use of that information can be differentially altered by nutritional input, and that the flexibility of epigenetic modifications underpins, profound shifts in developmental fates, with massive implications for reproductive and behavioral status.

During our lifetime, nutrients can modify physiologic and pathologic processes through epigenetic mechanisms that are critical for gene expression (summarized in Table 1). Modulation of these processes through diet or specific nutrients may prevent diseases and maintain health. However, it is very hard to delineate the precise effect of nutrients or bioactive food components on each epigenetic modulation and their associations with physiologic and pathologic processes in our body, because the nutrients also interact with genes, other nutrients, and other lifestyle factors. Furthermore, each epigenetic phenomenon also interacts with the others, adding to the complexity of the system [7].

	Nutrient or diet	**Epigenetic mechanism**
Embryonic development	Folate	DNA methylation, imprinting
	Choline	DNA methylation
	Protein restriction	DNA methylation, histone modifications
	Alcohol	DNA methylation
Stem cell	Butyrate	Histone acetylation, DNA methylation
	Retinoic acid	PRC
Aging	Folate	DNA methylation
	Calorie restriction	Histone acetylation
Immune function	Folate	DNA methylation
Cancer	Methyl-deficient diet	Histone modification, microRNA
	Genistein	DNA methylation, microRNA
	(-)-Epigallocatechin-3-gallate	DNA methylation, PRC
	Curcumin	microRNA
Obesity, insulin resistance	High-fat diet	DNA methylation, microRNA
	Methyl-deficient diet	DNA methylation
	Curcumin	Histone acetylation
Inflammation	Resveratrol	Histone acetylation
	AdoMet	Histone methylation
	Methyl-deficient diet	microRNA
Neurocognition	Choline	DNA methylation, histone methylation

Data in reference [7].

Table 1. Epigenetic roles of nutrition in physiologic and pathologic processes

2.1. Diet and genomic stability

Eukaryotic DNA replication starts at multiple sites throughout the genome and is necessarily coordinated with transcription, sister chromatid cohesion, nucleosome assembly and cell cycle progression. In addition to the complexity of the replication reaction it, during replication cells need to deal with DNA damage and stalled forks, originated inevitably by the action of exogenous and endogenous agents. The success of this process is crucial to preserve genome stability, and the inability to deal with DNA lesions during replication or to protect or restart stalled forks leads to DNA breaks, chromosomal rearrangements, and mutations that can cause the loss of cell viability, but in addition errors in DNA replication result in a large number of human syndromes, including premature aging, various cancer predispositions and genetic abnormalities. To solve or reduce these problems, cells use repair and detoxification pathways as well as surveillance mechanisms, called checkpoints, which serve to detect the problem and coordinate repair with chromosome segregation and progression through the cell cycle (see Figure 3. www.genomic-instability.org/).

Maintaining genomic stability in the face of replication and recombination requires a huge variety of different damage response proteins. A cell's ability to decide when and where to deploy this DNA repair kit is critical to prevent tumor development [11].

There is evidence that inappropriate nutrient supply can cause sizeable levels of genome mutation and alter expression of genes required for genome maintenance. Deficiencies in several micronutrients have been shown to cause DNA damage and are thought to be associated with a number of serious human diseases: folic acid, niacin, vitamin B6 and B12 deficiency may increase the risk of colon cancer, heart disease and neurological dysfunction due to chromosome breaks and disabled DNA repair [12]. On the other hand, as seen in reference [13], the authors believe that caloric restriction (CR) is an 'intervention' that alters the activation of specific 'stress response genes', key enzymes in DNA repair pathways, which then results in upregulation of 'DNA repair' capacity. Enhanced DNA repair reduces the levels of DNA damage, consequently reducing mutation frequency, which would result in maintenance of genomic stability.

Recommended dietary allowances (RDAs) of micronutrients have been traditionally defined as those levels necessary to prevent symptoms of deficiency diseases. There is increasing evidence that higher levels of many such micronutrients may be necessary for various DNA maintenance reactions, and that the current RDAs for some micronutrients may be inadequate to protect against genomic instability. Dietary imbalance may increase gene mutation and chromosome aberrations in human populations, similar to exposure to radiation, mutagens and carcinogens. Diet may well be a key factor in determining genomic stability since it impacts on all relevant pathways, i.e. exposure to dietary carcinogens, activation/detoxification of carcinogens, DNA repair, DNA synthesis and apoptosis, as mentioned previously. Many micronutrient minerals and vitamins act as substrates and/or co-factors in key DNA maintenance reactions, and the exact concentration of these in the cell may be critical. Sub-optimal levels of key micronutrients required for DNA maintenance will reduce genomic stability, producing similar effects to inherited genetic disorders or exposure to carcinogens [14].

http://dx.doi.org/10.5772/55429

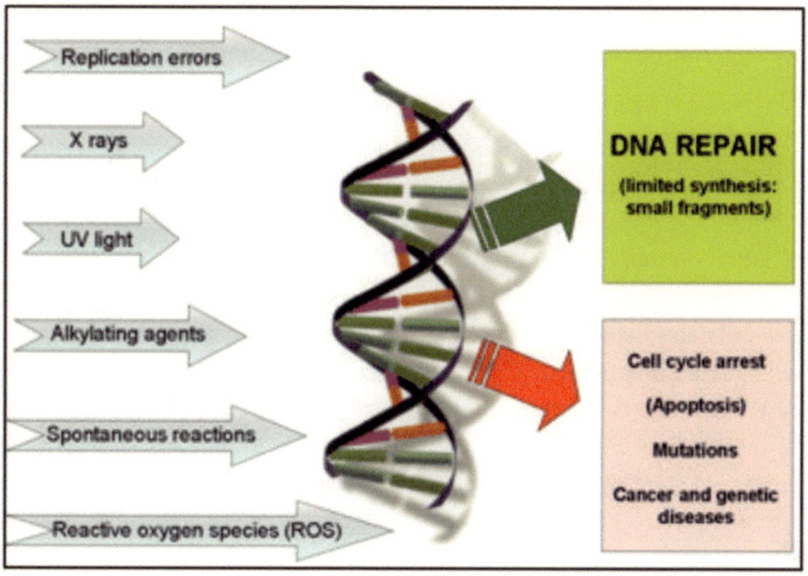

Figure 3. A general view of DNA insults and consequences on cell cycle and DNA repair (www.genomic-instability.org/).

3. Diet and cancer prevention

Current cancer models comprise those that are inherited through the germline and represent only ~5% of total cases of human cancers. These tumors originate because of mutational events. The remaining ~95% originate as sporadic events and evolve as a result of exposure to the environment, which includes exposure to both environmental contaminants and dietary agents. The multistage model of carcinogenesis identifies various phases, initiation, promotion, and progression, appears to be influenced by tissue microenvironment and organization. Significant opportunities in nutrition and cancer prevention exist in the early stages of initiation and promotion prior to clonal expansion of heterogeneous populations. Nutrigenomics represents a strategy that can be applied to the study and prevention of many diseases including cancer. DNA methylation and histone modifications are epigenetic events that mediate heritable changes in gene expression and chromatin organization in the absence of changes in the DNA sequence. The age-increased susceptibility to cancer may derive from accumulation of epigenetic changes and represents a potential target for therapies with bioactive compounds. Factors that mediate the response to dietary factors include nuclear receptors and transcription factors, which function as sensors to dietary components and determine changes in the profile of transcripts [15]. Milner and Romagnolo [15] affirm that the opportunity of targeting nutrients–gene interactions to influence the cancer process is modulated by genetic variations in human populations, epigenetic modifications that selectively and permanently alter gene expression, by complex interactions/associations among dietary components, and heterogeneity of cells within a certain tumor. Therefore, integration of information about gene polymorphisms, identification of gene targets that regulate cell and tissue specific pathways, and development of diagnostic strategies to control for clinical heterogeneity are important to understand how nutrigenomics may be used in cancer prevention.

Berrino, Krogh and Riboli [16] were made a review which showed an epidemiology studies on diet and cancer (see Table 2 that summarizes the results of the randomized studies published). The authors summarized (Table 3) the results of the World Cancer Research Fund (WCRF) evaluation on major foods and nutrients and major cancer sites. The 'probable' and 'possible' judgements provide a frame of hypotheses to be addressed in further studies. The overall pattern indicates that vegetarian food, except sugar and alcoholic beverages, is usually associated with cancer prevention, whereas animal food is frequently associated with cancer risk. The first WCRF dietary recommendation to reduce cancer, indeed, is: "Choose predominantly plant-based diets rich in a variety of vegetables and fruits, pulses (legumes) and minimally processed starchy staple foods". This seems to open a new perspective in nutrition and cancer research: from chemoprevention studies based on a single or a few micronutrients to an experimental strategy requiring a comprehensive modification of dietary habits.

Study and year of publication	Agent	Primary end point	Relative risk	Relative risk for secondary end points
ECPOS, 2000	Ispaghula fiber	Colon adenoma	1.67**	
APPP, 1995	Beta-carotene	Colon adenoma	1.50**	
CARET, 1996	Beta-carotene	Lung cancer	1.28**	
APPP, 1995	Cereal fibre	Colon adenoma	1.20	
TPPT, 1994	Cereal fibre*	Colon adenoma	1.20	
ATBC, 1994	Beta-carotene	Lung cancer	1.18**	0.98 for colon adenoma 1.05 for colorectal cancer 1.26 for stomach cancer 1.23 for prostate cancer
NPCS, 1996	Selenium	Skin, squamous cell	1.14	0.50** for all cancers
NPCS, 1996	Selenium	Skin, basal cell	1.10	
PPS, 1994	Vit C + Vit E	Colon adenoma	1.08	
SWCPS, 1997	Retinol	Skin, basal cell	1.06	
Linxian, China, 1993	Vit C + Mb	All cancers	1.06	1.10 for stomach cancer
SCPS, 1990	Beta-carotene	Skin	1.05	
PPS, 1994	Beta-carotene	Colon adenoma	1.01	

Study and year of publication	Agent	Primary end point	Relative risk	Relative risk for secondary end points
Linxian, China, 1993	Retinol + Zn	All cancers	1.00	0.96 for stomach cancer
EUROSCAN, 2000	Retinilpalmitate	Lung cancer	1.00	
Alberts et al., 2000	Cereal fiber	Colon adenoma	0.99	
ATBC, 1994	Alpha tocopherol	Lung cancer	0.99	0.64** for prostate cancer
				1.66** for colon adenoma
				0.83 for colorectal cancer
				1.26 for stomach cancer
				1.18** for stomach cancer
Linxian, China, 1993	14 vitamins + 12 minerals***	Esophagus/cardias	0.98	
PHS, 1996	Beta-carotene	All cancers	0.98	0.95 for lung cancer
Linxian, China, 1993	Riboflavin+niacin	All cancers	0.95	1.04 for stomach cancer
Linxian, China, 1993	Se + Vit E + beta-carotene	All cancers	0.93	0.79** for stomach cancer
				0.91** for total mortality
Baron et al., 1999	Calcium	Colon adenoma	0.83	
SWCPS, 1997	Retinol	Skin, squamous cell	0.74**	
ECPOS, 2000	Calcium	Colon adenoma	0.66	

*and low fat diet; **P < 0.05; ***including selenium, vitamin E and beta-carotene.
APPP, Australian Polyp Prevention Project; ATBC, Alpha Tocopherol Beta Carotene study; CARET, Carotene and Retinol Efficacy Trial; ECPOS, European Cancer Prevention Organisation Study Group; EUROSCAN, European Organization for Research and Treatment of Head and Neck Cancer and Lung Cancer Cooperative Group; NPCS, Nutritional Prevention of Skin Cancer; PHS, Physicians Health Study; PPS, Polyp Prevention Study Group; PPT, Polyp Prevention Trial; SCPS, Skin Cancer Prevention Study Group; SWCPS, Sothwest Skin Cancer Prevention Study; TPPT, Toronto Polyp Prevention Trial. Adapted from reference [16].

Table 2. Randomized controlled trials of dietary supplements to prevent cancer or colorectal adenomas, ordered by relative risk

American Cancer Society Guidelines on Nutrition and Physical Activity for Cancer Prevention [17] says that many epidemiologic studies have reported a modest but significant association

	Vegetables	Fruits	Grains, fibers	Tea	Sugar	Alcohol	Salt & salting	Meat	Eggs	Milk & dairy
Mouth, pharynx	–––	–––			+++					
Nasopharynx							+++			
Esophagus	–––	–––	+			+++				
Stomach	–––	–––	–	–			++			
Pancreas	––	––	–						+	
Gallbladder										
Liver	–					+++				
Colon, rectum	–––		–					++	+	
Larynx	––	––				+++				
Lung	–––	–––				+				
Breast	––	––	–			++		+		
Cervix	–	–								
Endometrium	–	–								
Ovary	–	–								
Prostate	–							+		+
Bladder	––	––								
Kidney	–							+		+
Thyroid	–									

Increased risk: +++, convincing; ++, probable; +, possible; decreased risk: –––, convincing; ––, probable; –, possible. Data adapted from reference [16].

Table 3. Matrix summary of the WCRF/AICR judgments on the role of various foods in the risk of cancer

between high intakes of processed meats (such as bacon, sausage, luncheon meats) and red meats (defined as beef, pork, or lamb) and increases in cancer incidence and mortality as well as death from other causes. The American Cancer Society says that current evidence supports approximately a 15% to 20% increased risk of cancers of the colon and/or rectum per 100 grams (g) of red meat or 50 g of processed meat consumed per day, while the evidence for some other cancers (those of the esophagus, stomach, lung, pancreas, breast, prostate, stomach, endometrium, renal, and ovarian) is considered limited and suggestive. According to American Cancer Society meat contains several constituents that could increase the risk of cancer. Mutagens and carcinogens (heterocyclic amines and polycyclic aromatic hydrocarbons) are produced by cooking meat at high temperatures and/or by charcoal grilling. Nitrates/nitrites and salt used to process meat contribute to the formation of nitrosamines, which are known mutagens and carcinogens in animals. Iron from the heme group of myoglobin in red meat may act as a catalyst to nitrosamine formation, and generate free radicals that may damage DNA. It is also possible that the fat content in meat contributes to risk through increasing the concentration of secondary bile acids and other compounds in the stool that could be carcinogens or promoters of carcinogenesis [17].

According to Davis [18] epidemiologic evidence suggests that regular consumption of fruits, vegetables, and whole grains may reduce cancer risk in some individuals. This association has been attributed to these foods being rich sources of numerous bioactive compounds. Plant foods contain a variety of components, including, but not limited to, essential nutrients, polyunsaturated fatty acids, and phytochemicals such as glucosinolates and flavonoids, many of which can inhibit cell proliferation and induce apoptosis, and which may act additively or synergistically when combined in the human diet.

3.1. Polyphenols

Polyphenols are common constituents of foods of plant origin and major antioxidants of our diet. The main dietary sources of polyphenols are fruits and beverages. Fruits like apple, grape, pear, cherry, and various berries contain up to 200–300 mg polyphenols per 100 g fresh weight. Typically, a glass of red wine or a cup of tea or coffee contains about 100 mg polyphenols. Cereals, chocolate, and dry legumes also contribute to the polyphenol intake [19]. Red wine polyphenols, which consisted of various powerful antioxidants such as flavonoids and stilbenes, have been implicated in cancer prevention and that promote human health without recognizable side effects. Experimental studies have shown that polyphenols from red wine, like resveratrol, quercetin, (+)-catechin and gallic acid, were potential cancer chemopreventive agents. However, red wine contains a wide range of different polyphenols and protective effects have not been assigned to a specific fraction or compound, so it is not yet clear which compounds present in red wine are endowed with protective activity [20]. Among the most highly cited class of polyphenols are the flavonoids, which comprise a large and diverse family of compounds synthesized by plants. Flavonoid subclasses include anthocyanidins in berries and grapes, flavanols in tea, flavanones in citrus fruits, flavonols in onions, flavones in herbs and peppers, and isoflavones in soy [21].

Zhou et al. [22] evaluated combined effects of soy phytochemical concentrate (SPC) and tea (green tea and black tea) components on the growth and metastasis of androgen-sensitive LNCaP human prostate cancer. The authors find that both black tea and green tea inhibited tumorigenicity rates of LNCaP tumors. For them the combination of soy phytochemicals and tea synergistically inhibited tumorigenicity, final tumor weight and metastasis to lymph nodes in vivo. This study supports further investigations using soy and tea combinations as effective nutritional regimens for prevention of prostate cancer. According to authors, studies of tea polyphenols suggest that epigallocatechin gallate (EGCG) is the major bioactive component in green tea and less is present in black tea. Black tea also contains other tea polyphenols such as theaflavins and thearubigins. They also affirm that chemopreventive properties of the soy isoflavone genistein have been the subject of extensive in vitro and in vivo.

Lambert and Yang [23] affirm that although numerous health benefits have been proposed for the consumption of tea, the effectiveness of tea as a cancer preventive agent in humans remains unclear. Animal models of carcinogenesis may be different from the human situation (e.g., the doses of tea and tea components used in animal studies are often much higher than those consumed by humans), and many confounding factors are involved in epidemiological studies. Interindividual variation in biotransformation and bioavailability may also affect the efficacy of tea as a cancer preventive agent. For them further studies on definitive mechanisms of cancer preventive activities of tea in animal models are needed. Although many possible mechanisms have been proposed, their relevance in vivo needs to be demonstrated. With some exceptions, the concentrations of catechins or theaflavins used in cell culture systems exceed the plasma concentrations obtained in animal studies by 10- to 100-fold. Mechanisms based on the use of such high concentrations may be relevant for cancers of the gastrointestinal tract but not for sites such as the lung, prostate and breast, which depend on systemic bioavailability. In spite of many in vitro and in vivo studies, the molecular mechanisms for the cancer preventive actions of these compounds are not clearly known. The relationship between tea consumption and cancer risk has not been conclusively demonstrated, and the relationship may become clearer if we consider the effects of specific types of tea, at defined doses, in populations with certain dietary patterns or genetic polymorphisms. Human intervention trials and large prospective studies are needed to further assess cancer preventive activities of tea constituents [24]. For the National Cancer Institute [25] more than 50 epidemiologic studies of the association between tea consumption and cancer risk have been published since 2006. The results of these studies have often been inconsistent, but some have linked tea consumption to reduced risks of cancers of the colon, breast, ovary, prostate, and lung. They also believe that the inconsistent results may be due to variables such as differences in tea preparation and consumption, the types of tea studied (green, black, or both), the methods of tea production, the bioavailability of tea compounds, genetic variation in how people respond to tea consumption, the concomitant use of tobacco and alcohol, and other lifestyle factors that may influence a person's risk of developing cancer, such as physical activity or weight status.

A double-blind intervention trial conducted in patients with oral mucosa leukoplakia using a mixed tea showed some direct evidence on the protective effects of tea on oral cancer. In this study developed by Li et al. [26] fifty-nine oral mucosa leukoplakia patients, diagnosed by established clinical and pathological criteria, were randomly divided into a treated group (3 g mixed tea oral administration and topical treatment) and a control group (placebo and glycerin treatment). After the 6-month trial, the size of oral lesion was decreased in 37.9% of the 29 treated patients and increased in 3.4%; whereas the oral lesion was decreased in 10.0% of the 30 control patients and increased in 6.7%.

3.2. Vitamins and micronutrients

Natural inhibitors of oxidizing agents that are found in the diet are important in preventing cancer and typically do not have the undesirable side effects of many xenobiotic compounds. Some vitamins, such as the antioxidant Vitamins A, E, and C, demonstrate these protective effects. The daily ingestion of antioxidants has the potential of not only protecting against cancer, but also cardiovascular disorders and neurological degenerative diseases [28]. Antioxidants nutrients such as vitamin E, vitamin C, vitamin A, and Beta-carotene are involved in detoxification of the Reactive oxygen species (ROS). Vitamin E, A, and Beta-carotene are lipophilic antioxidants whereas vitamin C is hydrophilic antioxidant. Vitamin E function as a free radical chain breaker particularly it interferes with the propagation step of lipid peroxidation. Vitamin A and Beta-carotene have actions by quenching both singlet oxygen and other free radicals generated by photochemical reactions [28].

The changes in the DNA by a deficiency of some micronutrients (folic acid, vitamin B12, vitamin B6, niacin, vitamin C, vitamin E, iron and zinc) are considered as the most likely cause of some types of cancer [29].

Studies investigating the interactions between dietary exposure and genetic polymorphisms have the potential to clarify mechanisms and identify susceptible subgroups so that preventative strategies can be focused on the subgroups for maximum benefit. Red meat or meat cooking methods such as frying and doneness levels have been associated with the increased risk of colorectal and other cancers [30]. It is not clear whether it is red meat intake or the way meat is cooked that is involved in the etiology of colorectal cancer, as stated above. Both cooking methods and doneness level of red meat are thought to be surrogates for heterocyclic amines (HCA) consumption [31]. Sinha and Caporaso [31] affirm that genetics polymorphisms may interact with various dietary components and thus define subgroups of individuals who may be at a higher risk of getting cancer. For them there are also other polymorphic enzymes that may interact with various dietary components and play a role in human carcinogenesis. The authors describe categories of susceptibility genes, potential dietary carcinogens and anticarcinogens, and cancer sites in which they may be involved (see Table 4). Many studies are currently investigating the role of circulating vitamin D metabolites and dietary calcium. Because the vitamin D receptor is involved in vitamin D and calcium metabolism, the vitamin D receptor polymorphisms may also be important for colorectal cancers. Martinez et al. [32] investigated the associations between the intake of calcium and vitamin D and the occurrence of colorectal cancer. They found that vitamin D is suggestive of an inverse association, particularly for total vitamin D in relation to rectal cancer. However, since most of the support for this protective effect was seen for total vitamin D. They not rule out the possibility that something other than vitamin D in multivitamin supplements contributes to this apparent effect. The relation between vitamin D and colorectal cancer may be better elucidated with additional dietary measurements and further follow-up. They conclude that available evidence does not warrant an increase in calcium intake to prevent colon cancer, but longer-term studies of both calcium and especially vitamin D in relation to colorectal cancer risk are needed.

Carotenoids are the pigments that give fruits and vegetables such as carrots, cantaloupe, sweet potato, and kale their vibrant orange, yellow, and green colors. Beta-carotene, lycopene, and lutein are all different varieties of carotenoids. They all act as antioxidants with strong cancer-fighting properties. Preclinical studies have shown that some carotenoids have potent antitumor effects both in vitro and in vivo, suggesting potential preventive and/or therapeutic roles for the compounds. Since chemoprevention is one of the most important strategies in the control of cancer development, molecular mechanism-based cancer chemoprevention using carotenoids seems to be an attractive approach [33]. Epidemiologic studies have shown an

Dietary component	Polymorphic gene/phenotype[1]	Cancer site
Carcinogens		
Heterocyclic amines	NAT2, (NAT1), CYP1A2 (CYP1A1)	Colorectal, breast, other sites
Polycyclic hydrocarbons	CYP1A1, GSTM1	Gastrointestinal tract Nasophyrangeal, stomach
Nitrosamines	CYP2E1	
Aflatoxins	GSTM1, EPHX	Liver
Alcohol	ADH (ALDH, CYP2E1)	Colorectal, oral
Anticarcinogens		
Cruciferous vegetables	CYP1A2, GST	Colorectal, other sites
Fruits and vegetables	CYP1A2, GST	Many sites
Calcium/vitamin D	Vitamin D receptor	Colorectal, prostate
Retinoids	Retinoic acid receptor Variant	Acute promylocytic Leukemia, skin, Head and neck, breast
Folate, methionine	MTHFR, Methionine Synthase	Colorectal, cervix

1 Abbreviations used: NAT, *N*-acetyltminsferase; CYP, cytochrome p450; GST, glutathione-S-transferase; EPHX, epoxide hydrolase; ADH, alcohol dehydrogenase; MTHFR, metheylenetetrahydrofolate reductase. Adapted from reference [31].

Table 4. Polymorphic genes, dietary components and cancer: possible candidates

inverse relationship between the presence of various cancers and dietary or blood carotenoid levels. According to Tanaka, Shnimizu and Moriwaki [33] the epidemiologic observations of the possible protective effects of high dietary (not supplemental) β-carotene intakes against cancer, along with what is known about carotenoid biochemical functions, has led to further study of the effect of β-carotene on cancer risk. Long-term large randomized intervention trials were designed to test the efficacy of high doses of β-carotene (20–30 mg/day) in the prevention of cancer. These results are summarized in Table 5.

Study Designs				
Studies	**Population**	**Intervention**	**Duration**	**Cancer outcome**
ATBC	29,133 Finish male smokers (50–69 years of age)	β-carotene, 20 mg/day; vitamin E, 50 mg/day	5–8 years	18% increase in lung cancer; 8% increase in mortality
CARET	18,314 men and women and asbestoss workers (45–74 years of age)	β-carotene, 30 mg/day; vitamin A, 25,000 IU	<4 years	28% increase in lung cancer; 17% increase in deaths
PHS	22,071 male physicians (40–84 years of age)	β-carotene, 50 mg on alternate days	12 years	No effect of supplementation in incidence of cancer
Linxian	29,584 men and women, vitamin and mineral deficient (40–69 years of age)	β-carotene, 15 mg/day; selenium, 50 mg/day; α-tocopherol, 30 mg/day	5 years	13% decrease in total cancers; 9% decrease in overall deaths
Women's Health Study	39,876 female health professionals (over 45 years of age)	β-carotene, 50 mg on alternate days	4.1 years (2.1 years' treatment and 2.0 years' follow-up)	No effect of supplementation in incidence of cancer

Data adapted from reference [33].
CARET, Beta-Carotene and Retinol Efficacy Trial; ATBC, Alpha Tocopherol and Beta-Carotene Cancer Prevention; PHS, Physicians' Health Study.

Table 5. β-Carotene supplementation trials.

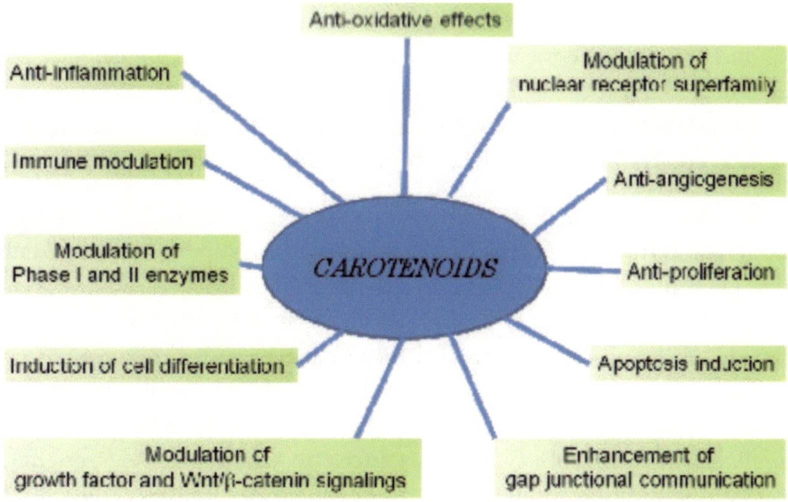

Figure 4. Proposed mechanisms by which certain carotenoids suppress carcinogenesis. Adapted from reference [33].

The authors [33] wrote an important review which showed a table (Table 6) about cancer prevention by means of carotenoids with dietary sources, function e effects. According to these authors the mechanisms underlying the anticancer and/or cancer chemopreventive activities of carotenoids may involve changes in pathways leading to cell growth or cell death. These include immune modulation, hormone and growth factor signaling, regulatory mechanisms of cell cycle progression, cell differentiation and apoptosis. In this sense the authors also showed an interesting figure proposing possible mechanisms by which certain carotenoids suppress carcinogenesis (see Figure 4 on the left).

Studies involving the use of vitamin C in cancer prevention are the most contradictory. Vitamin C is an essential vitamin the human body needs to function well. It is a water-soluble vitamin that cannot be made by the body, and must be obtained from foods or other sources. Vitamin C is found in abundance in citrus fruits such as oranges, grapefruit, and lemons, and in green leafy vegetables, potatoes, strawberries, bell peppers, and cantaloupe. American Cancer Society [34] wrote that many studies have shown a connection between eating foods rich in vitamin C, such as fruits and vegetables, and a reduced risk of cancer. On the other hand, evidence indicates that vitamin C supplements do not reduce cancer risk. This suggests that the activity of fruits and vegetables in preventing cancer is due to a combination of many vitamins and other phytochemicals and not to vitamin C alone. Clinical trials of high doses vitamin C as a treatment for cancer have not shown any benefit. High doses of vitamin C can cause a number of side effects.

According to Block [35] epidemiologic evidence of a protective effect of vitamin C for non-hormone-dependent cancers is strong. Of the 46 such studies in which a dietary vitamin C index was calculated, 33 found statistically significant protection, with high intake conferring approximately a twofold protective effect compared with low intake. 0f 29 additional studies that assessed fruit intake, 2 1 found significant protection. For cancers of the esophagus, larynx, oral cavity, and pancreas, evidence for a protective effect of vitamin C or some component in fruit is strong and consistent. For cancers of the stomach, rectum, breast, and cervix there is also strong evidence. Several recent lung cancer studies found significant protective effects of vitamin C or of foods that are better sources of vitamin C than of /3-carotene. It is likely that ascorbic acid, carotenoids, and other factors in fruits and vegetables act jointly.

Several lines of evidence suggest that vitamin C is a powerful antioxidant in biological systems in vitro. However, its antioxidant role in humans has not been supported by currently available clinical studies. Diets high in fruits and vegetables protect against cardiovascular disease and cancer, but such a protective effect cannot as yet be ascribed to vitamin C. In vivo markers of oxidative damage are being developed, and these have yet not shown major changes with vitamin C intake in humans [36]. The most important problem about vitamin C is that it can exert a pro-oxidant activity under certain conditions, particularly in the presence of transition metal ions or alkali. Thus, vitamin C *in vitro* reduces free ferric iron that generates hydrogen peroxide in the Fenton reaction and results in the production of hydroxyl radicals. The reactive hydroxyl radical quickly reacts with critical cellular macromolecules, including DNA, which may lead to mutagenesis and the initiation of cancer [37]. According to authors, the high

Carotenoids	Dietary Sources	Function	Effects
α-Carotene	Yellow-orange vegetables (carrots, sweet totatoes, pumpkin) and Dark-green vegetables (broccoli, green beans, spinach)	Provitamin A activity; Anti-oxidant	Immune- enhancement; Stimulate cell to cell communication; Decreases risk of some cancers
β-Carotene	Green leafy vegetables and orange and yellow fruits and vegetables (carrots, apricots, spinach, sweet potetoes, pumpkin, pepper, kale, cantaloupe)	Provitamin A activity; Antioxidant	Immune-enhancement; Decreases risk of some cancers and some cardiovascular events; high-dose supplementation may increase the risk of lung cancer among smokers
Lycopene	Tomatoes, water melon, apricot, peaches	Anti-oxidant	Decreases risk of some cancers and some cardiovascular events, diabetes, and osteoporosis
β-Cyptoxanthin	Orange fruits (mandarin orange and papaya, etc.), corn, peas, and egg yolks	Provitamin A activity; Anti-oxidant	Anti-inflammatory effects; Inhibits risks of some cancer and cardiovascular events; Immune enhancemen
Lutein/Zeaxanthin	Dark green leafy vegetables (spinach, kale), red peppers, maize, tomatoes, corn, and egg yolks	Anti-photosensitizing agent and photosynthetic pigment; Acts as antioxidants and blue light filters	Decrease age-related macular degeneration, cataract, and risk of cardiovascular disease and certain cancers
Astaxanthin	Green algae, salmon, trout, Crustacean	Antioxidant; Coloration	Prevent certain cancers, cataract, diabetes, and inflammatory neurodegenerative and cardiovascular diseases
Canthaxanthin	Salmon, crustacean	Antioxidant; Coloration	Immune enhancement; Decreases risk of some cancers
Focoxanthin	Brown algae, heterokonts	Antioxidant	Anti-cancer, anti-allergic, anti-obese, anti-inflammatory, and anti-osteoporotic activities

Adapted from reference [33].

Table 6. Sources, function, and effects of different carotenoids.

consumption of vitamin C–rich fruit and vegetables is not likely to be harmful. In general, data from in vitro and in vivo experiments and population-based studies do not indicate that high doses of vitamin C are linked to increased oxidative DNA damage or an elevated risk of cancer.

Lee et al. [37] believe that the cancer preventive effects of vegetables and fruit may result from multiple combined effects of various phenolic phytochemicals, vitamins, dietary fibers, indoles, allium compounds, and selenium rather than from the effect of a single active ingredient. For them, many dietary phenolic phytochemicals may have stronger antioxidant and antitumor promotion effects than do antioxidant vitamins, which may contribute to the chemopreventive effects of the phytochemicals in carcinogenesis. However, these authors suggest that the chemopreventive effects of vitamin C in carcinogenesis may be linked to the protective effects of vitamin C against epigenetic mechanisms, such as the inflammation and inhibition of gap junction intercellular communication (GJIC), as well as to antioxidant activities (see Figure 5).

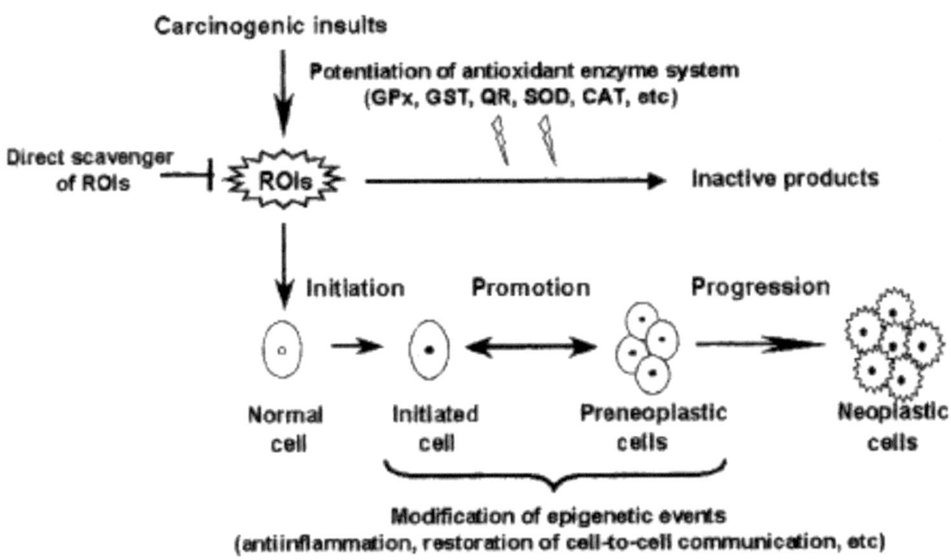

Figure 5. Possible chemopreventive mechanisms of vitamin C in carcinogenesis. ROIs, reactive oxygen intermediates; GPx, glutathione peroxidase; GST, glutathione *S*-transferase; QR, quinone oxidoreductase; SOD, superoxide dismutase; CAT, catalase. Adapted from reference [37].

Regarding the use of vitamin C in cancer patient the results were not promising. In a double-blind study 100 patients with advanced colorectal cancer were randomly assigned to treatment with either high-dose vitamin C (10 g daily) or placebo. Overall, these patients were in very good general condition, with minimal symptoms. None had received any previous treatment with cytotoxic drugs. Vitamin C therapy showed no advantage over placebo therapy with regard to either the interval between the beginning of treatment and disease progression or patient survival. Among patients with measurable disease, none had objective improvement. On the basis of this and our previous randomized study, it can be concluded that high-dose vitamin C therapy is not effective against advanced malignant disease regardless of whether the patient has had any prior chemotherapy [38].

The terms folic acid and folate are often used interchangeably for this water-soluble B-complex vitamin. Folic acid, the more stable form, occurs rarely in foods or the human body but is the form most often used in vitamin supplements and fortified foods. Folic acid is essential to numerous bodily functions ranging from nucleotide biosynthesis to the remethylation of homocysteine. The human body needs folate to synthesize DNA, repair DNA, and methylate DNA as well as to act as a cofactor in biological reactions involving folate.

Considerable epidemiological evidence suggests that a low-folate diet is associated with an increased risk of colorectal neoplasia. Much animal data support an antineoplastic effect of folate. However, in some animal studies, folate deficiency protects against, and supplementation increases, experimental carcinogenesis. Cole et al. [39] developed a double-blind, placebo-controlled, 2-factor, phase 3, randomized clinical trial conducted at 9 clinical centers between July 6, 1994, and October 1, 2004. Participants included 1021 men and women with a recent history of colorectal adenomas and no previous invasive large intestine carcinoma. Participants were randomly assigned in a 1:1 ratio to receive 1 mg/d of folic acid (n=516) or placebo (n=505), and were separately randomized to receive aspirin (81 or 325 mg/d) or placebo. Follow-up consisted of 2 colonoscopic surveillance cycles (the first interval was at 3 years and the second at 3 or 5 years later). In this double-blind, placebo-controlled, randomized clinical trial, was found that folic acid supplementation did not decrease the risk of adenoma occurrence among participants with a recent history of adenomas. The authors concluded that folate, when administered as folic acid for up to 6 years, does not decrease the risk of adenoma formation in the large intestine among individuals with previously removed adenomas. For them, the evidence for an increased risk of adenomas is equivocal and requires further research.

In March of 1996, the U.S. Food and Drug Administration mandated that all enriched flour and uncooked cereal grains sold in the United States should be fortified with 140 μg folic acid/100 g of flour no later than January of 1998. Following the institution of fortification population-based studies showed the effectiveness of this measure: plasma levels of folate in the adult population increased ~2-fold as a result and the incidence of births complicated by neural tube defects was variously reported to decline by 20% to 50%. However, analyses of several cereal grains that were purchased after the institution of fortification showed that in many instances the actual amount of folate was 150% to 300% greater than the mandate, suggesting that in this early era of fortification, manufacturers often included "overage" to ensure that they were meeting the minimal level of mandated fortification [40]. Thus, the authors hypothesize, by means of an epidemiological study, that the institution of folic acid fortification may have been wholly or partly responsible for the observed increase in colorectal cancer rates in the mid-1990s. The authors affirm that wish to highlight the potential complexity of the response to this nutrient and emphasize prior observations that have been made in both preclinical and clinical studies that indicate that administering high doses of folic acid to susceptible individuals or in an inappropriate time frame may accelerate the growth of existing neoplasms.

Vitamin C, also known as ascorbic acid, is a water-soluble vitamin. Unlike most mammals and other animals, humans do not have the ability to make their own vitamin C. Therefore, we must obtain vitamin C through our diet. Vitamin C is required for the synthesis of collagen, an important structural component of blood vessels, tendons, ligaments, and bone. Vitamin C also plays an important role in the synthesis of the neurotransmitter, norepinephrine. Neurotransmitters are critical to brain function and are known to affect mood. Vitamin C is also a highly effective antioxidant. Even in small amounts vitamin C can protect indispensable molecules in the body, such as proteins, lipids (fats), carbohydrates, and nucleic acids (DNA and RNA), from damage by free radicals and reactive oxygen species that can be generated during normal metabolism as well as through exposure to toxins and pollutants (e.g., cigarette smoke). In the U.S., the recommended dietary allowance (RDA) for vitamin C was revised in 2000 upward from the previous recommendation of 60 mg daily for men and women. The RDA continues to be based primarily on the prevention of deficiency disease, rather than the prevention of chronic disease and the promotion of optimum health. The recommended intake for smokers is 35 mg/day higher than for non-smokers, because smokers are under increased oxidative stress from the toxins in cigarette smoke and generally have lower blood levels of vitamin C (see Table 7 – reference [41]).

Life Stage	Age	Males (mg/day)	Females (mg/day)
Infants	0-6 months	40 (AI)	40 (AI)
Infants	7-12 months	50 (AI)	50 (AI)
Children	1-3 years	15	15
Children	4-8 years	25	25
Children	9-13 years	45	45
Adolescents	14-18 years	75	65
Adults	19 years and older	90	75
Smokers	19 years and older	125	110
Pregnancy	18 years and younger	-	80
Pregnancy	19 years and older	-	85
Breast-feeding	18 years and younger	-	115
Breast-feeding	19 years and older	-	120

Data from reference [41].

Table 7. Recommended Dietary Allowance (RDA) for Vitamin C

The relations between the intake of beta-carotene, vitamin C, selenium, and 25-yr mortality from lung cancer and total cancer were analyzed within the Zutphen Study, a cohort study on diet and chronic diseases [42]. The Zutphen Study is a prospective study on the relations between diet, other risk factors, and the incidence of chronic diseases. The results of this study suggest that vitamin C intake may be more important for prevention of lung cancer than beta-carotene. It can, however, not be ruled out that substances present in fruit other than vitamin C (eg, phenols, flavones, and terpenes) may also be of importance in lung cancer prevention. The results suggest that a vitamin C intake of ≥ 70 mg/d may be of importance in lung cancer prevention. Due to the role of vitamin C in the formation of N-nitrosocompounds, this may also be of importance for stomach cancer prevention. Another hand, 8 prospective studies does not suggest that intakes of vitamins A, C and E and folate reduce the risk of lung cancer. The results were similar with different analytic approaches and across studies, sex, smoking status and lung cancer cell type [43].

Data on intake of specific carotenoids and breast cancer risk are limited. Furthermore, studies of vitamins A, C, and E in relation to breast cancer risk are inconclusive. Zhang et al. [44] were made studies, using multivariate analysis, demonstrated associations between intakes of specific carotenoids, vitamins A, C, and E, consumption of fruits and vegetables, and breast cancer risk in a cohort of 83,234 women (aged 33-60 years in 1980). Through 1994, they identified 2,697 incident cases of invasive breast cancer (784 premenopausal and 1913 post-menopausal). The results demonstrated that intakes of beta-carotene from food and supplements, lutein/zeaxanthin, and vitamin A from foods were weakly inversely associated with breast cancer risk in premenopausal women. Strong inverse associations were found for increasing quintiles of alpha-carotene, beta-carotene, lutein/zeaxanthin, total vitamin C from foods, and total vitamin A among premenopausal women with a positive family history of breast cancer. An inverse association was also found for increasing quintiles of beta-carotene among premenopausal women who consumed 15 g or more of alcohol per day. Premenopausal women who consumed five or more servings per day of fruits and vegetables had modestly lower risk of breast cancer than those who had less than two servings per day (relative risk [RR] = 0.77; 95% confidence interval [CI] = 0.58-1.02); this association was stronger among premenopausal women who had a positive family history of breast cancer (RR = 0.29; 95% CI = 0.13-0.62) or those who consumed 15 g or more of alcohol per day (RR = 0.53; 95% CI = 0.27-1.04). The author concluded that consumption of fruits and vegetables high in specific carotenoids and vitamins may reduce premenopausal breast cancer risk [44].

In recent years, the intake of vitamins, minerals and herbs as a dietary supplement has increased dramatically. The supplementation with vitamins and minerals are used more often than the herbs. The most common supplements among users in the U.S. are multivitamins (75%), followed by vitamin C (38%), and iron (38%) [45]. Food supplementation with vitamins is a polemic question and it differs among authors. There are evidences that dietary supplementation with vitamin C may reduce the incidence of gastric cancer in certain populations, but it is unclear whether it was the antioxidant, vitamin or other property, responsible for this action [46]. However, the author states that it does not justify, in terms of cancer prevention to make a diet supplemented with vitamin C if the person has a good diet. Claycombe and Meydani [47] were made a review reporting the protective effect of vitamin E against chromosomal alterations induced by oxidation of DNA. However, the authors call attention to the careful supplementation, simultaneous with C vitamin E, considering a possible genotoxicity in the association of the two vitamins. Although most animal studies have shown cancer-preventive effects, a few recent studies suggest that soy phytoestrogens may stimulate breast cancer cell growth under certain circumstances. Before recommendations regarding phytoestrogen supplements can be safely made, we must have more information on the effects of the extracts on bone, heart and breast health. Until safety with respect to breast cancer is established, phytoestrogen supplements should not be recommended, particularly for women at high risk of breast cancer [48].

Cancer prevention can be done with a diet rich in vegetables, fruits, and low in red meat, saturated fats, salt and sugar. Carbohydrates should be consumed in the form of cereals - wheat bread and brown rice. The addition of fats should be in the form of fats dehydrogenated [49]. The types of vegetables or fruit that most often appear to be protective against cancer are allium vegetables, carrots, green vegetables, cruciferous vegetables, and tomatoes. Substances present in some vegetable and fruit may help cancer prevention and they include dithiolthiones, isothiocyanates, indole-3-carbinol, allium compounds, isoflavones, protease inhibitors, saponins, phytosterols, inositol hexaphosphate, vitamin C, D-limonene, lutein, folic acid, beta carotene, lycopene, selenium, vitamin E, flavonoids, and dietary fiber. Current US vegetable and fruit intake, which averages about 3.4 servings per day, is discussed, as are possible non-cancer-related effects of increased vegetable and fruit consumption, including benefits against cardiovascular disease, diabetes, stroke, obesity, diverticulosis, and cataracts [50].

4. Conclusion

Cancer incidence is projected to increase in the future and an effectual preventive strategy is required to face this challenge. Alteration of dietary habits is potentially an effective approach for reducing cancer risk. Assessment of biological effects of a specific food or bioactive component that is linked to cancer and prediction of individual susceptibility as a function of nutrient-nutrient interactions and genetics is an essential element to evaluate the beneficiaries of dietary interventions [51]. We know that diet is an important factor both to minimize, as to increase the risk of cancer development. But diet is not the only factor. There are several risk factors that can trigger a process of tumor formation. Sedentary life, environmental issues, viruses, smoking, alcohol in excess, are factors that contribute to and are also strategic points that should be worked in cancer prevention.

Author details

Júlio César Nepomuceno

Universidade Federal de Uberlândia/ Instituto de Genética e Bioquímica; Centro Universitário de Patos de Minas /Laboratório de Citogenética e Mutagênese, Brazil

References

[1] Pitot HC, Goldsworthy T., Moran S. The natural history of carcinogenesis: Implications of experimental carcinogenesis in the genesis of human cancer. Journal of Supramolecular Structure and Cellular Biochemistry. 2004;17: 133-146.

[2] Setlow RB. Human cancer: etiologic agents/dose responses/DNA repair/cellular and animal models. Mutat Res 2001;477(1-2): 1-6.

[3] Fujii T.M.M., Medeiros R. and Yamada R. Nutrigenomics and nutrigenetics: importante concepts for the nutrition science. J Brazilian Soc Food Nutr 2010;35(1): 149-166.

[4] Fogg-Johnson N and Kaput J. Nutrigenomics: An Emerging Scientific Discipline. Foodtechnology 2003;57(4): 60-67.

[5] Gabory A, Attig L and Junien C. Epigenetic mechanisms involved in developmental nutritional programming. World J Diabetes 2011;15; 2(10): 64-175.

[6] Phillips T. The role of methylation in gene expression; 2008 Nature Education http://www.nature.com/scitable/topicpage/the-role-of-methylation-in-gene-expression-107 (accessed 215 August 2012).

[7] Choi, Sang-Woon and Friso S. Epigenetics: A New Bridge between Nutritionand Health. Adv Nutr 2010;1: 8–16.

[8] Viré E, Brenner C, Deplus R, Blanchon L, Fraga M, Didelot C, Morey L, Van Eynde A, Bernard D, Vanderwinden JM, Bollen M, Esteller M, Di Croce L, de Launoit Y, Fuks F. The Polycomb group protein EZH2 directly controls DNA methylation. NATURE 2007;446(7137):824.

[9] Robertson KD. DNA methylation and human disease. Nat Rev Genet 2005;6(8): 597-610.

[10] Kucharski R, Maleszka J, Foret S, Maleszka R. Nutritional Control of Reproductive Status in Honeybees via DNA Methylation. Science 2008;319: 1827-1830.

[11] Scaplehorn N. Genome Instability, Cell 2011;145: 5-7.

[12] Ames BN and Wakimoto P. Are micronutrient deficiencies a major cancer risk? Nature Reviews Cancer 2002;2:694–704.

[13] Heydari AR, Unnikrishnan A, Lucente LV and Richardson A. Caloric restriction and genomic stability. Nucleic Acids Research 2007;35(22): 7485–7496.

[14] Fenech M and Ferguson LR. Vitamins/minerals and genomic stability in humans. Mutation Research/Fundamental and Molecular Mechanisms of Mutagenesis 2001;475:1-6

[15] Milner JA and Romagnolo DF. Nutrition and Health: Bioactive Compounds and Cancer, Edited by: J.A. Milner, D.F. Romagnolo, DOI 10.1007/978-1-60761-627-6_2, Humana Press. 824p., 2010.

[16] Berrino F, Krogh V and Riboli E. Epidemiology studies on diet and cancer. Tumori 2003;89: 581-585.

[17] Kushi LH, Byers T, Doyle C, Bandera EV, McCullough M, McTiernan A, Gansler T, Andrews KS and Thun MJ. Nutrition and Physical Activity Guidelines Advisory

Committee. American Cancer Society Guidelines on Nutrition and Physical Activity for Cancer Prevention Reducing the Risk of Cancer With Healthy Food Choices and Physical Activity. CA Cancer J Clin 2012;62:30–67.

[18] Davis CD. Nutritional Interactions: Credentialing of Molecular Targets for Cancer Prevention. Exp Biol Med 2007;232(2): 176-183.

[19] Scalbert A, Manach C, Morand C, Rémésy C, Jiménez L. Dietary Polyphenols and the Prevention of Diseases. Crit Rev Food Sci Nutr 2005;45(4): 287-306.

[20] He S, Sun C and Pan Y. Red Wine Polyphenols for Cancer Prevention. Int J Mol Sci 2008;9: 842-853.

[21] Dashwood RH. Frontiers in Polyphenols and Cancer Prevention. J Nutr 2007;137: 267S–269S.

[22] Zhou Jin-Rong, Yu L, Zhong Y and Blackburn GL. Soy Phytochemicals and Tea Bioactive Components Synergistically Inhibit Androgen-Sensitive Human Prostate Tumors in Mice. J Nutr 2003;133(2): 516-521.

[23] Lambert JD and Yang CS. Mechanisms of Cancer Prevention by Tea Constituents. Proceedings of the Third International Scientific Symposium on Tea and Human Health: Role of Flavonoids in the Diet. J Nutr 2003;133(10): 3262S-3267S.

[24] Yang, C S, Ju J, Lu G, Xiao H, Hao X, Sang S and Lambert JD (). Cancer prevention by tea and tea polyphenols. Asia Pac J Clin Nutr 2008;17(S1): 245-248.

[25] National Cancer Institute (2010) Tea and Cancer Prevention: Strengths and Limits of the Evidence. http://www.cancer.gov/cancertopics/factsheet/prevention/tea#r13 (accessed 20 August 2012).

[26] Li N, Sun Z, Han C, Chen J. The chemopreventive effects of tea on human oral precancerous mucosa lesions. Proceedings from the Society of Experimental Biology and Medicine 1999;220(4):218–224.

[27] Costa WF and Nepomuceno JC. Protective Effects of a Mixture of Antioxidant Vitamins and Minerals on the Genotoxicity of Doxorubicin in Somatic Cells of Drosophila melanogaster. Environmental and MolecularMutagenesis 2005;47(1):18-24.

[28] Nepomuceno, JC. Antioxidants in Cancer Treatment, Current Cancer Treatment: Intech, 2011. http://www.intechopen.com/books/current-cancer-treatment-novel-beyond-conventional-approaches/antioxidants-in-cancer-treatment (accessed 20 August 2012).

[29] Ames BN. DNA damage from micronutrient deficiencies is likely to be a major cause of cancer. Mutation Res 2001;475: 7-20.

[30] Glade MJ. Food, Nutrition and the Prevention of Cancer: A Global Perspective. American Institute for Cancer Research, Washington, DC, Nutrition 1997;15(6): 523-6.

[31] Sinha R and Caporaso N. Diet, Genetic Susceptibility and Human Cancer Etiology Symposium: Interactions of Diet and Nutrition with Genetic Susceptibility in Cancer. J Nutr 1999;129(2): 556S-559S.

[32] Martinez M, Giovannucci EL, Colditz GA, Stampfer M, Hunter DJ, Speizer FE, Wing A and Willet WC. Calcium, Vitamin D, and the Occurrence of Colorectal Cancer Among Women. J Natl Cancer Inst 1996;88:1375-82.

[33] Tanaka T, Shnimizu M and Moriwaki H. Cancer Chemoprevention by Carotenoids, Molecules 2012;17: 3202-3242.

[34] American Cancer Society. Vitamin C. http://www.cancer.org/Treatment/TreatmentsandSideEffects/ComplementaryandAlternativeMedicine/HerbsVitaminsandMinerals/vitamin-c (accessed 215 August 2012).

[35] Block G. Vitamin C and cancer prevention: the epidemiologic evidence. Am J Clin Nutr 1991;53: 270S-82S.

[36] Padayatty, S.J., Katz, A., Wang, Y., Eck, P., Kwon, O., Lee, J.H., Chen, S., Corpe, C., Dutta, A., Dutta, S.K. & Levine, M. (2003). Vitamin C as an Antioxidant: Evaluation of Its Role in Disease Prevention, J Am Coll Nutr 22(1):18-35.

[37] Lee KW, Lee HJ, Surh YJ and Lee CY. Vitamin C and cancer chemoprevention: reappraisal, Am J Clin Nutr 2003;78: 1074–8.

[38] Moertel CG, Fleming TR, Creagan ET, Rubin J, O'Connell MJ and Ames MM. High-Dose Vitamin C versus Placebo in the Treatment of Patients with Advanced Cancer Who Have Had No Prior Chemotherapy — A Randomized Double-Blind Comparison. N Engl J Med 1985;312:137-141

[39] Cole BF, Baron JA, Sandler RS, Haile RW, Ahnen DJ, Bresalier RS, McKeown-Eyssen G, Summers RW, Rothstein RI, Burke CA, Snover DC, Church TR, Allen JI, Robertson DJ, Beck GJ, Bond JH, Byers T, Mandel JS, Mott LA, Pearson LH, Barry EL, Rees JR, Marcon N, Saibil F, Ueland PM and Greenberg ER; Polyp Prevention Study Group. Folic Acid for the Prevention of Colorectal Adenomas - A Randomized Clinical Trial. JAMA 2007;297: 2351-2359.

[40] Mason JB, Dickstein A, Jacques PF, Haggarty P, Selhub J, Dallal G and Rosenberg IH. A Temporal Association between Folic Acid Fortification and an Increase in Colorectal Cancer Rates May Be Illuminating Important Biological Principles: A Hypothesis. Cancer Epidemiol Biomarkers Prev 2007;16: 1325-1329.

[41] Linus Pauling Institute. Micronutrient Information Center; Vitamin C. http://lpi.oregonstate.edu/infocenter/vitamins/vitaminC/ (accessed 12 September 2012).

[42] Kromhout D. Essential micronutrients in relation to carcinogenesis. Am J Clin Nutr May 1987;45(5):1361-1367.

[43] Cho E, Hunter DJ, Spiegelman D, Albanes D, Beeson WL, van den Brandt PA, Colditz GA, Feskanich D, Folsom AR, Fraser GE, Freudenheim JL, Giovannucci E, Gold-

bohm RA, Graham S, Miller AB, Rohan TE, Sellers TA, Virtamo J, Willett WC, Smith-Warner SA. Intakes of vitamins A, C and E and folate and multivitamins and lung cancer: a pooled analysis of 8 prospective studies. Int J Cancer 2006;118(4):970-8.

[44] Zhang S, Hunter DJ, Forman MR, Rosner BA, Speizer FE, Colditz GA, Manson JE, Hankinson SE, Willett WC. Dietary carotenoids and vitamins A, C, and E and risk of breast cancer. J Natl Cancer Inst 1999;91(6):547-56.

[45] Yu C. Contribution of Dietary Supplements to the Nutritional Status of College Students. (2011). Honors Scholar Theses. Paper 180. http://digitalcommons.uconn.edu/srhonors_theses/180

[46] Halliwell B. Vitamin C and genomic stability. Mutation Res 2001;475: 29-35.

[47] Claycombe KJ, Meydani SN. Vitamin E and genome stability. Mutat Res 2001;475(1-2):37-44.

[48] Kurzer MS. Phytoestrogen Supplement Use by Women. J Nutr 2003;133(6): 1983S-1986S.

[49] Willett WC. Diet and Cancer An Evolving Picture. JAMA 2005;293(2): 233-234.

[50] Steinmetz KA, Potter JD. Vegetables, fruit, and cancer prevention: a review. J Am Diet Assoc. 1996;96(10):1027-39.

[51] Ardekani AM and Jabbari S. Nutrigenomics and Cancer. Avicenna J Med Biotech 2009;1(1): 9-17.

Chapter 18

The Impact of Vitamin D in Cancer

Khanh vinh quoc Luong and Lan Thi Hoang Nguyen

Additional information is available at the end of the chapter

http://dx.doi.org/10.5772/55324

1. Introduction

The relationship between vitamin D and cancer has previously been reported in the literature. A systemic review and meta-analysis of prospective cohort studies revealed that a 20 nmol/L increase in the 25-hydroxyvitamin D_3 (25OHD) levels was associated with an 8% lower mortality in the elderly population (Schöttker et al., 2012). Oncology patients had significantly lower mean serum vitamin D levels than non-cancer primary care patients from the same geographic region (Churilla et al., 2011). In a community oncology experience, vitamin D deficiency is widespread in cancer patients and correlates with advanced stage disease (Churilla et al., 2012). A high prevalent of vitamin D deficiency has been associated with head and neck cancer (Orell-Kotikangas et al., 2011), breast cancer (Crew et al., 2009; Peppone et al., 2012), vulvar cancer (Salehin et al., 2012), prostate cancer (Varsavsky et al., 2011), pancreatic cancer (Wolpin et al., 2011), gastric cancer (Ren et al., 2012), colon and rectal cancer (Tangrea et al., 1997), ovarian cancer (Lefkowitz et al., 1994), oral cavity and esophagus cancers (Lipworth et al., 2009), myelo-proliferative neoplasms and myelo-dysplastic syndromes (Pardanani et al., 2011), multiple myeloma (Ng et at., 2009), non-Hodgkin's lymphoma (Drake et al., 2010), and chronic lymphocytic leukemia (Shamafelt et al., 2011). On the other hand, a serum 25OHD concentration of 25 nmol/L was associated with a 17% reduction in incidence of cancer, a 29% reduction in total cancer mortality, and a 45% reduction in digestive system cancer mortality (Giovannucci et al., 2006). Improving vitamin D status may also help lower the risk of colorectal cancer (Wu et al., 2011a). In a case-control study, a higher vitamin D intake is associated with a lower risk of esophageal squamous cell carcinoma (Launoy et al., 1998). A meta-analysis revealed that an increase of serum 25OHD by 50 nmol/L was associated with a risk reduction of 59% for rectal cancer and 22% for colon cancer (Yin et al., 2009). High 25OHD levels were associated with better prognosis in breast, colon, prostate cancer, and lung cancer relative to patients with lower 25OHD levels (Robsahm et al., 2004; Zhou et al., 2007). In a murine model, dietary vitamin D may play an important role as a preventive agent in androgen-insensitive human prostate tumor growth (Ray et al., 2012). The season in which patients were operated on seemed to have an effect on survival of patients undergoing resection of non-small cell lung cancer (Turna et al., 2012). The survival of patients who had surgery in winter was statistically significantly shorter than that of patients who underwent surgery in the summer. In Australia, prostate cancer mortality rates are inversely correlated with solar radiation exposure (Loke et al., 2011). Dietary vitamin D_3 and calcitriol have been shown to demonstrate equivalent anticancer activity in mouse xenograft models of breast and prostate cancers (Swani et al., 2012). The combination of calcitriol and dietary soy resulted in substantially greater inhibition of tumor growth than the inhibition achieved with either agent alone in a mouse xenograft model of prostate cancer (Wang et al., 2012a). Soy diets alone caused a modest elevation in serum calcitriol. Vitamin D_3 treatment significantly suppressed the viability of gastric cancer and cholangiocarcinoma cells and also had a synergistic effect with other anti-cancer drugs, such as paclitaxel, adriamycin, and vinblastine (Baek et al., 2011). The vitamin D analog, 19-Nor-2α-(3-hydroxypropyl)-1α,25-dihydroxyvitamin D_3, is a potent cell growth regulator with enhanced chemotherapeutic potency in liver cancer cells (Chiang et al., 2011). Alphacalcidol, a vitamin D analogue, has been demonstrated significant antitumor activity in patients with low-grade non-Hodgkin's lymphoma of the follicular, small-cleaved cell type (Raina et al., 1991). In patient with parathyroid cancer, vitamin D has been shown to prevent or delay the progression of recurrence (Palmieri-Sevier et al., 1993). In locally advanced or cutaneous metastatic breast cancer, topical calcipotriol treatment reduced the diameter of treated lesions that contained vitamin D receptor (*VDR*) (Bower et al., 1991). In a clinical trial, high-dose calcitriol decreased prostatic-specific antigen (PSA) levels by 50% and reduced thrombosis in prostate cancer patients (Beer et al., 2003 & 2006). In hepatocellular carcinoma, calcitriol and its analogs have been reported to reduce tumor volume, increase hepatocarcinoma cell apoptosis by 21.4%, and transient stabilize serum alpha-fetoprotein levels (Dalhoff et al., 2003; Luo et al., 2004; Morris et al., 2002). These findings suggested a relationship between vitamin D and cancer. In this chapter, we will discuss the role of vitamin D in cancer.

2. Genetic factors related to vitamin D and cancer

2.1. The Major Histocompatibility Complex (MHC) class II molecules

The major histocompatibility complex (MHC) class II molecules play an important role in the immune system and are essential in the defense against infection. The human MHC class II molecules are encoded by three different human leukocytic antigen (HLA) isotypes: HLA-DR, -DQ, and -DP. Studies have suggested that several genes within MHC region promote cancer susceptibility. A chimeric DR4 homozygous transgenic mouse line is reported to spontaneously develop diverse hematological malignancies at a high frequency (Raffegerst et al., 2009). Most of these neoplasms were highly similar to those found in human diseases. HLA-DR antigen expression was correlated with the histopathological type and to the degree of cell differentiation in cutaneous squamous cell carcinomas (Garcia-Plata et al., 1993). The DRB1*03 and DR-B1*13 alleles were significantly more frequent in patients with nasopharyngeal carcinoma compared with controls in southern Tunisia (Makni et al., 2010). The DR1 gene is strongly associated with thyroid carcinoma (Panza et al., 1982). The HLA-DR was also increased in poorly differentiated thyroid carcinoma, especially in the anaplastic type (Lindhorst et al., 2002). The DQA1*0102 and DPB1*0501 alleles were significantly more common in Chinese patients with hepatocellular carcinoma (HCC) (Donaldson et al., 2001). The frequency of DRB1*0404 allele was significantly higher in the gastric cancer group compared with the gastritis group in Koreans (Lee et al., 2009). However, the frequencies of the DRB1*0405 and DQB1*0401 alleles were increased in the Japanese patients with intestinal-type gastric cancer compared with controls (Ando et al., 2009). Somatic mutations affecting HLA class II genes may lead to loss of HLA class II expression due to the formation of microsatellites in unstable colorectal carcinomas (Michel et al., 2010). The DRB1*15 allele and the haplotype DRB1*15 DQB1*0602 were associated with human papillomavirus (HPV)-16 positive invasive cervical cancer in Mexican women (Hernández-Hernández et al., 2009). The DRB1*0410 allele was the susceptibility allele in Japanese patients with testicular germ cell carcinoma (Ozdemir et al., 1997). Furthermore, the frequencies of the DRB1*09 and DQB1*03 alleles were increased in patients with non-Hodgkin's lymphoma and diffuse large B cell lymphoma compared with normal controls (Choi et al., 2008). The frequencies of the DRB1*04 and DRB1*15 alleles were significantly higher in Turkish children with acute leukemia compared with controls (Ozdilli et al., 2010). The DRB1*16 allele was a marker for a signignificant risk of chronic myelogenous leukemia in Eastern Canada (Naugler and Liwski, 2009). The DRB1*04 and DRB5 alleles are associated with disease progression in Iranian patients with chronic lymphocytic leukemia (Hojattat-Farsangi et al., 2008). On the other hand, calcitriol is known to stimulate phagocytosis and suppress MHC class II antigen expression in human mononuclear phagocytes (Tokuda et al., 1992 & 1996), thereby preventing antigen-specific T cell proliferation. In addition, calcitriol exerts effects that opposes the effect of IL-4 on MHC class II antigen expression in human monocytes (Xu et al., 1993) and specifically modulates human monocyte phenotype and function by altering HLA-DR antigen expression and antigen presentation, while leaving lytic function intact (Rigby et al., 1990). Calcitriol also decreases interferon-γ-induced HLA-DR antigen expression in normal and transformed human keratinocytes (Tamaki et al., 1990-1991 & Tone et al., 1991) and reduces the levels of HLA-DR mRNA in cultured epithelial tumor cell lines (Tone et al., 1993). In addition, 1α-calcidol significantly modulates the expression of HLA-DR in human peripheral blood monocytes (Scherberich et al., 2005). These findings suggest that calcitriol may have an effect on cancer by suppressing the expression of MHC class II antigens.

2.2. Vitamin D Receptor (VDR)

The expression of VDR in a variety of cell lines, coupled with increased evidence of *VDR* involvement in cell differentiation, inhibition of cellular proliferation and angiogenesis in many tumor types, suggest that vitamin D plays a role in cancer (Luong and Nguyen, 2010 & Lương and Nguyễn, 2012). VDR ablation is associated with ductal ectasia of the primary mammary ducts, loss of secondary and tertiary branches and atrophy of the mammary fad pad (Welsh et al., 2011). Breast cancer patients with high VDR expression showed significant better in progression-free survival and overall survival than patients with moderate/negative VDR expression scores (Ditch et al., 2012). Certain allelic variations in the *VDR* may also be genetic risk factors for developing tumors. There are five important common polymorphisms within the *VDR* gene region that are likely to exert functional effects on *VDR* expression. The anti-carcinogenic potential of vitamin D might be mediated by VDR expression. The association between plasma 25OHD levels and colorectal adenoma was modified by the *Taq*I polymorphism of the VDR gene (Yamaji et al., 2011). There is a significant association between single nucleotide polymorphisms (SNPs) in the VDR gene and vitamin D intake in African Americans with colorectal cancer (Kupfer et al., 2011). The *Bsm*I polymorphism of the VDR gene also modified the association between dietary vitamin D intake and breast cancer (Rollison et al., 2012). The *AA* genotype of VDR is reported to be associated with colorectal cancer, with a stronger association in female patients (Mahmoudi et al., 2012). The *Fok*I and *Bsm*I genotypes of VDR gene are implicated in the pathogenesis of renal cell carcinoma (RCC) in a North Indian population (Arjumand et al., 2012). Altered VDR expression was associated with RCC carcinogenesis via the expression of epithelial Ca^{2+} channel transient receptor potential vanilloid subfamily 5 and 6 (TRPV5/6) (Wu et al., 2011b). There is a significant association between shorter progression-free survival time in patients with head and neck squamous cell carcinoma and the *Fok*I *TT* genotype, as well as the *Cdx2-Fox*I-*Apa*I haplotype (Hama et al., 2011). In Spanish children, osteosarcoma patients showed a significantly higher frequency of the *Ff* genotype of the *Fok*I *VDR* gene than the control group (Ruza et al., 2003). In a German population, the *AaTtBb* genotype of the VDR gene is associated with basal cell carcinoma risk, whereas the *aaTTbb* genotype is found at a high frequency in both basal cell carcinomas and cutaneous squamous cell carcinomas compared with controls (Köststner et al., 2012). In a systematic review, *Taq*I, *Bsm*I and *Fok*I polymorphisms of the VDR gene were found to be associated with malignant melanoma (Denzer et al., 2011). Furthermore, the presence of specific VDR *Bsm*I and *Taq*I alleles was associated with a higher C-reactive protein (CRP) level in cancer patients with cachectic syndrome (Punzi et al., 2012). In another prospective study, plasma 25OHD levels and common variation among several vitamin D-related genes (*CYP27A1, CYP2R1, CYP27B1, CYP24A1, GC, RXRA,* and *VDR*) were associated with lethal prostate cancer risk (Shui et al., 2012). Slattery et al. (2009) examined genetic variants that are linked to the pathway that contribute to colon cancer. They revealed that *Fox*I *VDR* polymorphism was associated with CpG Island methylator phenotype (CIMP) positive/Ki-ras mutated tumors, whereas the Poly *A* and *Cdx2 VDR* polymorphisms were associated only with Ki-ras mutated tumors.

2.3. MicroRNA (miRNA)

MiRNAs are endogenous noncoding RNAs that regulate gene expression through the translational repression or degradation of target mRNA (Bartel, 2004). Aberrant miRNA expression has been well characterized in cancer (Lu et al., 2005). Circulating miRNAs are suggested to be diagnostic and prognostic markers in breast cancer (Cortez et al., 2012). Circulating miRNA-125b expression is associated with chemotherapeutic resistance of breast cancer (Wang et al., 2012b). Several miRNAs are found to share 125b complementarity with a sequence in the 3'-unstranslated region of human VDR mRNA. The overexpression miRNA-125b significantly decreased the endogenous VDR protein level in human breast adenocarcinoma cells lines (MCF-7) to 40% of the control (Mohri et al., 2009). This miRNA is down-regulated in cancer tissue and causes high CYP24 protein expression, which catalyzes the inactivation of calcitriol (Komagata et al., 2009). Stress induced by serum starvation caused significant alteration in the expression of multiple miRNAs including miRNA-182, but calcitriol effectively reversed this alteration in breast epithelial cells (Peng et al., 2010). Vitamin D_3 up-regulated protein 1 (VDUP1) is regulated by miRNA-17-5p at the post-transcriptional levels in senescent fibroblasts (Zhuo et al., 2010). VDUP1 expression is increased in cancer cells (Takahashi et al., 2002; Dutta et al., 2005). In melanoma cell lines, the endogenous VDR mRNA level is inversely associated with expression of miRNA-125b (Essa et al., 2010), and calcitriol also reduced the miRNA-27b expression in these cell lines. In human colon cells, calcitriol induced miRNA-22 and may contribute to its antitumor action against this neoplasm (Alvarez-Diaz et al., 2012). Fifteen miRNAs are also differentially regulated by calcitriol in prostate cancer cells (LNCaP) (Wang et al 2011a). Furthermore, calcitriol regulated miRNA-32 and miRNA-181 expressions in human myeloid leukemia cells (Gocek et al., 2011; Zimmerman et al., 2011; Wang et al., 2009a).

2.4. Renin-Angiotensin System (RAS)

The primary function of the renin-angiotensin system (RAS) is to maintain fluid homeostasis and regulate blood pressure. The angiotensin converting enzyme (ACE) is a key enzyme in the RAS and converts angiotensin (AT) I to the potent vasoconstrictor AT II (Johnston, 1994). The local RAS may influence tissue angiogenesis, cellular proliferation, apoptosis, and inflammation (Deshayes and Nahmias, 2005). Epidemiological and experimental studies suggested that the RAS may contribute to the paracrine regulation of tumor growth. The renin levels are elevated in patients with liver cirrhosis and HCC and positively correlated with α-fetoprotein (Lotfy et al., 2010). The over-expression of ACE is reported in extrahepatic cholangiocarcinoma (Beyazit et al., 2011), leukemic myeloid blast cells (Aksu et al., 2006), and macrophages in the lymph nodes of Hodgkin's disease patients (Koca et al., 2007). The AT II receptors were also expressed in all human gastric cancer lines (Huang et al., 2008), pre-malignant and malignant prostate cells (Louis et al., 2007), human lung cancer xenografts (Feng et al., 2011a), and ovarian cancer (Ino et al., 2006). The RAS mutation in codon 61 was the most common genetic alteration in poorly differentiated thyroid carcinomas (Volante et al., 2009). The ACE *I/D* polymorphism is a possible target for developing genetic markers for breast cancer in Brazilian women (Alves Corrêa et al., 2009). The ACE *I/D* polymorphisms play an important role in breast cancer risk and disease-free survival in Caucasian postmenopausal women (González-Zuloeta Ladd et al., 2012). Carriers of the high-activity *DD* genotype had an increased risk of breast cancer compared with low activity *II/ID* genotype carriers (van der Knaap et al., 2008). The *DD* genotype was associated with patients with an aggressive stage of prostate cancer (Wang et al., 2011b). ACE2 expression was decreased in non-small-cell lung cancer and pancreatic ductal adenocarcinoma in which AT II levels were higher than those in controls (Feng et al., 2010; Zhou et al., 2009). ACE2 has been suggested as a potential molecular target for pancreatic cancer therapy (Zhou et al., 2011). The AT II concentration in gastric cancer region was significantly higher than those of normal region (Kinoshita et al., 2009). Furthermore, AT II receptor blockers (ARB) suppress the cell proliferation effects of AT II in breast cancer cells (Du et al., 2012). The addition of ACE inhibitor or ARB to platinum-based first line chemotherapy contributed to prolong survival in patients with advanced lung cancer (Wilop et al., 2009) and affected the prognosis of advanced pancreatic cancer patients receiving gemcitabine (Nakai et al., 2010). The RAS inhibitors also improved the outcome of sunitinib treatment in metastatic renal cell carcinoma (Keizman et al., 2011). On the other hand, the administration of ACE inhibitors in patients with the ACE *DD* genotype has been shown to decrease the level of calcitriol required (Pérez-Castrillón et al., 2006). In a hypertensive Turkish population, the presence of the ACE *D* allele, which correlates negatively with serum 25OHD levels, is linked to a higher left ventricular mass index value and elevated ambulatory blood pressure measurements (Kulah et al., 2007). In addition, genetic disruption of the *VDR* gene resulted in overstimulation of the RAS with increased renin and angiotensin II production, which lead to high blood pressure and cardiac hypertrophy. However, treatment with captopril reduced cardiac hypertrophy in VDR-knockout mice (Xiang et al., 2005), suggesting that calcitriol may function as an endocrine suppressor of renin biosynthesis. Moreover, calcitriol suppresses renin gene transcription by blocking the activity of the cyclic AMP response element in the renin core promoter (Yuan et al., 2007) and decreases ACE activity in bovine endothelial cells (Higiwara et al., 1988).

2.5. Toll-Like Receptor (TLR)

Toll-like receptors (TLRs) are a group of glycoproteins that functions as surface trans-membrane receptors and are involved in the innate immune responses to exogenous pathogenic microorganisms. Substantial evidence exists for an important role of TLRs in the pathogenesis and outcomes of cancer. TLR2 expression was significantly higher in sporadic colorectal cancerous tissue than in non-cancerous tissue (Nihon-Yanagi et al., 2012). The TLR5 play an important role in tumor progression of gastric cancer (Song et al., 2011). The TLR7 and TLR9 showed high expression in laryngeal carcinoma cells (Shikora et al., 2010). The over-expression of TLR9 was reported oral squamous cell carcinoma (Min et al., 2011), esophageal squamous cell carcinoma (Takala et al., 2011), and breast cancer cells (Qiu et al., 2011; Sandholm et al., 2012). The expression levels of TLR1, TLR2, TLR4, TLR5, TLR6, TLR8, and TLR10 are significantly higher in the human renal carcinoma cell line (780-6) than those in normal renal cell (HK-2) line (Yu et al., 2011). Chronic lymphocytic leukemia cells express all TLRs expressed by normal activated B cells, with a high expression of TLR9 and CD180 and an intermediate expression of TLR1, TLR6, and TLR10 (Arvaniti et al., 2011). The TLR4 polymorphisms are reported in patients with the risk of prostate cancer (Kim et al., 2012), head and neck squamous cell carcinomas (Bergmann et al., 2011), HCC (Minmin et al., 2011), and colon cancer (Eyking et al., 2011). Furthermore, multiple SNPs in TLR2 and TLR4 were associated with colon cancer survival (Slattery et al., 2012). On the other hand, vitamin D deficiency increases the expression of hepatic mRNA levels of TLR2, TLR4, and TLR9 in obese rats (Roth et al., 2011). However, calcitriol suppresses the expression of TLR2 and TLR4 protein and mRNA in human monocytes and triggers hypo-responsiveness to pathogen-associated molecular patterns (Sadeghi et al., 2006). Calcitriol has also been shown to down-regulate intracellular TLR2, TLR4 and TLR9 expression in human monocytes (Dickie et al., 2010). TLR activation results in the expression of the VDR and 1α-vitamin D hydroxylase in human monocytes (Liu et al., 2006). Additionally, calcitriol can cause the vitamin D-induced expression of cathelicidin in bronchial epithelial cells (Yim et al., 2007) and may enhance the production of cathelicidin LL-37 (Rivas-Santiago et al., 2008). The addition of a VDR antagonist has also been shown to inhibit the induction of cathelicidin mRNA by more than 80%, thereby reducing the protein expression of this antimicrobial agent by approximately 70% (Yim et al., 2007). Cathelicidin was abundant in tumor-infiltrating NK1.1$^+$ cells in mice. Cathelicidin knockout mice (*Camp*$^{-/-}$) permitted faster tumor growth than wild type controls; NK cells derived from *Camp*$^{-/-}$ mice showed impaired cytotoxic activity toward tumor targets compared with wild-type mice (Büchau et al., 2010). The human cathelicidin LL-37, which inhibits gastric cancer cell proliferation, is down-regulated in gastric adenocarcinomas (Wu et al., 2010). Gastrointestinal cancer cells lacked LL-37 expression; Cathelicidin expression is modulated by histone-deacetylase (HDAC) inhibitors in various gastrointestinal cells, including gastric and hepatocellular cells (Schauer et al., 2004). HDAC inhibitors enhance the acetylation of core proteins, which is linked to the formation of transcriptionally active chromatin in various cells. The expression of the LL-37/hCAP-18 gene was also reduced in some leukemia cells (Yang et al., 2003). In patients with acute myeloid leukemia, there was a marked reduction of LL-37/hCAP-18 expression in the peripheral blood compared with the level in healthy donors (An et al., 2005). In myeloid cells, cathelicidin gene is a direct target of the VDR and is strongly up-regulated by calcitriol (Gombart et al., 2005). The combination of TLR ligands (CpG oligodeoxynucleotides, CpG-ODN) LL-37 generated significantly better therapeutic tumor effects and enhanced survival in murine ovarian tumor-bearing mice compared with CpG-ODN or LL-37 alone (Chuang et al., 2009).

3. Role of vitamin D and its analog in cancer

3.1. The bacillus Calmette-Guerin (BCG) vaccination

The BCG vaccine was developed to provide protection against tuberculosis and has also been demonstrated to offer protection against cancer. The combination of BCG and ionizing radiation resulted in the induction of autophagy in colon cancer cells (Yuk et al., 2010). Intravesical BCG therapy has been demonstrated to reduce the recurrence rate and the risk of progression to muscle-invasive disease in patients with superficial bladder tumors (Herr et al., 1988). The BCG vaccination significantly prolongs the survival of patients with a malignant melanoma after initial surgical removed (Kölmel et al., 2005) and improved survival rates in patients with resected lung cancer (Repin, 1992). BCG inoculation delayed the tumor growth and prolonged the survival time in nude mice with leukemia (Wang et al., 2011c). BCG vaccination reduced the risk of lymphomas in a Danish population (Villumsen et al., 2009) and demonstrated to reduce the mortality, morbidity, and frequency of myeloic and chronic leukemia in children (Ambrosch et al., 1981). On the other hand, BCG-vaccinated infants are almost 6 times more likely to have sufficient vitamin D concentrations than unvaccinated infants 3 months after BCG vaccination, and this association remains strong even after adjusting for season, ethnic group and sex (Lalor et al., 2011). Among the vaccinated group, there was also a strong inverse correlation between the IFN-γ response to *M. tuberculosis* PPD and vitamin D concentration; infants with higher vitamin D concentrations had lower IFN-γ responses. Similarly, tuberculosis in cattle usually presents with a rapid transient increase in serum calcitriol within the first two weeks following infection (Rhodes et al., 2003). 1,25OHD-positive mononuclear cells were later identified in all of the tuberculous granulomas. During tuberculosis infection, alveolar macrophage-produced calcitriol plays a beneficial role by limiting inflammation-mediated tissue injury, potentiating NO production by stimulated monocytes/macrophages, inhibiting INF-γ production by stimulated $CD4^+$ cells, and suppressing the growth of *M. tuberculosis* (Ametaj et al., 1996; Rockett et al., 1998).

3.2. Matrix Metalloproteinase (MMPs)

MMPs are proteolytic enzymes responsible for extracellular matrix remodeling and the regulation of leukocyte migration through the extracellular matrix, which is an important step in inflammatory and infectious pathophysiology. MMPs are produced by many cell types including lymphocytes, granulocytes, astrocytes and activated macrophages. The MMP-1 expression is linked to sarcoma cell invasion (Garamszegi et al., 2011). MMP-2 expression is increased in gastric cancer cells (Partyka et al., 2012) and colorectal cancer (Dong et al., 2011). MMP-9 is expressed in many cancer cells, such as those associated with non-small-cell lung cancer (Peng et al., 2012), ovarian cancer invasion and metastasis (Zhang et al., 2011a), glioblastoma multiforme (Yan et al., 2011), and adamantinous craniopharyndioma (Xia et al., 2011). The MMP-2 and MMP-9 secreted by leukemic cells increase the permeability of blood brain barrier of the CNS by disrupting tight junction proteins (Feng et al., 2011b). In gastric cancer, MMP-2 and MMP-9 play an important role in tumor invasion and metastasis (Parsons et al., 1998). The risks for the development of hypophyseal adenoma and cervical neoplasia are greater in patients with MMP-1 polymorphisms (Altaş et al., 2010; Tee et al., 2012) than those with the wild-type allele. The MMP-2 polymorphism contributed to prostate cancer susceptibility in North India (Srivastava et al., 2012) and to the clinical outcome of Chinese patients with non-small cell lung cancer treated with first-line, platinum-based chemotherapy (Zhao et al., 2011). The MMP-7 polymorphisms are associated with esophageal squamous cell carcinoma and colorectal cancers (Manzoor et al., 2011; Dziki et al., 2011). The SPNs in the MMP-2 and MMP-9 region are associated with susceptibility to head and neck squamous cell carcinoma in an Indian population (Chaudhary et al., 2011). The SNPs of genes encoding MMPs (-1, -2, -3, -7, -8, -9, -12, -13, and -21) are related to breast cancer risk, progression, and survival (Wieczorek et al., 2012). Based on meta-analysis studies, the MMP-2 allele (-1306T) is a protective factor for digestive cancer risk (Zhang and Ren, 2011), the MMP-9 polymorphism is associated with a lower risk of colorectal cancer (Zhang et al., 2012a), and polymorphisms in the promoter regions of MMP-1, -3, -7, and -9 are associated with metastasis in some cancers (Liu et al., 2012). On the other hand, VDR-knock-out mice were shown to have an influx of inflammatory cells, phospho-acetylation of NF-κB, and up-regulated expression of MMP-2, MMP-9, and MMP-12 in the lung (Sundar et al., 2011). The *VDR TaqI* polymorphism is associated with decreased production of TIMP-1, a natural inhibitor of MMP-9 (Timms et al., 2002). In addition, calcitriol modulates tissue MMP expression under experimental conditions (Dean et al., 1996), down-regulates MMP-9 levels in keratinocytes, and may attenuate the deleterious effects of excessive TNF-α-induced proteolytic activity associated with cutaneous inflammation (Bahar-Shang et al., 2010). Calcitriol decreased the invasive properties of breast carcinoma cells and decreased MMP-9 levels in association with the increased levels of the tissue inhibitor of MMP-1 activity (Koli and Keshi-Oja, 2000). Calcitriol also inhibits endometrial cancer cell growth and is associated with decreased MMP-2 and MMP-9 expression

(Nguyen et al., 2011). Moreover, calciferol, calcitriol, and vitamin D analogs decreased MMP-2 and MMP-9 activities and inhibited prostate cancer cell invasion (Tokar and Webber, 2005; Schartz et al., 1997; Iglesias-Gato et al., 2011; Stio et al., 2011). A vitamin D analog has also been reported to reduce the expression of MMP-2, MMP-9, vascular endothelial growth factor (VEGF) and PTH-related peptide in Lewis lung carcinoma cells (Nakagawa et al., 2005). Taken together, these studies suggest that calcitriol may play an important role in the pathological processes in cancer by down-regulating the level of MMPs and regulating the level of TIMPs.

3.3. Wnt/β-catenin

The Wnt/β-catenin signaling pathway plays a pivotal role in the regulation of cell growth, cell development and the differentiation of normal stem cells. Wnt/β-catenin signaling is implicated in many human cancers, including gastrointestinal cancer, gastric cancer, colon cancer, melanoma, HCC, endometrial carcinoma, ovarian carcinoma, cervical cancer, papillary thyroid carcinoma, renal cell carcinoma, prostate cancer, parathyroid carcinoma, and hematological malignancies (White et al., 2012; Nuñez et al., 2011; Polakis, 2000; Li et al., 2012; Yoshioka et al., 2012; Guturi et al., 2012; Bulut et al., 2011; Gilber-Sirieix et al., 2011; Ueno et al., 2011; Svedlund et al., 2010; Ge and Wang, 2010). Calcitriol inhibits β-catenin transcriptional activity by promoting VDR binding to β-catenin and the induction of E-cadherin expression (Palmer et al., 2001). Paricalcitol, a vitamin D analog, suppressed β-catenin-mediated gene transcription and ameliorated proteinuria and kidney injury in adriamycin nephropathy (He et al., 2011). Most VDR variants fail to activate the vitamin D-responsive promoter and also fail to bind β-catenin or regulate its activity (Byers and Shah, 2007). VDR depletion enhances Wnt/β-catenin signaling and the tumor burden in colon cancer (Larriba et al., 2011). The action of cacitriol on colon carcinoma cells depends on the dual action of VDR as a transcription factor and a nongenomic activator of RhoA-ROCK and p38MAPK-MSK1, which are required for the inhibition of the Wnt/β-catenin signaling pathway and cell proliferation (Ordóñez-Morán et al., 2008). The *DICKKOFF*-4 gene induces a malignant phenotype, promotes tumor cell invasion, and angiogenesis in colon cancer cells and is repressed by calcitriol (Pendás-Franco et al., 2008a); whereas *DICKKOFF*-1 gene acts as a tumor suppressor in human colon cells and is up-regulated by calcitriol (Aguilera et al., 2007; Pendás-Franco et al., 2008b). The transcription factor TCF-4 acts as transcriptional repressor in breast and colorectal cancer cell growth. The TCF-4 and β-catenin binding partner are indirect targets of the VDR pathway. In the VDR knockout mouse, TCF-4 is decreased in the mammary gland when compared with a wild-type mouse. In addition, calcitriol increases TCF-4 RNA and protein levels in several human colorectal cancer cell lines (Beildeck et al., 2009). Furthermore, the Snail1 gene is associated with gastric cancer, melanoma, breast cancer, HCC, and colon carcinoma. Calcitriol inhibits the Wnt/β-catenin signaling pathway and is abrogated by Snail1 in human colon cancer cells (Larriba et al., 2007).

3.4. The Mitogen-Activated Protein Kinase (MAPK) pathways

The MAPK pathways provide a key link between the membrane bound receptors that receive these cues and changes in the pattern of gene expression, including the extracellular signal-regulated kinase (ERK) cascade, the stress activated protein kinases/c-jun N-terminal kinase

(SAPK/JNK) cascade, and the p38MAPK/RK/HOG cascade (Hipskind and Bilbe, 1998). In human colon cancer cells, calcitriol increases cytosolic Ca^{2+} concentration and transiently activates RhoA-ROCK, and then activates the p38MAPK-MSK signaling pathway (Ordóñez-Morán et al., 2008). In breast cancer cells, the MARK (JNK and p38) signaling pathway involved in calcitriol-induced breast cell death (Brosseau et al., 2010) and potentiated the cytotoxic action of calcitriol and TNF-α (Weitsman, et al., 2004). In murine squamous cell carcinoma cells, vitamin D induced apoptosis and selective induction of caspase-dependent MEK cleavage (McGuire et al., 2001). In an ovarian cancer animal model, vitamin D induced cell death and is mediated by the p38MAPK signaling pathway (Lange et al., 2010). In human promyeloblastic leukemia cells (HL60), vitamin D derivatives had anti-proliferative activity and activated MAPK signaling pathways (Ji et al., 2002). In human acute myeloid leukemia cells, calcitriol-induced differentiation is enhanced by the activation of MAPK signaling pathways (Zhang et al., 2011b).

3.5. The Prostaglandins (PGs)

Prostaglandins (PGs) play a role in inflammatory processes, and cyclooxygenase (COX) participates in the conversion of arachidonic acid in PGs. A variety studies have shown that prostaglandin signaling stimulates cancer cell growth and cancer progression. The regulation of PG metabolism and biological actions contribute to its anti-proliferation effects in prostate cells and calcitriol has been reported to regulate the expression of several key genes involved in the PG pathway, resulting in decreased PG synthesis (Moreno et al., 2005). The expression of the COX-2 gene is significantly increased in human gastric adenocarcinoma tissues compared with adjuvant normal gastric mucosal specimens (Ristimäki et al., 1997). There is inversely association between elevated COX-2 levels and decreased VDR expression in patients with breast and ovarian cancers compared with healthy women (Cordes et al., 2012). Calcitriol differentiated the human leukemic cell line (HL-60) and metabolized exogenous arachidonic acid to both COX products (predominantly thromboxane B_2 and PG E_2) and lipoxygenase products, including leukotriene B_4 (Stenson et al., 1988). In a mouse xenograft model of prostate cancer, the combination of cacitriol and dietary soy enhanced cacitriol activity in regulating target gene expression and increased the suppression of PG synthesis and signaling, such as COX-2, 15-hydroxyprostaglandin dehydrogenase (15-PGDH), and PG receptors. (Wang et al., 2012a). Calcitriol and its analogs have also been shown to selectively inhibit the activity of COX-2 (Aparna et al., 2008), and an inverse correlation exists between the expression of PG-metabolizing enzymes and reduced VDR expression in malignant breast cell lines (Thill et al., 2012). Taken together, these findings suggest that vitamin D may play a role in modulating the inflammatory process in cancer.

3.6. Oxidative stress

Reactive oxygen species (ROS) play a major role in various cell-signaling pathways. ROS activates various transcription factors and increases in the expression of proteins that control cellular transformation, tumor cell survival, tumor cell proliferation and invasion, angiogenesis, and metastasis. ROS has an important role in the initiation and progression of many cancers (Gupta et al., 2012; Marra et al., 2011; Zhang et al., 2011c; Wang et al., 2011c; Rogalska et al., 2011; Gupta-

Elera et al., 2012). Single nucleotide polymorphisms of antioxidant defense genes may significantly modify the functional activity of the encoded proteins. Women with genetic variability in the iron-related oxidative stress pathways may be at increased risk of post-menopausal breast cancer (Hong et al., 2007). The *ala* variant of superoxide dismutase (SOD) is associated with a moderately increased risk of prostate cancer (Woodson et al., 2003). Based on meta-analysis studies, manganese SOD (MnSOD) polymorphisms may contribute to cancer development (Val-9Ala) (Wang et al., 2009b), prostate cancer susceptibility (Val-16Ala) (Mao et al., 2010), but not to breast cancer susceptibility (Val-16Ala) (Ma et al., 2010a). Calcitriol can also protect nonmalignant prostate cells from oxidative stress-induced cell death through the prevention of reactive oxygen species (ROS)-induced cellular injuries (Bao et al., 2008). Vitamin D metabolites and vitamin D analogs have been reported to induce lipoxygenase mRNA expression, lipoxygenase activity and ROS in a human bone cell line (Somjen et al., 2011). Vitamin D can also reduce the extent of lipid peroxidation and induce SOD activity in the hepatic anti-oxidant system of rats (Sardar et al., 1996). Moreover, the activation of macrophage 1α-hydroxylase results in an increase in 1,25OHD, which inhibits iNOS expression and reduces nitric oxide (NO) production by LPS-stimulated macrophages (Chang et al., 2004). This calcitriol production by macrophages may provide protection against the oxidative injuries caused by the NO burst. Calcitriol is known to inhibit LPS-induced immune activation in human endothelial cells (Equil et al., 2005), and calcitriol has also been shown to enhance intracellular glutathione pools and significantly reduce the nitrite production induced by the LPS (Garcion et al., 1999). Furthermore, overproduction of ROS induces DNA damage and leads to carcinogenesis. In the mouse colon, there was an inverse relationship between VDR levels and colonic hyperproliferation; the expression of 8-hydroxy-2′-deoxyguanosine (8-OHdG), a maker of oxidative DNA damage, significantly increased with complete loss of VDR (Kállay et al., 2002). Vitamin D decrease 8-OHdG by 22% in the normal human colorectal mucosa (Fedirko et al., 2012). Calcitriol contributes to a reduction of the DNA intensify replication stress in lymphocytes (Halicka et al., 2012). In addition, vitamin D_3 up-regulated protein 1(VDUP1) is a regular for redox signaling and stress-mediated diseases (Chung et al., 2006). Taken together, these findings suggest that vitamin D modulates oxidative stress in cancer.

4. The use of vitamin D in cancer treatment

A number of clinical trials have used vitamin D_3 and calcitriol alone or in combination with anti-tumor agents. Most preclinical suggest that that the optimal anti-tumor effect of calcitriol and other analogs is seen with the administration of high dose calcitriol on intermittent schedule. A small number of single agent trials utilizing vitamin D_3 and calcitriol hace been conducted with limited success.

4.1. Vitamin D_3 trials

Fifteen patients were given 2,000 IU (50 microg) of cholecalciferol daily and monitored prospectively every 2-3 mo. There was a statistically significant decrease in the rate of PSA rise after administration of cholecalciferol compared with that before cholecalciferol. The median PSA doubling time increased from 14.3 months prior to commencing cholecalciferol to 25 months after commencing cholecalciferol. Fourteen of 15 patients had a prolongation of PSA doubling time after commencing cholecalciferol (Woo et al., 2005). Breast cancer patients with bone metastases received 10,000 IU of vitamin D_3 daily for 4 months. There was a significant reduction in the number of sites of pain (Amir et al., 2010). Arlet al. (2012) reported on an unexpected observation of a spectacular 13-month remission of chronic lymphocytic leukemia after the administration of cholecalciferol in an elderly patient. Dietary vitamin D_3 and calcitriol have been shown to demonstrate equivalent anticancer activity in mouse xenograft models of breast and prostate cancers (Swani et al., 2012).

4.2. Calcitriol trials — Single agent

In a clinical trial, high-dose calcitriol decreased prostatic-specific antigen (PSA) levels by 50% and reduced thrombosis in prostate cancer patients (Beer et al., 2003 & 2006). In hepatocellular carcinoma, calcitriol and its analogs have been reported to reduce tumor volume, increase hepatocarcinoma cell apoptosis by 21.4%, and transient stabilize serum alpha-fetoprotein levels (Dalhoff et al., 2003; Luo et al., 2004; Morris et al., 2002). The vitamin D analog, 19-Nor-2α-(3-hydroxypropyl)-1α,25-dihydroxyvitamin D_3, is a potent cell growth regulator with enhanced chemotherapeutic potency in liver cancer cells (Chiang et al., 2011). Alphacalcidol, a vitamin D analogue, has been demonstrated significant antitumor activity in patients with low-grade non-Hodgkin's lymphoma of the follicular, small-cleaved cell type (Raina et al., 1991). In patient with parathyroid cancer, vitamin D has been shown to prevent or delay the progression of recurrence (Palmieri-Sevier et al., 1993). Treatment with paricalcitol inhibited gastric cancer cell growth and peritoneal metastatic gastric cancer volume was significantly lower in paricalcitol treated mice (Park et al., 2012). Calcitriol treatment of breast cancer cell lines led to significantly fewer inflammatory breast cancer experimental metastases as compared to control (Hillyer et al., 2012).

4.3. Calcitriol trials — In combination

Calcitriol additively or synergistically potentiates the antitumor of other types of chemotherapeutic agents. Calcitriol enhances cellular sensitivity of human colon cancer cells to 5-fluorouracil (Liu et al., 2010). Combination of calcitriol and cytarabine prolonged remission in elderly patients with acute myeloid leukemia (AML) and myelodysplastic syndrome (MDS) (Slapak et al., 1992; Ferrero, et al., 2004). A renal cell carcinoma patient with multiple bone metastases that were almost completely resolved after treatment with vitamin D and interferon-α (Fujioka et al., 1988). In a prospective study, a combination of active vitamin D and α- interferon has shown to be effective in patients with metastatic renal cell carcinoma (Obara et al., 2008). Calcitriol promotes the anti-proliferative effects of gemcitabine and cisplatin in human bladder cancer models (Ma et al., 2010b), and also potentiates antitumor activity of paclitaxel and docetaxel (Hershberger et al., 2001; Ting et al. 2007). A phase II study showed that high-dose calcitriol with docetaxel may increase time to progression in patients with incurable pancreatic cancer when compared with docetaxel monotherapy (Blanke, 2009).Vitamin D_3 treatment significantly suppressed the viability of gastric cancer and cholangiocarcinoma cells and also had a synergistic effect with other anti-cancer drugs, such as paclitaxel, adriamycin, and vinblastine (Baek et al., 2011). In locally

http://dx.doi.org/10.5772/55324

advanced or cutaneous metastatic breast cancer, topical calcipotriol treatment reduced the diameter of treated lesions that contained vitamin D receptor (*VDR*) (Bower et al., 1991). Calcitriol potentiates both carboplatin and cisplatin-mediated growth inhibition in breast and prostate cancer cell lines (Cho et al., 1991; Moffatt et al., 1999). Tamoxifen and calcitriol or its analog used together to enhance growth inhibition in breast cancer cells than either agent alone (Vink-van Wijngaarden et al., 1994). Cacitriol sensitizes breast cancer cells to doxorubicin through the inhibition of the expression and activity of cytoplasmic antioxidant enzyme (Ravid et al., 1999). Calcitriol may increase cisplatin sensitivity in chemotherapy-resistant testicular germ cell cancer-derived cell lines (Jørgensen et al., 2012). Combination of retinoic acid and vitamin D analog exert synergistic growth inhibition and apoptosis induction on hepatocellular cancers cells (Zhang et al., 2012b). The combination of calcitriol and dietary soy resulted in substantially greater inhibition of tumor growth than the inhibition achieved with either agent alone in a mouse xenograft model of prostate cancer (Wang et al., 2012a).

5. Conclusion

Vitamin D has a role in the prevention and treatment of cancer. Genetic studies have provided the opportunity to determine what proteins link vitamin D to the pathology of cancer. Vitamin D also exerts its effect on cancer via non-genomic mechanisms. As a result, it is imperative that vitamin D levels in patients with cancer be followed. Many studies use the relationship between serum PTH and 25OHD to define the normal range of serum 25OHD. According to the report on Dietary Reference Intakes for vitamin D and calcium by the Institute of Medicine (IOM), persons are at risk of deficiency at serum 25OHD levels less than 30 nmol/L. Saliba et al. (2011) suggested that a 25OHD threshold of 50 nmol/L is sufficient for PTH suppression and prevention of secondary hyperparathyroidism in persons with normal renal function. It is necessary to check serum 25OHD$_3$ and parathyroid hormone (PTH) status in cancer patients. Serum levels of PTH have been reported to correlate with PSA levels and colorectal cancer (Skinner & Schwartz, 2009; Charalampopoulos et al., 2010). Some authors proposed that, in patients with normal calcium levels, the serum 25OHD$_3$ levels should be stored to > 55ng/ml in cancer patients (colon, breast, and ovary) (Garland et al., 2007). Calcitriol, 1,25OHD$_3$, is best used for cancer treatment, because of its active form of vitamin D$_3$ metabolite, suppression of PTH levels (acted as cellular growth factor), and their receptors presented in most of human cells. However, monitor of serum 25OHD$_3$ after taking calcitriol is not necessary because calcitriol inhibits the production of serum 25OHD$_3$ by the liver (Bell et al., 1984; Luong & Nguyen, 1996). The main limitation to the clinical widespread evolution of 1,25OHD$_3$ is its hypercalcemic side-effects.

Author details

Khanh vinh quoc Luong and Lan Thi Hoang Nguyen

Vietnamese American Medical Research Foundation, Westminster, California, USA

References

[1] Aguilera, O, Peña, C, García, J. M, Larriba, M. J, Ordóñez-morán, P, Navarro, D, & Barbáchano, A. López de Silanes I, Ballestar E, Fraga MF, Esteller M, Gamallo C, Bonilla F, González-Sancho JM, Muñoz A. The Wnt antagonist DICKKOPF-1 gene is induced by 1alpha,25-dihydroxyvitamin D_3 associated to the differentiation of human colon cancer cells. Carcinogenesis. (2007). Sep;, 28(9), 1877-84.

[2] Aksu, S, Beyazit, Y, Haznedaroglu, I. C, Canpinar, H, Kekilli, M, Uner, A, Sayinalp, N, Büyükasik, Y, Goker, H, & Ozcebe, O. I. Over-expression of angiotensin-converting enzyme (CD 143) on leukemic blasts as a clue for the activated local bone marrow RAS in AML. Leuk Lymphoma. (2006). May;, 47(5), 891-6.

[3] Ambrosch, F, Wiedermann, G, Krepler, P, Kundi, M, & Ambrosch, P. Effect of BCG vaccination of the newborn infant on the incidence and course of juvenile leukemias]. Fortschr Med. (1981). Sep 17;Article in German], 99(35), 1389-93.

[4] Ametaj, B, Beitz, D, Reihardt, T, & Nonnecke, B. (1996). dihydroxyvitamin D_3 inhibits secretion of interferon-gamma by mitogen- and antigen-stimulated bovine mononuclear leukocytes. Vet Immunol Imnunopathol. 52, 77-90., 1, 25.

[5] Amir, E, Simmons, C. E, Freedman, O. C, Dranitsaris, G, Cole, D. E, Vieth, R, Ooi, W. S, & Clemons, M. A phase 2 trial exploring the effects of high-dose (10,000 IU/day) vitamin D_3 in breast cancer patients with bone metastases. Cancer. (2010). Jan 15;, 116(2), 284-91.

[6] An, L. L, Ma, X. T, Yang, Y. H, Lin, Y. M, Song, Y. H, & Wu, K. F. Marked reduction of LL-37/hCAP-18, an antimicrobial peptide, in patients with acute myeloid leukemia. Int J Hematol. (2005). Jan;, 81(1), 45-7.

[7] Ando, T, Ishikawa, T, Kato, H, Yoshida, N, Naito, Y, Kokura, S, Yagi, N, Takagi, T, Handa, O, Kitawaki, J, Nakamura, N, Hasegawa, G, Fukui, M, Imamoto, E, Nakamura, C, Oyamada, H, Isozaki, Y, Matsumoto, N, Nagao, Y, Okita, M, Nakajima, Y, Kurokawa, M, Nukina, M, Ohta, M, Mizuno, S, Ogata, M, Obayashi, H, Park, H, Kitagawa, Y, Nakano, K, & Yoshikawa, T. Synergistic effect of HLA class II loci and cytokine gene polymorphisms on the risk of gastric cancer in Japanese patients with Helicobacter pylori infection. Int J Cancer. (2009). Dec 1;, 125(11), 2595-602.

[8] Altas, M, Bayrak, O. F, Ayan, E, Bolukbasi, F, Silav, G, Coskun, K. K, Culha, M, Sahin, F, Sevli, S, & Elmaci, I. The effect of polymorphisms in the promoter region of the MMP-1 gene on the occurrence and invasiveness of hypophyseal adenoma. Acta Neurochir (Wien). (2010). Sep;, 152(9), 1611-7.

[9] Alvarez-díaz, S, Valle, N, Ferrer-mayorga, G, Lombardía, L, Herrera, M, Domínguez, O, Segura, M. F, Bonilla, F, Hernando, E, & Muñoz, A. MicroRNA-22 is induced by vitamin D and contributes to its antiproliferative, antimigratory and gene regulatory effects in colon cancer cells. Hum Mol Genet. (2012). May 15;, 21(10), 2157-65.

[10] Alves Corrêa SA, Ribeiro de Noronha SM, Nogueira-de-Souza NC, Valleta de Carvalho C, Massad Costa AM, Juvenal Linhares J, Vieira Gomes MT, Guerreiro da Silva ID. Association between the angiotensin-converting enzyme (insertion/deletion) and angiotensin II type 1 receptor (A1166C) polymorphisms and breast cancer among Brazilian women. J Renin Angiotensin Aldosterone Syst. (2009). Mar;, 10(1), 51-8.

[11] Arjumand, W, Ahmad, S. T, Seth, A, Saini, A. K, & Sultana, S. Vitamin D receptor FokI and BsmI gene polymorphism and its association with grade and stage of renal cell carcinoma in North Indian population. Tumour Biol. (2012). Feb;, 33(1), 23-31.

[12] Arlet, J. B, Callens, C, Hermine, O, Darnige, L, Macintyre, E, Pouchot, J, & Capron, L. Chronic lymphocytic leukaemia responsive to vitamin D administration. Br J Haematol. (2012). Jan;, 156(1), 148-9.

[13] Arvaniti, E, Ntoufa, S, Papakonstantinou, N, Touloumenidou, T, Laoutaris, N, Anagnostopoulos, A, Lamnissou, K, Caligaris-cappio, F, Stamatopoulos, K, Ghia, P, Muzio, M, & Belessi, C. Toll-like receptor signaling pathway in chronic lymphocytic leukemia: distinct gene expression profiles of potential pathogenic significance in specific subsets of patients. Haematologica. (2011). Nov;, 96(11), 1644-52.

[14] Baek, S, Lee, Y. S, Shim, H. E, Yoon, S, Baek, S. Y, Kim, B. S, Oh, S. O, & Vitamin, D. regulates cell viability in gastric cancer and cholangiocarcinoma. Anat Cell Biol. (2011). Sep;, 44(3), 204-9.

[15] Bahar-shany, K, Ravid, A, & Koren, R. Upregulation of MMP-production by TNFalpha in keratinocytes and its attenuation by vitamin D. J Cell Physiol. (2010). , 222, 729-37.

[16] Bao, B. Y, Ting, H. J, Hsu, J. W, & Lee, Y. F. Protective role of 1α-dihydroxyvitamin D_3 against oxidative stress in nonmalignant human prostate epithelial cells. Int J Cancer. (2008). , 122, 2699-706.

[17] Bartel, D. P. (2004). MicroRNAs: genomics, biogenesis, mechanism, and function. Cell. , 116, 281-297.

[18] BeerTM; Lemmon, D; Lowe, BA; et al. ((2003). High-dose weekly oral calcitriol in patients with a rising PSA after prostatectomy or radiation for prostate carcinoma. Cancer. , 97, 1217-1224.

[19] BeerTM; Venner, PM; Ryan, CW; et al. ((2006). High dose calcitriol may reduce thrombosis in cancer patients. Br J Hematol. , 135, 392-394.

[20] Beildeck, M. E, Islam, M, Shah, S, Welsh, J, & Byers, S. W. Control of TCF-4 expression by VDR and vitamin D in the mouse mammary gland and colorectal cancer cell lines. PLoS One. (2009). Nov 17;4(11):e7872.

[21] Bell, N. H, Shaw, S, & Turner, R. T. Evidence that 1,25-dihydroxyvitamin D_3 inhibits the hepatic production of 25-hydroxyvitamin D in man. J Clin Invest. (1984). , 74, 1540-1544.

[22] Bergmann, C, Bachmann, H. S, Bankfalvi, A, Lotfi, R, Pütter, C, Wild, C. A, Schuler, P. J, Greve, J, Hoffmann, T. K, Lang, S, Scherag, A, & Lehnerdt, G. F. Toll-like receptor 4 single-nucleotide polymorphisms Asp299Gly and Thr399Ile in head and neck squamous cell carcinomas. J Transl Med. (2011). Aug 21;9:139.

[23] Beyazit, Y, Purnak, T, Suvak, B, Kurt, M, Sayilir, A, Turhan, T, Tas, A, Torun, S, Celik, T, Ibis, M, & Haznedaroglu, I. C. Increased ACE in extrahepatic cholangiocarcinoma as a clue for activated RAS in biliary neoplasms. Clin Res Hepatol Gastroenterol. (2011). Oct;, 35(10), 644-9.

[24] BlankeCD; Beer, TM; Todd; et al. ((2009). Phase II study of calcitriol-enhanced docetaxel in patients with previously untreated metastatic or locally advanced pancreatic cancer. *Investigational New Drugs.* , 27(4), 374-378.

[25] BowerM; Colston, KW; Stein, RC; et al. ((1991). Topical calcipotriol treatment in advanced breast cancer. Lancet. , 337(8743), 701-702.

[26] Brosseau, C. M, Pirianov, G, & Colston, K. W. Involvement of stress activated protein kinases (JNK and in 1,25 dihydroxyvitamin D3-induced breast cell death. Steroids. (2010). Dec 12;75(13-14):1082-8., 38.

[27] Büchau, A. S, Morizane, S, Trowbridge, J, Schauber, J, Kotol, P, Bui, J. D, & Gallo, R. L. The host defense peptide cathelicidin is required for NK cell-mediated suppression of tumor growth. J Immunol. (2010). Jan 1;, 184(1), 369-78.

[28] Bulut, G, Fallen, S, Beauchamp, E. M, Drebing, L. E, Sun, J, Berry, D. L, Kallakury, B, Crum, C. P, Toretsky, J. A, Schlegel, R, & Üren, A. Beta-catenin accelerates human papilloma virus type-16 mediated cervical carcinogenesis in transgenic mice. PLoS One. (2011). e27243.

[29] Byers, S, Shah, S, & Vitamin, D. and the regulation of Wnt/beta-catenin signaling and innate immunity in colorectal cancer. Nutr Rev. (2007). Aug;65(8 Pt 2):S, 118-20.

[30] Chang, J, Kuo, M, Kuo, H, Hwang, S, Tsai, J, et al. alpha,25-hydroxyvitamin D_3 regulates inducible nitric oxide synthase messenger RNA expression and nitric oxide release in macrophage-like RAW 264.7 cells. J Lab Clin Med. (2004). , 143, 14-22.

[31] Charalampopoulos A; Charalabopoulos, A; Batistatou, A; et al. ((2010). Parathormone and $1,25(OH)_2D_3$ but not $25(OH)D_3$ serum levels, in an inverse correlation, reveal an association with advanced stages of colorectal cancer. Clin Exp Med. , 10, 69-72.

[32] Chaudhary, A. K, Pandya, S, Mehrotra, R, Singh, M, & Singh, M. Role of functional polymorphism of matrix metalloproteinase-2 (-1306 C/T and-168 G/T) and MMP-9 (-1562 C/T) promoter in oral submucous fibrosis and head and neck squamous cell carcinoma in an Indian population. Biomarkers. (2011). Nov;, 16(7), 577-86.

[33] Chiang, K. C, Yeh, C. N, Chen, H. Y, Lee, J. M, Juang, H. H, Chen, M. F, Takano, M, Kittaka, A, & Chen, T. C. Nor-2α-(3-hydroxypropyl)-1α,25-dihydroxyvitamin D_3

(MART-10) is a potent cell growth regulator with enhanced chemotherapeutic potency in liver cancer cells. Steroids. (2011). Dec 11;, 76(13), 1513-9.

[34] Cho, Y. L, Christensen, C, Saunders, D. E, Lawrence, W. D, Deppe, G, Malviya, V. K, & Malone, J. M. Combined effects of 1,25-dihydroxyvitamin D_3 and platinum drugs on the growth of MCF-7 cells. Cancer Res. (1991). Jun 1;, 51(11), 2848-53.

[35] Choi, H. B, Roh, S. Y, Choi, E. J, Yoon, H. Y, Kim, S. Y, Hong, Y. S, Kim, D. W, & Kim, T. G. Association of HLA alleles with non-Hodgkin's lymphoma in Korean population. Int J Hematol. (2008). Mar;, 87(2), 203-9.

[36] Chuang, C. M, Monie, A, Wu, A, Mao, C. P, & Hung, C. F. Treatment with LL-37 peptide enhances antitumor effects induced by CpG oligodeoxynucleotides against ovarian cancer. Hum Gene Ther. (2009). Apr;, 20(4), 303-13.

[37] Chung, J. W, Jeon, J. H, Yoon, S. R, & Choi, I. Vitamin D upregulated protein 1 (VDUP1) is a regulator for redox signaling and stress-mediated diseases. J Dermatol. (2006). Oct;, 33(10), 662-9.

[38] Churilla, T. M, Lesko, S. L, Brereton, H. D, Klem, M, Donnelly, P. E, & Peters, C. A. Serum vitamin D levels among patients in a clinical oncology practice compared to primary care patients in the same community: a case-control study. BMJ Open. (2011). Dec 19;1(2):e000397.

[39] Churilla, T. M, Brereton, H. D, Klem, M, & Peters, C. A. Vitamin D Deficiency Is Widespread in Cancer Patients and Correlates With Advanced Stage Disease: A Community Oncology Experience. Nutr Cancer. (2012). Mar 27. [Epub ahead of print]

[40] Cordes, T, Hoellen, F, Dittmer, C, Salehin, D, Kümmel, S, Friedrich, M, Köster, F, Becker, S, Diedrich, K, & Thill, M. Correlation of prostaglandin metabolizing enzymes and serum PGE_2 levels with vitamin D receptor and serum $25(OH)_2D_3$ levels in breast and ovarian cancer. Anticancer Res. (2012). Jan;, 32(1), 351-7.

[41] Cortez, M. A, Welsh, J. W, & Calin, G. A. Circulating MicroRNAs as Noninvasive Biomarkers in Breast Cancer. Recent Results Cancer Res. (2012). , 195, 151-61.

[42] Crew, K. D, Shane, E, Cremers, S, Mcmahon, D. J, Irani, D, & Hershman, D. L. High prevalence of vitamin D deficiency despite supplementation in premenopausal women with breast cancer undergoing adjuvant chemotherapy. J Clin Oncol. (2009). May 1;, 27(13), 2151-6.

[43] Dalhoff K; Dancey, J; Astrup, L; et al. ((2003). A phase II study of the vitamin D analogue Seocalcitol in patients with inoperable hepatocellular carcinoma. *Br J Cancer.* , 89, 252-257.

[44] Dean, D. D, Schwartz, Z, Schmitz, J, Muniz, O. E, Lu, Y, et al. Vitamin D regulation of metalloproteinase activity in matrix vesicles. Connect Tissue Res. (1996). , 35, 331-6.

[45] Denzer, N, Vogt, T, & Reichrath, J. Vitamin D receptor (VDR) polymorphisms and skin cancer: A systematic review. Dermatoendocrinol. (2011). Jul;, 3(3), 205-10.

[46] Deshayes, F, & Nahmias, C. Angiotensin receptors: a new role in cancer? Trends Endocrinol Metab. (2005). Sep;, 16(7), 293-9.

[47] Dickie, L, Church, L, Coulthard, L, Mathews, R, Emery, P, & Mcdermott, M. Vitamin D downregulates intracellular toll-like receptor 9 expression and toll-like receptor 9-induced IL-6 production in human monocytes. Rheumatol. (2010). , 48, 1466-71.

[48] Ditsch, N, Toth, B, Mayr, D, Lenhard, M, Gallwas, J, Weissenbacher, T, Dannecker, C, Friese, K, & Jeschke, U. The association between vitamin D receptor expression and prolonged overall survival in breast cancer. J Histochem Cytochem. (2012). Feb;, 60(2), 121-9.

[49] Donaldson, P. T, Ho, S, Williams, R, & Johnson, P. J. HLA class II alleles in Chinese patients with hepatocellular carcinoma. Liver. (2001). Apr;, 21(2), 143-8.

[50] Dong, W, Li, H, Zhang, Y, Yang, H, Guo, M, Li, L, & Liu, T. Matrix metalloproteinase 2 promotes cell growth and invasion in colorectal cancer. Acta Biochim Biophys Sin (Shanghai). (2011). Nov;, 43(11), 840-8.

[51] Drake, M. T, Maurer, M. J, Link, B. K, Habermann, T. M, Ansell, S. M, Micallef, I. N, Kelly, J. L, Macon, W. R, Nowakowski, G. S, Inwards, D. J, Johnston, P. B, Singh, R. J, Allmer, C, Slager, S. L, Weiner, G. J, Witzig, T. E, & Cerhan, J. R. Vitamin D insufficiency and prognosis in non-Hodgkin's lymphoma. J Clin Oncol. (2010). Sep 20;, 28(27), 4191-8.

[52] Du, N, Feng, J, Hu, L. J, Sun, X, Sun, H. B, Zhao, Y, Yang, Y. P, & Ren, H. Angiotensin II receptor type 1 blockers suppress the cell proliferation effects of angiotensin II in breast cancer cells by inhibiting AT1R signaling. Oncol Rep. (2012). Jun;, 27(6), 1893-903.

[53] Dziki, L, Przybylowska, K, Majsterek, I, Trzcinski, R, & Sygut, M. A. A. G Polymorphism of the MMP-7 Gene Promoter Region in Colorectal Cancer. Pol Przegl Chir. (2011). Nov 1;, 83(11), 622-6.

[54] Equils, O, Naiki, Y, Shapiro, A. M, Michelsen, K, Lu, D, et al. hydroxyvitamin D_3 inhibits liposaccharide-induced immune activation in human endothelial cells. Clin Exp Immunol. (2005). , 143, 58-64.

[55] Essa, S, Denzer, N, Mahlknecht, U, Klein, R, Collnot, E. M, Tilgen, W, & Reichrath, J. VDR microRNA expression and epigenetic silencing of vitamin D signaling in melanoma cells. J Steroid Biochem Mol Biol. (2010). Jul;121(1-2):110-3.

[56] Essa, S, Reichrath, S, Mahlknecht, U, Montenarh, M, Vogt, T, & Reichrath, J. Signature of VDR miRNAs and epigenetic modulation of vitamin D signaling in melanoma cell lines. Anticancer Res. (2012). Jan;, 32(1), 383-9.

[57] Eyking, A, Ey, B, Rünzi, M, Roig, A. I, Reis, H, Schmid, K. W, Gerken, G, Podolsky, D. K, & Cario, E. Toll-like receptor 4 variant D299G induces features of neoplastic progression in Caco-2 intestinal cells and is associated with advanced human colon cancer. Gastroenterology. (2011). Dec;, 141(6), 2154-65.

[58] Fedirko, V, Bostick, R. M, Flanders, W. D, Long, Q, Shaukat, A, Rutherford, R. E, Daniel, C. R, Cohen, V, & Dash, C. Effects of vitamin D and calcium supplementation on markers of apoptosis in normal colon mucosa: a randomized, double-blind, placebo-controlled clinical trial. Cancer Prev Res (Phila). (2009). Mar;, 2(3), 213-23.

[59] Feng, Y, Wan, H, Liu, J, Zhang, R, Ma, Q, Han, B, Xiang, Y, Che, J, Cao, H, Fei, X, & Qiu, W. The angiotensin-converting enzyme 2 in tumor growth and tumor-associated angiogenesis in non-small cell lung cancer. Oncol Rep. (2010). Apr;, 23(4), 941-8.

[60] Feng, Y, Ni, L, Wan, H, Fan, L, Fei, X, Ma, Q, Gao, B, Xiang, Y, Che, J, & Li, Q. Overexpression of ACE2 produces antitumor effects via inhibition of angiogenesis and tumor cell invasion in vivo and in vitro. Oncol Rep. (2011). a Nov;, 26(5), 1157-64.

[61] Feng, S, Cen, J, Huang, Y, Shen, H, Yao, L, Wang, Y, & Chen, Z. Matrix metalloproteinase-2 and-9 secreted by leukemic cells increase the permeability of blood-brain barrier by disrupting tight junction proteins. PLoS One. (2011b). e20599.

[62] Ferrero, D, Campa, E, Dellacasa, C, et al. (2004). Differentiating agents + low-dose chemotherapy in the management of old/poor prognosis patients with acute myeloid leukemia or myelodysplastic syndrome. Haematologica. , 89, 619-620.

[63] Fujioka, T, Hasegawa, M, Ishikura, K, Matsushita, Y, Sato, M, & Tanji, S. Inhibition of tumor growth and angiogenesis by vitamin D3 agents in murine renal cell carcinoma. J Urol. (1998). , 160, 247-51.

[64] Garamszegi, N, Garamszegi, S. P, & Scully, S. P. Matrix metalloproteinase-1 contribution to sarcoma cell invasion. J Cell Mol Med. (2011). Jul 31. doi:j.x. [Epub ahead of print], 1582-4934.

[65] García-plata, D, Mozos, E, Carrasco, L, & Solana, R. HLA molecule expression in cutaneous squamous cell carcinomas: an immunopathological study and clinical-immunohistopathological correlations. Histol Histopathol. (1993). Apr;, 8(2), 219-26.

[66] Garcion, E, Sindji, L, Leblondel, G, Brachet, P, & Darcy, F. hydroxyvitamin D_3 regulates the synthesis of γ-glutamyl transpeptidase and glutathione levels in rat primary astrocytes. J Neurochem. (1999). , 73, 859-66.

[67] GarlandCF; Grant, WB; Mohr, SB; et al. ((2007). What is the dose-response relationship between vitamin D and cancer risk? *Nutr Rev.* Pt.2, , 65(8), S91-S95.

[68] Ge, X, & Wang, X. Role of Wnt canonical pathway in hematological malignancies. J Hematol Oncol. (2010). Sep 15;3:33

[69] Gilbert-sirieix, M, Makoukji, J, Kimura, S, Talbot, M, Caillou, B, Massaad, C, & Massaad-massade, L. Wnt/β-catenin signaling pathway is a direct enhancer of thyroid

transcription factor-1 in humanpapillary thyroid carcinoma cells. PLoS One. (2011). e22280.

[70] Giovannucci E; Liu, Y; Rimm, EB; et al. ((2008). Prospective study of predictors of vitamin D status and cancer incidence and mortality in men. J Natl Cancer Inst. , 98, 451-459.

[71] Gocek, E, Wang, X, Liu, X, Liu, C. G, & Studzinski, G. P. MicroRNA-32 upregulation by 1,25-dihydroxyvitamin D_3 in human myeloid leukemia cells leads to Bim targeting and inhibition of AraC-induced apoptosis. Cancer Res. (2011). Oct 1;, 71(19), 6230-9.

[72] Gombart, A. F, Borregaard, N, & Koeffler, H. P. Human cathelicidin antimicrobial peptide (CAMP) gene is a direct target of the vitamin D receptor and is strongly upregulated in myeloid cells by 1,25-dihydroxyvitamin D_3. FASEB J. (2005). Jul;, 19(9), 1067-77.

[73] González-Zuloeta Ladd AM, Arias Vásquez A, Sayed-Tabatabaei FA, Coebergh JW, Hofman A, Njajou O, Stricker B, van Duijn C. Angiotensin-converting enzyme gene insertion/deletion polymorphism and breast cancer risk. Cancer Epidemiol Biomarkers Prev. (2005). Sep;, 14(9), 2143-6.

[74] Gupta, S. C, Hevia, D, Patchva, S, Park, B, Koh, W, & Aggarwal, B. B. Upsides and Downsides of Reactive Oxygen Species for Cancer: The Roles of Reactive Oxygen Species in Tumorigenesis, Prevention, and Therapy. Antioxid Redox Signal. (2012). Jan 16. [Epub ahead of print]

[75] Gupta-elera, G, Garrett, A. R, Robison, R. A, & Neill, O. KL. The role of oxidative stress in prostate cancer. Eur J Cancer Prev. (2012). , 21, 155-62.

[76] Guturi, K. K, Mandal, T, Chatterjee, A, Sarkar, M, Bhattacharya, S, Chatterjee, U, & Ghosh, M. K. Mechanism of β-catenin mediated transcriptional regulation of EGFR expression in GSK3β inactivated prostate cancer cells. J Biol Chem. (2012). Apr 5. [Epub ahead of print]

[77] Hama, T, Norizoe, C, Suga, H, Mimura, T, Kato, T, Moriyama, H, & Urashima, M. Prognostic significance of vitamin D receptor polymorphisms in head and neck squamous cell carcinoma. PLoS One. (2011). e29634.

[78] Halicka, H. D, Zhao, H, Li, J, Traganos, F, Studzinski, G. P, & Darzynkiewicz, Z. Attenuation of constitutive DNA damage signaling by dihydroxyvitamin D_3. Aging (Albany NY). (2012). Apr 11. [Epub ahead of print], 1, 25.

[79] He, W, Kang, Y. S, Dai, C, & Liu, Y. Blockade of Wnt/β-catenin signaling by paricalcitol ameliorates proteinuria and kidney injury. J Am Soc Nephrol. (2011). Jan;, 22(1), 90-103.

[80] Hernández-hernández, D. M, Cerda-flores, R. M, Juárez-cedillo, T, Granados-arriola, J, Vargas-alarcón, G, Apresa-garcía, T, Alvarado-cabrero, I, García-carrancá, A, Salce-

do-vargas, M, & Mohar-betancourt, A. Human leukocyte antigens I and II haplotypes associated with human papillomavirus 16-positive invasive cervical cancer in Mexican women. Int J Gynecol Cancer. (2009). Aug;, 19(6), 1099-106.

[81] Herr, H. W, Laudone, V. P, Badalament, R. A, Oettgen, H. F, Sogani, P. C, Freedman, B. D, & Melamed, M. R. Whitmore WF Jr. Bacillus Calmette-Guérin therapy alters the progression of superficial bladder cancer. J Clin Oncol. (1988). Sep;, 6(9), 1450-5.

[82] Hershberger PA; Yu, WD; Modzelewski, RA; et al. ((2001). Calcitriol (1,25-dihydroxycholecalciferol) enhances paclitaxel antitumor activity in vitro and in vivo and accelerates paclitaxel-induced apoptosis. Clin Cancer Res. , 7, 1043-1051.

[83] Higiwara, H, Furuhashi, H, Nakaya, K, & Nakamura, Y. Effects of vitamin D_3 and related compounds on angiotensin converting activity of endothelial cells and on release of plasminogen activator from them. Chem Pharm Bull. (1988). , 36, 4858-64.

[84] Hillyer, R. L, Sirinvasin, P, Joglekar, M, Sikes, R. A, Van Golen, K. L, & Nohe, A. Differential effects of vitamin D treatment on inflammatory and non-inflammatory breast cancer cell lines. Clin Exp Metastasis. (2012). Dec;, 29(8), 971-9.

[85] Hipskind, R. A, & Bilbe, G. MAP kinase signaling cascades and gene expression in osteoblasts. Front Biosci. (1998). Aug 1;3:d, 804-16.

[86] Hojjat-farsangi, M, Jeddi-tehrani, M, Amirzargar, A. A, Razavi, S. M, Sharifian, R. A, Rabbani, H, & Shokri, F. Human leukocyte antigen class II allele association to disease progression in Iranian patients with chronic lymphocytic leukemia. Hum Immunol. (2008). Oct;, 69(10), 666-74.

[87] Hong, C. C, Ambrosone, C. B, Ahn, J, Choi, J. Y, Mccullough, M. L, Stevens, V. L, et al. Genetic variability in iron-related oxidative stress pathways (Nrf2, NQ01, NOS3, and HO-1), iron intake, and risk of postmenopausal breast cancer. Cancer Epidemiol Biomarkers Prev. (2007). , 16, 1784-94.

[88] Huang, W, Yu, L. F, Zhong, J, Qiao, M. M, Jiang, F. X, Du, F, Tian, X. L, & Wu, Y. L. Angiotensin II type 1 receptor expression in human gastric cancer and induces MMP2 and MMP9 expression in MKN-28 cells. Dig Dis Sci. (2008). Jan;, 53(1), 163-8.

[89] Ino, K, Shibata, K, Kajiyama, H, Yamamoto, E, Nagasaka, T, Nawa, A, Nomura, S, & Kikkawa, F. Angiotensin II type 1 receptor expression in ovarian cancer and its correlation with tumour angiogenesis and patient survival. Br J Cancer. (2006). Feb 27;, 94(4), 552-60.

[90] Iglesias-gato, D, Zheng, S, Flanagan, J. N, Jiang, L, Kittaka, A, Sakaki, T, Yamamoto, K, Itoh, T, Lebrasseur, N. K, Norstedt, G, & Chen, T. C. Substitution at carbon 2 of nor-1α,25-dihydroxyvitamin D_3 with 3-hydroxypropyl group generates an analogue with enhanced chemotherapeutic potency in PC-3 prostate cancer cells. J Steroid Biochem Mol Biol. (2011). Nov;127(3-5):269-75., 19.

[91] Ji, Y, Kutner, A, Verstuyf, A, Verlinden, L, & Studzinski, G. P. Derivatives of vitamins D_2 and D_3 activate three MAPK pathways and upregulate pRb expression in differentiating HL60 cells. Cell Cycle. (2002). Nov-Dec;, 1(6), 410-5.

[92] Johnston, C. I. Tissue angiotensin converting enzyme in cardiac and vascular hypertrophy, repair, and remodeling. Hypertension. (1994). , 23, 258-68.

[93] Jørgensen, A. Blomberg Jensen M, Nielsen JE, Juul A, Rajpert-De Meyts E. Influence of vitamin D on cisplatin sensitivity in testicular germ cell cancer-derived cell lines and in a NTera2 xenograft model. J Steroid Biochem Mol Biol. (2012). Oct 23. pii: S0960-0760(12)00208-7. doi:j.jsbmb.2012.10.008. [Epub ahead of print]

[94] Kállay, E, Bareis, P, Bajna, E, Kriwanek, S, Bonner, E, Toyokuni, S, & Cross, H. S. Vitamin D receptor activity and prevention of colonic hyperproliferation and oxidative stress. Food Chem Toxicol. (2002). Aug;, 40(8), 1191-6.

[95] Keizman, D, Huang, P, Eisenberger, M. A, Pili, R, Kim, J. J, Antonarakis, E. S, Hammers, H, & Carducci, M. A. Angiotensin system inhibitors and outcome of sunitinib treatment in patients with metastatic renal cell carcinoma: a retrospective examination. Eur J Cancer. (2011). Sep;, 47(13), 1955-61.

[96] Kim, H. J, Bae, J. S, Chang, I. H, Kim, K. D, Lee, J, Shin, H. D, Lee, J. Y, Kim, W. J, Kim, W, & Myung, S. C. Sequence variants of toll-like receptor 4 (TLR4) and the risk of prostate cancer in Korean men. World J Urol. (2012). Apr;, 30(2), 225-32.

[97] Kinoshita, J, Fushida, S, Harada, S, Yagi, Y, Fujita, H, Kinami, S, Ninomiya, I, Fujimura, T, Kayahara, M, Yashiro, M, Hirakawa, K, & Ohta, T. Local angiotensin II-generation in human gastric cancer: correlation with tumor progression through the activation of ERK1/2, NF-kappaB and survivin. Int J Oncol. (2009). Jun;, 34(6), 1573-82.

[98] Koca, E, Haznedaroglu, I. C, Uner, A, Sayinalp, N, Saglam, A. E, Goker, H, & Ozcebe, O. I. Angiotensin-converting enzyme expression of the lymphoma-associated macrophages in the lymph nodes of Hodgkin's disease. J Natl Med Assoc. (2007). Nov; 99(11):1243-4, 1246-7.

[99] Kölmel, K. F, Grange, J. M, Krone, B, Mastrangelo, G, Rossi, C. R, Henz, B. M, Seebacher, C, Botev, I. N, Niin, M, Lambert, D, Shafir, R, Kokoschka, E. M, Kleeberg, U. R, Gefeller, O, & Pfahlberg, A. Prior immunisation of patients with malignant melanoma with vaccinia or BCG is associated with better survival. An European Organization for Research and Treatment of Cancer cohort study on 542 patients. Eur J Cancer. (2005). Jan;, 41(1), 118-25.

[100] Komagata, S, Nakajima, M, Takagi, S, Mohri, T, Taniya, T, & Yokoi, T. Human CYP24 catalyzing the inactivation of calcitriol is post-transcriptionally regulated by miR-125b. Mol Pharmacol. (2009). Oct;, 76(4), 702-9.

[101] Koli, K, & Keski-oja, J. Alpha, 25-dihydroxyvitamin D and its analogues down-regulate cell invasion-associated proteases in cultured malignant cells. Cell Growth Differ. (2000). Apr;, 11(4), 221-9.

[102] Köstner, K, Denzer, N, Koreng, M, Reichrath, S, Gräber, S, Klein, R, Tilgen, W, Vogt, T, & Reichrath, J. Association of genetic variants of the vitamin D receptor (VDR) with cutaneous squamous cell carcinomas (SCC) and basal cell carcinomas (BCC): a pilot study in a German population. Anticancer Res. (2012). Jan;, 32(1), 327-33.

[103] Kulah, E, Dursun, A, Aktunc, E, Acikgoz, S, Aydin, M, et al. Effects of angiotensin-converting enzyme gene polymorphism and serum vitamin D levels on ambulatory blood pressure measurement and left ventricular mass in Turkish hypertensive population. Blood Press Monit. (2007). , 12, 207-13.

[104] Kupfer, S. S, Anderson, J. R, Ludvik, A. E, Hooker, S, Skol, A, Kittles, R. A, Keku, T. O, Sandler, R. S, Ruiz-ponte, C, Castellvi-bel, S, Castells, A, Carracedo, A, & Ellis, N. A. Genetic associations in the vitamin D receptor and colorectal cancer in African Americans and Caucasians. PLoS One. (2011). e26123.

[105] Ma, X, Chen, C, Xiong, H, Fan, J, Li, Y, Lin, H, et al. No association between SOD2 Val16Ala polymorphism and breast cancer susceptibility: a meta-analysis based on 9,710 cases and 11,041 controls. Breast Cancer Res Treat. (2010a). , 122, 509-14.

[106] Ma Y; Yu, WD; Trump, DL; et al. ((2010b). Enhances antitumor activity of gemcitabine and cisplatin in human bladder cancer models. *Cancer.*, 116, 3294-3303.

[107] Mahmoudi, T, Arkani, M, Karimi, K, Safaei, A, Rostami, F, Arbabi, E, Pourhoseingholi, M. A, Mohebbi, S. R, Nikzamir, A, Romani, S, Almasi, S, Abbaszadeh, M, Vafaei, M, & Zali, M. R. The-4817 G>A (rs2238136) variant of the vitamin D receptor gene: a probable risk factor for colorectal cancer. Mol Biol Rep. (2012). May;, 39(5), 5277-82.

[108] Makni, H, & Daoud, J. Ben Salah H, Mahfoudh N, Haddar O, Karray H, Boudawara T, Ghorbel A, Khabir A, Frikha M. HLA association with nasopharyngeal carcinoma in southern Tunisia. Mol Biol Rep. (2010). Jun;, 37(5), 2533-9.

[109] Malik, M. A, Sharma, K. L, Zargar, S. A, & Mittal, B. Association of matrix metalloproteinase-7 (-181A>G) polymorphism with risk of esophageal squamous cell carcinoma in Kashmir Valley. Saudi J Gastroenterol. (2011). Sep-Oct;, 17(5), 301-6.

[110] Mao, C, Qiu, L. X, Zhan, P, Xue, K, Ding, H, Du, F. B, et al. MnSOD Val16Ala polymorphism and prostate cancer susceptibility: a meta-analysis involving 8,962 subjects. J Cancer Res Clin Oncol. (2010). , 136, 975-9.

[111] Marra, M, Sordelli, I. M, Lombardi, A, Lamberti, M, Tarantino, L, Giudice, A, et al. Molecular targets and oxidative stress biomarkers in hepatocellular carcinoma: an overview. J Transl Med. (2011).

[112] Mcguire, T. F, Trump, D. L, & Johnson, C. S. Vitamin D induced apoptosis of murine squamous cell carcinoma cells. Selective induction of caspase-dependent MEK cleavage and up-regulation of MEKK-1. J Biol Chem. (2001). Jul 13;, 276(28), 26365-73.

[113] Michel, S, Linnebacher, M, Alcaniz, J, Voss, M, Wagner, R, Dippold, W, & Becker, C. von Knebel Doeberitz M, Ferrone S, Kloor M. Lack of HLA class II antigen expression in microsatellite unstable colorectal carcinomas is caused by mutations in HLA class II regulatory genes. Int J Cancer. (2010). Aug 15;, 127(4), 889-98.

[114] Min, R, Zun, Z, Siyi, L, Wenjun, Y, Lizheng, W, & Chenping, Z. Increased expression of Toll-like receptor-9 has close relation with tumour cell proliferation in oral squamous cell carcinoma. Arch Oral Biol. (2011). Sep;, 56(9), 877-84.

[115] Minmin, S, Xiaoqian, X, Hao, C, Baiyong, S, Xiaxing, D, Junjie, X, Xi, Z, Jianquan, Z, & Songyao, J. Single nucleotide polymorphisms of Toll-like receptor 4 decrease the risk of development of hepatocellular carcinoma. PLoS One. (2011). Apr 29;6(4):e19466.

[116] Moffatt, K. A, Johannes, W. U, & Miller, G. J. α Dihydroxyvitamin D_3 and platinum drugs act synergistically to inhibit the growth of prostate cancer cell lines. Clin Cancer Res. (1999). Mar;, 5(3), 695-703.

[117] Mohri, T, Nakajima, M, Takagi, S, Komagata, S, & Yokoi, T. MicroRNA regulates human vitamin D receptor. Int J Cancer. (2009). Sep 15;, 125(6), 1328-33.

[118] Moreno, J, Krishnan, A. V, Swami, S, Nonn, L, Peehl, D. M, & Feldman, D. Regulation of prostaglandin metabolism by calcitriol attenuates growth stimulation in prostate cancer cells. Cancer Res. (2005). Sep 1;, 65(17), 7917-25.

[119] Morris DL; Jourdan, JL; Finlay, I; et al. ((2002). Hepatic intra-arterial injection of 1,25-dihydroxyvitamin D_3 in lipiodol: pilot study in patients with hepatocellular carcinoma. *Int J Oncol.* , 21, 901-906.

[120] Nuñez, F, Bravo, S, Cruzat, F, Montecino, M, & De Ferrari, G. V. Wnt/β-catenin signaling enhances cyclooxygenase-2 (COX2) transcriptional activity in gastric cancer cells. PLoS One. (2011). Apr 6;6(4):e18562.

[121] Nakagawa, K, Sasaki, Y, Kato, S, Kubodera, N, & Okano, T. Oxa-1α,25-dihydroxyvitamin D_3 inhibits metastasis and angiogenesis in lung cancer. Carcinogenesis. (2005). , 26, 1044-54.

[122] Nakai, Y, Isayama, H, Ijichi, H, Sasaki, T, Sasahira, N, Hirano, K, Kogure, H, Kawakubo, K, Yagioka, H, Yashima, Y, Mizuno, S, Yamamoto, K, Arizumi, T, Togawa, O, Matsubara, S, Tsujino, T, Tateishi, K, Tada, M, Omata, M, & Koike, K. Inhibition of renin-angiotensin system affects prognosis of advanced pancreatic cancer receiving gemcitabine. Br J Cancer. (2010). Nov 23;, 103(11), 1644-8.

[123] Naugler, C, & Liwski, R. HLA risk markers for chronic myelogenous leukemia in Eastern Canada. Leuk Lymphoma. (2009). Feb;, 50(2), 254-9.

[124] Ng, A. C, Kumar, S. K, Rajkumar, S. V, & Drake, M. T. Impact of vitamin D deficiency on the clinical presentation and prognosis of patients with newly diagnosed multiple myeloma. Am J Hematol. (2009). Jul;, 84(7), 397-400.

[125] Nguyen, H, Ivanova, V. S, Kavandi, L, Rodriguez, G. C, Maxwell, G. L, & Syed, V. Progesterone and 1,25-dihydroxyvitamin D_3 inhibit endometrial cancer cell growth by upregulating semaphorin 3B and semaphorin 3F. Mol Cancer Res. (2011). Nov;, 9(11), 1479-92.

[126] Nihon-yanagi, Y, Terai, K, Murano, T, Matsumoto, T, & Okazumi, S. Tissue expression of Toll-like receptors 2 and 4 in sporadic human colorectal cancer. Cancer Immunol Immunother. (2012). Jan;, 61(1), 71-7.

[127] Lange, T. S, Stuckey, A. R, Robison, K, Kim, K. K, Singh, R. K, Raker, C. A, Brard, L, Lange, T. S, Stuckey, A. R, Robison, K, Kim, K. K, Singh, R. K, Raker, C. A, & Brard, L. Effect of a vitamin D_3 derivative (B3CD) with postulated anti-cancer activity in an ovarian cancer animal model. Invest New Drugs. (2010). Oct;, 28(5), 543-53.

[128] Lalor, M, Floyd, S, Gorak-stolinska, P, Weir, R, Blitz, R, Branson, K, et al. (2011). BCG vaccination: a role for vitamin D? PLos ONE. 6, 216709.

[129] Larriba, M. J, Valle, N, Pálmer, H. G, Ordóñez-morán, P, Alvarez-díaz, S, Becker, K. F, Gamallo, C, De Herreros, A. G, González-sancho, J. M, & Muñoz, A. The inhibition of Wnt/beta-catenin signalling by 1alpha,25-dihydroxyvitamin D_3 is abrogated by Snail1 in human colon cancer cells. Endocr Relat Cancer. (2007). Mar;, 14(1), 141-51.

[130] Larriba, M. J, Ordóñez-morán, P, Chicote, I, Martín-fernández, G, Puig, I, Muñoz, A, & Pálmer, H. G. Vitamin D receptor deficiency enhances Wnt/β-catenin signaling and tumor burden in colon cancer. PLoS One. (2011). e23524.

[131] Launoy, G, Milan, C, Day, N. E, Pienkowski, M. P, Gignoux, M, & Faivre, J. Diet and squamous-cell cancer of the oesophagus: a French multicentre case-control study. Int J Cancer. (1998). Mar 30;, 76(1), 7-12.

[132] Lee, H. W, Hahm, K. B, Lee, J. S, Ju, Y. S, Lee, K. M, & Lee, K. W. Association of the human leukocyte antigen class II alleles with chronic atrophic gastritis and gastric carcinoma in Koreans. J Dig Dis. (2009). Nov;, 10(4), 265-71.

[133] Lefkowitz, E. S, & Garland, C. F. Sunlight, vitamin D, and ovarian cancer mortality rates in US women. Int J Epidemiol. (1994). Dec;, 23(6), 1133-6.

[134] Li, Z. Q, Ding, W, Sun, S. J, Li, J, Pan, J, Zhao, C, Wu, W. R, & Si, W. K. Cyr61/CCN1 Is Regulated by Wnt/β-Catenin Signaling and Plays an Important Role in the Progression of Hepatocellular Carcinoma. PLoS One. (2012). e35754.

[135] Lindhorst, E, Schumm-draeger, P. M, Bojunga, J, Usadel, K. H, & Herrmann, G. Differences in tumor cell proliferation, HLA DR expression and lymphocytic infiltration in various types of thyroid carcinoma. Exp Clin Endocrinol Diabetes. (2002). Jan;, 110(1), 27-31.

[136] Lipworth, L, Rossi, M, Mclaughlin, J. K, Negri, E, Talamini, R, Levi, F, & Franceschi, S. La Vecchia C. Dietary vitamin D and cancers of the oral cavity and esophagus. Ann Oncol. (2009). Sep;, 20(9), 1576-81.

[137] Liu, P. T, Stenger, S, Li, H, Wenzel, L, Tan, B. H, Krutzik, S. R, et al. Toll-like receptor triggering of a vitamin D-mediated human antimicrobial response. Science. (2006). , 311, 1770-3.

[138] LiuG; Hu, X; Chakrabarty, S; et al. ((2010). Vitamin D mediates its action in human colon carcinoma cells in a calcium-sensing receptor-dependent manner: downregulates malignant cell behavior and the expression of thymidylate synthase and surviving and promotes cellular sensitivity to 5-FU. *Int J Cancer.* , 126, 631-639.

[139] Liu, D, Duan, W, Guo, H, Xu, X, & Bai, Y. Meta-analysis of associations between polymorphisms in the promoter regions of matrix metalloproteinases and the risk of colorectal cancer. Int J Colorectal Dis. (2011). Sep;, 26(9), 1099-105.

[140] Liu, D, Guo, H, Li, Y, Xu, X, Yang, K, & Bai, Y. Association between polymorphisms in the promoter regions of matrix metalloproteinases (MMPs) and risk of cancer metastasis: a meta-analysis. PLoS One. (2012). e31251.

[141] Loke, T. W, Sevfi, D, & Khadra, M. Prostate cancer incidence in Australia correlates inversely with solar radiation. BJU Int. (2011). Nov;108 Suppl , 2, 66-70.

[142] Lotfy, M. El-Kenawy Ael-M, Abdel-Aziz MM, El-Kady I, Talaat A. Elevated renin levels in patients with liver cirrhosis and hepatocellular carcinoma. Asian Pac J Cancer Prev. (2010). , 11(5), 1263-6.

[143] Louis, S. N, Wang, L, Chow, L, Rezmann, L. A, & Imamura, K. MacGregor DP, Casely D, Catt KJ, Frauman AG, Louis WJ. Appearance of angiotensin II expression in non-basal epithelial cells is an early feature of malignant change in human prostate. Cancer Detect Prev. (2007). , 31(5), 391-5.

[144] Lu, J, Getz, G, Miska, E. A, Alvarez-saavedra, E, Lamb, J, Peck, D, Sweet-cordero, A, Ebert, B. L, Mak, R. H, Ferrando, A. A, Downing, J. R, Jacks, T, Horvitz, H. R, & Golub, T. R. MicroRNA expression profiles classify human cancers. Nature. (2005). Jun 9;, 435(7043), 834-8.

[145] LuoWJ; Chen, JY; Xu, W; et al. ((2004). Effects of vitamin D analogue EB1089 on proliferation and apoptosis of hepatic carcinoma cells. *Zhonghua Yu Fang Yi Xue Za Zhi.* article in Chinese], 38, 415-418.

[146] Luong, K. V, & Nguyen, L. T. Coexisting hyperparathyroidism and primary hyperparathyroidism with vitamin D-deficient osteomalacia in a Vietnamese immigrant. Endocrine Practice. (1996). , 2, 250-254.

[147] Luong, K, & Nguyen, L. T. The beneficial role of vitamin D and its analogs in cancer treatment and prevention. Crit Rev Oncol Hematol. (2010). Mar;, 73(3), 192-201.

[148] Lương KVQNguyễn LTH. ((2012). Vitamin D and cancer. In "Advanced in Cancer Management". InTech Publishing Co. January 2012. , 1-16.

[149] ObaraW; Mizutani, Y; Oyama, C; et al. ((2008). Prospective study of combined treatment with interferon-alpha and active vitamin D_3 for Japanese patients with metastatic renal cell carcinoma. *Int J Urol.* , 15, 794-799.

[150] Ordóñez-Morán, P, Larriba, MJ, Pálmer, HG, Valero, RA, Barbáchano, A, Duñach, M, de Herreros, AG, Villalobos, C, Berciano, MT, Lafarga, M, & Muñoz, A. 1 mediate vitamin D effects on gene expression, phenotype, and Wnt pathway in colon cancer cells. J Cell Biol. 2008 Nov 17;183(4):697-710.

[151] Orell-kotikangas, H, Schwab, U, Osterlund, P, Saarilahti, K, Mäkitie, O, & Mäkitie, A. A. High prevalence of vitamin D insufficiency in patients with head and neck cancer at diagnosis. Head Neck. (2012). Jan 27. doi:hed.21954. [Epub ahead of print]

[152] Ozdemir, E, Kakehi, Y, Mishina, M, Ogawa, O, Okada, Y, Ozdemir, D, & Yoshida, O. High-resolution HLA-DRB1 and DQB1 genotyping in Japanese patients with testicular germ cell carcinoma. Br J Cancer. (1997). , 76(10), 1348-52.

[153] Ozdilli, K, Oguz, F. S, Anak, S, Kekik, C, Carin, M, & Gedikoglu, G. The frequency of HLA class I and II alleles in Turkish childhood acute leukaemia patients. J Int Med Res. (2010). Sep-Oct;, 38(5), 1835-44.

[154] Panza, N. Del Vecchio L, Maio M, De Felice M, Lombardi G, Minozzi M, Zappacosta S. ong association between an HLA-DR antigen and thyroid carcinoma. Tissue Antigens. (1982). Aug;, 20(2), 155-8.

[155] Pálmer, H. G, González-sancho, J. M, Espada, J, Berciano, M. T, Puig, I, Baulida, J, Quintanilla, M, Cano, A, De Herreros, A. G, Lafarga, M, Muñoz, A, & Vitamin, D. promotes the differentiation of colon carcinoma cells by the induction of E-cadherin and the inhibition of beta-catenin signaling. J Cell Biol. (2001). Jul 23;, 154(2), 369-87.

[156] Palmieri-SevierA; Palmieri, GM; Baumgartner, CJ; Britt, LG. ((1993). Case report: long-term remission of parathyroid cancer: possible relation to vitamin D and calcitriol therapy. *Am J Med Sci.* , 306(5), 309-312.

[157] Pardanani, A, Drake, M. T, Finke, C, Lasho, T. L, Rozell, S. A, Jimma, T, & Tefferi, A. Vitamin D insufficiency in myeloproliferative neoplasms and myelodysplastic syndromes: clinical correlates and prognostic studies. Am J Hematol. (2011). Dec;, 86(12), 1013-6.

[158] Park, M. R, Lee, J. H, Park, M. S, Hwang, J. E, Shim, H. J, Cho, S. H, Chung, I. J, & Bae, W. K. Suppressive effect of 19-nor-1α-25-dihydroxyvitamin D_2 on gastric cancer cells and peritoneal metastasis model. J Korean Med Sci. (2012). Sep;, 27(9), 1037-43.

[159] Parsons, S. L, Watson, S. A, Collins, H. M, Griffin, N. R, Clarke, P. A, & Steele, R. J. Gelatinase (MMP-2 and-9) expression in gastrointestinal malignancy. Br J Cancer. (1998). Dec;, 78(11), 1495-502.

[160] Partyka, R, Gonciarz, M, Jalowiecki, P, Kokocinska, D, & Byrczek, T. VEGF and metalloproteinase 2 (MMP 2) expression in gastric cancer tissue. Med Sci Monit. (2012). Apr 1;18(4):BR, 130-134.

[161] Pendás-franco, N, García, J. M, Peña, C, Valle, N, Pálmer, H. G, Heinäniemi, M, Carlberg, C, Jiménez, B, Bonilla, F, Muñoz, A, & González-sancho, J. M. DICKKOPF-4 is induced by TCF/beta-catenin and upregulated in human colon cancer, promotes tumour cell invasion and angiogenesis and is repressed by 1alpha,25-dihydroxyvitamin D_3. Oncogene. (2008). a Jul 24;, 27(32), 4467-77.

[162] Pendás-franco, N, Aguilera, O, Pereira, F, González-sancho, J. M, Muñoz, A, & Vitamin, D. and Wnt/beta-catenin pathway in colon cancer: role and regulation of DICKKOPF genes. Anticancer Res. (2008). Sep-Oct;28(5A):, 2613-23.

[163] Peng, X, Vaishnav, A, Murillo, G, Alimirah, F, Torres, K. E, & Mehta, R. G. Protection against cellular stress by 25-hydroxyvitamin D_3 in breast epithelial cells. J Cell Biochem. (2010). Aug 15;, 110(6), 1324-33.

[164] Peng, W. J, Zhang, J. Q, Wang, B. X, Pan, H. F, Lu, M. M, Wang, J, Peng, W. J, Zhang, J. Q, Wang, B. X, Pan, H. F, Lu, M. M, & Wang, J. Prognostic value of matrix metalloproteinase 9 expression in patients with non-small cell lung cancer. Clin Chim Acta. (2012). Jul 11;413(13-14):1121-6.

[165] Peppone, L. J, Rickles, A. S, Janelsins, M. C, Insalaco, M. R, Skinner, K. A, Peppone, L. J, Rickles, A. S, Janelsins, M. C, Insalaco, M. R, & Skinner, K. A. The Association Between Breast Cancer Prognostic Indicators and Serum OH Vitamin D Levels. Ann Surg Oncol. (2012). Mar 24. [Epub ahead of print], 25.

[166] Pérez-castrillón, J. L, Justo, I, Sanz, A, De Luis, D, & Dueñas, A. Effect of angiotensin converting enzyme inhibitors on $1,25(OH)_2$ D levels of hypertensive patients. Relationship with ACE polymorphisms. Horm Metab Res. (2006). , 38, 812-6.

[167] Polakis, P. (2000). Wnt signaling and cancer. Genes Dev , 14, 1837-1851.

[168] Punzi, T, Fabris, A, Morucci, G, Biagioni, P, Gulisano, M, & Ruggiero, M. Pacini S. C-reactive protein levels and vitamin d receptor polymorphisms as markers in predicting cachectic syndrome in cancer patients. Mol Diagn Ther. (2012). Apr 1;, 16(2), 115-24.

[169] Qiu, J, Shao, S, Yang, G, Shen, Z, & Zhang, Y. Association of Toll like receptor 9 expression with lymph node metastasis in human breast cancer. Neoplasma. (2011). , 58(3), 251-5.

[170] Raffegerst, S. H, Hoelzlwimmer, G, Kunder, S, Mysliwietz, J, Quintanilla-martinez, L, & Schendel, D. J. Diverse hematological malignancies including hodgkin-like lymphomas develop in chimeric MHC class II transgenic mice. PLoS One. (2009). Dec 31;4(12):e8539.

[171] RainaV; Cunninham, D; Gilchrist, N; Soukop, M. ((1991). Alphacalcidol is a nontoxic, effective treatment of follicular small-cleaved cell lymphoma. *Br J Cancer.* , 63, 463-465.

[172] Ray, R, Banks, M, Abuzahra, H, Eddy, V. J, Persons, K. S, Lucia, M. S, Lambert, J. R, & Holick, M. F. Effect of dietary vitamin D and calcium on the growth of androgen-insensitive human prostate tumor in a murine model. Anticancer Res. (2012). Mar;, 32(3), 727-31.

[173] Ravid, A, Rocker, D, Machlenkin, A, Rotem, C, Hochman, A, Kessler-icekson, G, Liberman, U. A, & Koren, R. Dihydroxyvitamin D_3 enhances the susceptibility of breast cancer cells to doxorubicin-induced oxidative damage. Cancer Res. (1999). Feb 15;, 59(4), 862-7.

[174] Ren, C, Qiu, M. Z, Wang, D. S, Luo, H. Y, Zhang, D. S, Wang, Z. Q, Wang, F. H, Li, Y. H, Zhou, Z. W, & Xu, R. H. Prognostic effects of hydroxyvitamin D levels in gastric cancer. J Transl Med. (2012). Jan 27;10:16., 25.

[175] Repin IuMBCG vaccine immunotherapy after radical operations for lung cancer]. Vestn Khir Im I I Grek. (1992). Jul-Aug;149(7-8):11-6. [Article in Russian]

[176] Rhodes, S. G, Terry, L. A, Hope, J, Hewinson, R. G, & Vordermeier, H. M. dihydroxy-vitamin D_3 and development of tuberculosis in cattle. Clin Diagn Lab Immunol. (2003). Nov;, 10(6), 1129-35.

[177] Ristimäki, A, Honkanen, N, Jänkälä, H, Sipponen, P, & Härkönen, M. Expression of cyclooxygenase-2 in human gastric carcinoma. Cancer Res. (1997). Apr 1;, 57(7), 1276-80.

[178] Rivas-santiago, B, Hernandez-pando, R, Carranza, C, Juarez, E, Contreras, J. L, et al. Expression of cathelicidin LL-37 during Mycobacterium tuberculosis infection in human alveolar macrophages, monocytes, neutrophils, and epithelial cells. Infect Immunity. (2008). , 76, 935-41.

[179] Robsahm, T. E, Tretli, S, Dahlback, A, Moan, J, & Vitamin, D. from sunlight may improve the prognosis of breast-, colon- and prostate cancer (Norway). Cancer Causes Control. (2004). Mar;, 15(2), 149-58.

[180] Rockett, K, Brookes, R, Udalova, I, Vidal, V, Hill, A, & Kwiatkowski, D. (1998). hydroxyvitamin D_3 induces nitric oxide synthase and suppresses growth of *Mycobacterium tuberculosis* in a human macrophage-like cell line. Infect Immun. 66, 5314-5321., 1, 25.

[181] Rogalska, A, Gajek, A, Szwed, M, Józwiak, Z, & Marczak, A. The role of reactive oxygen species in WP 631-induced death of human ovarian cancer cells: a comparison with the effect of doxorubicin. Toxicol In Vitro. (2011). , 25, 1712-20.

[182] Rollison, D. E, Cole, A. L, Tung, K. H, Slattery, M. L, Baumgartner, K. B, Byers, T, Wolff, R. K, & Giuliano, A. R. Vitamin D intake, vitamin D receptor polymorphisms,

and breast cancer risk among women living in the southwestern U.S. Breast Cancer Res Treat. (2012). Apr;, 132(2), 683-91.

[183] Roth, C. L, Elfers, C. T, Figlewicz, D. P, Melhorn, S. J, Morton, G. J, et al. Vitamin D deficiency in obese rats exacerbates NAFLD and increases hepatic resistin and toll-like receptor activation. Hepatol. (2011). Oct 12. [Epub ahead of print].

[184] Ruza, E, Sotillo, E, Sierrasesúmaga, L, Azcona, C, & Patiño-garcía, A. Analysis of polymorphisms of the vitamin D receptor, estrogen receptor, and collagen Ialpha1 genes and their relationship with height in children with bone cancer. J Pediatr Hematol Oncol. (2003). Oct;, 25(10), 780-6.

[185] Sadeghi, K, Wessner, B, Laggner, U, Ploder, M, Tamandl, D, et al. Vitamin D_3 down-regulates monocyte TLR expression and triggers hyporesponsiveness to pathogen-associated molecular patterns. Eur J Immunol. (2006). , 36, 361-70.

[186] Sandholm, J, Kauppila, J. H, Pressey, C, Tuomela, J, Jukkola-vuorinen, A, Vaarala, M, Johnson, M. R, Harris, K. W, & Selander, K. S. Estrogen receptor-α and sex steroid hormones regulate Toll-like receptor-9 expression and invasive function in human breast cancer cells. Breast Cancer Res Treat. (2012). Apr;, 132(2), 411-9.

[187] Salehin, D, Haugk, C, Thill, M, Cordes, T, William, M, Hemmerlein, B, & Friedrich, M. Serum 25-hydroxyvitamin D levels in patients with vulvar cancer. Anticancer Res. (2012). Jan;, 32(1), 265-70.

[188] Saliba, W, Barnett, O, Rennert, H. S, Lavi, I, & Rennert, G. The relationship between serum 25(OH)D and parathyroid hormone levels. Am J Med. (2011). , 124, 1165-70.

[189] Sardar, S, Chakraborty, A, & Chatterjee, M. Comparative effectiveness of vitamin D_3 and dietary vitamin E on peroxidation of lipids and enzymes of the hepatic antioxidant system in Sprague-Dawley rats. Int J Vitam Nutr Res. (1996). , 66, 39-45.

[190] Schauber, J, Iffland, K, Frisch, S, Kudlich, T, Schmausser, B, Eck, M, Menzel, T, Gostner, A, Lührs, H, & Scheppach, W. Histone-deacetylase inhibitors induce the cathelicidin LL-37 in gastrointestinal cells. Mol Immunol. (2004). Jul;, 41(9), 847-54.

[191] Scherberich, J, Kellermeyer, M, Ried, C, & Hartinger, A. alpha-calcidol modulates major human monocyte antigens and toll-like receptors TRL2 and TRL4 in vitro. Eur J Med Res. (2005). , 10, 179-82.

[192] Schöttker, B, Ball, D, Gellert, C, & Brenner, H. Serum hydroxyvitamin D levels and overall mortality. A systematic review and meta-analysis of prospective cohort studies. Ageing Res Rev. (2012). Feb 17. [Epub ahead of print], 25.

[193] Schwartz, G. G, Wang, M. H, Zang, M, Singh, R. K, & Siegal, G. P. alpha,25-Dihydroxyvitamin D (calcitriol) inhibits the invasiveness of human prostate cancer cells. Cancer Epidemiol Biomarkers Prev. (1997). Sep;, 6(9), 727-32.

[194] Shanafelt, T. D, Drake, M. T, Maurer, M. J, Allmer, C, Rabe, K. G, Slager, S. L, Weiner, G. J, Call, T. G, Link, B. K, Zent, C. S, Kay, N. E, Hanson, C. A, Witzig, T. E, & Cer-

han, J. R. Vitamin D insufficiency and prognosis in chronic lymphocytic leukemia. Blood. (2011). Feb 3;, 117(5), 1492-8.

[195] Shui, I. M, Mucci, L. A, Kraft, P, Tamimi, R. M, Lindstrom, S, Penney, K. L, Nimptsch, K, Hollis, B. W, Dupre, N, Platz, E. A, Stampfer, M. J, & Giovannucci, E. Vitamin D-Related Genetic Variation, Plasma Vitamin D, and Risk of Lethal Prostate Cancer: A Prospective Nested Case-Control Study. J Natl Cancer Inst. (2012). May 2;, 104(9), 690-699.

[196] Sikora, J, Frydrychowicz, M, Kaczmarek, M, Brzezicha, B, Mozer-lisewska, I, Szczepanski, M, & Zeromski, J. TLR receptors in laryngeal carcinoma- immunophenotypic, molecular and functional studies. Folia Histochem Cytobiol. (2010). Dec;, 48(4), 624-31.

[197] Skinner, H. G, & Schwartz, G. G. (2009). The relation of serum parathyroid hormone and serum calcium to serum levels of Prostatic-specific antigen: a population-based study. *Cancer Epidemiol Biomarkers Prev.* , 18(11), 2869-2873.

[198] Slapek, C. A, Desforges, J. F, Fogaren, T, et al. (1992). Treatment of acute myeloid leukemia in the elderly with low-dose cytarabine, hydroxyurea, and calcitriol. Am J Hematol. , 41, 178-183.

[199] Slattery, M. L, Wolff, R. K, Curtin, K, Fitzpatrick, F, Herrick, J, Potter, J. D, Caan, B. J, & Samowitz, W. S. Colon tumor mutations and epigenetic changes associated with genetic polymorphism: insight into disease pathways. Mutat Res. (2009). Jan 15;660(1-2):12-21.

[200] Slattery, M. L, Herrick, J. S, Bondurant, K. L, & Wolff, R. K. Toll-like receptor genes and their association with colon and rectal cancer development and prognosis. Int J Cancer. (2012). Jun 15;, 130(12), 2974-80.

[201] Somjen, D, Katzburg, S, Grafi-cohen, M, Knoll, E, Sharon, O, & Posner, G. H. Vitamin D metabolites and analogs induce lipoxygenase mRNA expression and as well as reactive oxygen species (ROS) production in human bone cell line. J Steroid Biochem Mol Biol. (2011). , 123, 85-9.

[202] Song, E. J, Kang, M. J, Kim, Y. S, Kim, S. M, Lee, S. E, Kim, C. H, Kim, D. J, & Park, J. H. Flagellin promotes the proliferation of gastric cancer cells via the Toll-like receptor 5. Int J Mol Med. (2011). Jul;, 28(1), 115-9.

[203] Srivastava, P, Lone, T. A, Kapoor, R, & Mittal, R. D. Association of Promoter Polymorphisms in MMP 2 and TIMP2 with Prostate Cancer Susceptibility in North India. Arch Med Res. (2012). Feb 25. [Epub ahead of print]

[204] Stenson, W. F, Teitelbaum, S. L, & Bar-shavit, Z. Arachidonic acid metabolism by a vitamin D_3-differentiated human leukemic cell line. J Bone Miner Res. (1988). Oct;, 3(5), 561-71.

[205] Stio, M, Martinesi, M, Simoni, A, Zuegel, U, Steinmeyer, A, Santi, R, Treves, C, & Nesi, G. The novel vitamin D analog ZK191784 inhibits prostate cancer cell invasion. Anticancer Res. (2011). Dec;, 31(12), 4091-8.

[206] Sundar, I, Hwang, J, Wu, S, Sun, J, & Rahman, I. Deletion of vitamin D receptor leads to premature emphysema/COPD by increased matrix metalloproteinase and lymphoid aggregates formation. Biochem Biophys Res Commun. (2011). , 406, 127-33.

[207] Swami, S, Krishnan, A. V, Wang, J. Y, Jensen, K, Horst, R, Albertelli, M. A, & Feldman, D. Dietary Vitamin D_3 and Dihydroxyvitamin D_3 (Calcitriol) Exhibit Equivalent Anticancer Activity in Mouse Xenograft Models of Breast and Prostate Cancer. Endocrinology. (2012). Mar 27. [Epub ahead of print], 1, 25.

[208] Svedlund, J, Aurén, M, Sundström, M, Dralle, H, Akerström, G, Björklund, P, & Westin, G. Aberrant WNT/β-catenin signaling in parathyroid carcinoma. Mol Cancer. (2010). Nov 15;9:294.

[209] Takala, H, Kauppila, J. H, Soini, Y, Selander, K. S, Vuopala, K. S, Lehenkari, P. P, Saarnio, J, & Karttunen, T. J. Toll-like receptor 9 is a novel biomarker for esophageal squamous cell dysplasia and squamous cell carcinoma progression. J Innate Immun. (2011). , 3(6), 631-8.

[210] Tamaki, K, Saitoh, A, & Kubota, Y. hydroxyvitamin D_3 decreases the interferon-gamma (IFN-gamma) induced HLA-DR expression but not intercellular adhesion molecule 1 (ICAM-1) on human keratinocytes. Reg Immunol. (1990). , 3, 223-7.

[211] Tangrea, J, Helzlsouer, K, Pietinen, P, Taylor, P, Hollis, B, Virtamo, J, & Albanes, D. Serum levels of vitamin D metabolites and the subsequent risk of colon and rectal cancer in Finnish men. Cancer Causes Control. (1997). Jul;, 8(4), 615-25.

[212] Tee, Y. T, Liu, Y. F, Chang, J. T, Yang, S. F, Chen, S. C, Han, C. P, Wang, P. H, & Liao, C. L. Single-Nucleotide Polymorphisms and Haplotypes of Membrane Type 1 Matrix Metalloproteinase in Susceptibility and Clinical Significance of Squamous Cell Neoplasia of Uterine Cervix in Taiwan Women. Reprod Sci. (2012). Apr 23. [Epub ahead of print]

[213] Thill, M, Hoellen, F, Becker, S, Dittmer, C, Fischer, D, et al. Expression of prostaglandin- and vitamin D-metabolising enzymes in benign and malignant breast cells. Anticancer Res. (2012). , 32, 367-72.

[214] Timms, P. M, Mannan, N, Hitman, G. A, Noonan, K, Mills, P. G, et al. Circulating MMP9, vitamin D and variation in the TIMP-1 response with VDR genotype: mechanisms for inflammatory damage in chronic disorders? Q J Med. (2002). , 95, 787-96.

[215] Ting HJ; Hsu, J; Bao,BY; Lee, YF. ((2007). Docetaxel-induced growth inhibition an apoptosis in androgen indepenpent prostate cancer cells are enhanced by 1alpha,25-dihydroxyvitamin D_3. Cancer Lett. , 247, 122-129.

[216] Tokar, E. J, & Webber, M. M. Cholecalciferol (vitamin D_3) inhibits growth and invasion by up-regulating nuclear receptors and 25-hydroxylase (CYP27A1) in human prostate cancer cells. Clin Exp Metastasis. (2005). , 22(3), 275-84.

[217] Tokuda, N, Mizuki, N, Kasahara, M, & Levy, R. B. hydroxyvitamin D_3 down-regulation of HLA-DR on human peripheral blood monocytes. Immunol. (1992). , 75, 349-54.

[218] Tokuda, N, & Levy, R. hydroxyvitamin D_3 stimulates phagocytosis but suppresses HLA-DR and CD13 antigen expression in human mononuclear phagocytes. Proc Soc Exp Biol Med. (1996). , 211, 244-50.

[219] Tone, T, Eto, H, Katsuoka, K, Nishioka, K, & Nishiyama, S. Suppression of gamma-interferon induced HLA-DR antigen expression on normal and transformed keratinocytes by 1,25 $(OH)_2$ vitamin D_3. Nippon Hifuka Gakkai Zasshi. (1991). Article in Japanese]., 101, 519-25.

[220] Tone, T, Eto, H, Katou, T, Otani, F, & Nishiyama, S. Alpha,25-dihydroxyvitamin D modulation of HLA-DR mRNA induced by gamma-interferon in cultured epithelial tumor cell lines. J Dermatol. (1993). , 20, 581-4.

[221] Turna, A, Pekçolaklar, A, Metin, M, Yaylim, I, & Gurses, A. The effect of season of operation on the survival of patients with resected non-small cell lung cancer. Interact Cardiovasc Thorac Surg. (2012). Feb;, 14(2), 151-5.

[222] Ueno, K, Hirata, H, Majid, S, Chen, Y, Zaman, M. S, Tabatabai, Z. L, Hinoda, Y, & Dahiya, R. Wnt antagonist DICKKOPF-3 (Dkk-3) induces apoptosis in human renal cell carcinoma. Mol Carcinog. (2011). Jun;, 50(6), 449-57.

[223] Wang, X, Gocek, E, Liu, C. G, & Studzinski, G. P. MicroRNAs181 regulate the expression of 27Kip1in human myeloid leukemia cells induced to differentiate by 1,25-dihydroxyvitamin D_3. Cell Cycle. (2009). a Mar 1;8(5):736-41.

[224] Wang, S, Wang, F, Shi, X, Dai, J, Peng, Y, Guo, X, et al. Association between manganese superoxide dismutase (MnSOD) Val-9Ala polymorphism and cancer risk- A meta-analysis. Eur J Cancer. (2009b). , 45, 2874-81.

[225] Wang, H. C, & Choudhary, S. Reactive oxygen species-mediated therapeutic control of bladder cancer. Nat Rev Urol. (2011). , 8, 608-16.

[226] Wang, W. L, Chatterjee, N, Chittur, S. V, Welsh, J, & Tenniswood, M. P. Effects of 1α, 25 dihydroxyvitamin D_3 and testosterone on miRNA and mRNA expression in LNCaP cells. Mol Cancer. (2011). a May 18;10:58.

[227] Wang, S, Wang, X, Wu, J, Lin, Y, Chen, H, Zheng, X, Zhou, C, & Xie, L. Association of vitamin D receptor gene polymorphism and calcium urolithiasis in the Chinese Han population. Urol Res. (2011). b Nov 25. [Epub ahead of print]

[228] Wang, Y. Y, Wang, L. Z, & Sun, L. R. Antitumor effect of BCG on growth of transplanted human myeloid leukemia HL-60 cells in nude mice]. Zhongguo Shi Yan Xue Ye Xue Za Zhi. (2011). c Jun;, 19(3), 725-9.

[229] Wang, J. Y, Swami, S, Krishnan, A. V, & Feldman, D. Combination of calcitriol and dietary soy exhibits enhanced anticancer activity and increased hypercalcemic toxicity in a mouse xenograft model of prostate cancer. Prostate. (2012). a Mar 27. doi:pros. 22516. [Epub ahead of print]

[230] Wang, H, Tan, G, Dong, L, Cheng, L, Li, K, Wang, Z, & Luo, H. Circulating MiR-125b as a Marker Predicting Chemoresistance in Breast Cancer. PLoS One. (2012b). e34210.

[231] Weitsman, G. E, Ravid, A, Liberman, U. A, & Koren, R. The role of MAP kinase in the synergistic cytotoxic action of calcitriol and TNF-alpha in human breast cancer cells. J Steroid Biochem Mol Biol. (2004). May;89-90(1-5):361-4., 38.

[232] Welsh, J, Zinser, L. N, Mianecki-morton, L, Martin, J, Waltz, S. E, James, H, & Zinser, G. M. Age-related changes in the epithelial and stromal compartments of the mammary gland in normocalcemic mice lacking the vitamin D_3 receptor. PLoS One. (2011). Jan 26;6(1):e16479

[233] White, B. D, Chien, A. J, & Dawson, D. W. Dysregulation of Wnt/β-catenin signaling in gastrointestinal cancers. Gastroenterology. (2012). Feb;, 142(2), 219-32.

[234] Wieczorek, E, Reszka, E, Gromadzinska, J, & Wasowicz, W. Genetic polymorphism of matrix metalloproteinases in breast cancer. Neoplasma. (2012). , 59(3), 237-47.

[235] Wilop, S, Von Hobe, S, Crysandt, M, Esser, A, Osieka, R, & Jost, E. Impact of angiotensin I converting enzyme inhibitors and angiotensin II type 1 receptor blockers on survival in patients with advanced non-small-cell lung cancer undergoing first-line platinum-based chemotherapy. J Cancer Res Clin Oncol. (2009). Oct;, 135(10), 1429-35.

[236] Wolpin, B. M, Ng, K, Bao, Y, Kraft, P, Stampfer, M. J, Michaud, D. S, Ma, J, Buring, J. E, Sesso, H. D, Lee, I. M, Rifai, N, Cochrane, B. B, Wactawski-wende, J, Chlebowski, R. T, Willett, W. C, Manson, J. E, Giovannucci, E. L, & Fuchs, C. S. Plasma 25-hydroxyvitamin D and risk of pancreatic cancer. Cancer Epidemiol Biomarkers Prev. (2012). Jan;, 21(1), 82-91.

[237] Woo, T. C, Choo, R, Jamieson, M, Chander, S, & Vieth, R. Pilot study: potential role of vitamin D (Cholecalciferol) in patients with PSA relapse after definitive therapy. Nutr Cancer. (2005). , 51(1), 32-6.

[238] Woodson, K, Tangrea, J. A, Lehman, T. A, Modali, R, Taylor, K. M, Snyder, K, et al. Manganese superoxide dismutase (MnSOD) polymorphism, alpha-tocopherol supplementation and prostate cancer risk in the alpha-tocopherol, beta-carotene cancer prevention study (Finland). Cancer Causes Control. (2003). , 14, 513-8.

[239] Wu, W. K, Sung, J. J, To, K. F, Yu, L, Li, H. T, Li, Z. J, Chu, K. M, Yu, J, & Cho, C. H. The host defense peptide LL-37 activates the tumor-suppressing bone morphogenetic

protein signaling via inhibition of proteasome in gastric cancer cells. J Cell Physiol. (2010). Apr;, 223(1), 178-86.

[240] Wu, K, Feskanich, D, Fuchs, C. S, Chan, A. T, Willett, W. C, Hollis, B. W, Pollak, M. N, & Giovannucci, E. Interactions between plasma levels of hydroxyvitamin D, insulin-like growth factor (IGF)-1 and C-peptide with risk of colorectal cancer. PLoS One. (2011a). e28520., 25.

[241] Wu, Y, Miyamoto, T, Li, K, Nakagomi, H, Sawada, N, Kira, S, Kobayashi, H, Zakohji, H, Tsuchida, T, Fukazawa, M, Araki, I, & Takeda, M. Decreased expression of the epithelial Ca2+ channel TRPV5 and TRPV6 in human renal cell carcinoma associated with vitamin D receptor. J Urol. (2011b). Dec;, 186(6), 2419-25.

[242] Yamaji, T, Iwasaki, M, Sasazuki, S, Sakamoto, H, Yoshida, T, & Tsugane, S. Association between plasma 25-hydroxyvitamin D and colorectal adenoma according to dietary calcium intake and vitamin D receptor polymorphism. Am J Epidemiol. (2012). Feb 1;, 175(3), 236-44.

[243] Yan, W, Zhang, W, Sun, L, Liu, Y, You, G, Wang, Y, Kang, C, You, Y, & Jiang, T. Identification of MMP-9 specific microRNA expression profile as potential targets of anti-invasion therapy in glioblastoma multiforme. Brain Res. (2011). Sep 9;, 1411, 108-15.

[244] Yang, Y. H, Zheng, G. G, Li, G, Zhang, B, Song, Y. H, & Wu, K. F. Expression of LL-37/hCAP-18 gene in human leukemia cells. Leuk Res. (2003). Oct;, 27(10), 947-50.

[245] Yim, S, Dhawan, P, Ragunath, C, Christakos, S, & Diamond, G. Induction of cathelicidin in normal and CF bronchial epithelial cells by 1,25-dihydroxyvitamin D_3. J Cys Fibros. (2007)., 6, 403-410.

[246] Yin, L, Grandi, N, Raum, E, Haug, U, Arndt, V, & Brenner, H. Meta-analysis: longitudinal studies of serum vitamin D and colorectal cancer risk. Aliment Pharmacol Ther. (2009). Jul 1;, 30(2), 113-25.

[247] Yoshioka, S, King, M. L, Ran, S, & Okuda, H. MacLean JA 2nd, McAsey ME, Sugino N, Brard L, Watabe K, Hayashi K. WNT7A regulates tumor growth and progression in ovarian cancer through the WNT/β-catenin pathway. Mol Cancer Res. (2012). Mar;, 10(3), 469-82.

[248] Yu, H, Xu, S. S, Cheng, Q. Q, He, L. M, & Li, Z. Expression and clinical significance of Toll-like receptors in human renal carcinoma cell 786-0 and normal renal cell HK-2]. Zhonghua Yi Xue Za Zhi. (2011). Jan 11;Article in Chinese], 91(2), 129-31.

[249] Yuan, W, Pan, W, Kong, J, Zheng, W, Szeto, F, et al. dihydroxyvitamin D_3 suppresses renin gene transcription by blocking the activity of the cyclic AMP response element in the renin gene promoter. J Biol Chem. (2007)., 282, 29821-30.

[250] Yuk, J. M, Shin, D. M, Song, K. S, Lim, K, Kim, K. H, Lee, S. H, Kim, J. M, Lee, J. S, Paik, T. H, Kim, J. S, & Jo, E. K. Bacillus calmette-guerin cell wall cytoskeleton enhan-

ces colon cancer radiosensitivity through autophagy. Autophagy. (2010). Jan;, 6(1), 46-60.

[251] Xia, Z, Liu, W, Li, S, Jia, G, Zhang, Y, Li, C, Ma, Z, Tian, J, & Gong, J. Expression of matrix metalloproteinase-9, type IV collagen and vascular endothelial growth factor in adamantinous craniopharyngioma. Neurochem Res. (2011). Dec;, 36(12), 2346-51.

[252] Xiang, W, Kong, J, Chen, S, Cao, L, Qiao, G, et al. Cardiac hypertrophy in vitamin D receptor knockout mice: role of the systemic and cardiac renin-angiotensin systems. Am J Phys Endocrinol Met. (2005). E, 125-32.

[253] Xu, H, Soruri, A, Gieseler, R. K, & Peters, J. H. dihydroxyvitamin D_3 exerts opposing effects to IL-4 on MHC class-II antigen expression, accessory activity, and phagocytosis of human monocytes. Scand J Immunol. (1993). , 38, 535-60.

[254] Zhao, X, Wang, X, Wu, W, Gao, Z, Wu, J, Garfield, D. H, Wang, H, Wang, J, Qian, J, Li, H, Jin, L, Li, Q, Han, B, Lu, D, & Bai, C. Matrix metalloproteinase-2 polymorphisms and clinical outcome of Chinese patients with nonsmall cell lung cancer treated with first-line, platinum-based chemotherapy. Cancer. (2011). Nov 9. doi:cncr. 26669. [Epub ahead of print]

[255] Zhang, L. Y, & Ren, K. W. Meta-analysis of MMP2-1306T allele as a protective factor in digestive cancer. Arch Med Res. (2011). Apr;, 42(3), 239-43.

[256] Zhang, W, Yang, H. C, Wang, Q, Yang, Z. J, Chen, H, Wang, S. M, Pan, Z. M, Tang, B. J, Li, Q. Q, & Li, L. Clinical value of combined detection of serum matrix metalloproteinase-9, heparanase, and cathepsin for determining ovarian cancer invasion and metastasis. Anticancer Res. (2011). a Oct;, 31(10), 3423-8.

[257] Zhang, J, Harrison, J. S, & Studzinski, G. P. Isoforms of gamma and delta contribute to differentiation of human AML cells induced by 1,25-dihydroxyvitamin D3. Exp Cell Res. (2011). b Jan 1;317(1):117-30., 38MAPK.

[258] Zhang, Q, Ma, Y, Cheng, Y. F, Li, W. J, Zhang, Z, & Chen, S. Y. Involvement of reactive oxygen species in 2-methoxyestradiol-induced apoptosis in human neuroblastoma cells. Cancer Lett. (2011c). , 313, 201-10.

[259] Zhang, L. F, Mi, Y. Y, Cao, Q, Wang, W, Qin, C, Wei, J. F, Zhou, Y. J, Li, Y. F, Tang, M, Liu, W. M, Zhang, W, & Zou, J. G. Update analysis of studies on the MMP-9-1562 C>T polymorphism and cancer risk. Mol Biol Rep. (2012). a Apr;, 39(4), 3435-41.

[260] Zhang, J, Zhang, H, Zhang, X, & Yu, Z. Synergistic effect of retinoic acid and vitamin D analog EBinduced apoptosis of hepatocellular cancer cells. Cytotechnology. (2012). b Oct 16. [Epub ahead of print], 1089.

[261] Zhou, W, Heist, R. S, Liu, G, Asomaning, K, Neuberg, D. S, Hollis, B. W, Wain, J. C, Lynch, T. J, Giovannucci, E, Su, L, & Christiani, D. C. Circulating 25-hydroxyvitamin D levels predict survival in early-stage non-small-cell lung cancer patients. J Clin Oncol. (2007). Feb 10;, 25(5), 479-85.

[262] Zhou, L, Zhang, R, Yao, W, Wang, J, Qian, A, Qiao, M, Zhang, Y, & Yuan, Y. Decreased expression of angiotensin-converting enzyme 2 in pancreatic ductal adenocarcinoma is associated with tumor progression. Tohoku J Exp Med. (2009). Feb;, 217(2), 123-31.

[263] Zhou, L, Zhang, R, Zhang, L, Yao, W, Li, J, & Yuan, Y. Angiotensin-converting enzyme 2 acts as a potential molecular target for pancreatic cancer therapy. Cancer Lett. (2011). Aug 1;, 307(1), 18-25.

[264] Zhuo de X, Niu XH, Chen YC, Xin DQ, Guo YL, Mao ZB. Vitamin D_3 up-regulated protein 1(VDUP1) is regulated by FOXO3A and miR-17-5p at the transcriptional and post-transcriptional levels, respectively, in senescent fibroblasts. J Biol Chem. (2010). Oct 8;, 285(41), 31491-501.

[265] Zimmerman, E. I, Dollins, C. M, Crawford, M, Grant, S, Nana-sinkam, S. P, Richards, K. L, Hammond, S. M, & Graves, L. M. Lyn kinase-dependent regulation of miR181 and myeloid cell leukemia-1 expression: implications for drug resistance in myelogenous leukemia. Mol Pharmacol. (2010). Nov;, 78(5), 811-7.

[266] Van Der Knaap, R, Siemes, C, Coebergh, J. W, Van Duijn, C. M, Hofman, A, & Stricker, B. H. Renin-angiotensin system inhibitors, angiotensin I-converting enzyme gene insertion/deletion polymorphism, and cancer: the Rotterdam Study. Cancer. (2008). Feb 15;, 112(4), 748-57.

[267] Varsavsky, M, Reyes-garcía, R, Cortés-berdonces, M, García-martin, A, Rozas-moreno, P, & Muñoz-torres, M. Serum 25 OH vitamin D concentrations and calcium intake are low in patients with prostate cancer. Endocrinol Nutr. (2011). Nov;, 58(9), 487-91.

[268] Vink-van Wijngaarden T, Pols HA, Buurman CJ, van den Bemd GJ, Dorssers LC, Birkenhäger JC, van Leeuwen JP. Inhibition of breast cancer cell growth by combined treatment with vitamin D_3 analogues and tamoxifen. Cancer Res. (1994). Nov 1;, 54(21), 5711-7.

[269] Villumsen, M, Sørup, S, Jess, T, Ravn, H, Relander, T, Baker, J. L, Benn, C. S, Sørensen, T. I, Aaby, P, & Roth, A. Risk of lymphoma and leukaemia after bacille Calmette-Guérin and smallpox vaccination: a Danish case-cohort study. Vaccine. (2009). Nov 16;, 27(49), 6950-8.

[270] Volante, M, Rapa, I, Gandhi, M, Bussolati, G, Giachino, D, Papotti, M, & Nikiforov, Y. E. RAS mutations are the predominant molecular alteration in poorly differentiated thyroid carcinomas and bear prognostic impact. J Clin Endocrinol Metab. (2009). Dec;, 94(12), 4735-41.

Chapter 19

The Treatment of Cancer: A Comprehensive Therapeutic Model Entailing a Complex of Interaction Modalities

R. Saggini and M. Calvani

Additional information is available at the end of the chapter

http://dx.doi.org/10.5772/55696

1. Introduction

Although an overall rise in cancer incidence has been observed over the past 300 years concomitantly with the industrial revolution, a more prominent increase has been recorded since the '30s, with a further acceleration during the last 2 decades.

Genetic factors are thought to account for 5-10% of all malignant neoplasms, even though hereditary susceptibility will be variably relevant depending on histotype, anatomic site, and epidemiologic context; additionally, a key role is played by environmental factors. Socioeconomic improvements have resulted in an increase in food availability as well as significant changes in lifestyle habits; with new technologies allowing for automation of manual work, an overall physical activity reduction has been observed leading to unbalances between caloric intake and energy expenditure.

Cancer is no longer a rapidly lethal disease for an increasing number of patients. Knowledge of the main risk factors for cancer development is essential for establishing a comprehensive and integrated treatment plan (tab 1).

Cancer patients receiving treatment combinations of surgery, radiation therapy and chemotherapy are prone to developing several treatment-related diseases.

Pain, heightened risk of infection, neural deficits, lymphedema, fatigue, nausea and vomiting, loss of flexibility, myopathies, muscle weakness, cachexia, dehydration, emotional distress, shortness of breath are common side-effects capable of negatively affecting patients' lifestyle and physical activities. Any combination of surgical treatments, chemotherapy, and radiotherapy must be integrated within a global therapeutic plan aimed to reduce the above-

1.	Obesity and overweight
2.	Low fruit and vegetable intake
3.	Physical inactivity
4.	Smoking
5.	Alcohol consumption
6.	Unprotected sex
7.	Urban air pollution
8.	Indoor air pollution due to household use of solid fuels
9.	Spread of bacterial and viral infections through unsafe health care procedures

Table 1. The 9 modifiable risk factors responsible for a third of all cancer deaths in the world

mentioned negative effects that may become apparent immediately as well as after several months or years.

Mullan (1985) classified the life of cancer survivors into three stages: 1) Acute Stage, spanning from diagnosis to the first year after primary treatment; 2) Extended Stage, until the 5th year after primary treatment; 3) Permanent Stage, from the 5th year after primary treatment onwards.

The first year after primary treatment should be considered just as the "tip of the iceberg", and it is crucial that any approach to cancer treatment is holistic and comprehensive, based on the assumption that cancer is a chronic illness rather than an acute condition.

The aim of this chapter is not to describe the specifics of early management of patients diagnosed with cancer; however, the authors' view is that such approach should be as integrative and comprehensive as possible.

It is essential that physicians in the process of planning specific therapeutic interventions (either actions specifically aimed to the primary disease or supportive therapies) extensively profile patients according to their physical status in order to establish an individual patient-tailored strategy.

The integrative management approach relies on a number of basic interventions, including:

1. Therapeutic changes of lifestyle habits and daily diet;
2. Specific physical exercises and walking prescriptions;
3. Physical therapies coupled with psychophysical techniques.

2. Therapeutic changes of lifestyle habits and daily diet

2.1. What do you know?

Up to 30-40% of all malignant cancers could be prevented by interventions on diet, physical activities, and daily lifestyle.

Calories intake directly correlates with risk of developing obesity as well as cancer.

Obesity *per se* is considered to be to blame for up to 14% and 20% of all men and women deaths.

Approximately 50% of all primary malignant cancers arise in tissues with a primary involvement in obesity physiopatology.

Cancer is responsible of approximately 25% of all deaths in the US.

According to recent predictions, by 2020 the global world population will have reached 7,5 billion, with a cancer incidence and disease-specific mortality of 15 million per year and 12 million per year, respectively.

At present the total US cancer survivors population is made of 5-y cancer survivors for up to 66%, and by 2020 it has been estimated that cancer survivors aged at least 65 years will have been increased by 42% compared to now.

The diet is responsible for approximately 30-35 % of total mortality in the US, with its impact on cancer development depending on histotype and anatomic location; nutrition may play a key role in up to 70% of colorectal cancer-related deaths.

Nowadays, men and women in Occidental countries are progressively increasing in body size, with average body-mass indexes (BMI, i.e. the ratio between weight and squared height) relentlessly soaring beyond the normal range (18.5-24.9); conversely, an increasing number of individuals is falling into the overweight range (25-29.9) as well as the overt obesity range (> 30).

Obesity is easily diagnosed by assessing the increase in horizontal body dimensions compared to height.

One method for measuring such imbalance is the BMI, i.e. the ratio between weight (kilograms) and squared height (centimeters^2). BMI ranges identifying malnutrition, normal weight, overweight and different obesity degrees (mild and severe) have been defined.

BMI, however, being frequently used in epidemiological studies to assess the effect of diet as a risk factor, may become a confounding factor; indeed, BMI is less reliable in elderly patients, with height being gradually reduced due to spinal degenerative processes. Likewise, children BMI measurements may be biased by different growth rates in different body areas. Additionally, BMI fail to provide any definite information regarding body composition, i.e. the percentage of lean body mass versus fat mass, bone mineralization status, and total body water, just to name a few examples.

The value of lean body mass is critical because it is the body component consuming higher energy values per weight unit, being therefore critical for any estimations of appropriate caloric intakes.

Any diet based on caloric restriction alone would be ineffective as well as potentially dangerous if no caloric intake assessment were to be calculated according to body composition and estimated energy requirements for performing daily physical activity (including walking, writing, or accomplishing ordinary housework actions).

Obesity plays a critical role in cancer promotion, progression, and therapy resistance; obesity oncogenic actions are thought to be mediated by dysregulation of hormonal networks (i.e., circulating insuline, IGF-1, testosterone, and estrogens levels) as well as through pro-inflammatory effects due to adipose tissues cytokines.

Increased BMI values correlate with circulating inflammatory cytokines levels, that appear to be related to insulin resistance.

A positive correlation between high BMI values (>30) and cancer risk is being observed in different areas worldwide, with significant increases in cancer risk being recorded for every 5 Kg/m^2-gain in BMI.

Obesity directly promotes tissue inflammation. Lipids intake should be proportional to that of other nutrients in order to reach an adequate energy balance; in this regard, it should be remembered that 1g of fat provides approximately 9 Kcal of energy, while 1g of carbohydrates or proteins only provides 4.5 Kcal. However, specific lipids significantly differ in their chemical structure and will result in different metabolic responses when given at equal calories levels. Increased amounts of fat per portion, a phenomenon commonly occurring in restaurant and cafèteria, leads to significant inflammatory response spikes, that can be quantified by assessing increases of circulating inflammatory factors; the latter are capable of inducing insulin resistance and free radicals production, resulting in oxidation of cell structures such as nucleic acids, proteins, and membrane lipids. Other lipids possess an anti-inflammatory activity. There is plenty of literature addressing the beneficial administration of omega-3 unsaturated lipids for lessening the inflammatory consequences of several chronic diseases. Omega-3 unsaturated lipids are available either as dedicated over-the-counter preparations or through several common foods, more prominently fish and dried fruit. Omega-3 lipids are unsaturated lipids, i.e. they are in liquid form at room temperature (oils); they can easily undergo oxidation if not protected by intrinsic animals antioxidant systems or by vitamin E addition in commercially available preparations. Their content in fish meat changes according to the species, the fishing site, temperature, type of feeding (algae or other kinds of food for livestock); these features make difficult to calculate the omega-3 unsaturated lipids daily dose. Many public health authorities have been encouraging increases in diet fish intake, but it is important to know diet fish origins because of the risk related to heavy metals; it is therefore necessary to avoid eating exceedingly large amounts fish. Of course, such details are hardly specified, if ever, in epidemiological studies assessing the effects of fish-based diets. Obesity results in a status of enduring subclinical inflammation within fat tissues. In obese individuals both visceral and subcutaneous adipose tissues are infiltrated by macrophages surrounding necrotic adipocytes forming the so-called crown-like structures (CLS). The infiltrating macrophages release inflammatory cytokines whose plasma levels in post-menopausal breast cancer patients were shown to correlate with cancer progression and disease-specific mortality. In both experimental animals and humans the CLS number is directly related to BMI values.

Diets with high concentration in saturated fatty acids (cafeteria food, sausages, dairy products, red meat) are becoming more and more frequent worldwide, leading to a global escalation in overnutrition-related diseases.

Diets rich in saturated fatty acids closely correlate with metabolic syndrome and inflammation, especially inflammation of the white adipose tissue, which is not only a storage organ for lipids but also an endocrine organ.

It has been known since 1885 that hyperglycemia is more frequent among cancer patients than in the healthy population.

Warburg in 1930 highlighted the abnormal glucidic metabolism occurring in cancer cells, i.e. the so-called aerobic glycolysis, defined as the tendency of the cancer tissues to produce lactic acid even in the presence of sufficient oxygen to sustain Krebs cycle and mitochondrial membrane oxidation processes.

Glucose intolerance is an established risk factor for several cancers (including colorectal, breast, prostatic, pancreatic, and gastric cancer). Obesity and glucose intolerance are part of the metabolic syndrome, a condition characterized by increased insulin levels both during fasting and after glucose load. Metabolic syndrome, first described by Reaven in 1988, is defined by the presence of at least three of the following components: intra-abdominal or visceral obesity, glucose intolerance, hypertension, low HDL blood levels, and high triglyceride levels. In 2001, the National Cholesterol Education Program developed an alternative definition, which required the presence of at least 3 of the following 5 factors: increased waist circumference, hypertriglyceridemia, low HDL cholesterol, hypertension, and high levels of fasting glycemic levels. At the roots of metabolic syndrome there are increase in visceral fat, excessive caloric intake, and low physical activity.

The prevalence of metabolic syndrome is steadily increasing all over the world together with the increase in several types of cancer.

In subjects with glucose intolerance (IGT), both the levels of glycemia and fasting insulin are increased. The latter are coupled until glycemia reaches the concentration of 7-8 mM, a level beyond which insulin does not show further increases and may even begin to decline as a result of functional failure of pancreatic β-cells (De Fronzo 1992). This is paralleled by the gradual increase in glycemia, starting with postprandial glycemia.

Many people with newly diagnosed cancer are obese, with further changes in body structure being induced by chemotherapy, surgery, and therapy-related physical inactivity.

Chemotherapy often changes, even a year later, body composition, increasing fat mass and reducing muscle mass, creating a phenotype that could be defined as post-cancer sarcopenic obesity; the latter appears to correlate with a high risk of cancer recurrence.

Modifications in body composition in cancer patients imply that many studies conducted through questionnaires, perhaps using only one scale, were affected by significant biases. The reduction in caloric intake as a strategy to reduce obesity should be assessed on a case by case basis, followed over time, and maintained proportional with nutritional needs of the whole body in order to prevent secondary nutritional deficiencies.

The caloric intake, however, should be calibrated according to the composition of energy sources (carbohydrates, lipids, proteins); the latter, in a typical Mediterranean diet, should be in the ratio of 60%, 25%, 15%, respectively.

The American Cancer Society guidelines suggests that carbohydrates should be in the ratio of 40-65% of the energy pool, the same as for healthy population, lipids in the ratio of 20-35%, of which <10% saturated fats, and proteins should be 10-35%.

Daily protein intake should not be less than 0.8-1 grams per Kg of body weight.

Nutrition does not mean only caloric intake, but also replenishment of the very primary elements that the body uses to live. Nutritionists from different countries define the optimal daily replenishment levels of micronutrients depending on gender, age, and functional status (i.e., pregnancy, sporting activities, etc.). However, patients suffering from cancer will be almost always exhibiting to nutritional deficiencies.

Obesity itself is a malnutrition disease characterized by several deficiencies, including vitamin D deficiency. Many other deficits can be induced by specific therapies (i.e., those impairing renal tubular reabsorption through tubular damage, or intestinal absorption through mucositis, anorexia, and vomiting) and by treatments for related comorbidities (cholesterol-lowering agents, diuretics, anti-hypertensive drugs, etc...) resulting in minerals and antioxidants loss. These events may worsen the peroxidation phenomena of several biological structures, that will have been already compromised by metabolic syndrome and administration of chemotherapy.

Obesity is also associated with insulin resistance, i.e. the insulin inability, despite being available in physiological concentrations, of exerting its metabolic tasks in different body districts.

Insulin resistance assessment is performed in specialized centers, at times requiring expensive and complex methods. Such assessment could be easier by evaluation of blood glucose levels and fasting insulin levels according to the HOMA-IR algorithm, with values above 2.5 being indicative of insulin resistance.

Diet should not cause any further increase in insulin levels, either basal or food-induced.

The daily intake of carbohydrates (i.e., glycemic load) should be proportional with the body composition, the energy percentage (calculated in relation with other energy sources), and the degree of physical activity (including daily activities as well as activities planned by the rehabilitation system to reduce overweight and improve muscular function).

Carbohydrates intake should be progressively reduced throughout the day in light of the circadian increase in insulin resistance, more prominently observed during the last day hours.

Last but not least, it is necessary to avoid foods with high glycemic index (GI). The GI is determined by comparing the post prandial glycemic response of a food with the postprandial glycemic response to the same amount of available carbohydrate from a standard food in the same individual.

Baseline plasma levels of cytokines in obese people return to normal values after weight loss.

3. Diet, caloric restriction and cooking: A therapeutic way

The nutritional sources of food themselves are different from those used by our ancestors. The production doesn't respect the proximity criteria (0 km), seasonality criteria, or crop rotation criteria, resulting in a loss of micro-elements in soil. Fruits and vegetables generally meet more the preservation criteria instead of those of maturation with the result of the unpredictability of their content in terms of micronutrients.

The taste for food has been gradually changing giving priority to a rapid food intake (fast food), high levels of fat, flour and refined sugar. The large use of sweetened drinks contributes to increase the excessive energy introduction.

As for oxygen free radicals (ROS) production, it is related to inflammation during oxidative stress.

In obese patients and in those with cancer the ROS problem has a special role; supplements or diets with high content of vegetables with antioxidant activity have been given. The use of fruits and vegetables showed positive results in reducing the risk for cancer and recurrences.

Data, however, are not univocal. Each vegetable contains many different compounds, their availability is not always in relation with their content (it is a typical example for Beta carotene of carrot), the contents of a type of antioxidant may differ for the production site, stage of maturation to collection, preservation, and preparation methods (tomato sauce contains more available lycopene than raw tomato). The availability of a substance may change in different individuals according to the integrity of the intestinal mucosa (often damaged by chemotherapy) or to the kind of intestinal flora (1-1,5 kg of bacteria). This condition can also modify the food chemical structure, producing harmful or healthy substances for our health as in the case of soy isoflavones transformed into the much more active Equol only in subjects with suitable bacteria. In our blood and urine there's a large amount of products of bacterial metabolism which may influence our health; it may differ depending on the breed, gender, functional states (pregnancy) and dietary habits: there's much more complexity in epidemiological studies with the use of the food or nutritional supplements than expected in the research protocol.

The real availability (absorption) of substances in food or in supplements has a good chance to be different from that hypothesized and calculated with questionnaires or bromatological tables.

Diet should not cause any further increase in insulin levels, either basal or food-induced.

The daily intake of carbohydrates (i.e., glycemic load) should be in proportional with the body composition, the energy percentage (calculated in relation with other energy sources), and the degree of physical activity (including daily activities as well as activities planned by the rehabilitation system to reduce overweight and improve muscular function).

Carbohydrates intake should be progressively reduced throughout the day according to the circadian increase in insulin resistance, more prominently observed during the last day hours.

Last but not least, it is necessary to avoid foods with high glycemic index (GI). The GI is determined by comparing the postprandial glycemic response of a food with the postprandial glycemic response to the same amount of available carbohydrate from a standard food in the same individual.

Often using fruit we take more attention to the amount (5 servings a day) and to the concentration in antioxidants rather than the sugar content, which brings us back to the problem of calories and metabolic syndrome (fructose plugged to lead to a lower insulin response, is indeed much more dangerous than glucose for the pathogenesis of metabolic syndrome).

Diet is often unbalanced, not respecting the right proportions between carbohydrates (60%), lipids (25%) and proteins (15%).

The use of processed foods induces a higher salt intake, with effects on blood pressure and 10 on the integrity of structures such as the gastric mucosa with possible susceptibility to cancer.

The use of sweetened drinks and refined flour, without fibers, which are characteristics of white bread and pasta, causes a rapid absorption of carbohydrates and a rapid elevation of blood glucose, followed by a massive insulin response. Insulin is a hormone with multiple activities involved in the regulation of blood glucose, the transport of amino acids, the mobilization of fat from their deposits, the monitoring of urine output and of cell proliferation.

Persistent high levels of insulin indicate a loss of activity of the hormone (insulin resistance) that goes together with obesity, dyslipidemia (low HDL cholesterol, high triglycerides), high blood pressure and, according to data, even the cancer.

Fast food diets, also known with the term "Cafeteria Diet", are often characterized by an excessive fat content, often saturated, (those who melt at higher temperatures) contained in marbled meat, so defined because at a thin shear it shows impregnation of lipids within the muscle structure, typical of those animals kept under movement restriction.

A high-fatty acids diet an altered ratio between saturated and unsaturated fats, an alteration in the ratio of unsaturated omega-6 (those that have a double bond in position 6 from terminal COOH) and omega-3 (those that have the double bond in position 3, typical of fish, nuts, etc.) causes increase in blood inflammatory markers. In a state of inflammation it leads to resistance to insulin receptors, which is the first step for obesity and metabolic syndrome.

Foods with sugar and refined flour should be reduced or abolished. Bread and pasta should be made with whole grain flours, that give them a distinctive dark color, rice should be strictly integral.

As for pasta it should be investigated whether the product is integral outset or if fibers have been added to starch in a second time. The difference is huge because the slow release of the starch in an originally integral flour can give an IG <40% than the refined flour = 75%. Rice and pasta should never be overcooked.

It is absolutely necessary to avoid using fructose as an alternative to sucrose.

Salt is an important part in the preparation and storage of food. It is blamed for stomach cancer, but may be also critical for its action on blood pressure and, indirectly, on the metabolic and inflammatory situation. Very often it is not calculated in nutritional epidemiological studies in oncology.

During the cooking process an improper use of heat can turn food into a non-profit element, even dangerous for health. The use of high temperatures for long periods can produce carcinogenic substances. The use of cooking helps the extraction of carotenoids from tomatoes and carrots, but degrades the antioxidants in cruciferous vegetables, often investigated for their anticancer properties. The problem regarding the cooking should be extended to the used instruments types (oven, microwave, fry, steam, etc.).

All food should be cooked with adequate methods, tools and cooking times. A typical example may be that of the french fries, for which the interest in compositional characteristics of nutritional caused a controversy about their potential toxicity, related to frying due to the formation of acrylamide.

4. Caloric restriction

Caloric restriction is an integral part of religion requirements in several countries (Islamic Ramadan, Orthodox Church abstinence during Christmas, Easter, Assumption, the Jewish tradition of Daniel's fasting, etc.).

Over the past 30 years there have been more and more studies addressing health benefits related to caloric intake reduction in animal models and in humans.

Data seem to show that maximum benefits may be achieved by applying the highest possible calory reduction without resulting in overt malnutrition, and by prolonging this status as long as possible.

In animal models, caloric reduction of not more than 10-40% of the normal calories intake exerts an anticancer effect which is directly related to its duration.

Caloric restriction induces changes in metabolic and hormonal status in a similar way among animals and humans.

Caloric restriction improves sensitivity to insulin and improves glucose metabolism.

Caloric restriction can reduce oxidative stress.

Caloric restriction can increase life expectancy in animals; however, the restriction of carbohydrates or lipids alone does not seem to influence this result, which instead appears to be related to the reduction in methionine intake by lowering consumption of animal proteins. One year-long caloric restriction alone, even without physical activity, can reduce several markers of inflammation in obese postmenopausal women, including C-reactive protein, serum amyloid, and IL-6.

Accordingly, the excess of caloric intake induces obesity and represents a risk factor for cancer.

From rodents to primates, including humans, caloric restriction has been shown to be one of the most powerful tools in the prevention of carcinogenesis.

However, epidemiological data deriving from forced restrictions during the events of II World War showed conflicting results.

Conversely, Norwegians with a mean caloric intake reduction of about 50%, maintaining a balanced diet, showed a reduction in the incidence of breast cancer compared to controls.

In the Netherlands, a caloric intake reduction (70% in adults, 50% children) was paralleled by an increase in breast cancer but not in other forms of cancer.

The survivors of German and Russian concentration camps showed a sharp increase in all forms of cancer.

This apparent inconsistency of results can be due, in our opinion, to the distinction between caloric restriction and forced malnutrition characterized by the presence of other factors such as emotional stress, infections, etc.

5. Physical exercise and walking prescriptions

5.1. What do you know?

About the component of physical exercise, the American Cancer Society recommends the exercise like part of a continuum of cancer survival care.

The physical exercise is able to reduce the risk to develop the breast cancer and colon on 25% and pulmonary cancer on 30%, uterine cancer and ovary cancer about on 20% and on 9% about the prostate cancer.

After the diagnosis and the treatment there is a reduction from 26 to 40% of recruitment of Brest cancer and of colon cancer with daily physical exercise and also good quality of life.

Also during the prostate cancer the aerobic and endurance physical activity can reduce the fatigue and improve the life's quality.

During the hematological cancer especially in non-Hodgkin lymphoma and multiple myeloma, the physical exercise can improve the quality of life with reduction of fatigue and also the aerobic capability in bone marrow transplantation.

The general benefits of physical exercise in cancer treatment are numerous and include: improved cardiac output, increased ventilation, improved flexibility and range of motion; increased muscular strength and endurance; decreased resting heart rate; improved stroke volume, vasodilatation, perfusion; improved metabolic efficiency; improved blood counts; improved psychological attitude to resist to the cancer disease. The cancer-specific benefits are related to cancer treatment toxicity especially to muscular degeneration with 1) fatigue and weakness, 2) neurotoxicity, 3) cardiotoxicity, 4) pulmonary toxicity.

Our therapeutic approach using the physical exercise and walking prescriptions is divided in 3 phases to: 1) recovery of residual capacity; 2) sensory-motor and functional recovery capacity; 3) the quality of life improvement.

The recovery of residual capacity is designed to recovery joint mobility and to increase the uninjured muscle tone after reprogram of flexibility.

In the cancer patient there is usually a marked reduction of the flexibility.

Flexibility is one of the physiological parameters involved in almost all forms of the human movement and is similar to aerobic capacity, strength, and neuromuscular endurance in being a trainable fitness parameter.

Flexibility has been defined as mobility compliance and, alternatively, as the reciprocal counterpart of stiffness. Most of the authors define flexibility either as range of motion at or about a joint. Another definition represents flexibility like the ability of a joint to move throughout its potential range of motion. Those definitions confuse the property of flexibility with the criterion able to measure the range of motion and using hardly synonymous; since potential range of motion is a variable factor among others in deterring flexibility, flexibility cannot be understood simple as relative to it.

We define flexibility like the disposition of body tissues to allow, without injury, excursions at a joint or set of joints. This property is measured by, but not equivalent to, range of motion. Both joint tissues and the surrounding soft tissues contribute to flexibility, although only the latter should be modified in order to enhance flexibility.

To increase this capability is possible to use yoga, slow / static and dynamic stretching techniques, Pilates method; in our experience we prefer anyway Elispheric Imoove method (fig. 5) and exercises deriving from proprioceptive neuromuscular facilitation (PNF). This last technique is designed as a manual, partner-assisted stretching; a partner is needed to provide the fixed resistance against which the lengthened agonist isometrical contracted at or near maximum (to use spindle facilitation).

Some factors that affect flexibility are modifiable, subject to voluntary control to some or large extent, others are not modifiable.

Flexibility decreases with age. In cancer patients, it suggests that regular activities, in order to maintain elasticity, or to do specific stretching programs, are important for aging.

Gender is another factor that influences flexibility. Females are generally more flexible than males especially during the same stretching program; probably women have a larger percentage of elastin in their miofascia.

Flexibility varies during the course of the day. There is greater flexibility of cervical spine during the late afternoon and evening hours and about the lower lumbar spine data show an improvement during daytime later hours.

About the anatomical constraints, the excessive fatty tissue limits range of motion related to the tightness of soft tissue structures. This problem is connected with some conditions of diseases like arthritis, diabetes mellitus, hemophilia and finally the cancer but also is correlated to bad posture in orthostasis or with seated flexed posture.

Other ways to improve flexibility: massage, warm-up and stretching are three basic techniques used to increase flexibility but neither massage or warm-up is as efficient as a proper stretching regimen in increasing flexibility.

The best method to realize stretching involves a series of less than maximal isometric contractions of the agonist muscles in a pre-lengthened state (to set up the stretch), followed by concentric contractions of the antagonist muscle group (to lengthen the agonist) in conjunction with light pressure from a partner when needed and with an instrumentation like sensorized postural bench system (TecnoBody, Italy).Though this mode the objectives are to alleviate muscle tension, to facilitate healing by increasing blood flow, to decrease muscle pain by reducing vasoconstriction. This work is to applied day by day using at the cancer patients home a specific personalized postural bench like Fleximat postural bench (fig. 1 DeltaDue, Italy).

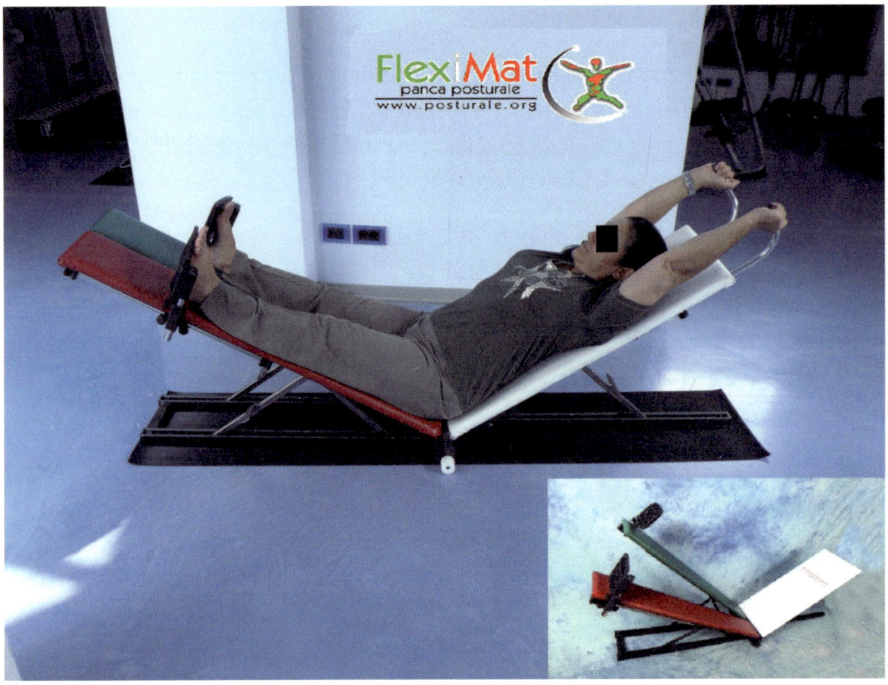

Figure 1. Fleximat

When it is not possible to get a flexibility increase in cancer treatment: there are specific contraindications, due to time and circumstances, where stretching should not be performed to get flexibility improvement. Especially when there are reduced joint receptor and pain sensation, when mobilization of tissue is not possible, for example in post-acute cancer surgical treatment or when stretching or tension in tissue elicits pain.

After the recovery the joint mobility with the flexibility replanning, the improvement of the uninjured muscle tone and strength should be possible using before focused vibratory acoustic stimulation at high intensity with Vissone (fig. 4 Vissman, Italy) and after anaerobic work with TRX system. Vibrations are able to induce muscular adaptions to the recovery of muscle tone at the 300 Hz, of frequency and to stimulate the upper motors centers in order to obtain a better performance of controls, responsible for the muscle recruitment. Is noted that so is possible to 1) activate the aerobic metabolism; 2) determine an analgesic effect; 3) increase local circulation and bone density; 4) finally increase the contractile capacity and elasticity of the muscle treated.

6. Walking prescriptions

To elicit the sensory-motor and functional recovery we need to get acceptable walking.

Human movement usually is defined by the walk and is not limited to bipedal locomotion; however, such locomotion is a fundamental part of daily life and is a prominent focus of public health physical activity guidelines.

The human gait is more complex; going one step forward, although it can start from the hip flexors of the Deep Frontal Line, especially the psoas and iliacus, afterwards, it involves the hip flexion, the knee extension, and the ankle dorsiflexion necessary to step forward, thanks to the myofascia of the Superficial Frontal Line. As the leg travels forward, the entire myofascia prepares to receive the weight of the body and the ground reaction.

Once the heel places on the ground and the step begins, the Superficial Back Line takes over as the back of leg engages into hip extension and plantar flexion. The abductors of Lateral Line, Ischio-Tibial-Tract, and the lateral compartment of the lower leg provide stability that prevents the hip adduction, while the adductor group and the other tissues of the Deep Frontal Line assist the flexion- extension motions and provide stability to the inner arch of the foot and up the inside of the leg. In the upper body, the common contralateral walking pattern involves the Functional Lines bringing the right shoulder forward to counterbalance the left leg when it swings forward and vice versa. Therefore the gist of walking capability is to improve the miofascial flexibility.

The walking objective monitoring evolution, using pedometer and accelerometer technology, offers an opportunity to perform guidelines, including recommendations for cancer patients.

All the studies in literature have used a variety of objective parameters using instruments that have been previously validated. The Yamax pedometer is considered a criterion research quality pedometer (Schneider et al., 2004), the Lifecorder's validity is well documented (Crouter et al., 2003; Schneider et al., 2004), and the ActiGraph has been adopted by national surveillance strategies (Troiano et al., 2008) and is probably the most utilized accelerometer in research today.

Therefore is possible to define with the pedometer the sedentary level into < 2,500 steps/ day (basally active) and into < 2,500 to 4,999 steps/day (limited activity); but using an established step-defined physical activity scale is possible to establish a level one for sedentary < 5,000 steps/day ; a level two >5,000 <7,499 steps/day for low active; a level three >7,500 <9,999 steps/day for somewhat active ; a level four >10,000 <12,499 steps/day for active; and a level five ≥ 12,500 steps/day for highly active.

We also noticed that healthy adults can perform between approximately 4,000 and 18,000 steps/day, and, in our opinion, also 7,500-9,9990 steps / day, resulting in between 50/ 85 steps /minute. That would be a reasonable target for the cancer patients in the first Mullan phase.

In order to get a better walking performance in the first phase of Mullan, and also in the second phase, we adopt two integrate procedures: 1) normalization of the foot-ground reaction forces using a personalized viscoelastic insoles to control vertical and shear forces on the foot during the stance phase without the obligatory use of athletic shoes; 2) use of the micrograviatary system S.P.A.D (fig. 2) that determine the sensory-motor and functional recovery of the posture during the walking in combination to the development of proprioceptive information from the periphery to the cortical central system.

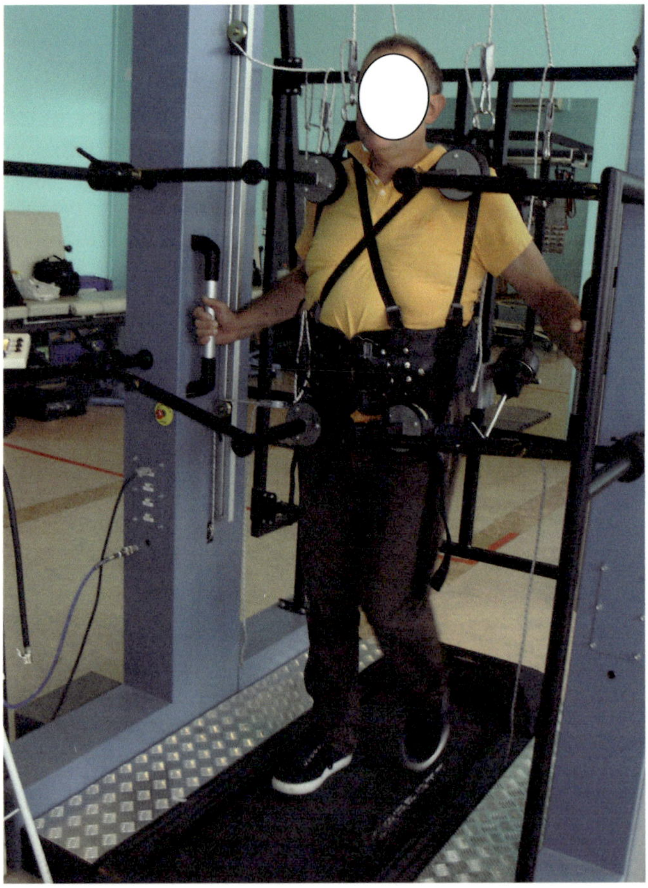

Figure 2. SPAD

7. Physical therapies connected with psychophysical techniques

During the first year after the cancer treatment the immune system shows some specific changes in patient with cancer especially in some specific T-cell populations.

There is no scientific evidence that physical therapies, like magnetic fields, are effective in the treatment of cancer itself. Global physics community perfectly knows what the extreme low frequencies and intensity of magnetic fields are. They also know how they provoke the resonance of ions (Ion Cyclotron Resonance), with the exact frequency in order to remove an ion from its orbit of rotation in order to escape.

Only in the last decades the studies in biophysics have shown that with the ion cyclotron resonance is possible to stimulate the passage of ions through the membranes of the cells of the living beings changing their permeability and therefore improving the ion exchange on both sides of the membrane itself. The increase of the bioavailability of the essential ions, makes better the efficiency of the cell itself to achieve its correct metabolism.

The role of electromagnetic fields for control of cancer pain and chemotherapy nausea-induced symptoms remains controversial but this theory is to be correlate to water coherence domains' theory (G. Preparata, E. Del Giudice, G. Talpo 1999).

The activities and the exchanges of the molecules in the body doesn't happen by chance, but they follow an "order" dictated by the magnetic field produced by the water, where all the elements fluctuate in phase in the those regions called coherence domains.

Only the molecules which react to the frequency of this magnetic field, interact with each other, starting in ordered way the correct chemical reactions necessary for life of the cell and the organism. An imbalance of this 'order' jeopardizes the functioning of the cell, with the consequence of the manifestations of the diseases.

The 40% of the water is coherent and it can receive and deliver electromagnetic information, while the remaining 60% is not coherent, equally essential for life; it represents the solvent of the ions and of the fundamental elements to the cellular economy.

Also Montagnier L. in 2009 has recognized the validity of the coherence domains, stating how the water is not an inert substance, but may take special configurations emitting electromagnetic waves that can become an not pharmacological instrument of the therapy and the adjustment, but always deeply medical care.

The cells' DNA emits extremely low frequency waves, from zero to a few hundred of Hertz. The studies were published on the unbalance of this "range" that disturbs the harmony of the cell, with the onset of the manifestations of diseases. Some chronic diseases such as Alzheimer's, Parkinson's, multiple sclerosis, rheumatoid arthritis, and the viral diseases such as HIV -AIDS, influenza A and hepatitis C, "inform" the water of our body (biological water) of their presence issuing a special electromagnetic signals that can then be "read and decoded".

With Ion Cyclotron Resonance we have the possibility to intervene in a not invasive, natural and precise adjustment mechanisms of the body's homeostasis, where the only pharmacological support can be not complete.

Therefore you get the possibility:

1. To rebalance subjective metabolism
2. To adjust the enzyme functions, the ion channels and the body pH
3. To strengthen the immune system
4. To encourage the bioavailability and absorption of nutrients for cell metabolism
5. To treat neuralgia, headaches and migraines
6. To stimulate healing in all kinds of wounds, even after surgery.
7. To balance the water retention
8. To enhance the effect of drugs and supplements
9. To detoxify and to allow antioxidant function against free radicals, metabolites, toxins
10. To stimulate a pain-killer function (acute and chronic)
11. To get muscle relaxation, from anxiety and stress
12. To improve the homeostasis recovery under stress (physiological micro trauma and muscle protein catabolism)
13. To improve the quality of life for cancer patients.

In a preliminary observational study of 43 cancer patient group, they were divided into 3 groups of 14 patients, using also the Ion Cyclotron Resonance with QUEC PHISIS QPS1 (fig. 3) we observed the initial and final values of d-ROMs Test.

The first group only used the QUEC PHISIS QPS1

The second group used the QUEC PHISIS QPS1 and the antioxidants.

The third group only used the antioxidants.

The study shows a significant improvement after 90 minutes before the beginning of the first treatment. The values are improved and consolidated in the time after a month about the end of the cycle of treatments with the values well below average.

http://dx.doi.org/10.5772/55696

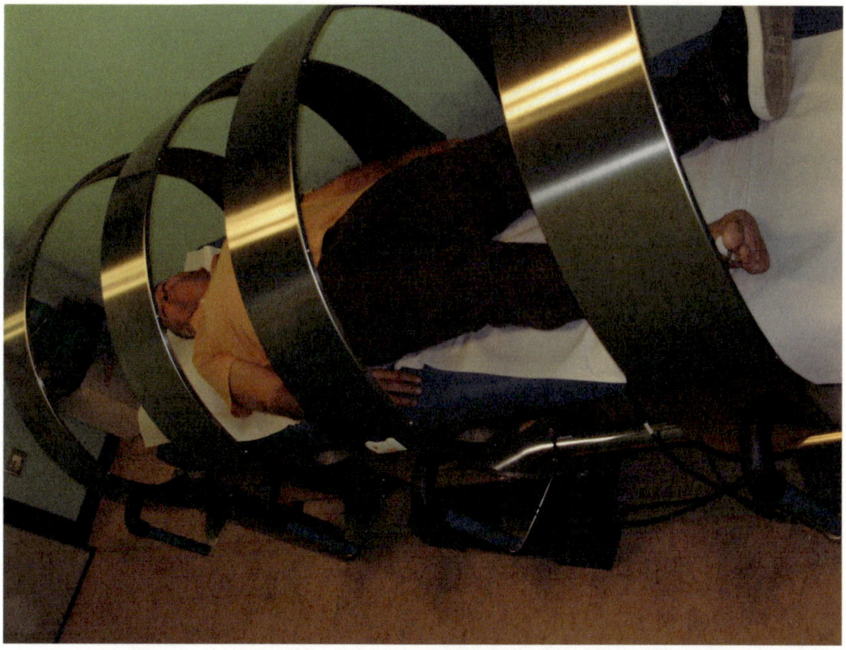

Figure 3. Qps 1

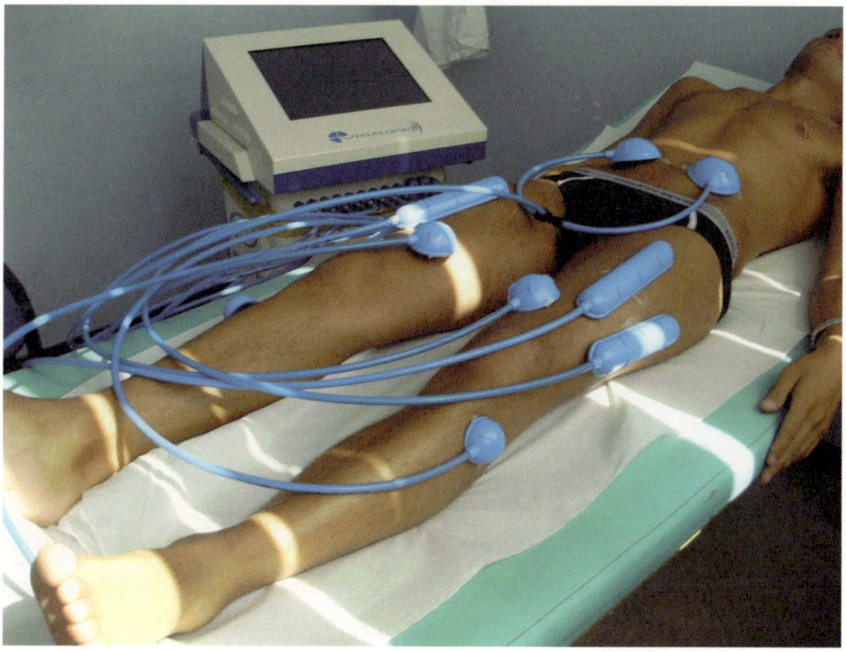

Figure 4. Viss

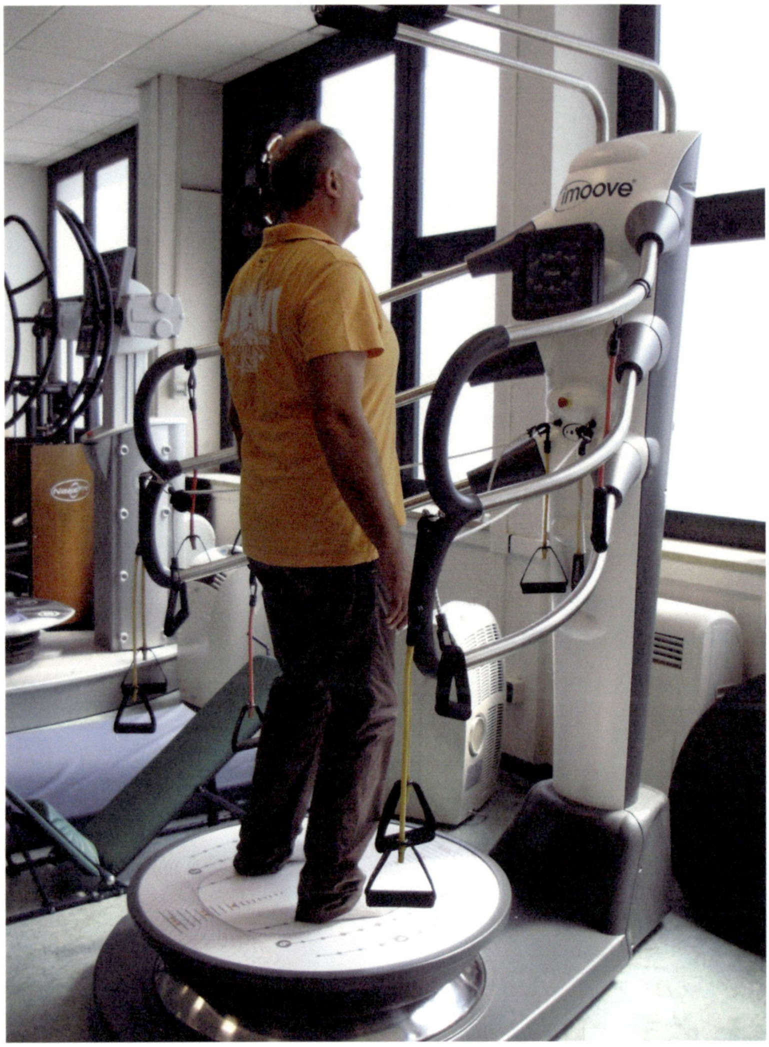

Figure 5. Imoove

8. Conclusion

The integration between the pharmacology, the biochemistry, the biophysics and the lifestyle with energetic modulation using therapeutic diet through the use of the information and the signals, probably will be able to restore a robust immune response in the tumor-bearing host or to promote by adoptive transfer of activated effector cells or tumor-specific antibodies into the tumor-bearing host.

http://dx.doi.org/10.5772/55696

Author details

R. Saggini[1,2] and M. Calvani[1,2]

1 Dept. of Neuroscience and Imaging, "G. d'Annunzio" University, Chieti, Italy

2 Specialitation school of Physical Medicine and Rehabilitation, "G. d'Annunzio" University, Chieti, Italy

References

[1] Amin Esfahani,, Julia M. W. Wong, Arash Mirrahimi, Korbua Srichaikul, David J. A. Jenkins, Cyril W. C. Kendall, Glycemic Index: Physiological Significance Journal of the American College of Nutrition, Vol. 28, No. 4, 439S–445S (2009).

[2] Amin Esfahani,, Julia M. W. Wong, Arash Mirrahimi, Korbua Srichaikul, David J. A. Jenkins, Cyril W. C. Kendall, Glycemic Index: Physiological Significance Journal of the American College of Nutrition, Vol. 28, No. 4, 439S–445S (2009).

[3] Arvidsson E, Viguerie N, Andersson I, Verdich C, Langin D, and Arner P. Effects of different hypocaloric diets on protein secretion from adipose tissue of obese women. *Diabetes* 53: 1966–1971, 2004.

[4] Bachelot T, Ray-Coquard I, Menetrier-Caux C, et al. Prognostic value of serum levels of interleukin 6 and of serum and plasmalevels of vascular endothelial growth factor in hormonerefractory metastatic breast cancer patients. *Br J Cancer*. 2003; 88:1721-1726.

[5] Balkau B, Barrett-Connor E, Eschwege E, et al. Diabetes and pancreatic carcinoma. Diabete Metab 1993;19:458–62.

[6] Bastard JP, Jardel C, Bruckert E, Blondy P, Capeau J, Laville M, Vidal H, and Hainque B. Elevated levels of interleukin 6 are reduced in serum and subcutaneous adipose tissue of obese women after weight loss. *J Clin Endocrinol Metab* 85: 3338–3342, 2000

[7] Bellomo R.G., Iodice P., Savoia V., Saggini A., Vermiglio G., Saggini R. (2009). Balance and posture in the elderly: an analysis of a sensorimotor rehabilitation protocol. *International journal of immunopathology and pharmacology*, vol. 22 No 3 (S), p. 37-44, ISSN: 0394-6320

[8] Bianchini F, Kaaks R, Vainio H. Overweight, obesity and cancer risk. Lancet Oncol 2002;3:565–74; Bray GA. The underlying basis for obesity: relationship to cancer. J Nutr 2002;132:3451S–5S)

[9] Caan B, Sternfeld B, Gunderson E, et al. Life After Cancer Epidemiology (LACE) Study: a cohort of early stage breast cancer survivors (United States). Cancer Causes Control 2005;16:545–556.

[10] Calle EE, Kaaks R. Overweight, obesity and cancer: epidemiological evidence and proposed mechanisms. Nat Rev Cancer 2004;4:579 –91.

[11] Calle EE, Rodriguez C, Walker-Thurmond K, Thun MJ. Overweight, obesity, and mortality from cancer in a prospectively studied cohort of U.S. adults. N Engl J Med 2003;348:1625–1638.

[12] Calle EE, Rodriguez C, Walker-Thurmond K, Thun MJ: Overweight,obesity, and mortality from cancer in a prospectively studied cohort of U.S. adults. *N Engl J Med* 2003, 348:1625-1638.)

[13] Camoriano JK, Loprinzi CL, Ingle JN, et al.Weight change in women treated with adjuvant therapy or observed following mastectomy for node-positive breast cancer. J Clin Oncol 1990; 8:1327–1334.

[14] Cancello R, Henegar C, Viguerie N, et al. Reduction of macrophage infiltration and chemoattractant gene expression changes in white adipose tissue of morbidly obese subjects after surgeryinduced weight loss. *Diabetes*. 2005;54:2277-2286

[15] Chao A, Connell CJ, Jacobs EJ, McCullough ML, Patel AV, Calle EE, Cokkinides VE, Thun MJ. Amount, type, and timing of recreational physical activity in relation to colon and rectal cancer in older adults: the Cancer Prevention Study II Nutrition Cohort. *Cancer Epidemiol Biomarkers Prev*. 2004 Dec;13(12):2187-2195.

[16] Chia-Ming Chang, Chien-Liang Wu and Yen-Ta Lu (2012). Cancer-associated immune deficiency: A form of accelerated immunosenescence? in Mohan R. (ed.) Topics in cancer survivorship pag 95-108. InTech Croatia isbn 978-953-307-894-6.

[17] Clement K, Viguerie N, Poitou C, Carette C, Pelloux V, Curat CA, Sicard A, Rome S, Benis A, Zucker JD, Vidal H, Laville M, Barsh GS, Basdevant A, Stich V, Cancello R, and Langin D. Weight loss regulates inflammation-related genes in white adipose tissue of obese subjects. *FASEB J* 18: 1657–1669, 2004

[18] Cnop M. Fatty acids and glucolipotoxicity in the pathogenesis of Type 2diabetes. Biochem Soc Trans. 2008;36:348–52.

[19] Coleman EA, Coon S, Hall-Barrow J, et al. Feasibility of exercise during treatment for multiple myeloma. Cancer Nurs 2003;26:410–419.

[20] Colleen Doyl; Lawrence H. Kushi; Tim Byers; Kerry S. Courneya; Wendy Demark-Wahnefried; Barbara Grant; Anne McTiernan; Cheryl L. Rock; Cyndi Thompson; Ted Gansler; Kimberly S. Andrews; for The 2006 Nutrition, Physical Activity and Cancer Survivorship Advisory Committee, Nutrition and Physical ActivityDuring and After Cancer Treatment: An American Cancer Society Guidefor Informed Choices CA Cancer J Clin 2006;56:323–353.

[21] Colman,R.J. et al. (2009) Caloric restriction delays disease onset and mortality in rhesus monkeys. Science, 325, 201–204.

[22] Courneya KS, Friedenreich CM, Arthur K, Bobick TM. Physical exercise and quality of life in postsurgical colorectal cancer patients. Psychology, Health and Medicine 1999;4:181–187.

[23] Courneya KS, Friedenreich CM, Quinney HA, et al. A randomized trial of exercise and quality of life in colorectal cancer survivors. Eur J Cancer Care (Engl) 2003;12:347–357.

[24] Courneya KS, Friedenreich CM. Relationship between exercise pattern across the cancer experience and current quality of life in colorectal cancer sur vivors. J Altern Complement Med 1997;3:215–226.

[25] Courneya KS. Exercise in cancer survivors: an overview of research. Med Sci Sports Exerc 2003;35:1846–1852.

[26] Cust AE (2011) Physical activity and gynecologic cancer prevention. In: Courneya KS, Friedenreich CM (eds) Physical activity and cancer: Recent results in cancer research, vol 186. *Springer*, Berlin Heidelberg.

[27] D.L. Roberts, C.Dive, A.G Renehan Biological mechanisms linking obesity and cancer risk: new perspectives, Annu Rev Med. 2010;61:301-16.

[28] Dandona P, Mohanty P, Ghanim H, Aljada A, Browne R, Hamouda W,Prabhala A, Afzal A, Garg R: The suppressive effect of dietary restriction and weight loss in the obese on the generation of reactive oxygen species by leukocytes, lipid peroxidation, and protein carbonylation. JClin Endocrinol Metab 2001, 86:355-362.

[29] Dandona P, Weinstock R, Thusu K, et al. Tumor necrosis factor alpha in sera of obese patients: fall with weight loss. *J Clin Endocrinol Metab*. 1998;83:2907-2910.

[30] Devesa SS, Blot WJ, Stone BJ, Miller BA, Tarone RE, Fraumeni JF Jr. Recent cancer trends in the United States. J Natl Cancer Inst 1995;87:175–82.

[31] Dimeo F, Bertz H, Finke J, et al. An aerobic exercise program for patients with haematological malignancies after bone marrow transplantation. Bone Marrow Transplant 1996;18:1157–1160.

[32] Dimeo FC, Tilmann MH, Bertz H, et al. Aerobic exercise in the rehabilitation of cancer patients after high dose chemotherapy and autologous peripheral stem cell transplantation. Cancer 1997;79:1717–1722.

[33] Elias S.G. et al. (2005) The 1944–1945 Dutch famine and subsequent overall cancer incidence. Cancer Epidemiol. Biomarkers Prev., 14, 1981–1985.

[34] Emaus A, Thune I (2011) Physical activity and lung cancer prevention. In: Courneya KS, Friedenreich CM (eds) Physical activity and cancer: Recent results in cancer research, vol 186. *Springer*, Berlin Heidelberg.

[35] Enger SM, Bernstein L. Exercise activity, body size and premenopausal breast cancer survival. Br J Cancer 2004;90:2138–2141.

[36] Enger SM, Bernstein L. Exercise activity, body size and premenopausal breast cancer survival. Br J Cancer 2004;90:2138–2141.

[37] Enger SM, Greif JM, Polikoff J, Press M. Body weight correlates with mortality in earlystage breast cancer. Arch Surg 2004;139:954–958; discussion 58–60.

[38] F. Brayand, and B. Moller. Predicting the future burden ofcancer. Nat. Rev. Cancer. 6:63–74 (2006))

[39] Flegal KM, Carroll MD, Ogden CL, Curtin LR. 2010. Prevalence and trends in obesity among US adults, 1999–2008. *JAMA* 303:235–41; World Cancer Res. Fund/Am. Inst. Cancer Res. 2007. *Food, Nutrition, Physical Activity, and the Prevention of Cancer: A Global Perspective.* Washington, DC: Am. Inst. Cancer Res.

[40] Freund E. Diagnosis des Carcinomas. Wiener Medizinische 1885; B1:268–268

[41] Friedenreich CM (eds) Physical activity and cancer: Recent results in cancer research. *Springer*, Berlin Heidelberg

[42] G. Danaei, S. Vander Hoorn, A. D Lopez, C. J L Murray, M. Ezzati, and the Comparative Risk Assessment collaborating group (Cancers), Causes of cancer in the world: comparative risk assessment of nine behavioural and environmental risk factors. Lancet 2005; 366: 1784–93.

[43] Galassetti PR, Nemet D, Pescatello A, Rose-Gottron C, Larson J, Cooper DM: Exercise, caloric restriction, and systemic oxidative stress. J Investig Med 2006, 54:67-75.

[44] Gapstur SM, Gann PH, Colangelo LA, et al. Postload plasmaglucose concentration and 27-year prostate cancer mortality (United States). Cancer Causes Control 2001;12:763–72.

[45] Gerber M, Corpet D. Energy balance and cancers. Eur J Cancer Prev1999;8:77– 89.

[46] Harvie MN, Campbell IT, Baildam A, Howell A. Energy balance in early breast cancer patients receiving adjuvant chemotherapy. Breast Cancer Res Treat 2004;83:201–210

[47] Haydon AM, Macinnis RJ, English DR, Giles GG. Effect of physical activity and body size on survival after diagnosis with colorectal cancer. Gut 2006;55:62–67.

[48] Hayes S, Davies PS, Parker T, et al. Quality of life changes following peripheral blood stem cell transplantation and participation in a mixedtype, moderate-intensity, exercise program. Bone Marrow Transplant 2004;33:553–558.

[49] Hayes SC, Rowbottom D, Davies PS, et al Immunological changes after cancer treatment and participation in an exercise program. Med Sci Sports Exerc 2003;35:2–9.

[50] Heilbronn L.K. et al. (2006) Effect of 6-month calorie restriction on biomarkers of longevity, metabolic adaptation, and oxidative stress in overweight individuals: a randomized controlled trial. JAMA, 295, 1539–1548.

[51] Holmes MD, Chen WY, Feskanich D, et al. Physical activity and survival after breast cancer diagnosis. JAMA 2005;293:2479–2486.

[52] Holmes MD, Chen WY, Feskanich D, et al. Physical activity and survival after breast cancer diagnosis. JAMA 2005;293:2479–2486

[53] Holt LE, Pelham TW, Campagna PD. Hemodynamics during a series of machine-aided and intensity-controlled proprioceptive neuromuscular facilitations. Can J Appl Physiol. 1995;20:407–416.

[54] Howell,A. et al. (2009) Energy restriction for breast cancer prevention. Recent Results Cancer Res., 181, 97–111

[55] Huntington MO 1985 Weight gain in patients receiving adjuvant chemotherapy for carcinoma of the breast. Cancer 56:472–474.

[56] Hursting SD, Berger NA. 2010. Energy balance, host-related factors, and cancer progression. *J. Clin. Oncol.* 28:4058–65.

[57] Hursting SD, Sarah M.Smith, LauraM.Lashinger, Alison E.Harvey and Susan N.Perkins; Calories and carcinogenesis: lessons learned from 30 years of calorie restriction. Research Carcinogenesis vol.31 no.1 pp.83–89, 2010.

[58] Hursting,S.D. et al. (2007) Energy balance and carcinogenesis: underlying pathways and targets for intervention. Curr. Cancer Drug Targets, 7, 484–491.

[59] I.Imayama, C. M. Ulrich, C.M. Alfano, C.Wang, L. Xiao, M. H. Wener, K. L. Campbell, C. Duggan, K. E. Foster-Schubert, A. Kong, C. E. Mason, C. Wang, G. L. Blackburn, C. E. Bain, H. J. Thompson, and A. McTiernan, Effects of a Caloric Restriction Weight Loss Diet and Exercise on Inflammatory Biomarkers in Overweight/Obese Postmenopausal Women: A Randomized Controlled Trial *Cancer Res May 1, 2012 72; 2314*

[60] Institute of Medicine. Dietary Reference Intakes for Energy, Carbohydrate, Fiber, Fat, Fatty ,Acids ,Cholesterol, Protein, and Amino Acids (Macronutrients). Washington, DC: National Academy Press; 2002

[61] Iodice Pierpaolo, Bellomo Rosa Grazia, Gialluca Glauco, Fanò Giorgio, Saggini Raoul (2011). Acute and cumulative effects of focused high-frequency vibrations on the endocrine system and muscle strength. EUROPEAN JOURNAL OF APPLIED PHYSIOLOGY, vol. 111(6), p. 897-904, ISSN: 1439-6319

[62] J. F Trepanowski, R. E Canale, K. E Marshall, M. M Kabir and R. J Bloomer. Impact of caloric and dietary restriction regimen on markers of health and longevity in humans and animals: a summary of available findings. Nutrition Journal 2011, 10:107-120

[63] Jemal R., Siegel E., Ward T., Murray J., Xu and M. J. Thun. Cancer statistics, 2007. CA Cancer J. Clin. 57:43–66 (2007).

[64] Jenkins DJ, Wolever TM, Taylor RH, Barker H, Fielden H, Baldwin JM, Bowling AC, Newman HC, Jenkins AL, Goff DV: Glycemic index of foods: a physiological basis for carbohydrate exchange. Am J C.

[65] Jenkins DJ, Wolever TM, Taylor RH, Barker H, Fielden H, Baldwin JM, Bowling AC, Newman HC, Jenkins AL, Goff DV: Glycemic index of foods: a physiological basis for carbohydrate exchange. Am J C.

[66] Johnson L, Mander A, Jones L, Emmett P, Jebb S. Energy-dense, lowfiber, high-fat dietary pattern is associated with increased fatness in childhood. Am J Clin Nutr. 2008;87:846–54.

[67] Jones LW, Courneya KS, Vallance JK, et al. Association between exercise and quality of life in multiple myeloma cancer survivors. Support Care Cancer 2004;12:780–788.

[68] K. M. Huffman, L. M. Redman, L. R. Landerman, C. F. Pieper, R. D. Stevens,M. J. Muehlbauer, B. R. Wenner, J. R. Bain, V. B. Kraus, C. B. Newgard, E. Ravussin, W. E. Kraus; Caloric Restriction Alters the Metabolic Response to Mixed-Meal: Results from a Randomized, Controlled Trial. PLoS ONE April 2012, Vol 7, Iss. 4.

[69] Kagawa,Y. (1978) Impact of Westernization on the nutrition of Japanese: changes in physique, cancer, longevity and centenarians. Prev. Med., 7, 205–217.

[70] Keinan-Boker,L. et al. (2009) Cancer incidence in Israeli Jewish survivors of World War II. J. Natl Cancer Inst., 101, 1489–1500.

[71] Kien CL, Bunn JY, Ugrasbul F. Increasing dietary palmitic acid decreases fat oxidation and daily energy expenditure. Am J Clin Nutr. 2005;82:320–6.

[72] Kim DJ, Gallagher RP, Hislop TG, et al. Premorbid diet in relation to survival from prostate cancer (Canada). Cancer Causes Control 2000;11: 65–77.

[73] Kim YI. Diet, lifestyle, and colorectal cancer: is hyperinsulinemia the missing link? Nutr Rev 1998;56:275–9.

[74] Knols R, Aaronson NK, Uebelhart D, et al. Physical exercise in cancer patients during and after medical treatment: a systematic review of randomized and controlled clinical trials. J Clin Oncol 2005;23:

[75] Koupil,I. et al. (2009) Cancer mortality in women and men who survived the siege of Leningrad (1941–1944). Int. J. Cancer, 124, 1416–

[76] Kroenke CH, Chen WY, Rosner B, Holmes MD. Weight, weight gain, and survival after breast cancer diagnosis. J Clin Oncol 2005;23:1370.

[77] L. S. A. Augustin, S. Gallus, E. Negri & C. La Vecchia, Glycemic index, glycemic load and risk of gastric cancer *Annals of Oncology* 15: 581–584, 2004

[78] Loi S, Milne RL, Friedlander ML, et al. Obesity and outcomes in premenopausal and postmenopausal breast cancer. Cancer EpidemiolBiomarkers Prev 2005;14:1686–1691.

[79] Lundman P, Boquist S, Samnega°rd A, Bennermo M, Held C, Ericsson CG, Silveira A, Hamsten A, Tornvall PA. high-fat meal is accompanied by increased plasma interleukin-6 concentrations. Nutr Metab Cardiovasc Dis. 2007;17:195–202.

[80] Lynch BM, Neilson HK, Friedenreich C (2011) Physical activity and breast cancer prevention. In: Courneya KS, Friedenreich CM (eds) Physical activity and cancer: Recent results in cancer research, vol 186. *Springer*, Berlin Heidelberg.

[81] McCarty MF, Barroso-Aranda J, Contreras F: The low-methionine content of vegan diets may make methionine restriction feasible as a life extension strategy. Med Hypotheses 2009, 72:125-128.

[82] Megna M., Amico A.P., Cristella G., Saggini R., Jirillo E., Ranieri M. (2012). *Effects of herbal supplements on the immune system in relation to exercise. International journal of immunopathology and pharmacology*, vol. 25, p. 43-50, ISSN: 0394-6320

[83] Meloni G, Proia A, Capria S, et al. Obesity and autologous stem cell transplantation in acute myeloid leukemia. Bone Marrow Transplant 2001;28:365–367.

[84] Meyerhardt JA, Giovannucci EL, Holmes MD, et al. Physical activity and survival after colorectal cancer diagnosis. J Clin Oncol 2006;24:3527–3534.

[85] Meyerhardt JA, Heseltine D, Niedzwiecki D, et al. Impact of physical activity on cancer recurrence and survival in patients with stage III colon cancer: findings from CALGB 89803. J Clin Oncol 2006;24:3535–3541.

[86] Michels,K.B. et al. (2004) Caloric restriction and incidence of breast cancer. JAMA, 291, 1226–1230.

[87] Miller RA, Buehner G, Chang Y, Harper JM, Sigler R, Smith-Wheelock M: Methionine-deficient diet extends mouse lifespan, slows immune and lens aging, alters glucose, T4, IGF-I and insulin levels, and increases hepatocyte MIF levels and stress resistance. Aging Cell 2005, 4:119-125.

[88] Morris PG, Hudis CA, Giri D, et al. Inflammation and increased aromatase expression occur in the breast tissue of obese women with breast cancer. *Cancer Prev Res (Phila)*. 2011;4:1021-1029.

[89] Mullan F. (1985).Seasons of Survival: Reflections of a Physician with Cancer N Engl J Med 1985; 313:270-273 July 25, 1985.

[90] Myers T.W. (2001). Anatomy Trains. Churchill Livingstone isbn 0-443-06351-6.

[91] N. Parekh, U. Chandranand E. V. Bandera. Obesity in Cancer Survival Annu. Rev. Nutr. 2012.32:311-342.

[92] Olefsky JM, Glass CK. Macrophages, inflammation, and insulin resistance. *Annu Rev Physiol*. 2010;72:219-246.

[93] Pan SY, Morrison H (2011) Physical activity and hematologic cancer prevention. In: Courneya KS, Friedenreich CM (eds) Physical activity and cancer: Recent results in cancer research, vol 186. *Springer*, Berlin Heidelberg.

[94] Parry C, Kent EE, Mariotto AB,AlfanoCM,Rowland JH. 2011. Cancer survivors: a booming population. *Cancer Epidemiol. Biomarkers Prev.* 20:1996–2005; Cancer Soc. 2011. *Cancer Facts & Figures 2011.* Atlanta, GA: Am. Cancer Soc. http://www.cancer.org/acs/groups/content/@epidemiologysurveilance/documents/document/acspc-029771)

[95] Patrick G. Morris, MD, MSc, Kotha Subbaramaiah, PhD,Andrew J. Dannenberg, MD, and Clifford A. Hudis, MD; Inflammation in the Pathogenesis and Progression of Breast Cancer educational summaries ?

[96] Pietrangelo T, Mancinelli R, Toniolo L, Cancellara L, Paoli A, Puglielli C, Iodice P, Doria C, Bosco G, D'Amelio L, di Tano G, Fulle S, Saggini R, Fanò G, Reggiani C. (2009). Effects of local vibrations on skeletal muscle trophism in elderly people: mechanical, cellular, and molecular events. International journal of molecular medicine, vol. 24, p. 503-512, ISSN: 1107-3756.

[97] R. A. De Fronzo, R C. Bonadonna, E. Ferrannini, Pathogenesis of NIDDM. A Balanced Overview. 1992 , Diabetes Care, 15:318-368.

[98] R. A. De Fronzo, R C. Bonadonna, E. Ferrannini, Pathogenesis of NIDDM. A Balanced Overview. 1992 , Diabetes Care, 15:318-368.

[99] R. Doll, and R. Peto. The causes of cancer: quantitative estimates of avoidable risks of cancer in the United States today. J. Natl. Cancer Inst. 66:1191–308 (1981); W. C. Willett. Diet and cancer. Oncologist. 5:393–404 (2000).

[100] R. J. Freedman, N. Aziz, D. Albanes, T. Hartman, D. Danforth, S. Hill, N. Sebring, J. C. Reynolds, And J. A. Yanovski Weight and Body Composition Changes during and after Adjuvant Chemotherapy in Women with Breast Cancer, The Journal of Clinical Endocrinology & Metabolism 89(5):2248–2253

[101] Reaven GM. Banting lecture 1988. Role of insulin resistance in human disease. Diabetes 1988;37:1595– 607.

[102] Redman,L.M. et al. (2009) Metabolic and behavioral compensations in response to caloric restriction: implications for the maintenance of weight loss. PLoS One, 4, e4377.

[103] Rise′rus U. Fatty acids and insulin sensitivity. Curr Opin Clin Nutr Metab Care. 2008;11:100–5.

[104] S. H. Saydah, C. M. Loria, M. S. Eberhardt, and F. L. Brancati. Abnormal Glucose Tolerance and the Risk of Cancer Death in the United State Am J Epidemiol 2003;157:1092–1100s.

[105] Saggini R. and Calvani M. (2012). Rehabilitation in cancer survivors: interaction between lifestyle and physical activity in Mohan R. (ed.) Topics in cancer survivorship pag 177-194. InTech Croatia isbn 978-953-307-894-6.

[106] Saggini R., Bellomo R.G., Iodice P., Lessiani G. (2009). Venous insufficiency and foot dysmorphism: effectiveness of visco-elastic rehabilitation systems on veno-muscle system of the foot and of the calf. *International journal of immunopathology and pharmacology*, vol. 22, No 3 (S), p. 1-8. ISSN: 0394-6320.

[107] Saggini R., Bellomo R.G., Saggini A., Iodice P., Toniato E. (2009). Rehabilitative treatment for lock pain with external pulsed electromagnetic fields. *International journal of immunopathology and pharmacology*, vol. 22 No 3 (S), p. 25-28, ISSN: 0394-6320

[108] Saggini R., Calvani M., Bellomo Rosa Grazia, Saggini Andrea (2008). Rehabilitation in cancer survivors: interaction between lifestyle and physical activity. *European journal of inflammation*, vol. 6, p. 99-104, ISSN: 1721-727.

[109] Schmitz KH, Holtzman J, Courneya KS, et al. Controlled physical activity trials in cancer survivors: a systematic review and meta-analysis. Cancer Epidemiol Biomarkers Prev 2005;14:1588–1595.

[110] Schoen RE, Tangen CM, Kuller LH, et al. Increased blood glucose and insulin, body size, and incident colorectal cancer. J Natl Cancer Inst 1999;91:1147–54.

[111] Segal RJ, Reid RD, Courneya KS, et al. Resistance exercise in men receiving androgen deprivation therapy for prostate cancer. J Clin Oncol 2003;21:1653–1659.

[112] Shaw JE, Hodge AM, de Courten M, et al. Isolated post-challenge hyperglycaemia confirmed as a risk factor for mortality. Diabetologia 1999;42:1050–4.

[113] Siegel R, Ward E, Brawley O, Jemal A. 2011. Cancer statistics, 2011: the impact of eliminating socioeconomic and racial disparities on premature cancer deaths. *CA Cancer J. Clin.* 61:212–36).

[114] Skrha J, Kunesova M, Hilgertova J, Weiserova H, Krizova J, Kotrlikova E: Short-term very low calorie diet reduces oxidative stress in obese type 2 diabetic patients. Physiol Res 2005, 54:33-39.

[115] Stoll BA. Western nutrition and the insulin resistance syndrome: a link to breast cancer. Eur J Clin Nutr 1999;53:83–7.

[116] Tretli,S. et al. (1996) Lifestyle changes during adolescence and risk of breast cancer: an ecologic study of the effect of World War II in Norway. Cancer Causes Control, 7, 507–512.

[117] Vallance JK, Courneya KS, Jones LW, Reiman T. Differences in quality of life between non- Hodgkin's lymphoma survivors meeting and not meeting public health exercise guidelines. Psychooncology 2005;14:979–991.

[118] Vallejo,E.A. (1957) [Hunger diet on alternate days in the nutrition of the aged.]. Prensa Med. Argent., 44, 119–120.

[119] van Kruijsdijk RC, van der Wall E, Visseren FL. Obesity and cancer: the role of dysfunctional adipose tissue. *Cancer Epidemiol Biomarkers Prev*. 2009;18:2569-2578.

[120] Vanio H, Bianchini F. IARC Handbooks of Cancer Prevention. Volume 6: Weight Control and Physical Activity. Lyon, France: International Agency for Research on Cancer; 2002.

[121] Vanio H, Bianchini F. IARC Handbooks of Cancer Prevention. Volume 6: Weight Control and Physical Activity. Lyon, France: International Agency for Research on Cancer; 2002.

[122] Vastag B: Obesity Is Now on Everyone's Plate. *Jama* 2004,291:1186-1188)

[123] Vozarova B, Weyer C, Hanson K, et al. Circulating interleukin-6 in relation to adiposity, insulin action, and insulin secretion. *Obes Res*. 2001;9:414-417).

[124] Walford RL, Mock D, MacCallum T, Laseter JL: Physiologic changes in humans subjected to severe, selective calorie restriction for two years in biosphere 2: health, aging, and toxicological perspectives. Toxicol Sci 1999, 52:61-65.

[125] Walford RL, Mock D, Verdery R, MacCallum T: Calorie restriction inbiosphere 2: alterations in physiologic, hematologic, hormonal, and biochemical parameters in humans restricted for a 2-year period. J Gerontol A Biol Sci Med Sci 2002, 57:B211-24.

[126] Warburg O. The metabolism of tumors. London, United Kingdom: Constable Press, 1930.

[127] WCRF/AICR: Food, nutrition and the prevention of cancer: aglobal perspective:. World Cancer Research Fund / American Institute for Cancer Research 1997.

[128] Weiss EP, Racette SB, Villareal DT, Fontana L, Steger-May K, Schechtman KB,Klein S, Holloszy JO, Washington University School of Medicine CALERIE Group: Improvements in glucose tolerance and insulin action induced by increasing energy expenditure or decreasing energy intake: a randomized controlled trial. Am J Clin Nutr 2006, 84:1033-1042.

[129] White E, Lee CY, Kristal AR. Evaluation of the increase in breast cancer incidence in relation to mammography use. J Natl Cancer Inst 1990;82:1546 –52.

[130] Windsor PM, Nicol KF, Potter J. A randomized, controlled tr ial of aerobic exercise for treatment-related fatigue in men receiving radical external beam radiotherapy for localized prostate carcinoma. Cancer 2004;101:

http://dx.doi.org/10.5772/55696

[131] Wolin KY, Tuchman H (2011) Physical activity and gastrointestinal cancer prevention. In: Courneya KS.

Section 5

Supportive Care for Cancer Patients

Chapter 20

Supportive and Palliative Care in Solid Cancer Patients

Bassam Abdul Rasool Hassan,
Zuraidah Binti Mohd Yusoff,
Mohamed Azmi Hassali and Saad Bin Othman

Additional information is available at the end of the chapter

http://dx.doi.org/10.5772/55358

1. Introduction

1.1. Cancer background

During this century, cancer has become one of the major problem and diseases which has caused predominant death and it will even surpass heart diseases. Many of the researchers begin to use the term lifetime risk for cancer patients which refer to the time that cancer will progress and developed or the time that the patient will die because of cancer. There are many problems (i.e., side effects) associated with cancer diseases either solid type or hematological type such as nausea, vomiting, diarrhea, constipation, hypercalcemia, pain, lost of appetite, anemia, fatigue, cachexia, leucopenia, neutropenia and thrombocytopenia. However the major problems are nausea and vomiting, neutropenia, anemia, thrombocytopenia and hypercalcemia. Hence due to these reasons cancer is consider as one of the major diseases that will effect on the quality of life for human [1-6].

1.2. Chemotherapy background

Chemotherapy was developed and used since the Word War I from the chemical weapon program of the United State of America (USA). Since then chemotherapy has became as one of the most important and significant treatment of cancer. Its main mechanism of action is by destroying the cancer cells which are characterized by their high multiplication and growth speed. However when comparing chemotherapy with other types of treatments, it still remain potentially high risk with many side effects which are difficult to manage. Chemotherapy used required the involvement of various clinical professionals during its various stages of administration and enormous patient health care is needed to overcome its side effects [7-8].

1.3. Chemotherapy side effects

The goal of chemotherapy is to be as effective as possible with tolerable side effects, since the dose of chemotherapy will be toxic to the cancer cells as well as to the normal cells. A proportion of the cancer patients suffer from only mild side effects whereas others may suffer from serious side effects. These side effects are classified as:

1. Acute, which develop within 24 hours after chemotherapy administration.
2. Delayed, which developed after 24 hours and up to 6 to 8 weeks after chemotherapy treatments.
3. Short term, combination of both acute and delayed effect.
4. Late/ long term, which developed after months or years of chemotherapy treatment.
5. Expected, which developed among 75% of the patients.
6. Common, occurred in 25%-75% of the patients.
7. Uncommon, happened is less than 15% of the patients.
8. Rare, occur in only 5% of the patients.
9. Very rare, occur with less than 1% of the patients.

Occurrence of specific side effects will vary according to the chemotherapy or medications used. The most common side effects experienced are nausea and vomiting, anemia, hair lost, bleeding (thrombocytopenia), hyperuricemia, neurotoxicity, cardiotoxicity, bone marrow depression, alopecia, nephrotoxicity, pulmonary toxicity, dehydration, cystitis and mucositis. So different parameters must be taken into consideration to prevent, reduce and overcome these side effects [8-10]. This chapter will focus on the main side effects caused by cancer disease and/ or chemotherapy.

2. Main problems caused by cancer disease itself and/ or chemotherapy treatment

2.1. Nausea and vomiting

Both nausea and vomiting are recognized as two separate and distinct conditions. Nausea is an unpleasant sensation of being vomit or urge to vomit which may or may not result in vomiting. While, vomiting or emesis is the process of expelling of undigested food through the mouth. Nausea and vomiting can arises from different or wide spectrum of etiologies which are either directly associated to cancer disease itself or to its treatment. According to the new ranking of chemotherapy side effects, nausea is the number one or the most disturbing side effect while vomiting is the third and sometimes the fifth disturbing chemotherapy side effects. Even so, not all cancer patients suffer from nausea and/ or vomiting because not all of them were treated with emetogenic chemotherapy [11-17].

2.1.1. Nausea and vomiting in solid cancer patients

Nausea and vomiting are two of the major problems that are associated with cancer patients and 50%-55% of cancer patients suffer from both nausea and vomiting even with the use of antiemetic drugs. The main causes for this are either due to the chemotherapy or because of the cancer progression. Some of the cancer patients who were treated with chemotherapy did not suffer from nausea or vomiting because the chemotherapy used were not significantly emetogenic. Nausea and vomiting still remain the major side effects that occur and are associated with chemotherapy and cancer diseases [11, 18-20].

2.1.2. Understanding nausea and vomiting in advanced solid cancer

Both nausea and vomiting are very common problems especially with advanced stages of solid cancer diseases like breast cancer and stomach cancer where 50 to 60% of the patients are mainly female under 65 years of age [21]. In this situation, nausea and vomiting occur because of the advanced stages of solid cancer diseases characterized by more severe complications than that caused by chemoradiotherapy or other treatments. The main causes for those problems are gastric stasis, obstruction of the intestine, opioid use, constipation caused by morphine uses, hypercalcemia, brain metastasis, renal failure, hyponatremia, increases in the intracranial pressure and tumor burden [21].

2.1.3. Pathophysiology of chemotherapy-induced nausea and vomiting

Chemotherapy cause nausea by stimulating the autonomic nervous system (ANS), while vomiting is triggered when afferent impulses from chemoreceptor trigger zone (CTZ), pharynx, cerebral cortex and vagal afferent fiber stimulate the vomiting center (VC) located in the medulla. The stimulation of the VC leads to contraction of muscles of abdomen, chest wall and diaphragm, so this will lead to an expulsion of stomach and intestine contents [11-20]. The main mechanism of chemotherapy induced vomiting is the stimulation of the entrochromaffin cells lining the wall of the gastrointestinal tract (GIT) hence causes the release of the serotonin. The serotonin will then bind to the vagal afferent 5-HT_3 receptors in the GIT which will send impulses to the CTZ and VC. Vomiting will be triggered when afferent impulses from CTZ, pharynx, cerebral cortex and vagal afferent fiber transfer impulses to the VC [22].

2.1.4. Major patients risk factors related with nausea and vomiting

1- Gender, 2-Age, 3- History of motion sickness and history of vomiting during pregnancy, 4- History of drinking alcohol, 5-Patient anxiety [11, 16, 18, 23-25]

2.1.5. Major chemotherapy factors responsible for incidence of nausea and vomiting

There are several chemotherapeutics factors that play a major role in the incidence and severity of both nausea and vomiting which are:

1- Emetogenic potential of the drug, 2- Dosage level, 3- Schedule of administration, 4- Route of administration, 5- History of previous chemotherapy, 6- Rate of I.V infusion [11, 16, 18, 23, 26].

2.1.6. Classification of chemotherapy induced nausea and vomiting

This classification is based on the emetogenic potential of the chemotherapeutic drug.

1. Severe (90% of the patients will experience nausea and vomiting) Example: Carmustine I.V ≥ 250 mg/ m^2, Cisplatin I.V ≥ 50 mg/ m^2, Cyclophosphamide I.V > 1500 mg/ m^2, Dacarbazine, Mechlorethamine, Nitrogen mustard and Streptozocin.

2. High (60%-90%) Example: Carboplatin, Carmustine I.V ≤ 250 mg/ m^2, Cisplatin I.V < 50 mg/ m^2, Cyclophosphamide I.V 750 mg/ m^2 to 1500 mg/ m^2, Cytarabine I.V > 1gm/ m^2, Dactinomycin, Daunorubicin, Doxorubicin I.V > 60 mg/ m^2, Irinotecan, Methotrexate I.V > 1 gm/ m^2 and Procarbazine PO dose.

3. Moderate (30%-60%) Example: Altretamine I.V PO dose, Asparginase, Cyclophosphamide (I.V) ≤ 750 mg/ m^2, Cyclophosphamide PO dose, Doxorubicin (I.V) 20 to 60 mg/ m^2, Epirubicin I.V, Idarubicin, Ifosfamide, Lomustine PO dose, Methotrexate (I.V) 250-1000 mg/ m^2, Mitoxantrone (I.V) < 15 mg/ m^2, Pemetrexed, Raltitrexed, Temozalamide and Topotecan.

4. Low (10%-30%) Example: Aldesleukin, Amsacrine, Bortezomib, Capecitabine, PO dose, Docetaxel, Doxorubicin liposomal, Etoposide all dose I.V or PO, Erlotrinib PO dose, Fluorouracil, Gefitinib PO dose, Gemcitabine, Methotrexate (I.V) 50-250 mg/ m^2, Mitomycin, Paclitaxel, Porfimer, Teniposide and Trastuzumab.

5. Very low (less than 10%) Example: Bleomycin, Busulfan PO dose, Chlorambucil PO dose, Cladribine, Fludaradine, Hydroxyurea PO dose, Interferon, Levamisole, Melphalan PO dose, Methotrexate < 50mg/ m^2, Rituximab, Thalidomide, Thioguanine, Thiotepa, Vinblastine, Vincristine, Vinorelbine and Vindesine [25, 27].

2.1.7. Classification and incidence of chemotherapy induced nausea and vomiting

CINV are clinically classified as:

1- Acute chemotherapy related nausea and vomiting, 2- Delayed emesis, 3- Anticipatory emesis [11, 16, 18, 28].

2.1.8. Nausea and vomiting treatment options

The main goal of the antiemetic treatment is to abolish nausea and vomiting which in the last twenty years consider as an inevitable chemotherapy side effect. This prevention is focused on the entire period of emetic risk which is 4 days for patients who received highly or moderately emetogenic chemotherapy [22, 29]. This could be perfectly achieved by understanding the mechanisms of these antiemetic drugs either alone or in combination so as to get their maximum benefit [30]. Modern antiemetic treatments help in preventing 70%-80% of nausea and vomiting problems. Combination antiemetic treatment becomes the standard regimen used for the control of nausea and vomiting caused by chemotherapy [30]. The different types of treatments are as follows: Serotonin-receptor antagonists ($5\text{-}HT_3$), Dopamine-2-receptor antagonists, Corticosteroids, Neurokinin-1-recptor antagonists, Cannabinoids & Benzodiazepines [29].

2.1.9. *Genetic polymorphism and incidence of nausea and vomiting*

Interindividual diversity in drug metabolism is caused by many factors including environmental factors, cultural factors related with type of diet, concomitant drug therapy as well as genetic factors i.e., ethnic variation. All of these variations play an important role in changing pharmacokinetic and pharmacodynamic properties, volume of distribution, elimination, disposition and clinical effect for many drugs [31, 32]. Much of this distinction has shown to be caused by genetic polymorphisms of the human cytochrome P450 enzymes (CYP) [32]. CYP is the most vital enzymatic system concerned with drug metabolism. Approximately 65% of common drugs used are metabolized by cytochrome P450 enzymes and half of them are mediated by the CYP3A subfamily [32].

2.2. Anemia

This is a condition characterized by lack of blood or in other word a reduction of total quantity of erythrocyte (red blood cells, RBC) or hemoglobin in the circulation which are necessary for normal function. This is caused by the inability of the bone marrow to replace the erythrocyte lost. The normal level of RBC for the male is 5.4×10^6 cell/ µl and for female is 4.8×10^6 cell/ µl [11, 33-35]. It is considered as one of the most frequent hematological demonstration of malignant diseases, which will lead to momentous impairment in every tissues and organs of cancer patients and put them under serious stress. This major problem may arise because of the underlining diseases (i.e., cancer diseases) or radiotherapy or chemotherapy treatment received [36, 37].

2.2.1. *Red blood cell (RBC) and iron*

The large proportion of body iron (20 mg per day) is used in the synthesis of erythrocyte cells. The body absorbed about 1 mg of iron per day from the gut to compensate the amount of daily iron lost. After the transition from erythroblast to reticulocyte, it will then remain for 3 to 4 days in the bone marrow after which being released into the blood circulation and circulate for about 100-120 days. Red blood cell (RBC) has no mitochondria so are totally dependent on ATP generated during glycolysis process. In the circulation RBC loss about 20% of its hemoglobin and shows physiological steps of aging. They will be phagocytes by the macrophage leading to destruction of the erythrocyte and the removal of the iron from the hemoglobin (Hb) which will be released into the plasma and redistributed again [38].

2.2.2. *Types of anemia*

There are different types of anemia as follows:

1- Iron deficiency anemia, 2- Folic acid deficiency anemia, 3- Vitamin (Vit) B_{12} deficiency anemia, 4- Vit C deficiency anemia, 5- Hemolytic anemia. It is an acquired type of anemia, 6- Thalassemias, 7- Sickle cell anemia, 8- Anemia of chronic diseases (ACD) [36, 37].

2.2.3. *Erythropoietin (EPO) description and action*

EPO is a glycoprotein hormone consists of 165 amino acid with a peptide mass of 18.2 kDa. It is mainly produce by the liver during fetal stage but after birth the kidneys become the primary production sites. It has been realized that most of EPO in the circulation comes and produce from the cortex of the kidney [39]. EPO production is mainly controlled by the feedback system between kidney and bone marrow. The kidneys mainly depend on the renal oxygen sensor for EPO production. Kidney cells response greatly towards hypoxia by increasing the EPO production. Serum level of EPO ranges between 10 to 20 mU/ mL and for normal situation the observed EPO concentration/ predictive EPO concentration (O/P) ratio must range between 0.8-1.2 [41]. EPO maintain erythropoiesis is by preventing the colony forming unit-erythroid (CFU-E) from death by apoptosis process. By this way these progenitor cells will keep proliferating and differentiating to produce erythrocyte [39].

2.2.4. *Causes of anemia of chronic diseases (ACD)*

Anemia remain as one of the serious and frequent problem of cancer mainly cancer of the gastrointestinal, liver, head and neck, ovarian and cervix. This is mainly caused by cytokines including interlukine-1, interlukine-6, interferon-γ and tumor necrosis factor-α produced by these cancer diseases. These cytokines caused impairment of erythropoietin (EPO) synthesis, reduce erythrocytes life span and prevent normal iron utilization. Other direct effect of tumor that cause anemia is bone marrow replacement which is associated with inhibition of the body ability for the production of RBC. This condition of bone marrow suppression is associated with specific types of cancers like breast, prostate, myeloma, lymphoma and acute leukemia. Also bone marrow suppression is mainly caused by chemotherapy and radiotherapy which are the main treatment for cancer. Mainly in cancer patients the major risk factors responsible for incidence and severity of anemia are the form of cancer as well as type and dose of chemotherapy administered to the cancer patients. [11, 33-36, 40, 41].

2.2.5. *Diagnosis of anemia*

Several parameters need to be checked for anemia diagnosis since each one is considered important and they are as follow: Family history, laboratory tests, X-ray, biopsy and bone examination [33, 35, 42].

2.2.6. *Grades of anemia (levels)*

The grades or severity of anemia will depend on several factors like hemoglobin level, velocity of onset of anemia, age, co-morbidities, extent of the underlining malignancy, intensity of treatment and the biological function of the patients organ. Anemia grades as follows:

Normal level (women Hb= 12.0 g/ dL-16.0 g/ dL, men Hb= 14.0 g/ dL- 18.0 g/ dL)

Mild Anemia Hb= 10g/ dL

Moderate Anemia Hb= 8.0 g/ dL- 10.0 g/ dL

Severe Anemia Hb= 6.5 g/ dL- 7.9 g/ dL

Life Threatening Anemia Hb= < 6.5 g/ dL [33, 36, 43].

2.2.7. Clinical signs and symptoms of anemia in cancer patients

The severity of signs and symptoms of anemia depend on several factors like Hb level, age, extent of the underlining malignant, comorbidity, rate of anemia onset, biological activity of patients vital organs and intensity of treatment used for anemia. Generally in elderly patients the clinical signs and symptoms appear with Hb level higher than that in younger patients. These symptoms usually appear gradually, starting with fatigue which is considered as one of the major signs happing in 60% to more than 90% of the anemic patients. Lethargy and lost of concentration will also take place as the Hb becomes lower than 12 g/ dL. When anemia becomes severe and chronic this will lead to decompensation of cadiorespiratory and impairment of several body organs and activities [36, 46].

2.2.8. Role of cancer patients ages

It has been found that the incidence of anemia and cancer increases as the age of the patient increases too. Anemia is much more related and significantly present as the age became higher than 60 years old and with steeper increases after age 80 years. Many studies showed that the hemoglobin levels remain stable between age 60 to 98 years old but there are several causes for the high incidence of anemia in the old age since there were high comorbidity, hematopoietic stress and reduce in function of many vital organs. For this reason there will be great association and increases in occurrence of anemia in elderly patients [44].

2.2.9. Cancer patients gender and anemia

As mention above anemia highly occur in patients older than 60 years old, but it has been found that among women, anemia happen at a younger age. The main difference between men and women are the presence of menstrual cycle i.e., blood loss and childbearing iron loss which make incidence and association of anemia higher in younger women as compared to men [44]. Besides that men and women who do not have menstruation, the amount of iron lost in one day is 1 mg. While, in women still with menstrual, the loss is about 0.6 to 2.5 times more than previous mentioned amount. The amount of iron lost during each menstruation cycle depends on the severity of bleeding. The standard iron lost per menstrual cycle for woman weighting about 60 kg is about 10 mg. So all of these evidences showed that anemia is associated with female as a gender more than male [45].

2.2.10. Cancer patients race

Race also play an important role in incidence of anemia since it is consider as one of the risk factor which play role in its occurrence. The prevalence of anemia in USA among white women is 7.1% and 25.1% among black women even after adjustment of iron level. Besides that black women are characterized by lower mean hemoglobin level compared to white women. Also black woman has a wide standard deviation in mean of hemoglobin than the white one has [45].

2.2.11. Mechanisms of anemia in cancer patients

2.2.11.1. Role of cancer disease

Occurrence and association of anemia with cancer depends on several factors including patients age, stage of cancer, presence or absence of infection and other comorbidities. Anemia prevalence is highly associated especially with lymphomas, genitourinary tumor, lung and multiply myeloma. The incidence of mild to moderate anemia with solid tumor is higher than incidence of severe anemia which occurs highly with hematological cancers than solid one [36, 46, 47]. The main mechanism whereby cancer causes anemia is by producing cytokines which are mainly tumor necrosis factor (TNF-α) and interleukin-1 and they have the ability to hamper EPO production and action, reduce the life span of RBC and preclude ordinary utilization of iron. Other mechanisms which will cause association of anemia with cancer will be separated from the cancer itself like Vit B_{12}, folic acid and iron deficiency. Renal, endocrinal disorders splenomegaly, clonogenic and cachexia occurrence with cancer also play a major role in occurrence of anemia [36].

2.2.11.2. Role of chemotherapy

Anemia is one of the common side effect of chemotherapy especially with the myelosuppressive type. Incidence and severity of anemia depend on several different factors which are the chemotherapy type, schedule and intensity as well as type of cancer. Chemotherapy cycles also play an important role in increasing the severity of anemia since multiply cycles will cumulatively inhibit or reduce erythropoiesis. It has been found by the European Cancer Anaemia Survey (ECAS) that the incidence of anemia after the first cycle is 19.5% and after second cycle is 34.3% while after the third the incidence was more than 40%. Also single or combination chemotherapy play a serious and major role in anemia incidence and severity since the use of combination chemotherapy regimen will leads to severe anemia more than the use of single chemotherapy drug [48-50]. Besides chemotherapy myelosuppression, anemia can take place as a result of direct destruction of the RBC (i.e., direct effect on the erythropoiesis in the bone marrow) or reduced erythropoietin production (i.e., impact on EPO production). When this chemotherapy drug or other drugs used repetitively this may lead to prolong production of anemia. Also the results that obtained from clinical trials showed that the probability of mild anemia incidence after the use of chemotherapy is 100%, while the probability of severe anemia incidence after chemotherapy is 80%. From these results and data it has been proven that chemotherapy is the major impact factor for anemia onset and severity in cancer patients [41, 48, 51-53].

2.2.12. Indications and options for anemia treatments

Anemia and its related symptoms have serious negative effects on patients quality of life (QOL) and anticancer treatment since it will leads to treatment delay. These effects may be tolerated in young patients even with very low hemoglobin levels. While in patients with multimorbidity would not be able to tolerate this and as a result of that many severe clinical signs and symptoms will developed even with minor reduction in the Hb levels [36, 54, 55]. The treatment strategies of anemia mainly based on the clinical situation, clinical signs and symptoms and on the underlining cause of anemia. These treatments will include red blood cell transfusion, corticosteroids, VitB12 and Epoetin alfa (recombinant human erythropoietin, rHuEPO). All these treatments were used to overcome anemia related signs, symptoms and to improve the anemic patients (QOL) [36].

2.3. Thrombocytopenia

Thrombocytopenia is a term used to denote abnormal decrease or drop in platelets numbers. The main function of these platelets is clot formation during bleeding in order to prevent blood lost. Thus a decrease in platelet number will leads to bleeding condition which ranges from mild bleeding from small blood vessels to severe bleeding from large blood vessels. Severe bleeding in the presence of severe thrombocytopenia or when is coupled with other clotting disorders can leads to serious morbidity or death. Thrombocytopenia is a common problem experience by cancer patients, which usually resulted from the use of conventional chemotherapy and at times is a dose limiting factor for chemotherapy administration. The incidence of thrombocytopenia among solid cancer patients is rather low i.e., ranging between 10%-25% among breast cancer, ovarian and germ cell cancer patients who were treated with intensive chemotherapy. However thrombocytopenia incidence is high among acute leukemia patients [56-63].

2.3.1. Platelets morphology and structure

Platelets or thrombocytes are irregular, disc shaped cells which are considered as the smallest cells in the blood (0.5 to 3.0 μm diameter). They are usually produce from the megakaryocytes which are large cells (80 to 150 μm diameter) found specifically in the spongy center of long bones by the stimulation of thrombopoietin (TPO) by process called endomitosis whereby each megakaryocyte cell produce about 2000 platelets. These platelets shared a characteristic of having a very short life span (five to nine days only) so the bone marrow of healthy individual continuously keep producing new platelets cells to replace the old dead ones. The thrombopoietin hormone is mainly synthesis and produce by the liver and plays a major role in stimulation of proliferation and maturation of platelets. The circulating platelets have no nucleus but they have alpha granules and dense granules [57, 64, 65]. Physiologically the platelets are removed from the blood circulation by two mechanisms. The first is being used at common sites of vascular injury like in the microcirculation, secondly to be phagocyte by macrophages cells predominantly in the spleen and liver [66].

2.3.2. Platelets function

Platelets have vital functions in immunity, wound repair and homeostasis. These functions mainly depend on platelets concentration in blood circulation. Platelets prevent bleeding by either sealing the hole in the blood vessel wall or by forming haemostatic plug or by liberating several chemicals that will activate more clotting formation by breaking down more of the platelets. The main steps for platelets action to form clot are the following:

1. Adhesion (Step 1): This reaction is mediated by release of granules and characterized by shape change of the platelets from disc shape to spiny spheres after their adhesion to collagen. The aggregation of the platelets in this face is reversible.

2. Aggregation (Step 2): In this step more of platelets adhere to each other and there will be an obvious shape change of these platelets. The main factors that stimulate this step are the chemical changes.

3. Release (Step 3): Here the aggregation caused by the dense granules released by the platelets themselves is irreversible. In addition vasoconstriction will take place as a result of thromboxane A_2 released by the platelets.

4. Stabilization of the clot (Step 4): This is the main reaction which is responsible for the thrombus formation, whereby the aggregate platelets will release factor V that will accelerate the aggregation of other platelets and this will lead to stabilized clot formation [64, 67].

From this it is clear that thrombocytopenia which is associated with decrease in platelets count in the blood of cancer patients such as leukemic patients is considered as a very serious problem. Thrombocytopenia prevalence in hematological patients is very high. While in case of solid tumor, thrombocytopenia happens because of chemotherapy uses and thus the incidence is rather low. However in some subgroups the incidence is higher than 20% and it still remain as a serious and dangerous problem [62].

2.3.3. Thrombopoietin hormone (TPO)

It is a single 353- amino acid protein, synthesized primarily in the liver. Its level will increase during thrombocytopenia and keep increasing in response to the decline in platelet mass. For this reason most of the studies found that when platelets is transfused to the thrombocytopenic patients the TPO level will decreased. TPO mainly act by increasing the numbers of megakaryocyte colony forming cells (Meg-CFC), increases their ploidy, size and growth to produce more of the platelets. Moreover, it will stimulate the hematopoietic stem cell of the bone marrow and it has been found that high doses of TPO will lead to reactivation of the mature platelets to some aggregation stimuli [61].

2.3.4. Main causes of thrombocytopenia

The main causes leading to occurrence of thrombocytopenia are:

1. Chemotherapy drugs.

2. Solid cancer.
3. Blood cancer (Leukemia).
4. Spleen cancer.
5. Anemia.
6. Hemorrhage which will lead to increases loss of platelets.
7. When the rate of platelets destruction is higher than the rate of bone marrow platelets production [57, 59, 65].

2.3.5. Role of age and gender

Repetto (2003) mentioned that anemia is highly prevalent and happened in the elderly cancer patients who receive chemotherapy. This is specifically because their senescent cells have low ability to repair DNA and their low mass of the hematopoietic stem cell causing slowing of their recovery ability. Repetto also mentioned in his study that the occurrence of grade 3 thrombocytopenia is highly associated with older female suffering from breast cancer and found that there is an association between age and gender with thrombocytopenia. While others retrospective studies of solid tumor patients found that there is no association between age and myelosuppression i.e., neutropenia, anemia and thrombocytopenia occurrence [68].

2.3.6. Chemotherapy and thrombocytopenia

Thrombocytopenia is a detrimental side effect of chemotherapy since it will lead to hemorrhage from vital organ particularly the brain specifically within solid cancer patients who were treated with chemotherapy. These chemotherapies caused thrombocytopenia by different mechanisms either by suppressing megakaryopoiesis leading to prevention of platelets production or by direct damaging of the platelets. Chemotherapies like antimetabolites and alkylating agents induced severe thrombocytopenia due to their ability in causing bone marrow suppression and specifically after the first cycle of chemotherapy [62, 69, 70, 71].

2.3.7. Mechanism of thrombocytopenia in solid cancer

The association between bleeding and thrombocytopenia in patient suffering from leukemia was first described in 1962. Later in 1878 and 1984 this was reported happening among patient suffering from solid cancer [72]. Thrombocytopenia as a serious side effect is usually associated with solid cancer as a result of its metastasis to bone marrow. Theoretically most of solid tumors can metastasis to bone marrow but the most frequent are breast, lung and prostate cancers. These cancers when metastasized to bone marrow will lead to bone marrow suppression resulting in neutropenia and thrombocytopenia with serious morbidity and mortality (Kilickap *et al.*, 2007). Besides that Elting and his colleagues mentioned that solid cancer patients are characterized by several things which are poor performance status, low baseline for platelets count and bone marrow metastasis. Despite that the bleeding situation among solid cancer patients remain poor compare with hematological malignant unless all the above characteristic are all present [62].

2.3.8. Diagnosis of thrombocytopenia

Different parameters are taken into consideration in order to diagnose thrombocytopenia such as medical history and laboratory test. Platelets count which is considered as part of the complete blood count (CBC) is the main key for the diagnosis of thrombocytopenia. It measures the exact numbers of platelets in a measured volume of blood. If the test shows low number of platelets then a careful examination for spleen and bone marrow biopsy must be done since both have a direct association with thrombocytopenia occurrence. Usually in adults when the platelets count is less than 100,000 cell/ microliter it is considered low but sometimes this happen without any symptoms. Other important tests which are used to diagnose thrombocytopenia are the prothrombin time (PT), activated partial thromboplastin time (aPTT) and thrombin time (TT). The results of these tests play a critical role in the diagnosis and certification of the presence of thrombocytopenia. In addition to liver enzymes test, renal function test, erythrocyte sedimentation rate (ESR), Vit B_{12} and folic acid levels are also carried out [57, 59, 64, 65, 73, 74].

2.3.9. Grades of thrombocytopenia

The normal range of the platelets is between 150,000 and 450,000 cells per microliter of blood (i.e., 150-450×10^9/ L) while thrombocytopenia could be classified into three levels as follows:

1. Mild thrombocytopenia if platelets count < 150 and ≥ 100 × 10^9/ L.
2. Moderate thrombocytopenia if platelets count < 100 and ≥ 50 × 10^9/ L.
3. Severe thrombocytopenia if platelets count < 20 × 10^9/ L [75, 76].

2.3.10. Clinical signs and symptoms of thrombocytopenia

There are several signs and symptoms which occasionally happen with thrombocytopenia. These are bloody stool, dizziness, headache, hemorrhage, oral bleeding, nose bleeding, vaginal bleeding, black stool and petechiae (reddish purple spots in the skin) [57, 58, 74].

2.3.11. Options for thrombocytopenia treatments

There are different options for thrombocytopenia treatment but the selection will mainly depends on the etiology and severity of thrombocytopenia. Sometimes with asymptomatic thrombocytopenia treatment is not required like that in children with viral infection. But if thrombocytopenia incidence is because of spleen enlargement then splenectomy will be beneficial and effective in increasing the platelets counts. While for thrombotic thrombocytopenic purpura (TTP) treatment is needed since it can leads to renal failure. In case of idiopathic thrombocytopenic purpura (ITP) the treatment depends on severity of the case and the platelets counts. In the case of heparin induce thrombocytopenia and thrombosis (HITT) the treatment is by stopping heparin administration. If the cause of thrombocytopenia is due to patient's immune system causing destruction to the platelets then the use of corticosteroids is very effective so as to suppress immune response. While if the cause is due to chemotherapy then the decision to either continue the treatment with low chemotherapy doses or use of alternative drugs or use of platelets growth factors (i.e., thrombopoietic growth factor) (Oprelvekin, Neumega®) should be made. Recombinant human interleukin-11 (rhIL-11) will stimulate megakaryocyte maturation and proliferation and maintain platelets production. It has been proven by the Food and Drug Administration (FDA) that rhIL-11 is very effective in reducing and preventing of severe thrombocytopenia as well as it will decrease the need for platelet transfusions especially after myelosuppressive chemotherapy which could be continue with the same doses. In the case of severe thrombocytopenia (i.e., platelet level ≤ 20,000/ μL) which is due to intensive chemotherapeutics drugs treatment of hematological and solid cancer patients, in this case platelet transfusion is needed. At this point, patient will suffer from severe bleeding and the laboratory tests signify that platelets transfusion is very important and a required treatment. Platelets transfusion is one of the most important treatments for acute and severe thrombocytopenia, but there are some limitations to its use which are: the availability of the blood products since it must be freshly taken and used within 5 days, cost, refractoriness, transfusion reaction and diseases transmission [57-59, 63, 76, 77].

2.3.12. *Thrombocytopenia and neutropenia*

Acute thrombocytopenia has been described in patients given Hematopoietic Growth Factors. The main factor which play role in this incidence is neutropenia treatments which are either GM-CSF and/ or G-CSF. This rapid incidence for thrombocytopenia in association with these treatments is mainly because these treatments sometimes target the platelets or caused their destruction. But the main mechanism which is responsible for the incidence of neutropenia with thrombocytopenia together has not been defined yet [78].

2.4. Hypercalcemia

Hypercalcemia is a life threatening situation in which serum calcium level is elevated greater than 10.5 mg/ dl, while albumin concentration is lower than 4 g/ dl. It is a serious problem that occurs in about 10%-20% of all cancer patients especially lung, breast, head and neck cancer patients. While, in hematological cancer hypercalcemia also takes place specifically in the advanced phases of both myeloma and lymphoma. Besides that a very important point is that hypercalcemia is mainly caused by cancer without any effect or role from anticancer treatments. So many references consider hypercalcemia as a very serious and dangerous complication that caused a significant morbidity and mortality frequently in breast cancer patients. It can occur in patients with and without bone metastasis and the main cause of hypercalcemia is the pathological bone resorption. Bone resorption is caused by the secretion of cytokine like parathyroid hormone-related protein (PTHrP) leading to activation and differentiation of osteoclast cell. In normal condition normal breast cells also secreted PTHrP during lactation so as to stimulate bone resorption and skeletal calcium release which will be used in milk synthesis. In this situation hypercalcemia is asymptomatic since the elevation of calcium level is mild, but when serum calcium elevation became very high it will leads to significant morbidity and mortality. Hypercalcemia is highly associated with breast cancer more than other types of cancers [78-83].

2.4.1. Calcium homeostasis

Calcium in human body has multiply functions, it is one of the major components and mineral of the body skeleton and its concentration is maintained by influx and efflux to the extracellular fluid from kidney, bone and gut. This vital process is regulated by two hormones which are parathyroid hormone (PTH) and 1, 25 dihydroxyvitamin D. Serum calcium consist of calcium bounded to albumin 37%, bounded with globulin (10%), biologically active calcium (47%) i.e., ionized form and calcium complex with anion (10%) (like: phosphate, citrate, bicarbonate). The ionized serum calcium is the only form metabolically active and is regulated by homeostatic mechanisms [87, 90, 98]. Calcium also has other important role in regulation of the cellular metabolism function, since it is a co-factor for many of body enzymes reactions. Also, calcium is needed for cell adhesion, cell death, an important component of cellular electrical current and has a very important function in muscular contraction process [84, 85].

2.4.2. Kidney role in calcium homeostasis

Kidney plays a very important role in regulation of calcium concentration in the extracellular fluid and its capacity to clear the calcium is about 600 mg per day (15 mmol/ day). In adult approximately 98% of calcium is resorbed by kidney. This process of calcium absorption is mainly controlled by PTH and 65% of total reabsorbed calcium happens at the proximal tubules, 20-25% in the ascending loop of Henle, while only 10% in the distal convoluted tubules [86].

2.4.3. Gut role in calcium homeostasis

The daily amount of calcium absorbed ranges between 150-200 mg/ day and this is send to the extracellular fluid. This process of absorption is mainly regulated by 1, 25 dihydroxyvitamin D hormone and calcium concentration in the blood circulation. Besides that the amounts of calcium absorbed from the daily diet is affected by the amount of calcium in the diet and presence of other dietary components which may serve to increase (lactose, fatty acid) or decreases (oxalate, phosphate and phytate) calcium absorption. The absorption of calcium from the daily diet varies even in healthy adult from 20% to 70%. The main parts responsible for absorption are the ileum (65%) and jejunum (17%). This is because these parts are the longest parts and hence the longest time calcium will be absorbed [87].

2.4.4. Bone role in calcium homeostasis

Bone consider as the main storehouse of calcium which store 99% of the body calcium. The role of bone in calcium homeostasis is important in normal conditions since the process of bone formation is tightly coupled with processes of bone resorption i.e., the velocity of calcium influx and efflux between the extracellular fluid and bone. The extracellular calcium concentration will be disturbed when the rates of bone resorption increase more than the rate of bone formation. This is seen in cases of advanced cancer diseases which caused activation of the osteoclast cell of the bone marrow leading to increase in bone marrow destruction and increase in calcium efflux. This mainly happy when the cancer disease metastasis to bone marrow and is usually consider as a catastrophic situation. Metastasis to bone marrow happens in 30% of breast cancer patients and causing disturbances in the plasma calcium concentration. Thus it is clear that bone play a critical role in the maintenance of serum calcium level [86, 88].

2.4.5. Main hormones responsible for calcium control

The extra cellular calcium concentration is maintained in a narrow range of 8.5-10.2 mg/ dL (2.1-2.55 mmol/ L) by two main hormones which are:

1. Parathyroid hormone (PTH)
2. 1,25-dihydroxy-vitamin D [1,25 $(OH)_2$ D]

Both act on the three main organs which are kidney, gut and skeleton but PTH is more important since it regulate calcium level from minute to minute (i.e., very rapid effect), PTH it is consists of 84 amino acid single chain polypeptides and is mainly secreted by the chief cells of the four parathyroid glands besides the thyroid gland in the neck. PTH secretion is regulated by the serum calcium level of the extracellular fluid. When calcium concentration increases, the PTH secretion will be suppressed and when the calcium concentration decreases, PTH secretion increases. PTH mainly regulates the calcium transportation between extracellular fluids and kidney, bone and gut. PTH has a direct effect on bone and plays a critical role in increasing the rate of bone formation and turnover. Its effect on bone came from its stimulation and activation for the osteoclast cells which will lead to increase in bone turnover and it also increases the rate for bone formation. This effect has been found to be dependent on the presence of other hormones like 1, 25-dihydroxyvitamin D. PTH effect on kidney will leads to an increase in distal tubules reabsorption of calcium. Here its effect is enhanced by 1, 25-dihydroxyvitamin D, but it has no direct effect on the gut [78, 85, 88]. 1, 25 dihydroxyvitamin D is the major biological active metabolite of vitamin D. This steroid-like metabolite is derived either from skin during its exposure to ultraviolet light (i.e., sun light) or from plant ergosterol after its ingestion in the gut. It increases the absorption of calcium and phosphorus from the gut by active transport as well as it increases the bone resorption. 1, 25 dihydroxyvitamin D is characterized by its slower action than PTH but it is more effective than PTH in long term control of the serum calcium level [83, 86, 89]. Besides these two hormones, calcitonin which is 32 amino acid peptide also is involved in calcium content. It is synthesis and secreted by parafollicular cells of the thyroid gland. Its main action is by inhibition of the osteoclast cell from resorption of the bone by causing their dissolution to mononuclear cells [85].

2.4.6. Causes of hypercalcemia

The main causes of hypercalcemia during solid or hematological malignancy are as follows:

1. The direct effect of cancer diseases on the bone by causing bone destruction such as with breast cancer, lung cancer, multiply myeloma and leukemia. Hypercalcemia occurs in about 10%-20% of all cancer patients during specific stages of their malignant diseases. Lung and breast cancers are highly associated with hypercalcemia incidence beside head

and neck cancer. While myeloma and lymphoma are the most common hematological types of cancers associated with hypercalcemia.

2. Some cancers diseases lead to production of parathyroid hormone-related protein (PTHrP) which is mainly associated with solid cancer but not with malignant cancer.

3. Some cancer diseases decrease the ability of the kidneys to remove excess calcium also leading to decreases in the urination.

4. Dehydration due to nausea and vomiting which will lead to difficulties of the kidneys to remove excess calcium from the blood.

5. Decreases in the movement and activity of cancer patients which will lead to breakdown of the bone and hence increase in the release of the calcium into the blood [90-94].

2.4.7. Hypercalcemia diagnosis

Diagnosis of hypercalcemia is made based on serum calcium level and also on levels of phosphate, chloride, PTH and alkaline phosphates. Other tests for kidney function especially urea level, creatinine level and albumin level tests also performed because in hypercalcemia these are elevated. Bone scan, prospective computed tomography (CT) scan for neck, chest and magnetic resonance imaging (MRI) may help to determined whether the tumor has metastasized to the bone [95].

2.4.8. Hypercalcemia levels

Normal level of calcium in the blood ranges between 8.7 – 10.4 mg/ dl. Correct calcium level in the blood could be determined by using the following equation:

Corrected calcium (mg/ dl) = measured calcium + ([4- albumin (g/ dl)] × 0.8).

Serum calcium ranging between 10.5 – 12.0 mg/ dl indicates mild hypercalcemia.

Moderate hypercalcemia is being diagnosed when serum calcium is between 12.0 – ≤ 14.0 mg/ dl.

Severe hypercalcemia (hypercalcemia crisis) occurs when serum calcium is higher than 14.0 mg/ dl and is associated with acute signs and symptoms [87, 90-96].

2.4.9. Signs and symptoms of hypercalcemia

Since calcium has a wide range of physiological actions so it has a myriad of clinical effects on multi organs. On central nervous system (CNS), hypercalcemia will cause fatigue, depression, confusion, headache, difficulty in thinking and stupor. Cardiovascular system effects manifestation will range from abnormal electrocardiogram to arrhythmias. Gastrointestinal system signs will involve constipation, nausea and vomiting. Hypercalcemia will cause impaired kidney function and as a consequence will lead to decrease in the renal excretion of calcium and thus increase in the severity of hypercalcemia. Dehydration, bone pain and lost of appetite has also been observed. The hypercalcemia due to primary hyperparathyroidism is usually mild or moderate and the patient will be asymptomatic or only suffer from minor clinical signs mentioned above. While hypercalcemia occurs as a result of breast cancer is usually acute or subacute and the calcium level will be highly elevated and many of the clinical signs mentioned above will be manifested. While mild hypercalcemic patients will be asymptomatic and hypercalcemia will be detected fortuitously during routine laboratory screening [83, 97-99].

2.4.10. Hypercalcemia treatments and options

There are different types of treatments used for hypercalcemic patients whereby some are often use for daily cases and some others used for emergency cases of hypercalcemia:

1. Bisphosphonates (Etidronate, Clodronate and Pamidronate):
2. Plicamycin (Mithramycin)
3. Calcitonin (Calcimar®)
4. Zoledronic acid (Zometa®)
5. Glucocorticoids (Prednisone)

While for emergency cases with calcium level exceeding 13 mg/ dl the following treatments are preferred:

1. Normal saline 200-400 ml/ hour I.V.
2. Furosemide (Lasix®) 200-400 ml/ hour [83, 86, 87, 97-99].

2.4.11. Role of age and gender

Hypercalcemia is usually seen in aged female patients more than male where the main characteristic is the presence of hypercalcemia without any symptoms. The main cause is either malignant disease or hyperparathyroidism [83, 86].

2.4.12. Mechanisms of hypercalcemia occurrence with malignancy

Mechanism of hypercalcemia incidence in solid cancer patients can be divided into two groups. In the first group, hypercalcemia may or may not be associated with bone metastasis and the main factor is the solid cancer itself since it will produce systematic circulating humoral factors which will ultimately cause loss of calcium from the bone i.e., bone resorption. Moreover these factors will lead to increase in calcium reabsorption from renal tubules. So this group is named as humoral hypercalcemia of malignancy (HHM) which include lung, ovarian, head and neck, pancreas and kidney cancer but the most frequent are the lung and head and neck cancers. The main factors produced by the cancer cells responsible for this situation are PTH, PTH-like factors, transforming growth factors, colony stimulating factors and leukocyte cytokines. In the second group, hypercalcemia is mainly caused or produced by extensive bone metastasis (i.e., extensive localized bone destruction) which include breast cancer. Breast cancer is considered as the highest and the most frequent solid cancer associated with hypercalcemia caused by bone metastasis. This hypercalcemia is called local osteolytic hypercalcemia (LOH). The main difference is that in LOH, hypercalcemia is caused by localized bone destruction resulting from bone metastasis by the solid cancer, while in HHM the systematic humoral factor is the sole responsible factor and that hypercalcemia is unrelated to the extent of bone metastasis. In LOH, hypercalcemia is produced by direct effect of the solid cancer cells on the bone i.e., by acting like osteoclast cell producing acid protease (lysosomal enzymes) and collagens responsible for removing of mineral from bone and mainly lead to resorption of bone matrix and causing an increase in cAMP and inhibition of microtubule assembly by agents like colchicine. Resorption could also happened or take place independently of osteoclast cell activity. While for hematological cancers i.e., myeloma the main causes for hypercalcemia are increase bone resorption and glomerular filtration impairment. The main cause of hypercalcemia during lymphoma is bone resorption associated with increase in absorption of calcium from the gut [82, 86, 100].

2.4.13. Relation of hypercalcemia with nausea and vomiting

The main mechanism of hypercalcemia incidence in solid cancer is the metastasis of the cancer to the bone. Breast cancer which is the highest type of the LOH has shown to cause bone marrow destruction leading to hypercalcemia. Hypercalcemia will lead to many side effects mainly nausea and vomiting and there are studies indicating that hypercalcemia is one of the main risk factor for nausea and vomiting [16, 101].

2.5. Neurotoxicity

Neurotoxicity which induced by chemotherapy can occurs because of the direct or indirect effect and/ or damage that chemotherapy will cause to the central nervous system (CNS) or peripheral nervous system or any combination of these [102]. It is a critical matter to distinct between the two components of the nervous system. The CNS consists from the brain and the spinal cord. CNS mainly responsible for controlling neurological function of mental status, level of consciousness, motor power, sensory function, cerebral function and cranial nerve function. While for the peripheral nervous system it consists of peripheral nerves, this system mainly responsible for sensing pain, temperature and sensation [103].

This side effect i.e., neurological toxicity remain as one of the major critical side effect of chemotherapy treatment. Its clinical presentation varies significantly as a result of that it became very difficult to confirm the diagnosis [104].

2.5.1. General signs and symptoms of neurotoxicity

Symptoms associated with neurotoxicity may include cerebellar effects i.e., (tremor, loss of balance and fine motor movements), confusion, visual impairment, peripheral neuropathy, somnolence and auditory [102].

It has been found that neurotoxicity problems usually temporary i.e., resolving once treatment is completed, even so sometimes permanent neurological deficits may happened [102].

2.5.2. Blood-brain barrier and it's role in protecting CNS

Blood-brain barrier consider as a very efficient part of the nervous system that determine whether a chemotherapy agent is able to reach the nervous system or not. This barrier has the ability to block certain chemotherapy agents from entering nervous system at the cellular level [105]. Blood-brain barrier which surrounding the CNS varies from the one which surrounding the peripheral nervous system, as a result of this variation some chemotherapy agents such as vincristine significantly affect the peripheral nervous system but not the CNS. Chemotherapy agent will produce neurotoxic effects only if it has the ability to cross the blood-brain barrier [106].

2.5.3. Neurotoxicity and chemotherapy

Chemotherapy agents that significantly associated with neurotoxicity include the following: 1- Platinum compounds, 2- Taxanes, 3- Vinca alkaloid [104].

2.5.4. Factors associated with the incidence of neurotoxicity

There are many factors play role in the incidence of neurotoxicity but the most critical factors are the following::

1. Chemotherapy doses.

2. Route of chemotherapy administration [107].

2.5.5. Other factors

The incidence of neurotoxicity can be related to factors other than chemotherapy, these factors are:

1. Primary or secondary tumor deposits, which may involve the nervous system.

2. Metabolic or electrolyte imbalance which will leads to neurological disturbance.

3. Neurological deficits [108].

2.5.6. Neurotoxicity evaluation and management

Treatment used for neurotoxicity that caused by chemotherapy agents is limited. The focus of care should be on early recognition of neurotoxicity and careful monitoring of patients at high risk of toxicity [109]. There are various agents that either block the development and/ or incidence of neurotoxicity that caused by chemotherapy agents. Even so the mechanisms of action for these agents still mysterious [110]. Example for agent used as antidote for encephalopathy cause by ifosfamide is the methylene blue [111], besides that amifostine and adrenocorticotropic hormone analogues have also been found to be an effective neuroprotective agents. But farther investigation still required to clarifying the role of these agents in overcoming and/ or preventing neurotoxicity problem which leads to either delay in chemotherapy schedule, reduction in chemotherapy doses or substitution with an alternative agent [104].

2.6. Cardiotoxicity

The major function of the heart is to pump the blood to the whole body to supply body organs with adequate oxygen and nutrition they need. This process will happened by contracting muscular walls of the left ventricle [112]. There are various factors which can leads to cardiac injury in the cancer patients. This may happened as a result of either infiltration of metastases to infections and/ or because of chemotherapy toxicity [112].

2.6.1. Major factors which cause cardiac damage in cancer patients

a-Cardiac tumors, b-Bacterial infections, c-Chemotherapy induce toxicity, e-Radiation induce toxicity, f-Fungal and/ or viral infection [113, 114].

Chemotherapy effects will be classified into two types: acute and chronic effects.

2.6.2. Acute toxic effect

Acute cardiotoxicity caused by doxorubicin came from combination of factors which are: mitochondrial changes, cellular degeneration and a loss of myocardial fibrils. The incidence of cardiotoxicity will be either during or after doxorubicin administration, this cardiotoxicity will leads to cardiac abnormalities which include: ST and T wave changes, sinus tachycardia, atrial and ventricular ectopics, complete heart block, supraventricular tachycardia and ventricular tachycardia [116, 117].

Although doxorubicin cause cardiotoxicity there is no specific treatment for this condition, but there is only a supportive treatments. Researchers and clinicians keep on using of cardioprotective agents that allow chemotherapy agents specifically anthracycline to be used at a higher dose without causing cardiotoxicity [114]. Example for these cardioprotective agents are dexrazoxane and amifostine [118].

2.6.3. Chronic toxicity

This type of toxicity is one of the most common toxicity caused by doxorubicin it is characterized by chronic dilated cardiomyopathy. This condition i.e., cardiomyopathy usually happened either at late of chemotherapy cycle or shortly after the end of it [119]. Cardiomyopathy is significantly attenuated by the chelation of iron. Moreover, cardiomyopathy has been diagnosed among the survivors of cancer patients who have been treated with doxorubicin during their childhood [120].

2.7. Pulmonary toxicity

It is one of the main side effects of chemotherapy, which become clinically obvious after weeks, months or even years of termination of chemotherapy. It usually associated with several clinical symptoms which are: dry cough, dyspnoea and progressive worsening of symptoms with a poor prognosis for recovery [121].

2.7.1. Chemotherapy and pulmonary toxicity

Chemotherapeutic agents will be divided into three groups, this will mainly based on their effects on pulmonary function:

1. Hypersensitive pulmonary reaction: Bleomycin, 6-mercaptopurine, methotrexate, mitomycin and procarbazine. This condition take place as a result of either desquamative interstitial pneumonitis or an eosinophilic pneumonitis [122, 123].

2. Non-cardiogenic pulmonary oedema: Cyclophosphamide, cytarabine and methotrexate. This condition will take place after few days of strating using of chemotherapy treatment.

3. Chronic pulmonary fibrosis: Bleomycin, busulfan, carmustine, cyclophosphamide, fludarabine, ifosfamide, methotrexate and mitomycin [122, 123]. This clinical condition will take place within months of using chemotherapy treatment.

Besides that it has been found that when mitomycin used in combination with vinca alkaloids and/ or gemcitabine with docetaxel or when the later two agents i.e., gemcitabine and docetaxel used alone they can cause pulmonary toxicity [124, 125, 126, 127].

2.7.2. Assessment of pulmonary function

It is very important to assess patients pulmonary function before start administration of chemotherapy, the assessment will include the following:1- Chest X-ray 2- Lung biopsy required to differentiate chronic fibrosis from lung metastasis [121].

2.7.3. Treatments used for pulmonary toxicity cases

Managements used for pulmonary problems i.e., toxicity will include the following: 1- Bronchodilator, 2- Corticosteroid 3- Expectorant 4- Oxygen 5- Antibiotics 6- Nebulised saline 7- Aminophylline and theophylline [128-129].

3. Conclusion

Cancer has become a major killer in the world which almost surpasses the cardiovascular diseases and will become the main lethal cause in this century. Although the global war against cancer leads to remarkable gain in understanding the main molecular mechanism for the cancer cell, this progress is still consider as slow and not enough especially in case of treatment of common solid tumor in adults. Besides that there are so many types of serious side effects caused by the tumor itself or because of its chemotherapy treatment.

Therefore it is an obligate for all the clinicians and physicians to focus on these main side effects that emerged as a result of cancer itself or its treatment and working to built and develop treatment guidelines to overcome or palliate these major side effects.

Acknowledgements

I would like to show and express my great appreciation and heartfelt thanks to my main supervisor Associate Prof. Dr. Zuraidah Mohd Yusoff, for her great support and guidance. Moreover, I'd like to express my great appreciation for my co-supervisors Associate Prof. Saad Bin Othman and Associate Prof. Dr Mohamed Azmi Hassali for their creative advice and guidance.

Also I'd like to express my grateful appreciation to Universiti Sains Malaysia and a special thanks to the School of Pharmaceutical Sciences. I'd like to thank those who represent the greatest support in my whole life, those who fill my life with all of colorful beauties of hope and nature, who always by their skillful advice made the correct scope for my life, my family specifically my great and marvelous father (Abdul Rasool), mother (Basma) and my daughter (Shams).

Author details

Bassam Abdul Rasool Hassan[1*], Zuraidah Binti Mohd Yusoff[1], Mohamed Azmi Hassali[2] and Saad Bin Othman[1]

*Address all correspondence to: bassamsunny@yahoo.com

1 Clinical Pharmacy Discipline, School of Pharmaceutical Sciences, Universiti Sains Malaysia, Minden, Penang, Malaysia

2 Discipline of Social and Administrative Pharmacy, School of Pharmaceutical Sciences, Universiti Sains Malaysia, Minden Penang, Malaysia

References

[1] Carson-DeWitt RCancer. In: Longe JL. (ed.) The Gale Encyclopedia of Medicine Farmington Hills. Gale Group; (2002). , 631-638.

[2] Markman, M. Principles of cancer screening. In: Aziz K., & Wu GY. (ed.) Cancer screening A Practical Guide for Physicians. New Jersey: Humana Press; (2002). , 170-189.

[3] Dolan, S. Thrombocytopenia. In: Brighton D., Wood M. (ed.) The Royal Marsden Hospital Handbook of Cancer Chemotherapy. London: Churchill Livingstone; (2005). , 231-247.

[4] Henry, L. Malnutrition. In: Brighton D., Wood M. (ed.) The Royal Marsden Hospital Handbook of Cancer Chemotherapy. Churchill Livingstone: Elsevier; (2005). , 177-184.

[5] Sitamvaram, R. Gastrointestinal effects In: Brighton D., Wood M. (ed.) The Royal Marsden Hospital Handbook of Cancer Chemotherapy. Churchill Livingstone: Elsevier; (2005). , 161-164.

[6] Stephens, M. Nausea and Vomiting. In: Brighton D., Wood M. (ed.) The Royal Marsden Hospital Handbook of Cancer Chemotherapy. Churchill Livingstone: Elsevier; (2005). , 155-160.

[7] Weir-hughes, D. Foreword. In: Brighton D., Wood M. (ed.) The Royal Marsden Hospital Handbook of Cancer Chemotherapy. London: Elsevier / Churchill Livingstone; (2005). p ix.

[8] Rizzo, T, & Cloos, R. Chemotherapy. In: Thackery E. (ed.) The Gale Encyclopedia of Cancer. Detroit: Gale Group; (2002). , 225-233.

[9] Abrams, A. C. Drugs Used in Oncologic Disorders. In: Repchinsky C. (ed.) Clinical Drug Therapy. 36 ed. Ontario: Canadian Pharmacists Association; (2001). , 17-29.

[10] Koda-Kimble LYYWayne A., Kradjan BJG., Brain KA., Robin LC. Applied Therapeutics the Clinical Use of Drugs. In: Troy D. (ed.) Hand Hook of Applied Therapeutics. Philadelphia: Lippincott Williams & Wilkins; (2002). , 212-234.

[11] Haggerty, M. Nausea and Vomiting. In: Donna O., Christine J., Karen B. (ed.) The Gale Encyclopedia of Medicine. Farmington Hills: Gale Research; An International Thomson company; (1999). , 21-34.

[12] Oberleitner, M. G. Nausea and Vomiting In: Ellen T. (ed.) The Gale Encyclopedia of Cancer. Detroit: Gale group; (2002). , 37-52.

[13] Coates, A, Abraham, S, & Kaye, S. B. On The Receiving End-Patient Perception of The Side-Effects of Cancer Chemotherapy. European Journal of Cancer & Clinical Oncology (1983). , 19, 203-208.

[14] Lebourgeois, J. P, Mckenna, C. J, & Coster, B. Efficacy of an Ondansetron Orally Disintegrating Tablet: A Novel Oral Formulation of This 5-HT3 Receptor Antagonist in The Treatment of Fractionated Radiotherapy-Induced Nausea and Emesis. Clinical Oncology (1999). , 11, 340-347.

[15] Morrow, G. R, Hickok, J. T, Roscore, J. A, & Matteson, S. A Biobehavioral Perspective of Nausea and Emesis In: Hesketh PJ. (ed.) Management of Nausea and Vomiting in Cancer and Cancer Treatment. Mississauga: Jones and Barlett; (2005). , 119-146.

[16] Hesketh, P. J. Management of Nausea and Vomiting in Cancer Treatment: Introduction, Scope of The Problem. In: Hesketh PJ. (ed.) Management of Nausea and Vomiting in Cancer and Cancer Treatment. Mississauge: Jones and Bartlett; (2005). , 1-14.

[17] Rudd, J. A. Andrews PLR. Mechanisms of Acute, Delayed and Anticipatory Emesis Induced by Anticancer Therapies In: Hesketh PJ. (ed.) Management of Nausea and Vomiting in Cancer and Cancer Treatment. Mississauge: Jones and Bartlett; (2005)., 1-14.

[18] Oberleitner, M. G. Nausea and Vomiting In: Ellen T. (ed.) The Gale Encyclopedia of Cancer. Detroit: Gale group; (2002)., 71-89.

[19] Mitchell, E. P, & Schein, P. S. Gastrointestinal Toxicity of Therapeutics Agents. In: Perry MC., Yarbro JW. (ed.) Toxicity of Chemotherapy. Orlando: Grune & Stratton; (1984)., 55-65.

[20] Bartlett, N, & Koczwara, B. Review: Control of Nausea and Vomiting After Chemotherapy: What is The Evidence?. Internal Medicine Journal (2002)., 32, 401-407.

[21] Molassiotis, A, & Börjeson, S. Nausea and Vomiting In: Kearney N., Richardson A., editor. Nursing Patients With Cancer/ Principles and Practice. Philadelphia: Churchill Livingstone; (2006)., 415-437.

[22] Navari, R. M. Overview of The Updated Antiemetic Guidelines for Chemotherapy-Induced Nausea and Vomiting. Community Oncology (2007)., 4(4), 3-11.

[23] Hesketh, P. J. Potential Role of The NK1 Receptor Antagonists in Chemotherapy-Induced Nausea and Vomiting. Supportive Care in Cancer. (2001)., 9, 350-354.

[24] Osoba, D, Zee, B, Warr, D, Latreille, J, Kaizer, L, & Pater, J. Effect of Postchemotherapy Nausea and Vomiting on Health-Related Quality of Life. Support Care Cancer (1997)., 5, 307-313.

[25] Rubenstein, E. The Role of Prognostic Factors in Chemotherapy Induced Nausea and Vomiting In: Hesketh PJ. (ed.) Management of Nausea and Vomiting in Cancer and Cancer Treatment. Mississauga: Jones and Bartlett; (2005)., 87-97.

[26] Ballatori, E, & Roila, F. Methodological Issues in The Assessment of Nausea and Vomiting. In: Hesketh PJ. (ed.) Management of Nausea and Vomiting in Cancer and Cancer Treatment Mississauga: Jones and Bartlett; (2005)., 67-85.

[27] Hesketh, P. J. Comparative Review of 5-HT3 Receptor Antagonists in The Treatment of Acute Chemotherapy-Induced Nausea and Vomiting. Cancer Invest (2000)., 18, 163-73.

[28] Kris, M. G, Gralla, R. J, & Clark, R. A. Incidence, Course and Severity of Delayed Nausea and Vomiting Following the Administration of High-Dose Cisplatin. Journal of clinical oncology (1985)., 3, 1379-84.

[29] Jordan, K, Kasper, C, & Schomll, H-J. Chemotherapy-Induced Nausea and Vomiting: Current and New Standards in The Antiemetic Prophylaxis and Treatment. European Journal of Cancer (2005)., 41, 199-205.

[30] Grunberg, S. M, & Dugan, M. Integrated Therapy of Nausea and Vomiting. In: Hesketh PJ. (ed.) Management of Nausea and Vomiting in Cancer and Cancer Treatment. Mississauga: Jones and Bartlett; (2005). , 147-160.

[31] Gross, S. A, Bridge, S, & Shenfield, G. M. Pharmacokinetic of Tolbutamide in Ethnic Chinese. Journal of Clinical Pharmacology (1999). , 47, 151-6.

[32] Ruzilawati, A. B. Mohd Suhaimi AW, Gan SH. Genetic Polymorphisms of CYP3A4: CYP3A4*18 Allele is Found in Five Healthy Malaysian subjects. Clinica Chimica Acta (2007). , 383, 158-162.

[33] Haut, A. Anemia. In: Weil J, Blumel D, Tylor R, Geller E. (ed.) Encyclopedia of Science and Technology. New York McGraw-Hill; (2007). , 12-31.

[34] Blaser, L. Anemia. In: Mcgrath KA, Lachford SB. (ed.) The Gale Encyclopedia of Science. Farmington Hills: Gale group; (2001). , 201-211.

[35] Brown, T, & Olde, T. G. Anemia. In: Longe JL. (ed.) The Gale Encyclopedia of Cancer2. Detroit Gale group; (2005). , 341-352.

[36] Pohl, G, & Ludwig, H. Positive Effects of Correction of Anemia in Malignant Diseases. In: Weiss G., Gordeuk VR., Hershko C. (ed.) Anemia of Chronic Disease. New York: Taylor & Francis; (2005). , 489-557.

[37] Gordeuk, V. R. Iron Therapy and the Anemia of Chronic Disease In: Weiss GG VR., Hershko C. (ed.) Anemia of Chronic Disease New York Taylor & Francis Group; (2005). , 381-395.

[38] Marx JJMErythrophagocytosis and Decreased Erythrocyte Survival In: Weiss G., Gordeuk VR., Hershko C. (ed.) Anemia of Chronic Disease New York: Taylor & Francis group; (2005). , 201-227.

[39] Metzen, E, & Jelkmann, W. Erythropoietin and Erythropoiesis In: Weiss GG., Gordeuk VR., Hershko C. (ed.) Anemia of Chronic Disease New York: Taylor & Francis Group; (2005). , 61-85.

[40] Gordon, M. S. Managing Anemia in The Cancer Patient: Old Problems, Future Solutions. Oncologist. (2002). , 7, 331-41.

[41] Beguin, Y. Endogenous Eryhthropoietin in The Anemia of Chronic Disorders In: Weiss G., Gordeuk VR., Hershko C. (ed.) Anemia of Chronic Disease. New York: Taylor & Francis group; (2005). , 145-200.

[42] Punnonen, K, & Rajamaki, A. Usefulness of Old and New Diagnostic Test in ACD. In: Weiss GG., Gordeuk VR., Hershko C. (ed.) Anemia of Chronic Disease New York: Taylor & Francis Group; (2005). , 349-364.

[43] Pronzato, P. Cancer-Related Anaemia Management in The 21st Century. Cancer Treatment Reviews. (2006). , 32, 1-3.

[44] Balducci, L. Anemia, cancer, and aging. Cancer Control. (2003). , 10(6), 478-86.

[45] Killip, S, Bennett, J. M, & Chambers, M. D. Iron deficiency anemia. American Family Physician. (2007). , 75, 671-678.

[46] Reed, W. R, Hussey, D. H, & Degowin, R. L. Implications of The Anemia of Chronic Disorders in Patients Anticipating Radiotherapy. The American Journal of Medical Sciences. (1994). , 308, 9-15.

[47] Ludwig, H, & Fritz, E. Anemia in Cancer Patients. Semin Oncol. (1998). , 25, 2-6.

[48] Groopman, J. E, & Itri, L. M. Chemotherapy-Induced Anemia in Adults: Incidence and Treatment. Journal of the National Cancer Institute (1999). , 91(19), 1616-34.

[49] Barrett-lee, P. J, Ludwig, H, Birgegård, G, Bokemeyer, C, Gascón, P, Kosmidis, P. A, & Krzakowski, M. Nortier JWR, Kongable G, Schneider M, Schrijvers D, Van Belle SJ. Independent Risk Factors for Anemia in Cancer Patients Receiving Chemotherapy: Results From the European Cancer Anaemia Survey. Oncology (2006). , 70, 34-48.

[50] Ruggiero, A, Attinà, G, Haber, M, Coccia, P, Lazzareschi, I, & Riccardi, R. Assessment of Chemotherapy-Induced Anemia in Children with Cancer. Central European Journal of Medicine (2008). , 3(3), 341-345.

[51] Glaspy, J, Jadeja, J. S, & Justice, G. A dose-Finding and Safety Study of Novel Erythropoiesis Stimulating Protein (NESP) For The Treatment of Anaemia in Patients Receiving Multicycle Chemotherapy. British Journal of Cancer (2001). , 84(1), 17-23.

[52] Cazzola, M. Mechanisms of Anaemia in Patients With Malignancy: Implications For The Clinical Use of Recombinant Human Erythropoietin. Medical Oncology (2000). , 17(1), 11-16.

[53] Danova, M, Aglietta, M, & Pierelli, L. The Use of Erythropoietin Alpha in Programs of High Dose Chemotherapy. Recenti Prog Med (2000). , 91, 681-9.

[54] Manegold, C. The Causes and Prognostic Significance of Low Hemoglobin Levels in Tumor Patients. Strahlenther Onkol (1998). , 174(4), 17-19.

[55] Sabbatini, P. The Relationship Between Anemia and Quality of Life in Cancer Patients. Oncologist (2000). , 5(2), 19-23.

[56] Dolan, S. Thrombocytopenia. In: Brighton D., Wood M. (ed.) The Royal Marsden Hospital Handbook of Cancer Chemotherapy. London: Churchill Livingstone; (2005). , 15-28.

[57] De Bellis, D. Thrombocytopenia. In: Olendorf D., Jeryan C., Boyaden K. (ed.) The Gale Encyclopedia of Medicine. Farmington Hills: Gale Research, An international Thomson company; (1999). , 75-88.

[58] Miller, B, & De Bellis, D. Thrombocytopenia. In: Longe JL. (ed.) The Gale Encyclopedia of Cancer 2. Detroit: Gale group; (2005). , 115-123.

[59] Dolan, S. Haemorrhagic problems. In: Grundy M. (ed.) Nursing in Haematological Oncology. London: Bailliere Tindall; (2000). , 11-19.

[60] Terranova, L, Gerli, G, & Cattaneo, M. Platelet Disorders in The Elderly. In: Bladucci L., Ershler W., de Gaetano G. (ed.) Blood Disorders in The Elderly. Cambridge: University Press; (2007). , 420-431.

[61] Kuter, D. J. Thrombopoietin: Biology and Potential Clinical Applications In: McCrae KR. (ed.) Thrombocytopenia New York: Taylor & Francis Group; (2006). , 17-51.

[62] Elting, L. S, Rubenstein, E. B, Martin, C. G, Kurtin, D, Rodriguez, S, Laiho, E, Kanesan, K, Cantor, S. B, & Benjamin, R. S. Incidence, Cost, and Outcomes of Bleeding and Chemotherapy Dose Modification Among Solid Tumor Patients With Chemotherapy-Induced Thrombocytopenia. Journal of Clinical Oncology (2001). , 19(4), 1137-1146.

[63] Cantor, S. B, Elting, L. S, Hudson, D. V, & Rubenstein, E. B. Pharmacoeconomic Analysis of Oprelvekin (Recombinant Human Interleukin-11) For Secondary Prophylaxis of Thrombocytopenia in Solid Tumor Patients Receiving Chemotherapy. American Cancer Society (2003). , 97(12), 3099-3106.

[64] Castellone, D. Overview of Hemostasis and Platelet Physiology. In: Ciesla B. (ed.) Hematology in practice. Philadelphia: F. A. Davis Company; (2007). , 229-244.

[65] Miller, B, & De Bellis, D. Thrombocytopenia. In: Longe JL. (ed.) The Gale Encyclopedia of Cancer 2. Detroit: Gale group; (2005). , 315-322.

[66] Mckenzie, S, & Reilly, M. Platelet Clearance In: McCrae KR. (ed.) Thrombocytopenia New York: Taylor & Francis group; (2006). , 101-114.

[67] Groeger, J. S. Critical Care of The Cancer Patient. St Louis: Mosby Year Book; (1991).

[68] Repetto, L. Greater Risks of Chemotherapy Toxicity in Elderly Patients With Cancer. The Journal of Supportive Oncology (2003). , 1(2), 18-24.

[69] Zeuner, A, Signore, M, Martinetti, D, Bartucci, M, Peschle, C, & De Maria, R. Chemotherapy-Induced Thrombocytopenia Derives From the Selective Death of Megakaryocyte Progenitors and can be Rescued by Stem Cell factor. Cancer Research (2007). , 67(10), 4767-4773.

[70] Margaglione, M. Congenital Platelet Disorders. In: Hoffbrand AV., Catovsky D., & Tuddenham EGD. (ed.) Postgraduate Haematology. Massachusetts: Blackwell Publishing Ltd; (2005). , 925-936.

[71] Avvisati, G, Tirindelli, M. C, & Annibali, O. Thrombocytopenia and Hemorrhagic Risk in Cancer Patients. Critical Reviews in Oncology/ Hematology (2003). , 48, 13-16.

[72] Elting, L. S, Cantor, S. B, Martin, C. G, Hamblin, L, Kurtin, D, Rivera, E, Vadhan-raj, S, & Benjamin, R. S. Cost of Chemotherapy-Induced Thrombocytopenia Among Pa-

tients with Lymphoma or Solid Tumors. American Cancer Society (2003). , 97(6), 1541-1550.

[73] Betrosian, A. P, Theodossiades, G, & Lambroulis, G. Heparin-Induced Thrombocytopenia with Pulmonary Embolism and Disseminated Intravascular Coagulation Associated with Low-Molecular-Weight. American Journal of Medicine Sciences (2003). , 325, 45-7.

[74] WikipediaThrombocytopenia Wikipedia the Free Encyclopedia: WKIPEDIA. http://en.wikipedia.org/wiki/updated (2008). cited] (accessed 17th August 2008).

[75] Lea, B, Anna, P, Shakuntala, N, & Rajeev, M. Thrombocytopenia Related Neonatal Outcome in Preterms. Indian Journal of Pediatrics (2007). , 74, 269-74.

[76] Mcclure, M. W, Berkowitz, S. D, Sparapani, R, Tuttle, R, Kleiman, N. S, Berdan, L. G, Lincoff, A. M, Deckers, J, Diaz, R, Karsch, K. R, Gretler, D, Kitt, M, Simoons, M, Topol, E. J, Califf, R. M, & Harrington, R. A. Clinical Significance of Thrombocytopenia During a non-ST-Elevation Acute Coronary Syndrome The Platelet Glycoprotein IIb/IIIa in Unstable Angina: Receptor Suppression Using Integrilin Therapy (PURSUIT) Trial Experience. Journal of the American Heart Association (1999). , 99, 2892-2900.

[77] Milman, E, Berdon, W. E, Garvin, J. H, Cairo, M. S, Bessmertny, O, & Ruzal-shapiro, C. Periostitis Secondary to Interleukin-11 (Oprelvekin, Neumega) Treatment for Thrombocytopenia in Pediatric Patients. Pediatr Radiol (2003). , 33, 450-452.

[78] Mcfarlane-parrott, S. Oprelvekin. In: Thsckery E. (ed.) The Gale Encyclopedia of Cancer: Farmington Hills; (2002). , 33-47.

[79] Aster, R. H, & George, J. N. Drug-Induced Thrombocytopenia. In: McCrae KR. (ed.) Thrombocytopenia New York: Taylor & Francis Group; (2006). , 145-177.

[80] Helft, P. R, & Rudin, C. M. Metabolic and Electrolyte Complications of Malignancy In: Vokes EE., Golomb HM. (ed.) Oncologic Therapies Chicago: Springer-Verlag Berlin Heidelberg (1999). , 244-257.

[81] Dolan, S. Electrolyte abnormalities In: Brighton D., Wood M. (ed.) The Royal Marsden Hospital Handbook of Cancer Chemotherapy Churchill Livingstone Elsevier (2005). , 205-208.

[82] Swartout-corbeil, D. Hypercalcemia In: Thackery E. (ed.) Gale Encyclopedia of Cancer Detroit: Gale group; (2002). , 516-518.

[83] Swartout-corbeil, D. Hypercalcemia In: Longe JL. (ed.) Gale Encyclopedia of Cancer 2. Detroit: Gale group; (2005). , 579-581.

[84] Ericson, K. Hypercalcemia. In: Olendorf D., Jeryan C., Boyaden K. (ed.) Gale Encyclopedia of Medicine. Farmington Hills: Gale Research, An International Thomson company; (1999). , 1500-1503.

[85] Broadus, A. E. Mineral balance and homeostasis. In: Favus MJ. (ed.) Primer on The Metabolic Bone Diseases and Disorders of Mineral Metabolism. Washington: Asbmr; (2003). , 702-744.

[86] Juppner, H. W, Gardella, T. J, Brown, E. M, Kronenberg, H. M, & Potts, J. T. Parathyroid Hormone and Parathyroid Hormone Related Peptide in The Regulation of Calcium Homeostasis and Bone Development. In: Degroot LJ., Jameson JL. (ed.) Endocrinology. Philadelphia: WB Saunders; (2001). , 557-569.

[87] Mundy, G. R. Calcuim Homeostasis: Hypercalcemia and Hypocalcemia/ General Concepts of Calcuim Homeostasis.. Dunitz M. (ed.) Cambridge: The University Press; (1990). , 75-89.

[88] Mundy, G. R. Calcuim Homeostasis-Role of The Gut, Kidney and Bone. Dunitz M. (ed.) Cambridge: The University Press; (1990). , 103-121.

[89] Mundy, G. R. Mechanisms of Bone Metastasis/ Skeletal Complications of Malignancy. Cancer supplement (1997). , 80(8), 1546-1556.

[90] De Mauro, S, & Wysolmerski, J. Hypercalcemia in Breast Cancer: An Echo of Bone Mobilization During Lactation? Journal of Mammary Gland Biology and Neoplasia (2005). , 10, 157-67.

[91] Edelson, G. W, & Kleerekoper, M. Hypercalcemic Crisis. Medical Clinical of North America (1995). , 79, 79-92.

[92] Walls, J, Ratcliffe, W. A, Howell, A, & Bundred, N. J. Parathyroid hormone and parathyroid hormone-related protein in the investigation of hypercalcaemia in two hospital populations. Clinical Endocrinology (Oxford) (1994). , 41, 407-413.

[93] Gurbuz, A. T, & Peetz, M. E. Giant Mediastinal Parathyroid Cyst: An Unusual Cause of Hypercalcemic Crisis-Case Report and Review of The Literature. Surgery (1996). , 120, 795-800.

[94] Potts, J. J. Hyperparathyroidism and Other Hypercalcemic Disorders. Advance in Internal Medicine (1996). , 41, 165-212.

[95] Hiraki, A, Ueoka, H, Takata, I, Gemba, K, Bessho, A, Segawa, Y, Kiura, K, Eguchi, K, Yoneda, T, Tanimoto, M, & Harada, M. Hypercalcemia-leukocytosis syndrome associated with lung cancer. Lung Cancer (2004). , 43, 301-307.

[96] Bilezikian, J. P. Clinical review 51: Management of Hypercalcemia. Journal of Clinical Endocrinology Metabolism (1993). , 77, 1445-1449.

[97] Bushinsky, D. A, & Monk, R. D. Calcium. Lancet (1998). , 352, 306-311.

[98] Ariyan, C. E, & Sosa, J. A. Assessment and Management of Patients with Abnormal Calcium. Critical Care Medicine (2004). , 32, 146-154.

[99] Leboff, M. S, & Mikulec, K. H. Hypercalcemia: Clinical Manifestations, Pathogenesis, Diagnosis and Management. In: Favus MJ. (ed.) Primer on The Metabolic Bone Diseases and Disorders of Mineral Metabolism. Washington ASBMR (2003)., 631-651.

[100] Swartout-corbeil, D. Hypercalcemia In: Longe JL. (ed.) Gale Encyclopedia of Cancer 2. Detroit: Gale group; (2005)., 579-581.

[101] Wysolmerski, J. J, & Broadus, A. E. Hypercalcemia of Malignancy: The Central Role of Parathyroid Hormone-Related Protein. Annual Review of Medicine (1994)., 45, 189-200.

[102] Molassiotis, A, & Börjeson, S. Nausea and Vomiting In: Kearney N., Richardson A. (ed.) Nursing Patients With Cancer/ Principles and Practice Philadelphia Churchill Livingstone (2006)., 415-437.

[103] Groenwald, S. Hansen Frogge M., Goodman M. Cancer Nursing: Principles and Practice. 4th edn. Boston: Jones and Bartlett; (1997).

[104] Armstrong, T, Rust, D, & Kohtz, J. Neurologic, Pulmonary and Cutaneous Toxocities of High Dose Chemotherapy. Oncology Nursing Forum (1997)., 24(1), 23-33.

[105] Merien-bennett, R. Chemotherapy-Induced Neurological Toxicities. In: Brighton D. (ed.) The Royal Marsden Hospital Handbook of Cancer Chemotherapy. New York: Churchill Livingstone; (2005)., 213-215.

[106] Cline, M. J, & Haskel, C. M. Cancer Chemotherapy. Philadelphia: WB Saunders; (1980).

[107] Holmes, S. Cancer Chemotherapy. A Guide For Practice. Surrey: Asset Books; (1997).

[108] Kaplan, R, & Wiernik, P. Neurotoxicity of Antineoplastic Drugs. Seminars in Oncology (1982)., 16-103.

[109] Wilson, J, & Marsarryk, T. Neurological Emergencies in The Cancer Patient. Seminars in Oncology Journal (1989)., 16, 490-503.

[110] Cameron, J. Ifosfamide Neurotoxicity: A Challenge For Nurse, A Potential Nightmare For Patients. Cancer Nursing Journal (1993)., 16(1), 40-46.

[111] Gilbert, M. Neurologic Complications. In: Abeloff M, Armatige J., Lichter A. (ed.) Clinical Oncology. 2nd Edition. Edinburgh: Churchill Livingstone; (2000)., 1000-1020.

[112] Kupfer, A, Aeschlimann, C, & Cerny, T. Methylene Blue and The Neurotoxic Mechanisms of Ifosfamide Encephalopathy. European Journal of Clinical Pharmacology (1996)., 50(4), 249-259.

[113] Dolan, S. Cardiac Effects. In: Brighton D. (ed.) The Royal Marsden Hospital Handbook of Cancer Chemotherapy. New York: Churchill Livingstone; (2005)., 217-219.

[114] Zennhausern, R, Tobler, A, & Leoncini, L. Fatal Cardiac Arrhythmia After Infusion of Dimethyl Sulfoxide-Cryopreserved Hematopoietic Stem Cells in a Patient With Se-

vere Primary Cardiac Amyloidosis and End-Stage Renal Failure. Annals of Hematology (2000). , 79(9), 523-526.

[115] Whedon, M. B, & Wujcik, D. Blood and Marrow Stem Cell Transplantation. Boston: Jones and Bartlett (1997).

[116] Groeger, J. S. Critical Care of The Cancer Patient. St Louis: Mosby Year Book; (1991).

[117] Von Herbay, A, Drorken, B, & Mall, G. Cardiac Damage in Autologous Bone Marrow Transplant Patients: An Autopsy Study. Klinische Wochenschrift (1988). , 66, 1175-1181.

[118] Nelson, M. A, Frishman, W. H, & Seiter, K. Cardiovascular Considerations With Anthracycline Use in Patients With Cancer. Heart Disease Journal (2001). , 3(3), 157-168.

[119] Lefrak, E. A, Pitha, J, & Rosenheim, S. A Clinicopathologic Analysis of Adriamycin Cardiotoxicity. Cancer (1973).

[120] Ferrans, V. J, Clark, J. R, & Zhang, J. Pathogenesis and Prevention of Doxorubicin Cardiomyopathy. Tsitologiia (1997). , 39(10), 928-937.

[121] Stephens, M. Pulmonary Effects. In: Brighton D. (ed.) The Royal Marsden Hospital Handbook of Cancer Chemotherapy. New York: Churchill Livingstone; (2005). , 221-223.

[122] Rosenow, E. C, & Limper, A. H. Drug-Induced Pulmonary Disease. Semin Respir Infect Journal (1995). , 10, 86-95.

[123] Helman Dl Jr, Byrd JC, Ales NC. Fludarabine-Related Pulmonary Toxicity: A Distinct Clinical Entity in Chronic Lymphoproliferative Syndromes. Chest (2002). , 122(3), 785-790.

[124] Dunsford, M. L, Mead, G. M, & Bateman, A. C. Severe Pulmonary Toxicity in Patients Treated With Combination of Docetaxel and Gemcitabine for Metastatic Transitional Cell Carcinoma. Annals of Oncology (1999). , 10(8), 943-947.

[125] Rivera, M. P, Kris, M. G, & Gralla, R. J. Syndrome of Acute Dyspnea Related to Combined Mitomycin Plus Vinca Alkaloid Chemotherapy. American Journal of Clinical Oncology (1995). , 18(3), 245-250.

[126] Lanzowsky, P. Manual of Pediatric Hematology and Oncology. 3rd edition. San Diego: Academic Press; (2000).

[127] Stover, D. E. Pulmonary Toxicity. In: DeVita VT, Hellman SH, Rosenberg SA. Cancer; Principles and Practice of Oncology. 4th edition. Philadelphia: Lippincott; (1993). , 1993, 2362-2370.

[128] Bruera, E, Macmillan, K, & Pither, J. Effects of Morphine on The Dyspnea of Terminal Cancer Patients. Journal of Pain and Symptoms Management (1990). , 5, 341-344.

[129] Filshi, J, Penn, K, & Ashley, S. Acupuncture For The Relief of Cancer-Related Breathlessness. Palliative Medicine (1996). , 10, 145-150.

Chapter 21

Impact of Cancer Treatment on Reproductive Health and Options for Fertility Preservation

Kenny A. Rodriguez-Wallberg

Additional information is available at the end of the chapter

http://dx.doi.org/10.5772/55980

1. Introduction

1.1. Cancer in patients of reproductive age

Cancer is in general regarded as a disease of elderly people. Nevertheless, although age is the most significant risk factor for cancer in both sexes, young adults and children may also develop cancer diseases. Overall, men have a 45% risk of developing cancer at some time during their lives. For women, this risk is a bit lower, approximately 37% [1] and thus, in many cases, male and female cancer patients would be young and may not have been started building their families at the time of diagnosis. In people younger than 39 years, the risk of cancer is of about 1/72 for men and 1/51 for women. This risk increases with aging and between 40-59 years, 1/12 men and 1/11 women will develop cancer [1].

The majority of children, adolescents, and young adults diagnosed with cancer today will become long-term survivors. One primary concern of cancer survivors will be the ability to reproduce and have children. Detrimental effects on the reproductive system following cancer treatment have shown to negatively affect quality of life[2], [3]. Large studies of women and men with cancer have reported that the risk of infertility related to their treatments may be an important issue for those who have not yet started or completed their family size [2], [4].

2. Cancer treatment modalities with impact in reproductive health

Cancer surgery may have impact in fertility by removing reproductive organs or damaging structures needed for reproduction. Chemotherapy and radiotherapy have toxic effects on the gonads and may in certain cases induce ovarian and testicular failure, affecting thus all aspects of reproductive health, including pubertal development, impairment of hormone production and sexual function in adults. Effects of cancer biological therapy on gametes and reproductive organs are not yet established.

3. Cancer surgery may cause infertility

Surgery is currently the most effective treatment for cancer and eventually up to 100% of patients may be cured when complete removal of the tumor is achieved. Surgery may also be indicated for cancer prophylaxis, such as the case of premalignant disease of the cervix in female patients. In those very early stages of cervix cancer, the conization of a significant part of the cervix, may offer to patients a complete disease-free survival. However, in case of loop excisions, even if they are small, surgery of the cervix may induce subfertility by affecting the normal functioning of the cervix and its glandular secretion. Infertility induced by those interventions may be overcomed by using assisted reproductive technologies, such as treating the patient with intrauterine insemination or performing In Vitro Fertilization, IVF.

Surgery may also affect future fertility if there is removal or damage of the reproductive organs. In male patients, surgery for pelvic cancer such as for prostate, bladder or colon cancer may damage nerves and affect potency or ejaculation. Further on, surgical adjuvant treatment by removing the gonads may be indicated in female and male patients with hormone sensitive tumors.

In case of large tumors, neo-adjuvant chemotherapy and radiation may be indicated as first line treatment aiming to a reduction of tumor size and control of subclinical metastatic disease before surgical treatment. Neo-adjuvant therapy is usually planned before surgery in female patients with stage III breast cancer and young male cancer patients with bulky testicular cancer.

3.1. Cancer surgery aiming at preserving fertility

Fertility-sparing surgery may be an option for selected patients who wish to retain the ability to achieve a pregnancy. In many cases, pregnancies will occur spontaneously, nevertheless, causes of subfertility may be present in some patients, and a number of those may further require assisted reproduction treatments [5]. In gynecologic and urologic oncologic surgery, there has been a gradual development of fertility-sparing surgery aiming at preserving reproductive organs without compromising survival. Indications for fertility-sparing surgery include, in general, a well-differentiated low-grade tumor in its early stages or with low malignant potential.

3.2. Fertility sparing surgery in female patients

Table 1 presents a compilation of current data on fertility sparing surgery for young female patients with gynaecological cancer. In cases of selected ovarian tumors i.e. borderline tumors, young female patients may be offered a single oophorectomy aiming at preserving the uterus and the contralateral ovary[6].

Diagnosis	Type of surgery	Description	Obstetric outcome	Oncologic outcome
Cervical cancer stage IA1,1A2,1B1	Radical vaginal trachelectomy	Laparoscopic pelvic lymphadenectomy. Vaginal resection of the cervix and surrounding parametria keeping the corpus of the uterus and the ovaries intact	Spontaneous pregnancies described in up to 70%. Risk of second trimester pregnancy loss and preterm delivery	Rates of recurrence and mortality are comparable to those described for similar cases treated by means of radical hysterectomy or radiation therapy
Borderline ovarian tumors FIGO stage I	Unilateral oophorectomy	Removal of the affected ovary only, keeping in place the unaffected one and the uterus	Pregnancies have been reported and favorable obstetric outcome	Oncologic outcome is comparable with the more radical approach of removing both ovaries and the uterus. Recurrence 0-20% vs 12-58% when only cystectomy was performed
Ovarian epithelial cancer stage I, grade 1	Unilateral oophorectomy	Removal of the affected ovary only, keeping in place the unaffected one and the uterus	Pregnancies have been reported and favorable obstetric outcome	7% recurrence of the ovarian malignancy and 5% deaths
Malignant ovarian germ cell tumors/sex cord stromal tumors	Unilateral oophorectomy	Removal of the affected ovary only	Pregnancies have been reported and favorable obstetric outcome	Risk of recurrence similar to historical controls
Endometrial adenocarcinoma Grade 1, stage 1A (without myometrial or cervical invasion)	Hormonal treatment with progestational agents for 6 months	Follow-up with endometrial biopsies every 3 months	Pregnancies have been reported	Recurrence rate 30-40%. Five percent recurrence during progesterone treatment

Table 1. Fertility-sparing interventions in female patients. Reprinted, with permission from Rodriguez-Macias Wallberg et al, *J Pediatric Blood & Cancer, 2009*, Ref [6].

The most established surgical procedure for fertility preservation of women is the radical trachelectomy described first by Dargent in 1994 [7]. It is currently offered in cases of invasive cervical cancer in early stages to patients interested in preserving fertility. About 500 cases have been reported worldwide, most of them in European countries, Japan, U.S.A, Canada and China [8-12].

The global utilization of fertility-sparing surgery in female patients is currently unknown. A recent European study collecting data from several countries demonstrated a low incidence of those procedures and it raised concerns on the need to centralize fertility sparing treatments of gynaecological cancer at accredited units, to ensure a sufficient number of patients at each center aiming at maintaining thus healthcare quality [13].

3.3. Cervical cancer and fertility sparing surgery during pregnancy

In pregnant women, the gynaecological cancer most commonly diagnosed is also the cancer of the cervix, usually detected at an early stage in those patients. The treatment of pregnant women should be established in the same way as in non-pregnant patients, based on the stage of the disease according to the International Federation of Gynecology (FIGO). Nevertheless, individualization of the treatment should be considered based on the desire to continue the pregnancy, the gestational age and the risks of modifying or delaying cancer treatment during the pregnancy. Clinical practice guidelines by the European Society for Medical Oncology ESMO are available on this respect [14]. Both abdominal radical trachelectomy [15] and vaginal trachelectomy [16] with lymphadenectomies have been reported during pregnancy to preserve an ongoing pregnancy and female fertility.

3.4. Fertility sparing surgery in males

In men, a partial orchidectomy has become an established method to preserve hormonal and sperm production in carefully selected patients. This method, originally developed for treatment of benign teratomas in prepubertal patients, has shown good results when adopted for treatment of testicular malignancies in adults [17]. Data from The German Testicular Cancer Study Group reported a 98.6% disease-free survival rate at 7 years follow-up after conservative surgery of tumors <2 cm [18].

4. Radiotherapy treatments and their impact in reproductive health

Radiation therapy is a component of curative therapy for a number of diseases, including those presenting frequently in young patients such as breast cancer, Hodgkin's disease, head and neck cancer and gynecologic cancers. It is often indicated for the treatment of prostate cancer as well.

It is known that cancer cells present with defects in their ability to repair sub-lethal DNA whereas normal cells have the ability to recover. Although radiation therapy is aimed to a loco-regional application and although cancer cells are the target, radiation may also induce damage to normal cells in the tissues.

The response to radiation therapy depends on various factors such as the phase of cell cycle the cells are (cells in late G1 and S are more resistant), the degree of cell ability to repair the DNA damage and other factors such as hypoxia (hypoxic cells are more resistant), tumor mass and growth fraction. Non-dividing cells are more resistant than dividing cells.

http://dx.doi.org/10.5772/55980

Except for the bone marrow, the most sensitive organs to radiation therapy in the body are the gonads, both the male testis and the female ovary. The extent of damage in the female and male gonads depends on the dose, fractionation schedule and irradiation field [19] [20]. Radiation therapy can be administered as teletherapy, which aims at treating a large volume of tissue. For small volumes of tissue, such as in the case of cervix cancer in the female, radiation therapy can be administered in encapsulated sources of radiation that can be implanted directly into or adjacent to tumor tissue.

Whenever female reproductive organs are involved in the irradiated field, i.e., the ovaries, the uterus and the vagina may be compromised and damaged by direct irradiation. Scattered radiation may also damage reproductive organs. In the female, radiation therapy results in dose-related damage of the gonads by the destruction of primordial follicles, which constitute the nonrenewable follicle pool. In women, the degree and persistence of the damage is also influenced by age at the time of exposure to radiotherapy and due to a reduced reserve of primordial follicles in older women, the number of follicles remaining may be also be reduced at older ages [21]. Table 2 presents a compilation of current knowledge on the impact of radiation doses and age at radiotherapy in male and female gonadal function [22]. In general, a dose of about 2 Gy applied to the gonadal area destroys up to 50 % of the ovarian follicle reserve. In pediatric patients, failure in pubertal development may be the first sign of gonadal failure in both sexes. Total body irradiation (TBI) given in conjunction with myeloablative conditioning prior to bone marrow transplantation is one of the most toxic treatments for the gonads and it is highly related to gonadal failure in both sexes [23] [24].

High risk of prolonged azoospermia in men or amenorrhea in women
Total Body Irradiation (TBI) for bone marrow transplant/stem cell transplant (9,15,16)
Testicular radiation dose "/>2.5 Gy in adult men (9,17)
Testicular radiation dose ≥ 6 Gy in pre-pubertal boys (18,19)
Pelvic or whole abdominal radiation dose ≥ 6 Gy in adult women (20,21,22)
Pelvic or whole abdominal radiation dose ≥ 10 Gy in post-pubertal girls (21,22,23,24)
Pelvic radiation or whole abdominal dose ≥ 15 Gy in pre-pubertal girls (21,22,23,24)
Intermediate risk
Testicular radiation dose 1-6 Gy from scattered pelvic or abdominal radiation (13,16)
Pelvic or whole abdominal radiation dose 5-10 Gy in post-pubertal girls (21,24)
Pelvic or whole abdominal radiation dose 10-15 Gy in pre-pubertal girls (21,22,24)
Craniospinal radiotherapy dose ≥ 25 Gy (14)

Table 2. Radiotherapy protocols with high or intermediate impact on ovarian and testicular function. Reprinted, with permission from Rodriguez-Wallberg and Oktay, *J Ped Hematol Oncol*, 2010, Ref [22].

In men, the gonadal stem cells responsible for the continual differentiation and production of mature spermatozoa, the spermatogoniae, are extremely sensitive to radiation. The Leydig cells, which are responsible for the hormonal production of testosterone, are on the contrary more resistant to radiotherapy and adult patients may thus preserve hormonal production although becoming infertile. In prepubertal boys, the sensitivity to radiation therapy of Leydig cells is greater than that of older males at very high doses [25]. Prepubertal patients may retain Leydig cell function after radiation therapy during childhood and in those cases they will present with normal pubertal development and well-preserved sexual function later in life. Nevertheless, most of those patients present at adulthood with reduced testicular size, impaired spermatogenesis and infertility.

4.1. Gonadal shielding and ovarian transposition

The standard medical procedure currently offered to reduce scatter radiation to reproductive organs and preserve fertility in male and female patients, both adult and prepubertal, is the use of shielding. When shielding of the gonadal area is not possible, the surgical fixation of the ovaries in females far from the radiation field known as oophoropexy (ovarian transposition) may be considered. It is estimated that this procedure significantly reduces the risk of ovarian failure by about 50% and those patients may retain some menstrual function and fertility [26]. Scattered radiation and damage of the blood vessels that supply the ovaries are related to the failure of this procedure [26].

4.2. Radiotherapy of the uterus

Radiotherapy of the uterus in young women and girls has shown to induce tissue fibrosis, restricted uterine capacity, restricted blood flow and impaired uterine growth during pregnancy, as shown by follow-up of cancer survivors [27] [28]. The uterine damage seems to be more pronounced in the youngest patients at the time of radiotherapy. As a consequence, radiotherapy-treated female patients present with a high risk of unfavorable pregnancy outcomes such as spontaneous abortion, premature labor and low birth weight offspring [27] [28]. Irradiation of the vagina is related to fertility and sexual issues due to loss of lubrication, anatomical impairments and in some cases vaginal stenosis.

4.3. Cranial irradiation and hormonal dysfunction

Cranial irradiation may induce disruption of the hypothalamic-pituitary-gonadal axis, which is a recognized potential complication that can lead to infertility in both female and male patients. Follow-up of female patients treated for brain tumors with cranial irradiation post- and pre-pubertally has evidenced a high incidence of primary hypothalamic and pituitary dysfunction with consecuent disturbance in gonadotropin secretion. In some cases, precocious puberty may also be induced by cranial irradiation in childhood, which has been attributed to cortical disruption and loss of inhibition by the hypothalamus.

5. Impact of chemotherapy in reproductive health

Chemotherapy given as only treatment may be curative for a series of cancer presenting in young adults and children. In a vast majority of cancer treatments, chemotherapy protocols combine several agents and there is a possibility of a synergistic gonadotoxic effect[29]. In the female, primordial ovarian follicles including their oocytes and granulosa cells are particularly sensitive to alkylating agents, which induce apoptosis, as demonstrated in vitro [26], and in vivo using human ovarian tissue xenotransplanted in SCID mouse [30]. Ovarian failure is thus common after alkylating treatment [22].

Because of a high ovarian reserve with high numbers of follicles in young women, the risk of developing ovarian failure and permanent infertility after a cancer treatment is lower in younger than in older women [21]. Younger patients at the time of cancer treatment have thus a higher chance of recovering ovarian function following chemotherapy, nevertheless their fertility window might be reduced, and they should be recommended not to delay childbearing for too long [31].

5.1. Clinical evaluation of ovarian reserve

The development of amenorrhea should be considered unfavorable as it may be due to permanent gonadal failure. On the other hand, the presence of cycles should not be interpreted as proof of fertility. In the clinical setting, a gynecological examination including ultrasonography and estimation of antral follicle counts together with the determination of hormones such as follicle-stimulating hormone (FSH) and estradiol, inhibin and anti-mullerian hormone (AMH), may help the clinician in evaluating patient's remaining ovarian reserve after a cancer treatment and providing counseling on her chances to obtain a pregnancy.

5.2. Conception following chemotherapy

Due to toxicity of cancer treatments on growing oocytes, patients should be advised to avoid conception in the 6 -12 month period immediately following completion of chemotherapy treatment [32]. There is a high risk of teratogenesis during or immediately following chemotherapy, nevertheless DNA integrity has shown to return over time after a cancer treatment and thus no increase in childhood malignancies or genetic malformations have been shown in a large follow-up of more than 4000 children of cancer survivors [33].

5.3. Chemotherapy in males

In male patients, prepubertal status does not provide protection from gonadal damage and alkylating agents at high doses induce germ cell injury although Leydig cell function is commonly preserved [29]. Because most chemotherapy agents are given as part of a combination regimen, it has been difficult to quantify the gonadotoxicty of individual drugs.

Table 3 summarizes the gonadotoxic impact of chemotherapy agents on the female ovary and male testis.

High risk of prolonged azoospermia in men or amenorrhea in women
Cyclophosphamide
Ifosphamide
Melphalan
Busulfan
Nitrogen mustard
Procarbazine
Chlorambucil
Intermediate risk
Cisplatin with low cumulative dose
Carboplatin with low cumulative dose
Adriamycin
Low risk
Treatment protocols for Hodgkin lymphoma without alkylating agents
Bleomycin
Actinomycin D
Vincristine
Methotrexate
5 fluorouracil

Table 3. Chemotherapy agents with high or intermediate gonadotoxic impact in women and men

6. Options to preserve fertility by using cryopreservation methods

In 2006, an expert panel commissioned by the American Society of Clinical Oncology ASCO published guidelines for fertility preservation for male and female patients [26]. Established cryopreservation methods for fertility preservation available for adult female and male cancer patients before starting cancer treatments included sperm freezing for male patients and embryo cryopreservation following ovarian stimulation with gonadotropins and In Vitro Fertilization, IVF for females. All remaining options were still considered experimental at that time and they included the freezing of unfertilized oocytes for adult women and the cryopreservation of gonadal tissue, ovarian or testicular, both methods still under development which constitute the only options that can be offered to pre-pubertal children (Figure 1).

Recently, by the end of 2012, the methods for cryopreservation of oocytes by vitrification techniques have markedly improved and thus freezing of unfertilized eggs is currently becoming an established clinical option for female patients.

http://dx.doi.org/10.5772/55980

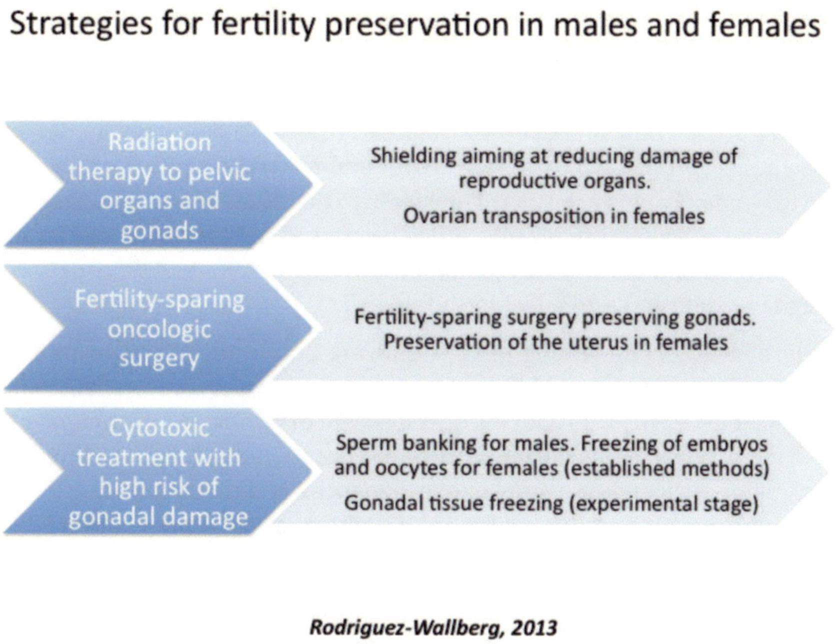

Figure 1. Strategies for fertility preservation in males and females

6.1. Sperm banking for male patients

As many children are born after fertility treatments using frozen-thawed sperm, the cryopreservation of ejaculated semen is regarded as an established fertility preservation method in adult patients and pubertal boys. Although spermatogenesis starts in the pre-pubertal period and mature spermatozoa can be found at a Tanner III stage with a testis volume above 5 ml, spermatozoa production is generally effective only at the age of 13-14 years [33]. Sperm cryopreservation has been reported in adolescent patients from the age of 13 years with a high prevalence of normal sperm counts and semen volumes [34] [35]. Traditionally, sperm banking by cryopreservation of at least three semen samples with an abstinence period of at least 48 hours in between the samples has been recommended for adult males desiring to preserve their fertility [36].

In the situation of ejaculation failure, the search for spermatozoa in a urine sample could be proposed. When failure in obtaining a semen sample in young men and adolescents, a testicular sperm extraction TESE can be performed to retrieve spermatozoa [35]. Other methods described to retrieve spermatozoa in adolescents include penile vibratory stimulation and electro ejaculation.

6.2. Cryopreservation of embryos or oocytes after controlled ovarian stimulation in females

Adult women wishing to preserve fertility may undergo controlled ovulation stimulation with gonadotropins, for retrieval of matured oocytes and egg freezing, or, if the woman wishes, for in vitro fertilization (IVF) of the retrieved eggs and freezing of embryos. In general, controlled ovarian stimulation with gonadotropins for IVF may require only two weeks to achieve, as it has been shown that a random-start in the stimulation cycle, independently of cycle day, does not have a negative impact on the number and quality of oocytes retrieved.

Oocyte retrieval is undertaken usually by vaginal ultrasound assistance under sedation or general anaesthesia. Fertilization of the oocytes for embryo cryopreservation has traditionally been offered to woman having a partner. Transfer of frozen/thawed embryos today is a clinical routine in fertility clinics worldwide and it has been used for over 25 years. Intact embryos after thawing have similar implantation potential as fresh embryos and this treatment can lead to a 59% pregnancy rate and a 26% live birth rate [37].

Freezing unfertilized oocytes aiming at later thawing and fertilizing them by IVF is also a promising option to preserve fertility today. As the methods for cryopreservation of eggs have notably developed in recent years with the development of vitrification techniques, improving success in oocyte survival and fertilization rates has been achieved, approaching that of fresh oocytes. Worldwide, an increasing number of pregnancies and children born after fertilization of frozen-thawn oocytes has been reported and although overall pregnancy rates are still relatively lower than those with embryo freezing [38-40], pregnancy rates and livebirths after thawing and fertilizing frozen eggs are currently reaching those obtained after embryo cryopreservation [41].

6.3. Ovarian stimulation using aromatase inhibitors to maintain low systemic estradiol levels in case of breast cancer

Ovarian stimulation with gonadotropins before egg retrieval aims at obtaining more than one oocyte per cycle and it is a key component of the success of IVF.

In women with an estrogen-sensitive tumor, the elevation of circulating estradiol levels during ovulation stimulation is undesirable and it has been regarded as potentially harmful. Therefore, hormone positive breast cancer patients have been largely excluded of the option to preserve fertility aiming at freezing eggs or embryos [42].

Alternative protocols, including natural cycle IVF (without hormone stimulation) or inducing ovulation by using Selective Estrogen Receptor Modulators (SERMs) and aromatase inhibitors alone or in combination with gonadotropins have been proposed, as they might be potentially safer. Natural cycle IVF gives only one oocyte or embryo per cycle and this treatment protocol has a high rate of cycle cancellation.

Both tamoxifen and letrozole can be administered alone or alongside with gonadotropins to increase the number of oocytes yielded for cryopreservation. Stimulation protocols using letrozole alongside with gonadotropins have shown to be most effective resulting in higher number of oocytes obtained and fertilized when compared to tamoxifen protocols [43]. The short-term follow-up of breast cancer patients having undergone ovarian stimulation with letrozole for fertility preservation has not shown any detrimental effects on survival [44].

Although aromatase inhibitors are contraindicated during pregnancy, data indicate that fertility treatments with letrozole are safe and the use of letrozole before conception does not induce any increased risks for the fetus [45]. Letrozole is currently used in the treatment of anovulatory infertility in many countries.

6.4. Cryopreservation of immature oocytes obtained without hormonal stimulation

Freezing immature oocytes is also an option for female fertility preservation in case of patients having a contraindication for hormonal stimulation or when there is not time available for stimulation. The oocytes are retrieved in the natural cycle and frozen at an immature stage or after maturation *in vitro* (IVM) [46]. Immature oocytes survive cryopreservation better than mature metaphase II oocytes [47]. After thawing they can be matured in vitro and fertilized. In vitro maturation of oocytes is at an experimental stage and needs further development. Only few fertility centers worldwide offer treatments using this technique.

6.5. Ovarian tissue freezing for prepubertal and adult patients

As the vast majority of eggs making up the ovarian reserve are within primordial follicles in the ovarian cortex, small cortical ovarian biopsies may provide a high number of eggs to be preserved. This procedure is usually performed by laparoscopy, can be planned immediately after the diagnosis of malignant disease and does not require hormonal stimulation. In cases when the patient needs to undergo abdominal surgery for the treatment of cancer, the ovarian tissue can be harvested during the same surgical procedure. Although it is preferable to carry out cryopreservation of ovarian tissue before a gonadotoxic treatment, young women, adolescents and girls have normally an abundant number of primordial follicles in their ovaries and attempts to harvest ovarian tissue for cryopreservation may still be worthwhile after the first courses of chemotherapy, if the procedure was not possible before [6].

Cryopreservation of ovarian tissue is the only option in prepubertal girls, as sexual maturity is not required. As this procedure does not cause any significant delay to initiation of cancer treatment and it does not require ovarian stimulation, some adult female patients also prefer to preserve fertility by this method.

6.6. Ovarian tissue transplantation

Transplantation of frozen-thawn ovarian cortex has shown to be a new promising method for recovery of ovarian function [48] and in some cases sufficient to restore fertility [49-51]. Ovarian tissue can be transplanted orthotopically, i.e. at the anatomical intrapelvic ovarian site or heterotopically, i.e. at other places including extrapelvic sites [52, 53].

There have been hundreds of patients undergoing ovarian tissue freezing but only a small percentage of these have returned for ovarian transplantation.

Autotransplantation is only possible if absence of malignant cells in the graft is confirmed. Methods for detection of cancer cells in the ovarian tissue of patients having suffered from hematological malignancies are under development including immunohistochemistry or the polymerase chain reaction applied to the tissue [54]. The investigation of residual malignant cells in the ovarian tissue may also be performed by xeno-transplantation to immunodeficient SCID mouse. Autotransplantation of ovarian tissue in patients having suffered from systemic hematological malignancies is not recommended due to the high risk of retransmission of malignancy and only patients with cancer diagnosis associated with a negligible or no risk of ovarian compromise should be considered for future autotransplantation [55]. Ovarian tissue cryopreservation and transplantation has shown not to interfere with proper genomic imprinting in mice pups [56] but additional studies in other animal models are needed.

6.7. In vitro culture of ovarian follicles

Although many improvements have been reported on the in vitro culture of follicles at early stages aiming at developing them into competent mature follicles, those methods are still on development [57-59]. Follicles cultured isolated or within a piece of thawed tissue will be the option for patients with hematological and ovarian malignancies. The normality of imprinted genes of cryobanked oocytes cultured and matured in vitro has yet to be verified experimentally.

6.8. Testicular tissue cryopreservation

This technique involves removal of testicular tissue from the male patient before cytotoxic therapy is initiated. In prepubertal boys, as there is absence of spermatozoa and spermatids, studies have been going on to cryopreserve the testicular totipotent precursors, i.e. the spermatogonial stem cells. Success has been reported in cryopreservation methods of testicular tissue [60] but more research is still needed in how to use the frozen-thawed tissue and obtain mature spermatozoa in vitro. Research suggests that in vitro spermatogenesis is likely to be the safest option for boys suffering from haematological malignancies, which might be re-transmitted by retransplantation, but this technique is still to be fully developed [61]. Although there are promising results in experimental animal studies of autologous retransplantation of spermatogonial stem cells showing re-colonization of seminiferous tubules generating complete spermatogenesis and mature germ cells and thus restoring natural fertility, the technique is still experimental in humans [61].

Cryopreservation of gonadal tissue offers hope to childhood cancer survivors, however it also raises several medical and ethical questions. Experimental methods for fertility preservation should only be offered to patients at specialized centers working with ethics board-approved research protocols and only in case when the recognized risks associated to the procedure are minimal.

6.9. Ovarian suppression to prevent gonadal damage

It has been hypothesized that suppressing the gonadal function transiently during chemotherapy could prevent ovarian follicle destruction in female patients by maintaining the follicles dormant. However, the pool of primordial follicles is normally non-proliferating. Those follicles lack FSH receptors [62] and their initial recruitment is not controlled by gonadotropins [63], therefore hormonal manipulation by suppressing gonadotropin release is not likely to affect them [64]. The vast majority of available studies having investigating gonadal protection by gonadotropin-releasing hormone analogues (GnRHa) agonists or antagonists during chemotherapy in females have been small, retrospective and uncontrolled. A significant number of those studies had used resumption of menses as a surrogate marker for fertility and many of them had reported higher frequency of resumption of menses in women having received GnRHa but none has demonstrated a beneficial effect regarding fertility recovery. Although data indicate that infertility is increased after a chemotherapy treatment, even if menstrual cycles are resumed [65], studies suggesting a beneficial effect of GnRHa co-treatment on preserving menstruation have had a great impact in the medical community and the empirical use of GnRHa for ovarian protection during chemotherapy is currently widely spread [26].

7. Counseling and prompt referal increase the chances to preserve fertility

Despite the fact that fertility issues are recognized in young people with cancer, health care professionals still report never referring cancer patients of reproductive age to a reproductive specialists for fertility preservation, indicating that many patients still do not receive adequate and timely information [66] [67]. This contrasts to data indicating that approximately three out of four cancer patients younger than 35 years and childless at the time of cancer treatment may be interested in having children in the future [2]. Because incidence of most cancers increases with age, the trend of delaying childbearing in Western societies will naturally result in more female cancer patients interested in fertility preservation.

In despite of this, recent data indicate that female cancer patients are still poorly informed on fertility threats of cancer treatment and options to preserve fertility in comparison with their gender counterparts. A recent Swedish survey found that less than half of female patients recalled having received appropriate information on reproductive threats of cancer therapy whereas 80% of male patients recalled having had an appropriate discussion [67]. Only a small number of female patients used fertility preservation methods compared to a rate >70% of sperm freezing in male patients in that study. Urgency to start cancer treatment and lack of appropriate time, lack of knowledge on fertility preservation and awareness of the costs of assisted reproduction methods are recognized barriers to counseling and referring patients to fertility preservation [68].

8. Conclusion

Infertility due to gonadal failure is one of the major consequences of cancer therapy, particularly in patients who receive aggressive chemotherapy and/or radiotherapy treatment. Many surveys of cancer survivors have found that those patients are at increased risk of emotional distress if they become infertile as a result of their treatment. Evidence suggests that long-term survival after treatment for cancer during childhood is associated with increased risk of impaired quality of life and higher frequency of psychosocial problems often related to infertility issues. Adolescent cancer survivors have increased anxieties about body image and dating, and pediatric cancer survivors are less likely to marry than matched controls. Although cancer survivors can become parents by adoption or gamete donation, most would prefer to have biological parenthood and biologically related children.

Oncologists should thus be prepared to discuss the negative impact of cancer therapy on reproductive potential with their patients in the same way as any other risks of cancer treatment are discussed. Furthermore, patients interested in fertility preservation should be promptly referred to a reproductive medicine expert to offer timely and appropriate counseling and improve success of fertility preservation. Close collaboration between the oncology team and the reproductive endocrinologists should be encouraged.

Author details

Kenny A. Rodriguez-Wallberg[1,2,3]

Address all correspondence to: kenny.rodriguez-wallberg@karolinska.se

1 Clinical Responsible of Fertility Preservation Programme, Karolinska University Hospital, Stockholm, Sweden

2 Karolinska Institutet, Department of Clinical Science, Intervention and Technology, Division of Obstetrics and Gynecology, Sweden

3 Karolinska University Hospital Huddinge, Fertility Unit, Stockholm, Sweden

References

[1] SEER Cancer Statistics Review 1975-2007, N.C.I., updated January 7, 2011 2011.

[2] Schover, L.R., et al., *Having children after cancer. A pilot survey of survivors' attitudes and experiences.* Cancer, 1999. 86(4): p. 697-709.

[3] Rosen, A., K.A. Rodriguez-Wallberg, and L. Rosenzweig, *Psychosocial distress in young cancer survivors.* Semin Oncol Nurs, 2009. 25(4): p. 268-77.

[4] Schover, L.R., et al., *Knowledge and experience regarding cancer, infertility, and sperm banking in younger male survivors.* Journal of clinical oncology : official journal of the American Society of Clinical Oncology, 2002. 20(7): p. 1880-9.

[5] Wong, I., et al., *Assisted conception following radical trachelectomy.* Human reproduction (Oxford, England), 2009. 24(4): p. 876-9.

[6] Wallberg, K.A., V. Keros, and O. Hovatta, *Clinical aspects of fertility preservation in female patients.* Pediatr Blood Cancer, 2009. 53(2): p. 254-60.

[7] Dargent, D., et al., *La trachelectomie elargie(te), une alternative a l'hysterectomie radicale dans le traitement des cancer infiltrants developpes sur la face externe du col uterin.* 1994. 2: p. 285-292.

[8] Morice, P., et al., *[Effects of radiotherapy (external and/or internal) and chemotherapy on female fertility].* Bull Acad Natl Med, 2010. 194(3): p. 481-92; discussion 492-4, 529-30.

[9] Liou, W.S., et al., *Innovations in fertility preservation for patients with gynecologic cancers.* Fertil Steril, 2005. 84(6): p. 1561-73.

[10] Abu-Rustum, N.R. and Y. Sonoda, *Fertility-sparing surgery in early-stage cervical cancer: indications and applications.* J Natl Compr Canc Netw, 2010. 8(12): p. 1435-8.

[11] Plante, M., et al., *The vaginal radical trachelectomy: An update of a series of 125 cases and 106 pregnancies.* Gynecologic oncology, 2011. 121(2): p. 290-7.

[12] Li, J., et al., *Radical abdominal trachelectomy for cervical malignancies: Surgical, oncological and fertility outcomes in 62 patients.* Gynecologic oncology, 2011. 121(3): p. 565-70.

[13] Kesic, V., et al., *Fertility Preserving Management in Gynecologic Cancer Patients: The Need for Centralization.* International Journal of Gynecological Cancer, 2010. 20(9): p. 1613-9.

[14] Pentheroudakis, G., et al., *Cancer, fertility and pregnancy: ESMO Clinical Practice Guidelines for diagnosis, treatment and follow-up.* Ann Oncol, 2010. 21 Suppl 5: p. v266-73.

[15] Ungar, L., et al., *Abdominal radical trachelectomy during pregnancy to preserve pregnancy and fertility.* Obstet Gynecol, 2006. 108(3 Pt 2): p. 811-4.

[16] Sioutas, A., et al., *Three cases of vaginal radical trachelectomy during pregnancy.* Gynecologic oncology, 2011. 121(2): p. 420-1.

[17] Sabanegh, E.S. and A.M. Ragheb, *Male fertility after cancer.* Urology, 2009. 73(2): p. 225-31.

[18] Heidenreich, A., et al., *Organ sparing surgery for malignant germ cell tumor of the testis.* The Journal of urology, 2001. 166(6): p. 2161-5.

[19] Gosden, R.G., et al., *Impact of congenital or experimental hypogonadotrophism on the radiation sensitivity of the mouse ovary.* Human reproduction (Oxford, England), 1997. 12(11): p. 2483-8.

[20] Speiser, B., P. Rubin, and G. Casarett, *Aspermia following lower truncal irradiation in Hodgkin's disease.* Cancer, 1973. 32(3): p. 692-8.

[21] Wallace, W.H.B., R.A. Anderson, and D.S. Irvine, *Fertility preservation for young patients with cancer: who is at risk and what can be offered?* The lancet oncology, 2005. 6(4): p. 209-18.

[22] Rodriguez-Wallberg, K.A. and K. Oktay, *Fertility preservation medicine: options for young adults and children with cancer.* Journal of pediatric hematology/oncology : official journal of the American Society of Pediatric Hematology/Oncology, 2010. 32(5): p. 390-6.

[23] Sklar, C., *Growth and endocrine disturbances after bone marrow transplantation in childhood.* Acta paediatrica (Oslo, Norway : 1992) Supplement, 1995. 411: p. 57-61; discussion 62.

[24] Thibaud, E., et al., *Ovarian function after bone marrow transplantation during childhood.* Bone marrow transplantation, 1998. 21(3): p. 287-90.

[25] Shalet, S.M., et al., *Vulnerability of the human Leydig cell to radiation damage is dependent upon age.* The Journal of endocrinology, 1989. 120(1): p. 161-5.

[26] Lee, S.J., et al., *American Society of Clinical Oncology recommendations on fertility preservation in cancer patients.* Journal of clinical oncology : official journal of the American Society of Clinical Oncology, 2006. 24(18): p. 2917-31.

[27] Wo, J.Y. and A.N. Viswanathan, *Impact of radiotherapy on fertility, pregnancy, and neonatal outcomes in female cancer patients.* International journal of radiation oncology, biology, physics, 2009. 73(5): p. 1304-12.

[28] Green, D.M., et al., *Ovarian failure and reproductive outcomes after childhood cancer treatment: results from the Childhood Cancer Survivor Study.* Journal of clinical oncology : official journal of the American Society of Clinical Oncology, 2009. 27(14): p. 2374-81.

[29] Hudson, M.M., *Reproductive outcomes for survivors of childhood cancer.* Obstetrics and gynecology, 2010. 116(5): p. 1171-83.

[30] Oktem, O. and K. Oktay, *A novel ovarian xenografting model to characterize the impact of chemotherapy agents on human primordial follicle reserve.* Cancer research, 2007. 67(21): p. 10159-62.

[31] Wallberg, K.A.R.-M., V. Keros, and O. Hovatta, *Clinical aspects of fertility preservation in female patients.* Pediatric blood & cancer, 2009. 53(2): p. 254-60.

[32] Meirow, D., et al., *Administration of cyclophosphamide at different stages of follicular maturation in mice: effects on reproductive performance and fetal malformations.* Human reproduction (Oxford, England), 2001. 16(4): p. 632-7.

[33] Guerin, J.F., *[Testicular tissue cryoconservation for prepubertal boy: indications and feasibility].* Gynecol Obstet Fertil, 2005. 33(10): p. 804-8.

[34] Bahadur, G., et al., *Semen quality and cryopreservation in adolescent cancer patients.* Hum Reprod, 2002. 17(12): p. 3157-61.

[35] Menon, S., et al., *Fertility preservation in adolescent males: experience over 22 years at Rouen University Hospital.* Hum Reprod, 2009. 24(1): p. 37-44.

[36] Meseguer, M., et al., *Sperm cryopreservation in oncological patients: a 14-year follow-up study.* Fertil Steril, 2006. 85(3): p. 640-5.

[37] Marrs, R.P., J. Greene, and B.A. Stone, *Potential factors affecting embryo survival and clinical outcome with cryopreserved pronuclear human embryos.* Am J Obstet Gynecol, 2004. 190(6): p. 1766-71; discussion 1771-2.

[38] Oktay, K., A.P. Cil, and H. Bang, *Efficiency of oocyte cryopreservation: a meta-analysis.* Fertility and sterility, 2006. 86(1): p. 70-80.

[39] Practice Committee of the American Society for Reproductive Medicine, P.C.o.t.S.f.A.R.T., *Ovarian tissue and oocyte cryopreservation.* Fertil Steril, 2008. 90: p. 134-5.

[40] Medicine, P.C.o.t.A.S.f.R., *ASRM Practice Committee response to Rybak and Lieman: elective self-donation of oocytes.* Fertil Steril, 2009. 92(5): p. 1513-14.

[41] Noyes, N., E. Porcu, and A. Borini, *Over 900 oocyte cryopreservation babies born with no apparent increase in congenital anomalies.* Reprod Biomed Online, 2009. 18(6): p. 769-76.

[42] Rodriguez-Wallberg, K.A. and K. Oktay, *Fertility preservation in women with breast cancer.* Clinical obstetrics and gynecology, 2010. 53(4): p. 753-62.

[43] Oktay, K., et al., *Fertility preservation in breast cancer patients: a prospective controlled comparison of ovarian stimulation with tamoxifen and letrozole for embryo cryopreservation.* Journal of clinical oncology : official journal of the American Society of Clinical Oncology, 2005. 23(19): p. 4347-53.

[44] Azim, A.A., M. Costantini-Ferrando, and K. Oktay, *Safety of fertility preservation by ovarian stimulation with letrozole and gonadotropins in patients with breast cancer: a prospective controlled study.* Journal of clinical oncology : official journal of the American Society of Clinical Oncology, 2008. 26(16): p. 2630-5.

[45] Tulandi, T., et al., *Congenital malformations among 911 newborns conceived after infertility treatment with letrozole or clomiphene citrate.* Fertil Steril, 2006. 85(6): p. 1761-5.

[46] Chian, R.C., et al., *Live birth after vitrification of in vitro matured human oocytes.* Fertil Steril, 2009. 91(2): p. 372-6.

[47] Boiso, I., et al., *A confocal microscopy analysis of the spindle and chromosome configurations of human oocytes cryopreserved at the germinal vesicle and metaphase II stage.* Hum Reprod, 2002. 17(7): p. 1885-91.

[48] Oktay, K. and G. Karlikaya, *Ovarian function after transplantation of frozen, banked autologous ovarian tissue.* The New England journal of medicine, 2000. 342(25): p. 1919.

[49] Andersen, C.Y., et al., *Two successful pregnancies following autotransplantation of frozen/thawed ovarian tissue.* Hum Reprod, 2008. 23(10): p. 2266-72.

[50] von Wolff, M., et al., *Cryopreservation and autotransplantation of human ovarian tissue prior to cytotoxic therapy--a technique in its infancy but already successful in fertility preservation.* European journal of cancer (Oxford, England : 1990), 2009. 45(9): p. 1547-53.

[51] Oktay, K., I. Turkcuoglu, and K.A. Rodriguez-Wallberg, *Four spontaneous pregnancies and three live births following subcutaneous transplantation of frozen banked ovarian tissue: what is the explanation?* Fertility and sterility, 2011. 95(2): p. 804 e7-10.

[52] Oktay, K., et al., *Embryo development after heterotopic transplantation of cryopreserved ovarian tissue.* Lancet, 2004. 363(9412): p. 837-40.

[53] Sonmezer, M. and K. Oktay, *Orthotopic and heterotopic ovarian tissue transplantation.* Best Pract Res Clin Obstet Gynaecol, 2010. 24(1): p. 113-26.

[54] Meirow, D., et al., *Searching for evidence of disease and malignant cell contamination in ovarian tissue stored from hematologic cancer patients.* Hum Reprod, 2008. 23(5): p. 1007-13.

[55] Ajala, T., et al., *Fertility preservation for cancer patients: a review.* Obstet Gynecol Int, 2010. 2010: p. 160386.

[56] al, S.e., *Immature cryopreserved ovary restores puberty and fertility in mice without alteration of epigenetic marks.* PLoS One, 2008.

[57] Telfer, E.E., et al., *A two-step serum-free culture system supports development of human oocytes from primordial follicles in the presence of activin.* Hum Reprod, 2008. 23(5): p. 1151-8.

[58] Smitz, J., et al., *Current achievements and future research directions in ovarian tissue culture, in vitro follicle development and transplantation: implications for fertility preservation.* Hum Reprod Update, 2010. 16(4): p. 395-414.

[59] Telfer, E.E. and M. McLaughlin, *In vitro development of ovarian follicles.* Semin Reprod Med, 2011. 29(1): p. 15-23.

[60] Keros, V., et al., *Methods of cryopreservation of testicular tissue with viable spermatogonia in pre-pubertal boys undergoing gonadotoxic cancer treatment.* Hum Reprod, 2007. 22(5): p. 1384-95.

[61] Jahnukainen, K., et al., *Intratesticular transplantation of testicular cells from leukemic rats causes transmission of leukemia.* Cancer Res, 2001. 61(2): p. 706-10.

[62] Rice, S., et al., *Stage-specific expression of androgen receptor, follicle-stimulating hormone receptor, and anti-Mullerian hormone type II receptor in single, isolated, human preantral follicles: relevance to polycystic ovaries.* J Clin Endocrinol Metab, 2007. 92(3): p. 1034-40.

[63] McGee, E.A. and A.J. Hsueh, *Initial and cyclic recruitment of ovarian follicles.* Endocr Rev, 2000. 21(2): p. 200-14.

[64] Oktay, K., D. Briggs, and R.G. Gosden, *Ontogeny of follicle-stimulating hormone receptor gene expression in isolated human ovarian follicles.* The Journal of clinical endocrinology and metabolism, 1997. 82(11): p. 3748-51.

[65] Letourneau, J.M., et al., *The prevalence of self-reported reproductive impairment in young female cancer survivors throuhgout California.* Fertil Steril, 2010. 94(4): p. 510 (Abstract).

[66] Forman, E.J., C.K. Anders, and M.A. Behera, *Pilot survey of oncologists regarding treatment-related infertility and fertility preservation in female cancer patients.* J Reprod Med, 2009. 54(4): p. 203-7.

[67] Armuand, G.M., Rodriguez-Wallberg K.A. et al., *Sex differences in fertility-related information received by young adult cancer survivors.* J Clin Oncol, 2012. 30(17): p. 2147-53.

[68] Quinn, G.P., et al., *Patient-physician communication barriers regarding fertility preservation among newly diagnosed cancer patients.* Soc Sci Med, 2008. 66(3): p. 784-9.

Section 6

Perspectives in Cancer Biology and Modeling

Chapter 22

Sialyl Salivary–Type Amylase Associated with Ovarian Cancer

Takanori Moriyama

Additional information is available at the end of the chapter

http://dx.doi.org/10.5772/55452

1. Introduction

1.1. Review of related literature

Studies of tumor-producing amylase originated with Weiss et al.'s 1951 report illustrating a case of bronchogenic carcinoma associated with elevated serum amylase levels [1]. Since then, many reports have focused on lung cancer-producing amylase [2-11], and there have been similar reports in pancreatic [12], stomach [13], uterine [14], and ovarian cancers [15, 16]. Moreover, there have been reports of non-epithelial amylase-producing osteosarcoma [17] and multiple myeloma [18-20]. In these cases, the amylase had the salivary phenotype. However, pancreatic-type amylase has been reported in one case of uterine cancer [21] and two cases of breast cancer [22, 23]. Among those reported cases, determine of the total amylase activity in the sera and amylase isoenzyme electrophoretic analysis have been contributed much to the diagnosis and treatment.

In contrast, Sudo and Kanno [24] reported so-called sialic-acid-containing amylase in the sera of patients with lung and pancreatic cancer. It was similarly detected in the sera of patients with IgA-type [25] and IgD-type multiple myeloma [26], and identified to be sialyl salivary-type amylase by electrophoretic study with neuraminidase treatment and immunological characterization [26]. In 2004, Shigemura et al. [27] demonstrated, using cell culture and immunohistochemical techniques, that sialyl salivary-type amylase, together with normal salivary amylase (defined by electrophoretic characteristics), was produced by myeloma cells. In 2006, Yokouchi et al. [28] also detected the same type of amylase in culture medium from the amylase-producing lung adenocarcinoma cell line IMEC-2. In 2008, the author reported that the characterization of sialyl salivary-type amylase associated with ovarian cancer using conserved sera that were obtained from a retrospective study of amylase zymograms [29]. That by this paper, universally seen sialyl salivary-type amylase has been revealed in the patients' sera with those malignancies.

1.2. Ovarian cancer–producing amylase

When you focus on ovarian cancer-producing amylase, many studies have been published so far [30-46]. In these reports, the important thing is the following three points.

1. Amylase is directly produced from tumor cell and it can be thought of as of one of the important tumor marker.
2. Serum levels of amylase is decreased after removal the tumor and/or treatments.
3. The phenotype has been deflected to the salivary-type.

In those reports [30-46], in 1988, Henriksen and Brock had been already reported about "fast-migrated amylase isoenzymes" in the patient's serum, cyst fluid, and tumor tissue. They reported that electrophoretic separation of the amylase revealed fast-migration forms in serum 10 of 47 (21.3%) patients with malignant ovarian neoplasms. Unfortunately, they did not characterize the fast-migrating amylase isoenzyme forms [45], however, it is considered in the perspective of today think and as "sialyl salivary-type amylase" similar to our reports [25, 28, 29]. In the following, describe the research results that led to the identification of the amylase found in the sera with ovarian cancer.

2. Materials and methods

2.1. Subjects

Three patients' sera were chosen from strictly retrospective observation of routine amylase isoenzyme electrophoresis data, 2,850 specimens, which were analyzed from April 1988 to March 1999 in the Clinical Laboratory, Asahikawa Medical College Hospital, Hokkaido, Japan. The criteria were: a S3 to S2 ratio of over 1.0 and/or acidic fast-migrated sub-bands from S4 to S6. The sera were stored at -80ºC until required.

A sample with a normal amylase isoenzyme electrophoretic pattern was used as control in the analyses of neuraminidase treatment, reaction with anti-salivary monoclonal antibody, and size-exclusion HPLC.

2.2. Measurement of total amylase activity

Total serum amylase activity was measured on a Hitachi 7170 automated analyzer with G4-CNP as substrate (Toyobo, Osaka, Japan) at 37ºC. The reference interval of total serum amylase activity was from 40 to 160 U/L.

2.3. Amylase isoenzyme electrophoresis

The electrophoresis was performed for 60 min at 300 V using a cellulose acetate membrane (Titan III lipo, Helena Labs, Beaumont, TX, USA) with discontinuous buffer system [47]. Amylase activity was detected by blue starch staining, according to the technique described by Leclerc and Forest [48]. This electrophoretic technique is the most convenient way to have a high resolution.

2.4. Treatment with neuraminidase

Neuraminidase from *Arthrobacter ureafaciens* (specificities: α-2→3, α-2→6 and α-2→8) and *Clostridium perfringens* (specificities: α-2→3 and α-2→6) were purchased from Nakalai Tesque (Kyoto, Japan) and Sigma (St. Louis, MO, USA), respectively. Neuraminidase treatment was performed at 37ºC for 1 h and the treated sample was analyzed by amylase isoenzyme electrophoresis. It was confirmed, using samples from previous reports that the results of both treatments did not differ between whole serum and a purified amylase fraction sample obtained by size-exclusion chromatography [25, 26]. Whole sera were used for this treatment and the next reaction with monoclonal antibody, because the sample volumes were very low.

2.5. Reaction with anti-human salivary monoclonal antibody

Inhibitory monoclonal antibody against human salivary amylase was obtained from an amylase isoenzyme PNP kit (Roche Diagnostics, Tokyo, Japan) based on the method of Gerber et al. [49]. The monoclonal antibody solution was concentrated 5-fold with Minicon B15 clinical sample concentrators (Millipore, Billerica, MA, USA). The monoclonal antibody binds specifically to salivary amylase and inhibits *ca*. 90% of total activity. The whole serum was mixed with this antibody, and incubated at 37°C for 1 h then at 4°C for 18 h. After the reaction, amylase isoenzyme electrophoresis of the mixture was performed.

2.6. High performance liquid chromatography (HPLC)

Size-exclusion HPLC analysis was carried out on a Pharmacia (Uppsala, Sweden) fast-protein liquid chromatography (FPLC) apparatus with a Superose 12 HR column (30 cm 1.0 cm) [50]. The serum (100 μL) was eluted with a phosphate buffer (50 mmol/L, pH 7.2) containing NaCl (150 mmol/L). The volume of each fraction was 0.8 mL. Protein was monitored by absorbance at 280 nm, and amylase activity (absorbance at 600 nm) was monitored with an amylase test kit purchased from Iatoron Labs, Tokyo, Japan.

3. Results

3.1. Ages, serum total amylase activities, amylase isoenzyme electrophoretic analyses, and clinical diagnoses of selected sera

Three specimens came from female patients, and afterward it was found out that they had been diagnosed with ovarian cancer based on medical histories. The patients' ages, total serum amylase activities, and amylase isoenzyme electrophoretic data at the time of amylase electrophoretic analysis are summarized in Table 1. Their total amylase activities were 300, 772, and 798 U/L and the ratios of activity to the upper reference interval were 1.88, 4.20, and 4.99, respectively. Amylase isoenzymes with abnormal anodic migration were detected in all three patients' sera and are shown in Fig. 1A (lane 3), B (lane 3), and C (lane 3). Table 1 gives the ratios of total fast-migrated isoenzymes to S1 and S2 isoenzymes ((S3+S4+S5+S6)/(S1+S2)) and of S3 to S2 (S3/S2). These ratios approximately indicate the proportion of sialyl salivary-type amylase in the total salivary amylase fraction. In cases 2 and 3, the S3 sub-bands were slightly more dominant than the S2 sub-bands, but the ratio of S3 to S2 was below 1.00 only in case 1. The ratio of abnormal anodic bands (from S3 to S6) to normal salivary sub-bands (S1 and S2) was highest for case 3. Unfortunately, these cases were not recognized as having an abnormal amylase pattern in the routine electrophoretic analyses. It was considered that the S3 sub-bands were obviously dominant over the S2 sub-band in previous cases of multiple myeloma [25, 26]; this was less pronounced in the cases here.

3.2. Neuraminidase treatment

The serum samples of the three cases were treated with neuraminidase and submitted to electrophoretic analyses. The results using neuraminidase from *Arthrobacter ureafaciens* are shown in Fig. 1A (lane 2), 1B (lane 2), and 1C (lane 2). The abnormal anodic bands (from S3 to S6) showed a reduction of electrophoretic mobility compared with those in untreated sera, and shifted to the cathodic side corresponding to normal salivary isoenzymes in all cases. Both S1 and S2 bands were resultantly stained more strongly, respectively. These densitometric data are shown in Table 1 together with original amylase isoenzyme data. Neuraminidase from *Clostridium perfringens* had similar effects (data not shown). Therefore, it was considered that the binding pattern of the sialic acid residue was α-2→3 or α-2→6 in those cases. It has been previously confirmed that normal serum shows no change in electrophoresis under the same neuraminidase treatment conditions [25].

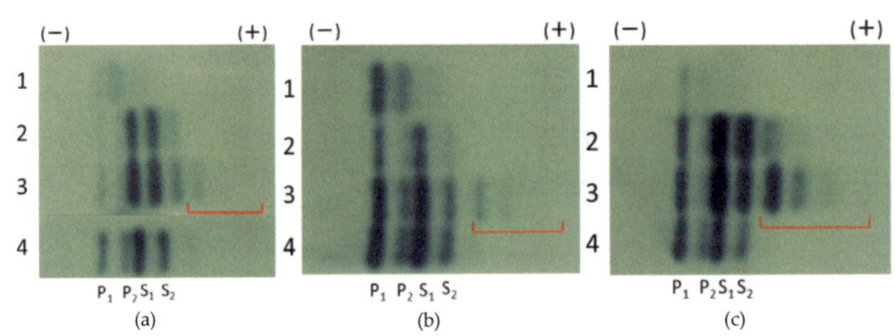

A, Case 1; B, Case 2; C, Case 3. 1, After reaction with anti-salivary amylase monoclonal antibody; 2, after neuraminidase treatment; 3, patient's original serum; 4, normal serum. The fast-migrated amylase isoenzymes were indicated by the bracket.

Figure 1. Amylase isoenzyme electrophoretic analysis of three patients' sera treated with anti-salivary monoclonal antibody and neuraminidase.

3.3 Reaction with an anti-salivary amylase monoclonal antibody

The fast-migrating bands found in the three cases disappeared from the electrophoretic patterns, together with residual normal salivary bands, on reaction with the anti-salivary amylase monoclonal antibody, and a faint broad band of amylase activity was observed on the original patterns. Formation of the faint broad band is evidence that the fast-migrating amylase reacted completely with the monoclonal antibody [25]. These results are shown in Fig. 1A (lane 1) 1B (lane 1), and 1C (lane 1), respectively. It was confirmed previously that the salivary amylase bands in normal serum disappeared from the electrophoretic pattern following similar treatment [25].

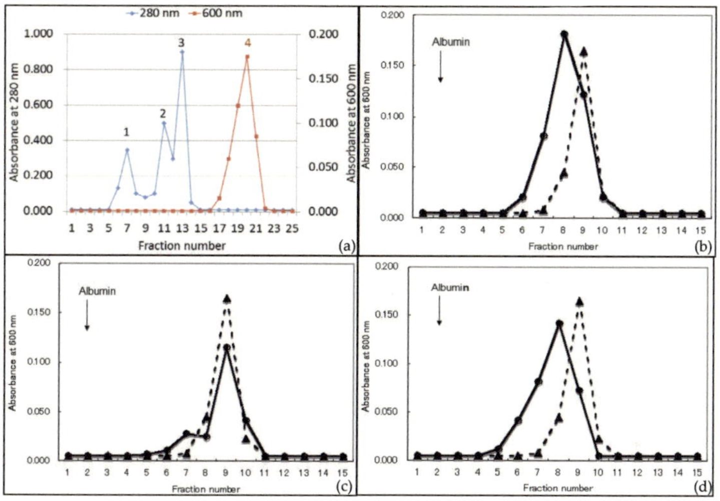

A, Elution profile of normal serum amylase. Protein concentration and amylase activity were monitored at 280 nm (blue line) and 600 nm (red line), respectively. Peak 1, IgM; peak 2, IgG; peak 3, alubumin; peak 4, normal amylase. B, Elution profile of amylase in the serum of case 1; C, that of case 2; D, that of case 3. Amylase activity was monitored at 600 nm. Amylase activities of normal and patient were indicated by the broken line and solid line, respectively. In case 1 and 3, amylase activity was eluted in a broad peak. In case 2, amylase activity was eluted in two peaks. Fraction numbers 7 and 9 correspond to the peak of sialyl salivary-type amylase and the normal serum amylase, respectively.

Figure 2. Elution profiles of amylase from normal serum and three patients' sera by HPLC on a Superose 12 HR column.

3.4. HPLC analysis

Normal serum and the patients' sera were subjected to HPLC using a Superose 12 column, and the elution patterns are shown in Fig. 2. Typically, normal serum amylase is eluted as a single peak far from sharp in the low-molecular-weight albumin, indicated in Fig. 2A. From Fig. 2B to 2D, elution patterns of the three cases are shown in comparison with normal amylase peak. Normal serum amylase eluted in fraction number 9, illustrated with a broken line. In contrast, two amylase activity peaks were noted in case 2, in fractions 7 and 9 (Fig. 2C). In cases 1 and 3, the amylase activity eluted in a large peak, fraction number 8 (Fig. 2B and D). It has been confirmed using isoamylase electrophoretic characterization that fraction 9 corresponds to normal salivary and pancreatic amylase, fraction 8 corresponds to a mixture of fast-migrating abnormal amylases with normal amylases, and fraction 7 corresponds to the fast-migrating abnormal amylase [25].

4. Discussion

The fast-migrating amylase isoenzyme bands found in the three cases of ovarian cancer were determined to be a sialyl salivary-type amylase from the following results:

1. The isoenzyme bands showed reduced electrophoretic mobility to the cathodic side following neuraminidase treatment.
2. The isoenzyme bands disappeared from the amylase zymograms, and faint broad bands were formed, on reaction with anti-human salivary amylase monoclonal antibody.
3. The isoenzyme bands could be separated by Superose 12 HR size-exclusion HPLC. Thus, an apparent extra high-molecular-mass peak was observed on the chromatogram.

These characteristics of sialyl salivary-type amylase were also demonstrated in the author's first report of myeloma [25]. The three characteristics above were considered simultaneously as strict criteria to detect sialyl salivary-type amylase. The author would like to recommend that, in the future, at least neuraminidase treatment and size-exclusion HPLC analysis should be used for identification.

Many investigators have reported amylase-producing ovarian cancer and reported that serum amylase is an important tumor marker [15, 30-44]. In particular, amylase isoenzyme electrophoresis has been helpful [6, 32] in making an early diagnosis and distinguishing from pancreatitis; the amylase phenotype was generally salivary. In contrast, there have been a few unique reports [30, 40, 44, 45] describing acidic amylase and/or fast-migrating amylase found in the sera or ascites associated with ovarian cancer. Unfortunately, neuramidase treatment and characterization of other properties were not performed in these studies. The author considers those amylases, from the findings of this and previous reports [25-28], to be most likely sialyl salivary-type. It seems likely that sialylated salivary-type amylase is directly produced together with normal salivary amylase by ovarian cancer cells, as in multiple mylelona cells [27] and lung cancer cells [28].

In contrast, acidic amylase from ovarian cystic fluids [51, 52] can be distinguished clearly from sialyl salivary-type amylase because the cystic amylases are unaffected by treatment with neuraminidase. These amylases are thought to result from aging transformation of cystic amylase, as reported by Warshaw and Lee [53], and Weaver et al.[54]. Therefore, neuraminidase treatment is expected to provide a very important and useful means of distinguishing between aging salivary amylase and sialyl salivary-type amylase. For contrast, we previously published the electrophoretic pattern of aging sialyl salivary-type amylase in pleural effusion with IgD-type multiple myeloma [26].

Size-exclusion HPLC characteristic is another important means of distinguishing sialyl salivary-type amylase from normal salivary amylase. The molecular mass of sialyl salivary-type amylase from myeloma was determined by immunoblotting to be approximately 60,000 Da, the same as normal salivary amylase [25]. Unfortunately, the equivalent experiment could not be repeated in this study, owing to the small serum sample sizes, but as the elution profiles in this report were the same as in previous reports [25-28], the molecular mass is assumed to be the same. However, the sialyl salivary-type amylases were well separated by Superose 12 HPLC analyses. Moreover, the peak of the amylases did not change following neuraminidase treatment; such elution behavior can probably be explained by the unusual protein conformation of this abnormal salivary-type amylase [25].

Recently, Shigemura et al.[55] reported that sialyl salivary-type amylase was detected in serum from 7 out of 11 (63.6%) subjects with multiple myeloma. It was emphasized that sialyl salivary-type amylase is a useful marker of disease activity in multiple myeloma, and that sialylation of the amylase molecule might be concerned with oncogenic transformation or chromosomal abnormalities. Moreover, it was disclosed that sialyl salivary-type amylases could be detected in the serum of patients with a normal serum amylase level and apparently normal electrophoretic patterns. In our cases, although even cases 2 and 3 were not recognized at the time of the samples were taken, the electrophoretic pattern of case 1 was close to normal. However, there certainly were some (small) abnormal fast-migrating sub-bands; those observations were extremely significant. Accordingly, if amylase isoenzyme electrophoresis is more widely and carefully applied to hyperamylasemia with ovarian cancer, it seems likely that more cases will be detected. Serum sialyl salivary-type amylase will no doubt prove a useful marker of ovarian cancer, as for multiple myeloma [55].

In this study, a case of salivary amylase genetic variant [56] might be experienced by unexpectedly. In amylase zymogram of case 1, S2 sub-band was equal or dominant to S1 sub-band. However, further studies could not be performed in this study and there are no evidences. Isoamylase analysis of saliva and/or tumor extract should been carried out to characterize the variant [57].

Sialyl salivary-type amylase has been found in the sera of patients with lung cancer [24, 28], pancreatic cancer [24], multiple myeloma [25], and ovarian cancer [29]. Therefore, it is expected that the sialyl salivary-type amylase will be found generally in patients with amylase-producing tumors. The author especially recommends that amylase isoenzyme electrophoresis should be applied to hyperamylasemia with malignancies, in place of immunological amylase isoenzyme analysis [49] or that a rapid immunological technique for sialyl salivary-type amylase should be developed in future.

Zakrzewska and Pietrynczak [58] had already elucidated that the total serum and urinary amylase activity and salivary isoenzyme were significantly decreased after surgical removal of the tumor with different types of ovarian cancer. Moreover, they demonstrated that those activities in the serum of the patients with ovarian carcinoma with various types were significantly decreased after radiotherapy [59]. Although the frequency of salivary amylase and/or sialyl salivary-type amylase in ovarian cancer has not been revealed those amylase could be definitely considered as a nonspecific tumor maker [60]. Therefore, the author would like to propose that this old and new amylase should be added with standard tumor marker CA125 [61, 62] in the routine treatment and surgery in ovarian cancer

5. Conclusion

Sialyl salivary-type amylase was detected in the sera of the patients with ovarian cancer. The amylase was considered to have been directly produced together with salivary-type amylase from tumor cells. These studies have contributed to the research into amylase-producing tumors, particularly into amylase-producing ovarian cancer.

Acknowledgements

The author extremely grateful to the deceased Professor Tatsuo Tozawa, Department of Laboratory Medicine, Hyogo College of Medicine, Nishinomiya, Hyogo, Japan, for encouragement and helpful discussions.

Author details

Takanori Moriyama

Address all correspondence to: moriyama@hs.hokudai.ac.jp

Medical Laboratory Science, Faculty of Health Sciences, Hokkaido University, Kitaku, Sapporo, Japan

References

[1] Weiss MJ, Edmondson HA, Wertman M. Elevated serum amylase associated with bronchogenic carcinoma; report of case. Am J Clin Pathol. 1951 Nov;21(11):1057-61.

[2] Ammann RW, Berk JE, Fridhandler L, Ueda M, Wegmann W. Hyperamylasemia with carcinoma of the lung. Ann Intern Med. 1973 Apr;78(4):521-6.

[3] Gomi K, Kameya T, Tsumuraya M, Shimosato Y, Zeze F, Abe K, et al. Ultrastructural, histochemical, and biochemical studies of two cases with amylase, ACTH, and beta-MSH producing tumor. Cancer. 1976 Oct;38(4):1645-54.

[4] Yokoyama M, Natsuizaka T, Ishii Y, Ohshima S, Kasagi A, Tateno S. Amylase-producing lung cancer: ultrastructural and biochemical studies. Cancer. 1977 Aug;40(2): 766-72.

[5] Morohoshi T, Nakamura N, Hayashi K, Kanda M. Amylase producing lung cancer. Electronmicroscopical and biochemical studies. Virchows Arch A Pathol Anat Histol. 1980;387(2):125-32.

[6] Maeda M, Otsuki M, Yuu H, Saeki S, Yamasaki T, Baba S. Salivary-type hyperamylasemia in primary lung cancer: observation of a possible precursor of the salivary-type isoamylase. Eur J Cancer Clin Oncol. 1982 Feb;18(2):123-8.

[7] Yoshida Y, Mori M, Sonoda T, Sakauchi F, Sugawara H, Suzuki A. Ultrastructural, immunohistochemical and biochemical studies on amylase and ACTH producing lung cancer. Virchows Arch A Pathol Anat Histopathol. 1985;408(2-3):163-72.

[8] Tomita N, Matsuura N, Horii A, Emi M, Nishide T, Ogawa M, et al. Expression of alpha-amylase in human lung cancers. Cancer Res. 1988 Jun 1;48(11):3292-6.

[9] Tsukawaki M, Izawa M, Yoshida M, Araki N, Hashiba Y, Nakagawa H, et al. A case of amylase-producing lung cancer. Intern Med. 1992 Jan;31(1):60-3.

[10] Grove A. Amylase in lung carcinomas. An ultrastructural and immunohistochemical study of two adenocarcinomas, and a review of the literature. APMIS. 1994 Feb; 102(2):135-44.

[11] Lenler-Petersen P, Grove A, Brock A, Jelnes R. alpha-Amylase in resectable lung cancer. Eur Respir J. 1994 May;7(5):941-5.

[12] Shimamura J, Fridhandler L, Berk JE. Nonpancreatic-type hyperamylasemia associated with pancreatic cancer. Am J Dig Dis. 1976 Apr;21(4):340-5.

[13] Nomura H, Tokumitsu SI, Takeuchi T. Ultrastructural, cytochemical, and biochemical characterization of alpha-amylase produced by human gastric cancer cells in vitro. J Natl Cancer Inst. 1980 May;64(5):1015-24.

[14] Ueda G, Yamasaki M, Inoue M, Tanaka Y, Inoue Y, Nishino T, et al. Immunohistochemical demonstration of amylase in endometrial carcinomas. Int J Gynecol Pathol. 1986;5(1):47-51.

[15] Corlette MB, Dratch M, Sorger K. Amylase elevation attributable to an ovarian neoplasm. Gastroenterology. 1978 May;74(5 Pt 1):907-9.

[16] Nakayama T HY, Kitamura M, editor. Onco-developemental gene expression. New York: Academic Press; 1976: 455-62.

[17] Masiar PJ. Serum amylase and isoamylases in malignant bone tumors. Neoplasma. 1984;31(3):351-9.

[18] Hata H, Matsuzaki H, Tanaka K, Nomura H, Kagimoto T, Takeya M, et al. Ectopic production of salivary-type amylase by a IgA-lambda-type multiple myeloma. Cancer. 1988 Oct 15;62(8):1511-5.

[19] Fujii H, Yashige H, Kanoh T, Urata Y. Amylase-producing multiple myeloma. Arch Pathol Lab Med. 1991 Sep;115(9):952-6.

[20] Delannoy A, Hamels J, Mecucci C, Fally P, Wallef G, de Fooz C, et al. Amylase-producing IgD-type multiple myeloma. J Intern Med. 1992 Nov;232(5):457-60.

[21] Matsuyama M, Inoue T, Ariyoshi Y, Doi M, Suchi T, Sato T, et al. Argyrophil cell carcinoma of the uterine cervix with ectopic production of ACTH, beta-MSH, serotonin, histamine, and amylase. Cancer. 1979 Nov;44(5):1813-23.

[22] Weitzel JN, Pooler PA, Mohammed R, Levitt MD, Eckfeldt JH. A unique case of breast carcinoma producing pancreatic-type isoamylase. Gastroenterology. 1988 Feb; 94(2):519-20.

[23] Inaji H, Koyama H, Higashiyama M, Noguchi S, Yamamoto H, Ishikawa O, et al. Immunohistochemical, ultrastructural and biochemical studies of an amylase-producing breast carcinoma. Virchows Arch A Pathol Anat Histopathol. 1991;419(1):29-33.

[24] Sudo K, Kanno T. Sialic acid containing abnormal amylases in human sera. Clin Chim Acta. 1975 Nov 3;64(3):303-6.

[25] Moriyama T, Tozawa T, Yamashita H, Onodera S, Nobuoka M, Makino M. Separation and characterization of sialic acid-containing salivary-type amylase from patients' sera with immunoglobulin A-type myeloma. J Chromatogr. 1991 Nov 15;571(1-2):61-72.

[26] Moriyama T, Tozawa T, Nobuoka M, Ikeda H. Sialyl salivary-type amylasemia associated with immunoglobulin D-type multiple myeloma. Clin Chim Acta. 1995 Jan 16;233(1-2):127-34.

[27] Shigemura M, Moriyama T, Endo T, Shibuya H, Suzuki H, Nishimura M, et al. Myeloma cells produce sialyl salivary-type amylase. Clin Chem Lab Med. 2004;42(6): 677-80.

[28] Yokouchi H, Yamazaki K, Asahina H, Shigemura M, Moriyama T, Takaoka K, et al. Establishment and characterization of amylase-producing lung adenocarcinoma cell line, IMEC-2. Anticancer Res. 2006 Jul-Aug;26(4B):2821-7.

[29] Moriyama T. Sialyl salivary-type amylase associated with ovarian cancer. Clin Chim Acta. 2008 May;391(1-2):106-11.

[30] Sandiford JA, Chiknas SG. Hyperamylasemia and ovarian carcinoma. Clin Chem. 1979 Jun;25(6):948-50.

[31] Cramer SF, Bruns DE. Amylase-producing ovarian neoplasm with pseudo-Meigs' syndrome and elevated pleural fluid amylase: case report and ultrastructure. Cancer. 1979 Nov;44(5):1715-21.

[32] Norwood SH, Torma MJ, Fontenelle LJ. Hyperamylasemia due to poorly differentiated adenosquamous carcinoma of the ovary. Arch Surg. 1981 Feb;116(2):225-6.

[33] Takeuchi T, Fujiki H, Kameya T. Characterization of amylases produced by tumors. Clin Chem. 1981 Apr;27(4):556-9.

[34] Shapiro R, Dropkin R, Finkelstein J, Aledort D, Greenstein AJ. Ovarian carcinomatosis presenting with hyperamylasemia and pleural effusion. Am J Gastroenterol. 1981 Oct;76(4):365-8.

[35] Hodes ME, Sisk CJ, Karn RC, Ehrlich CE, Lehrner LM, Roth LM, et al. An amylase-producing serous cystadenocarcinoma of the ovary. Oncology. 1985;42(4):242-7.

[36] Hayakawa T, Kameya A, Mizuno R, Noda A, Kondo T, Hirabayashi N. Hyperamylasemia with papillary serous cystadenocarcinoma of the ovary. Cancer. 1984 Oct 15;54(8):1662-5.

[37] Yagi C, Miyata J, Hanai J, Ogawa M, Ueda G. Hyperamylasemia associated with endometrioid carcinoma of the ovary: case report and immunohistochemical study. Gynecol Oncol. 1986 Oct;25(2):250-5.

[38] Teshima H, Kitamura H, Mizoguchi Y, Hino S, Mizutani K, Mori H, et al. Immunohistochemical and immunoelectron microscopic study of an amylase-producing, CA19-9 positive ovarian mucinous cystadenocarcinoma. Gynecol Oncol. 1988 Jul; 30(3):372-80.

[39] Schlikker I, Nakad A, Gerbaux A, Azzouzi K, Kadou J, Lezaire P, et al. Hyperamylasemia with papillary serous cystadenocarcinoma of the ovary. Acta Clin Belg. 1989;44(4):255-8.

[40] Brophy CM, Morris J, Sussman J, Modlin IM. "Pseudoascites" secondary to an amylase-producing serous ovarian cystadenoma. A case study. J Clin Gastroenterol. 1989 Dec;11(6):703-6.

[41] Tohya T, Shimajiri S, Onoda C, Yoshimura T. Complete remission of ovarian endometrioid adenocarcinoma associated with hyperamylasemia and liver metastasis treated by paclitaxel and carboplatin chemotherapy: a case report. Int J Gynecol Cancer. 2004 Mar-Apr;14(2):378-80.

[42] Srivastava R, Fraser C, Gentleman D, Jamieson LA, Murphy MJ. Hyperamylasaemia: not the usual suspects. BMJ. 2005 Oct 15;331(7521):890-1.

[43] Kavitha S, Balasubramanian R. Elderly lady with ascites. J Assoc Physicians India. 2006 Apr;54:325-6.

[44] Kosches DS, Sosnowik D, Lendvai S, Bank S. Unusual anodic migrating isoamylase differentiates selected malignant from nonmalignant ascites. J Clin Gastroenterol. 1989 Feb;11(1):43-6.

[45] Henriksen R, Brock A. Amylase activity and fast-migrating amylase isoenzymes in serum and cyst fluid from patients with ovarian neoplasms. Acta Obstet Gynecol Scand. 1988;67(1):65-70.

[46] Bruns DE, Mills SE, Savory J. Amylase in fallopian tube and serous ovarian neoplasms: immunohistochemical localization. Arch Pathol Lab Med. 1982 Jan;106(1): 17-20.

[47] Kohn J. Separation of haemoglobins on cellulose acetate. J Clin Pathol. 1969 Jan;22(1): 109-11.

[48] Leclerc P, Forest JC. Electrophoretic determination of isoamylases in serum with commercially available reagents. Clin Chem. 1982 Jan;28(1):37-40.

[49] Gerber M, Naujoks K, Lenz H, Gerhardt W, Wulff K. Specific immunoassay of alpha-amylase isoenzymes in human serum. Clin Chem. 1985 Aug;31(8):1331-4.

[50] Moriyama T YK, Takebe T, Makino I, Nobuoka M, Makino M. Purification of the pancreatic stone protein by high-performance liquid chromatography. J Chromatogr. 1989;493:164-9.

[51] Zakowski JJ, Bruns DE. Improved DEAE-Sephadex column chromatography in measuring amylase in serous ovarian neoplasms, and results for 13 cases. Clin Chem. 1982 Oct;28(10):2095-8.

[52] Zakowski JJ, Gregory MR, Bruns DE. Amylase from human serous ovarian tumors: purification and characterization. Clin Chem. 1984 Jan;30(1):62-8.

[53] Warshaw AL, Lee KH. Aging changes of pancreatic isoamylases and the appearance of "old amylase" in the serum of patients with pancreatic pseudocysts. Gastroenterology. 1980 Dec;79(6):1246-51.

[54] Weaver DW, Bouwman DL, Walt AJ, Clink D, Sessions S, Stephany J. Aged amylase: a valuable test for detecting and tracking pancreatic pseudocysts. Arch Surg. 1982 May;117(5):707-11.

[55] Shigemura M, Moriyama T, Shibuya H, Obara M, Endo T, Hashino S, et al. Multiple myeloma associated with sialyl salivary-type amylase. Clin Chim Acta. 2007 Feb; 376(1-2):121-5.

[56] Ward JC, Merritt AD, Bixler D. Human salivary amylase: genetics of electrophoretic variants. Am J Hum Genet. 1971 Jul;23(4):403-9.

[57] Moriyama T NM, Ikeda H. Properties of dominant amylase-2 found in routine electrophoreric analysis. Jpn J Electroph. 1995;39:195-200.

[58] Zakrzewska I, Pietrynczak M. [Changes in activity of alpha amylase and its salivary isoenzyme in serum and urine after surgical treatment of ovarian neoplasms]. Ginekol Pol. 1996 Oct;67(10):504-9.

[59] Zakrzewska I, Pietrynczak M. The alterations in the activity of amylase and its salivary isoenzyme in the serum of patients with ovarian carcinoma, submitted to radiotherapy. Rocz Akad Med Bialymst. 1997;42(1):229-35.

[60] Seyama K, Nukiwa T, Takahashi K, Takahashi H, Kira S. Amylase mRNA transcripts in normal tissues and neoplasms: the implication of different expressions of amylase isogenes. J Cancer Res Clin Oncol. 1994;120(4):213-20.

[61] Bast RC, Jr., Xu FJ, Yu YH, Barnhill S, Zhang Z, Mills GB. CA 125: the past and the future. Int J Biol Markers. 1998 Oct-Dec;13(4):179-87.

[62] Bast RC, Jr., Badgwell D, Lu Z, Marquez R, Rosen D, Liu J, et al. New tumor markers: CA125 and beyond. Int J Gynecol Cancer. 2005 Nov-Dec;15 Suppl 3:274-81.

Chapter 23

Role of CREB Protein Family Members in Human Haematological Malignancies

Francesca D'Auria and Roberta Di Pietro

Additional information is available at the end of the chapter

http://dx.doi.org/10.5772/55368

1. Introduction

Cyclic AMP Response Element Binding (CREB) protein is a member of the CREB/ATF (Activating Transcription Factor) family of transcription factors playing an important role in the nuclear responses to a variety of external signals that lead to proliferation, differentiation, apoptosis and survival. Other authors' evidences have highlighted a critical role of CREB in the regulation of normal haematopoiesis and leukemogenesis due to the interaction with target genes crucially involved in the cell cycle machinery. Recent findings of our research group have demonstrated that CREB and ATF-1 phosphorylation levels are related to a different sensitivity of T leukaemia cell clones to the cytotoxic action of TNF-related apoptosis inducing ligand (TRAIL) and that low dose radiation treatment of erythroleukaemia cells (K562) can trigger CREB activation and deliver a survival signal. Since one fundamental problem of most malignancies, including those of haematological origin, is the development of multiple mechanisms of resistance, which progressively reduce or suppress the therapeutic efficacy of anticancer treatment, the early identification of biological markers of responsiveness/unresponsiveness and the follow-up of individual response are highly desirable to adjust therapeutic treatments. In light of all these considerations and of the complex molecular interactions involving CREB/ATF family members, the present chapter is aimed at revising literature focusing, in particular, on the involvement of CREB/ATF family members in leukemogenesis and lymphomagenesis, in order to gain more insight into this matter that could result useful to the treatment of leukaemia and lymphoma diseases.

2. CREB family members

The CREB or CREB/ATF multigenic family is composed by several nuclear transcription factors. The prototype of this family is CREB, a 43 kDa – basic-region leucine zipper (bZIP) transcription factor that elicits responses to a variety of extracellular signals, including stress and growth factors, and that is involved in several cellular processes such as glucose homeostasis, proliferation, ageing and differentiation, survival and apoptosis, memory and learning [1]. The CREB/ATF family of transcription factors includes three homologous genes: cAMP response element binding (*CREB)*, cAMP response element modulator (*CREM*), and activating transcription factor-1 (*ATF-1*), whose structure domains are illustrated in a recent review [2]. These genes generate a group of highly homologous proteins that have been named after their prototypes: CREB, CREM, and ATF-1, respectively [3].

CREB/ATF proteins were initially identified for their binding to the cyclic AMP response element (CRE) in various gene promoters that contain the octanucleotide consensus sequence TGACGTCA [4]. Over the years, cDNA clones encoding identical or homologous proteins have been isolated. Up to now, at least 20 different mammalian proteins with the prefix CREB or ATF have been characterized and grouped into subgroups on the basis of their amino acid similarity [5, 6]. CREB/ATF family members include CREB-1 (also known as CREB), CREB-2 (recently named ATF-4), CREB-3, CREB-5, CREM, ATF-1 (also known as TREB36), ATF-2 (also known as CRE-BP1), ATF-3, ATF-4 (previously named CREB-2), ATF-5 (also known as ATFX), ATF-6, ATF-7 and B-ATF subgroups [7, 8]. Proteins belonging to this class represent a large group of bZIP transcription factors containing highly divergent N-terminal domains, but sharing a C-terminal leucine zipper domain. The basic region in the bZIP domain is rich in basic amino acids and is responsible for specific DNA binding, while the leucine zipper region contains leucine residues and is responsible for dimerization of the proteins by resembling a zipper. Based on the sequence of each bZip domain, these proteins form homodimers or heterodimers both with other members of the family and with other bZIP containing proteins like the activator protein-1 (AP-1), C/EBP, Fos, Jun or Maf family proteins [8]. That implies the expansion of the repertoire and different opportunities of target gene regulation that are further increased by the alternative splice products of *CREB* and *CREM* genes that show repressor or activator properties [5, 7]. Whereas CREB, CREM, and ATF-1 are relatively well characterized and known to regulate gene transcription via binding to CRE sites, ATF-2, ATF-3, and ATF-4 are structurally more distant and their functional properties remain poorly understood. Rather than being activated by the cAMP cascade, ATF-2 is activated by c-Jun N-terminal kinase (JNK) and can dimerize with members of the AP-1 family such as c-Jun to bind to CRE or AP-1 sites [9, 10]. Additionally, ATF-2 homodimers and ATF-2/c-Jun heterodimers can bind to certain CRE-like sites that are insensitive to CREB [11]. ATF-3 and ATF-4 also dimerize with various Jun species and can shift c-Jun DNA binding site preferences from AP-1 to CRE, thereby promoting crosstalk among AP-1 and CREB protein families [9]. In addition, ATF-4 is able to dimerize with Nrf1 (NF-E2 related factor 1) and Nrf2 (NF-E2 related factor 2) and then interact with the antioxidant responsive element (ARE) present in the promoters of many antioxidant genes [12]. ATF-2, ATF-3, and ATF-4 have been considered as cellular stress response proteins [5, 13, 14] but recently they have been also involved in non-stress adaptations. In fact, extensive studies have demonstrated that ATF-3 is an adaptive response gene that is activated by a wide variety of signals including those initiated by cytokines, genotoxic agents or physiological stresses [15]. Interestingly, unlike other ATF family members, emerging evidences have implicated ATF-3 in the host defence against invading pathogens and cancer. These processes are controlled by the efficient coordination of cell responses and genetic regulatory networks which allow this key transcription factor to modulate the expression of a diverse set of target genes, depending on the cell type and/or the nature of the stimuli [16, 17].

While both CREBs and ATF-1 are ubiquitously expressed, CREMs are mainly present in spermatids [6] and in the neuroendocrine system [18]. Interestingly, a recently published paper on the effects of traumatic brain injury demonstrated the nuclear co-localization of CREM-1 and active caspase-3 in the ispilateral cortex of adult rats, suggesting a possible role for CREM-1 in neuronal apoptosis [19]. In a recent report of our research group on Jurkat leukaemia cells [20], we observed a different cell compartmentalization of CREB protein in dependence of the TRAIL dose employed and induced cytotoxicity. Indeed, both under normal or low serum culture conditions an evident nuclear translocation of phospho-CREB was detected after 1 h treatment only with the lower dose of TRAIL (100 ng/mL) and prevented in the presence of PI3K/Akt and p38 mitogen-activated protein kinase (MAPK) specific inhibitors [20]. In another model under investigation in our laboratories and represented by K562 erythroleukaemia cells induced to differentiation [21], the nuclear localization of the active form of CREB was clearly evident after only 1 h treatment with haemin. Interestingly, CREB positive nuclei resembled the features of apoptotic nuclei, suggesting that CREB phosphorylation is possibly required to determine the nuclear structural changes occurring during erythroblast maturation [21, 22]. Concerning other family members, it has been recently shown that ATF-2 is a nucleocytoplasmic shuttling protein and that its subcellular localization is regulated by AP-1 dimerization [23]. ATF-3 is ubiquitously expressed and localized in the nucleus but maintained at low levels in the absence of cellular stresses. Instead, it is rapidly transcriptionally induced under different conditions, among which hypoxia, DNA damage (induced by UV radiation, ionizing radiation, etoposide), heat or cold shock, serum starvation or stimulation [13, 15]. ATF-4 is of particular interest since it has been demonstrated to translocate from the cytoplasmic membrane to the nucleus in neuronal cells upon γ aminobutyric acid (GABA) receptor activation, to be likely involved in neuronal plasticity by coupling receptor activity to gene expression [24]. Finally, a number of immunofluorescent and cell fractionation experiments indicate that ATF-6 is linked to the endoplasmic reticulum (ER) chaperone Bip/Crp78 and localizes in the precursor form on the ER membrane [25]. Upon ER stress induced by prolonged nutrient deprivation, it translocates to the Golgi where it is cleaved by resident proteases to liberate its active N-terminal domain. In this active form it translocates to the nucleus where it up-regulates a number of target genes involved in energy homeostasis [25].

3. CREB binding proteins

The human CREB-binding protein (CBP) and its paralogue, p300, are highly related proteins that are well conserved amongst mammals. Due to their high degree of sequence similarity, these two proteins are most often functionally interchangeable although they also possess unique functions [26, 27]. CBP was initially recognized as an interaction partner for CREB nuclear transcription factor [28], whereas p300 cDNA was cloned encoding the 300 kDa protein known to be associated with the adenoviral protein E1A [29]. Though encoded by different genes, CBP/p300 share several conserved regions that constitute most of their known functional domains [for details see 27]. Both CBP and p300 have originally been described as transcriptional co-activators that bridge DNA-binding transcription factors to components of the basal transcriptional machinery, including the TATA-box-binding protein (TBP) [30], TFIIB [31] and, via RNA helicase A, also RNA polymerase II [32]. Due to the huge size of over 2400 amino acids, CBP/p300 can also behave as a scaffold, bridging together a variety of cofactor proteins at the same time and leading to the assembly of multi-competent co-activator complexes [26, 27]. In addition, CBP/p300 interact with protein kinases such as the MAPKs and the cyclin E-Cdk2 complex, thus mediating the phosphorylation of CBP/p300-interacting transcription factors such as ER81 and E2F family members. Both CBP and p300 have been found originally to possess histone acetyltransferase (HAT) activity [33]. This acetyltransferase function has profound consequences for nucleosomal structure and the activity of transcription factors, and thereby affects gene activity in multiple ways. In fact, it is well known that acetylation of multiple sites in the histone tails has been directly associated with transcriptional up-regulation, whereas de-acetylation correlates with transcriptional repression. Mechanistically, histone acetylation promotes the accessibility of DNA to transcription protein complexes, by facilitating the "unwiring" of the chromatin structure. During the last years, both CBP and p300 have been regarded as protein acetyltransferases rather than only HAT since they have shown the capacity to acetylate a number of non-histone nuclear proteins, including the tumour suppressor protein p53, dTCF, EKLF (erythroid Kruppel-like factor), GATA-1, NF-Y and other basal transcription factors [34, 35]. Thus, in light of the number of proteins interacting with CBP/p300, it is not surprising to find that many physiological processes, including cell growth, cell division, cell differentiation, cell transformation, embryogenesis and apoptosis, are dependent on CBP/p300 function [27, 28, 34]. Moreover, the importance of CBP/p300 is underscored by the fact that genetic alterations as well as their functional dysregulation are strongly linked to human diseases [36, 37].

Previous studies have shown that CBP and p300 play distinct roles in haematopoiesis and act non-redundantly in microenvironment-mediated haematopoietic regulation in spite of their high homology [38-40]. It has been widely documented that both proteins interact with crucial transcriptional regulators in virtually all haematopoietic lineages. Intriguingly, CBP/p300 can promote, on one hand, normal differentiation and cell cycle arrest (by cooperating with GATA-1) and, on the other hand, cell cycle progression and transformation by cooperating with c-Myb and PU.1, an Ets family transcription factor. It is conceivable that an overexpressed oncoprotein might compete with differentiation-inducing factors for CBP/p300 function. Furthermore, during normal development, CBP/p300 could differentially partition among transcriptional regulators with opposing functions, thus controlling the balance between proliferation and differentiation. As an example, the down-modulation of the proto-oncoproteins PU.1 and c-Myb during the erythroleukaemia MEL cell line maturation might increase availability of CBP/p300 for differentiation-associated factors such as GATA-1, NF-E2 and EKLF. Moreover, besides the involvement in erythroid cell lineage differentiation, CBP and, very likely, p300 target a broad range of myeloid and lymphoid expressed transcription factors [38-40].

Because of its central role in transcription, it is not surprising that aberrations in *CREBBP* can affect many tissues [17]. In humans, chromosomal translocations involving the *CREBBP* gene have been observed in leukaemia and myelodysplastic syndrome [38]. Mutations of *CREBBP* in the germline have been associated to the Rubinstein-Taybi syndrome (RTS), an autosomal dominant disease characterized by mental retardation, skeletal abnormalities and a high propensity to develop cancer, including leukaemia [36]. Similarly, *CREBBP*(+/-) mice show abnormalities in bone, haematopoietic tissues and neural tissues and an increased tendency to develop haematological malignancies with age [41]. In earlier studies, in *CREBBP*(+/-) HSCs (haematopoietic stem cells) a number of cell-intrinsic defects have been described, including diminished HSC self-renewal and excessive myeloid differentiation [42]. The combination of skeletal and haematopoietic defects in *CREBBP*(+/-) mice suggests the involvement of the bone marrow (BM) microenvironment in the haematopoietic phenotype of these mice. One of the genes whose transcription is directly regulated by CBP is matrix metalloproteinase 9 (MMP9) that was reported to be a microenvironmental regulator of haematopoiesis [43]. Interestingly, *CREBBP* heterozygosity in the BM microenvironment results in reduced levels of MMP9 and soluble kit ligand (KITL) and increased expression of endothelial cell adhesion molecule 1 (ESAM1) and cadherin 5 (CDH5) on a subset of endothelial cells. In addition, it has been reported that the loss of a single *CREBBP* allele is deleterious for the BM microenvironment, leading to defective haematopoiesis. In fact, the *CREBBP*(+/-) microenvironment poorly supports HSCs, promotes excessive myelopoiesis and reduces lymphopoiesis. Furthermore, it has been reported that *CREBBP*(+/-) mice have reduced bone volume due to increased osteoclastogenesis. A concomitant reduction in CFU-fibroblasts (CFU-Fs) and osteoblasts per tissue area was also identified and likely contributes to fewer HSC niches [41]. Thus, all these findings reveal the importance of CBP in the development and function of the BM microenvironment and underscore the multiple levels at which this protein acts to regulate haematopoiesis. Indeed, half of the normal complement of *CREBBP*, but not of *EP300*, in the BM microenvironment has a deleterious effect on haematopoiesis via multiple mechanisms, leading to the development of excessive myelopoiesis, disrupting the proper architecture of the BM and resulting in poor maintenance of HSC number and quality.

4. CREB physiological roles and signalling pathways

CREB is a multi-functional transcriptional activator that is involved in many signalling pathways under normal and pathologic conditions. CREB mediates its transcriptional responses following phosphorylation at Ser133 [7] and the consequent association with the 256 kDa co-activator CBP [28] or related family members like p300 [29]. Both Ser133 phosphorylation and CBP association play an essential role for gene transactivation mediated by an octanucleotide CRE consensus sequence placed in the promoters of many cellular genes [29]. In more detail, CREB transactivation domain, that is the site able to interact with other nuclear factors, contains a constitutive glutamine rich domain termed Q2 and an inducible domain, termed the kinase-inducible domain (KID), regulated by cellular kinases [2]. The Q2 domain interacts with a TATA binding protein-associated factor and is constitutively active; instead, the KID region promotes isomerization by recruiting the co-activator factors CBP and p300 to the gene promoters and is active only when it is phosphorylated at Ser133 by a variety of cellular kinases. Recent studies using a genome-wide analysis showed that the number of putative target genes for CREB is about 5000, among which immediate-early genes, including *c-FOS*, *AP-1/JunB* and early growth response protein 1 (*EGR-1*) [44], as well as genes crucially involved in the cell cycle machinery, namely *Cyclin A1* and *D1* [7]. In this respect, it has been found that Cyclin A is up-regulated in cell lines, transgenic mice and patient bone marrow that show increased CREB levels [44]. It is still to unravel whether this occurs through a direct or indirect mechanism. To address this issue or, in other words, to determine whether CREB overexpression results in target gene activation through increased occupancy of binding sites or by altering levels of Ser133 phosphorylation, several authors proposed to use chromatin immunoprecipitation assays. Moreover, microarray analysis of potential CREB target genes will help in understanding the downstream pathways through which CREB contributes to normal and aberrant haematopoiesis. By interacting with its huge number of target genes CREB plays a critical role in the regulation of various biological processes including haematopoiesis, liver gluconeogenesis, pituitary gland physiology, circadian rhythm, spermatogenesis, learning and memory [1, 45, 46]. Concerning haematopoiesis, CREB is a downstream target of haematopoietic growth factor signalling activated by granulocyte-macrophage–colony stimulating factor (GM-CSF) and interleukin-3 (IL-3), thus resulting a crucial factor for normal myelopoiesis [44]. In addition, it appears to play a role in primary erythroblast differentiation [47] as well as in megacaryocyte differentiation where it is activated in a MAPK-dependent manner [48]. More recently, it has also been involved in HSC and uncommitted progenitor proliferation and survival through its effects on cell cycle control [45, 46]. A growing body of evidences is unravelling the role of CREB in the regulation of the immune system [49]. Indeed, several immune-related genes contain a cAMP responsive element, as in the case of IL-2, IL-6, IL-10 and TNF-α. In monocytes and macrophages CREB exerts anti-apoptotic survival effects. Moreover, CREB promotes normal B and T cell survival and proliferation when it is phosphorylated in response to signalling by the B-cell receptor or different kinases [49]. Particularly well characterized is the regulatory role that CREB plays in the nervous system. Actually, numerous papers have demonstrated CREB involvement in promoting neuronal survival, precursor proliferation, neurite outgrowth and neuronal differentiation in certain neuronal populations [50], highlighting the importance of CREB signalling in learning and memory processes in several organisms [2, 51].

In the late 1980s, it was discovered that cAMP mediates the hormonal stimulation of several cellular processes by regulating the phosphorylation of critical proteins among which CREB transcription factor [52]. Although it was initially identified as a target of the cAMP signalling pathway, studies on activation of immediate-early genes revealed that CREB is a substrate for kinases other than cAMP-dependent protein kinase A (PKA) and that various signalling routes converge on CREB and CREM, controlling their function by modulating their phosphorylation states [52, 53]. As above mentioned, almost all the signalling pathways that activate CREB lead to the phosphorylation of Ser133, which is required for CREB-induced gene transcription, but additional sites on CREB or on linked proteins can be phosphorylated exerting a modulation of CREB activity [35]. For example, Ser133 phosphorylation primes CREB for phosphorylation by Glycogen synthase kinase 3 (GSK-3) at Ser129. However, unlike Ser133 phosphorylation, the physiologic consequences of Ser129 phosphorylation are not well defined, although evidence suggests that it is also linked to CREB activation [54]. In different systems a number of different kinases have been shown to stimulate CREB phosphorylation and several CREB kinase candidates have been identified so far. PKA, which is activated by cAMP, is the major kinase that targets Ser133 in many processes [1, 3]. Other signalling molecules responsible for CREB Ser133 phosphorylation include mitogen- and stress-activated kinase 1 (MSK-1), extracellular signal-regulated kinase (ERK), calcium/calmodulin-dependent kinases (CaMKs), p90 ribosomal S6 kinase (RSK), MAPKs and Akt/protein kinase B (PKB) [1, 3, 7, 55, 56]. Both MAPK and Akt have been shown to enhance the survival of cultured cells by stimulating CREB-dependent target gene expression [56]. CREB activity is also regulated by a family of cytoplasmic co-activators known as transducers of regulated CREB activity (TORCs) and including TORC1, TORC2 and TORC3. TORCs are activated by extracellular stimuli represented by nutrients (glucose) and hormones. Once activated, they translocate into the nucleus where they bind to the bZIP domain of CREB exerting its activation through a phospho-Ser133-independent mechanism. All TORCs are regarded as strong activators of CREB-dependent transcription [57].

In Fig. 1 the main factors and signalling molecules leading to CREB activation in haematopoietic cells are schematically represented.

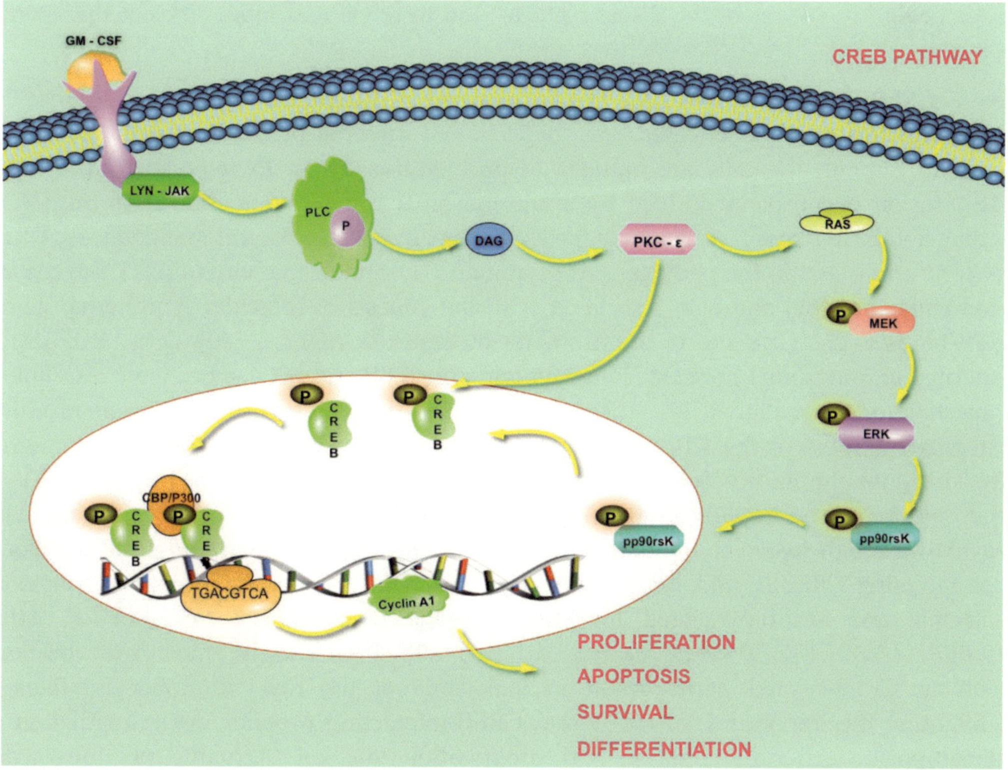

Figure 1. Schematic representation of the main factors and signalling molecules leading to CREB activation in haematopoietic cells. A various array of extracellular stimuli promote CREB activation through phosphorylation or through interaction with CREB co-activators to enhance the expression of CREB responsive genes. CREB target genes, including Cyclin A1, are able to mediate effects on cellular proliferation, apoptosis, survival and differentiation. PLC: phospholipase-C; DAG: 1,2-diacylglycerol; PKC-ε: protein kinase C-ε.

5. CREB family members and leukemogenesis

Recent data suggest that CREB acts as a proto-oncogene in haematopoietic cells and contributes to the leukaemia phenotype [37, 38, 45, 46]. It has been shown anyway that CREB is able to promote tumour formation only when other oncogenes are also activated. In fact, its overexpression is not sufficient to induce acute leukaemia *in vivo*. This is consistent with similar observations obtained with translocations, such as AML1-ETO (Acute Myeloid Leukaemia Eight-Twenty-One), a chimeric protein that requires additional mutations to develop leukaemia in mouse models [58]. In previous works different strategies have been delineated to identify the oncogenes cooperating with CREB to drive leukemogenesis: one way is represented by crossing different transgenic mice of known oncogenes such as *K-RAS*, *MEIS 1*, *PML/RARα* etc. to *CREB* transgenic mice; another approach consists in infecting *CREB* transgenics with a retrovirus such as the Molony murine leukaemia virus to insertionally activate cooperating oncogenes. The latter approach has also the potential to identify novel collaborators of CREB besides the already known CBP and p300. Identifying novel oncogenic alterations that cause leukaemia and discovering the signalling pathways involved will be of great value to gain a better knowledge of the disease and to lead to novel and more efficient therapeutic measures.

Several CREB family members have been implicated in different malignant conditions. The first malignancy to be discovered was the clear cell sarcoma of the soft tissue (CSST). In this solid tumour, the cells are induced to proliferation by an Ewing's Sarcoma (EWS)-ATF-1 fusion oncoprotein derived by a chromosomal translocation that fuses the DNA-binding and bZip domain of ATF-1 to the EWS gene. In haematological malignancies, CREB has been implicated in the pathogenesis of human T lymphotropic virus I (HTLV-I) related T-cell leukaemia [59] and also associated with the genesis of follicular lymphoma, where CREB binds to the CRE site in the promoter of translocated Bcl-2 [46]. Other leukaemia-associated chromosomal translocations involving the CBP and p300 genes were also linked to haematological malignancies. These translocations generally result in fusion products that preserve most of the CBP and p300 molecules, suggesting that the disease mechanism does not simply involve loss of function of CBP, as is the case in Rubinstein-Taybi syndrome, but often implies an altered cofactor function (dominant positive or dominant negative) through fusion to another molecule. The most frequent chromosomal translocations targeting *CREBBP* and *EP300* have been described in specific subtypes of myeloid leukaemia and are represented by Mixed-Lineage Leukaemia 1 (*MLL)-EP300*, *MLL-CREBBP*, *MOZ-CREBBP* and *MOZ-EP300* [37, 60]. Interestingly, most translocations involving CREB-related genes result in leukaemia of the myeloid/monocytic lineage, highlighting the importance of CREB and CREB-interacting proteins in the regulation of haematopoietic cell differentiation and proliferation [45, 46]. Actually, previous work demonstrated that bone marrow cells from patients with acute myeloid or lymphoid leukaemia expressed higher levels of CREB compared to patients not affected by leukaemia or with normal bone marrow [60]. Moreover, it appears that an elevated CREB expression is associated with an increased risk of relapse or persistent disease and decreased event-free survival [45]. This is consistent with the observation that leukaemia cell lines expressing CREB at elevated levels show an increased growth/proliferation rate in normal conditions and an increased survival when exposed to stress like serum starvation [61]. On the contrary, down-regulation of endogenous CREB in leukaemia cell lines by siRNA resulted in reduced cell viability [20, 45], indicating that CREB is a critical regulator of growth and survival in both myeloid and lymphoid leukaemia cells. Unfortunately, chromosomal translocations have also been involved in drug-induced leukaemia. For instance, the involvement of 11q23-balanced translocations in acute leukaemia after treatment with drugs that inhibit the function of DNA topoisomerase II (topo II) is being recognized with increasing frequency. It has been shown that the gene at 11q23, involved in all of these treatment-related leukaemias, is *MLL* (also called ALL1, Htrx, and HRX). In general, the translocations occurring in these leukaemias are the same as those occurring in *de novo* leukaemia [eg. t(9;11), t(11;19), and t(4;11)]. Interestingly, the t(11;16)(q23;p13.3) has been cloned and has been shown to involve both *MLL* and *CREBBP* [62]. Besides chromosomal translocations, another way for CREB to contribute to tumorigenesis is through the suppression of cellular genes either by competing with or binding to sites occupied by other transcription factors or by confiscating the transcriptional machinery [63].

5.1. Acute myeloid leukaemia

Acute leukaemia derives from the clonal expansion of haematopoietic stem/progenitor cells that have lost their ability to undergo terminal differentiation. Since transcription factors control HSC production and differentiation, it is conceivable that disorders of the haematopoietic system often involve alterations of the regulatory network of transcription factors. In haematological malignancies transcription factors can be overexpressed, involved in chromosomal translocations or become targets of somatic mutations that disrupt their normal function [37, 60-63]. Previous studies have demonstrated that *CREB* is a proto-oncogene whose overexpression promotes cellular proliferation in haematopoietic cells [1, 3]. The abnormal proliferation and survival of myeloid cells *in vitro* and *in vivo* appears to be due to the up-regulation of CREB target genes such as *Cyclin A1* [60, 63]. Transgenic mice that overexpress CREB in myeloid cells develop a myeloproliferative disease with splenomegaly and aberrant myelopoiesis. However, CREB overexpressing mice do not spontaneously develop acute myeloid leukaemia (AML) [61]. To identify genes that accelerate leukaemia in CREB transgenic mice retroviral insertional mutagenesis has been used. The mutagenesis screen identified several integration sites, including oncogenes *Gfi1*, *Myb*, and *Ras*. Among transcription factors, *Sox4* was identified with the screen as a gene that cooperates with *CREB* in myeloid leukemogenesis by contributing to increased proliferation of haematopoietic progenitor cells [64]. Moreover, chromatin immunoprecipitation assays have demonstrated that *CREB* is a direct target of *Sox4*. In fact, it has been shown that the transduction of *CREB* transgenic mouse bone marrow cells with a Sox4 retrovirus increases survival and self-renewal of cells *in vitro* and results in increased expression of CREB target genes. Consistently, leukaemia blasts from the majority of AML patients have higher levels of CREB, phospho-CREB, and Sox4 protein expression in the bone marrow [64]. The increase in both CREB protein and mRNA levels in primary AML cells is possibly due to *CREB* gene amplification in the blast cells. Furthermore, a higher level of CREB has been found to correlate with a less favourable prognosis and an increased risk of relapse and decreased event-free survival in a small cohort of AML patients [45, 61]. Generally, AML in adults has a 20% five-year disease free survival despite treatment with aggressive cytotoxic chemotherapy and two thirds of AML patients do not experience significant periods of remission. Therefore, in light of its important role in the pathogenesis of leukaemia, CREB has been indicated as a potential prognostic marker of disease progression in AML and a molecular target for future treatment of leukaemia.

Clinical and experimental findings underline that AML is induced by numerous functionally cooperating genetic alterations, including chromosomal translocations that lead to the expression of fusion proteins often behaving as aberrant transcription factors. Several AML-associated lesions target chromatin regulators like histone methyltransferases or histone acetyltransferases, including MLL1 or CBP/p300 [65]. As already mentioned, CBP is an adapter protein that is involved in regulating transcription and histone acetylation, through which it is thought to contribute to an increased level of gene expression. The *CBP* gene was recently identified as a partner gene in the t(8;16) that occurs in *de novo* acute myelomonocytic leukaemia (AML-M4) and rarely in treatment-related AML [66]. The fusion gene could alter the CBP protein so that it becomes constitutively active or, alternatively, it could modify the chromatin-association functions of *MLL* gene [38, 40]. *MLL* and *HOXB4*, a member of the homeobox domain transcription factors, have been identified as regulators of HSC maturation during early haematopoiesis [67]. *HOXB4* belongs to the *HOX* genes, a family of oncogenes implicated in the pathogenesis of various human cancers and highly expressed in the majority of AML. In a recent report Wang et al. [54] demonstrated the association of CREB and its co-activators TORC and CBP with homeodomain protein MEIS1, a HOX DNA-binding cofactor and critical downstream mediator of the *MLL* oncogenic program. This MEIS-CREB nexus is regulated by GSK-3, a multi-functional serine/threonine kinase that impairs the proliferation and induces the differentiation of a variety of cancers, including leukaemias, induced by *MLL* oncogenes. This kinase mediates CREB activation through phosphorylation at Ser129. In fact, CREB Ser129 mutation antagonizes *HOX/MEIS* activity and decreases colony-forming abilities of *HOX/MEIS* or *MLL* transformed cells. These and other similar observations provide a molecular rationale for targeting *HOX*-associated transcription through GSK-3 inhibition in a subset of leukaemias.

Myelodysplastic syndromes (MDS) include a heterogeneous group of clonal haematopoietic stem cell malignancies with significant morbidity and high mortality. The incidence of MDS increases markedly with age and the disease is most prevalent in individuals who are white and male. Because of an ageing population and an improving awareness of the disease, the documented disease burden is expected to worsen in the near future. Due to the poor survival of individuals with MDS, it is important to identify prognostic factors to better risk-stratify patients for more effective treatments [68]. Genomic instability is associated with progression of the disease so that a part of patients develops AML. It has been reported that an increased incidence of haematological malignancies occurs in *CREBBP* heterozygous mice and other authors have shown that *CREBBP* is one of the genes altered by chromosomal translocations in patients suffering from therapy-related myelodysplastic syndrome [69]. Moreover, it has been demonstrated that *CREBBP*(+/-) mice invariably develop myelodysplastic/myeloproliferative neoplasm within 9-12 months of age. They are also hypersensitive to ionizing radiation and show a marked decrease in poly(ADP-ribose) polymerase-1 activity after irradiation. In addition, protein levels of XRCC1 (X-ray repair complementing defective repair in Chinese hamster cells 1) and APEX1 (APEX nuclease), key components of base excision repair machinery, are reduced in un-irradiated *CREBBP*(+/-) cells or upon targeted knockdown of *CREBBP* levels. These results provide validation of a new myelodysplastic/myeloproliferative neoplasm mouse model and, more importantly, point at a defective repair of DNA damage as a contributing factor to the pathogenesis of this currently incurable disease [46].

5.2. Acute lymphoblastic leukaemia

Acute lymphoblastic leukaemia (ALL) is a heterogeneous disease characterized by the predominance of immature haematopoietic cells, in which malignant cells express phenotypes of either T-cell or B-cell lineages [61]. ALLs account for the 25-30% of all cancer diagnoses in children. CREB involvement in the molecular events related to *in vitro* and *in vivo* lymphoblastic proliferation is still little known, whereas a lot of evidences disclose a role of *CREB* as a proto-oncogene in haematopoiesis and in AML. *CREB* can be overexpressed in the 84% of ALL patients (73/86) at diagnosis but neither in remission nor in non-leukaemia samples [70]. By contrast, the parallel expression of the cAMP early inducible repressor (*ICER*), which represses CREB activity by competing for the CRE consensus site, appears down-regulated at diagnosis but neither in remission nor in control samples [70]. Thus, it is presumable that *CREB* overexpression leads to target gene up-regulation and increase in cell proliferation and survival that are not counteracted by the insufficient level of *ICER* expression. Besides this hypothesis, Pigazzi et al. [71] have also demonstrated the co-expression of miR34b in *CREB* overexpressing myeloid leukaemia cells providing new information about myeloid transformation and therapeutic strategies. Despite the apparently good prognosis, the 15% of high hyper-diploid (HD) childhood ALL cases relapse [72, 73]. Relapsed ALL is a leading cause of death due to disease in young people, but the molecular mechanisms of treatment failure are still to be elucidated. Genome-wide profiling of structural DNA alterations in ALL identified multiple sub-microscopic somatic mutations targeting key cellular pathways and demonstrated evolution in genetic alterations from diagnosis to relapse [74]. Many of the mutations that have been identified concern the transcriptional co-activators *CREBBP* and *NCOR1*, the transcription factors *ERG*, *SPI1*, *TCF4* and *TCF7L2*, components of the Ras signalling pathway, histone genes, genes involved in histone modification (*CREBBP* and *CTCF*) and genes target of DNA copy number alterations [74]. The parallel analysis of an extended cohort of diagnosis-relapsed cases and acute leukaemia cases that did not relapse showed that the 18.3% of relapsed cases had sequence or deletion mutations of *CREBBP* [72, 74]. *CREBBP* is expressed in leukaemia cells and normal B-cell progenitors, and the mutant *CREBBP* alleles are expressed in ALL cell lines harbouring mutations. Mutations at diagnosis or acquired at relapse consist in truncated alleles or deleterious substitutions in conserved residues of the histone acetyltransferase domain, impairing histone acetylation and transcriptional regulation of *CREBBP* targets, including glucocorticoid responsive genes. In mice the homozygous deletion of *CREBBP* or *EP300* is lethal due to developmental abnormalities whereas *CREBBP*(+/−) mice show defects in B lymphoid development and an increased incidence of haematopoietic tumours [75]. Both *CREBBP* and *EP300* sequence mutations have been reported in solid tumours and, more recently, also in haematological malignancies, whereas rare *EP300* mutations have been detected in an ALL cell lines and myelodysplasia [74, 76]. A lot of detected mutations at relapse, the same identified at diagnosis in other clones, prove that mutations confer resistance to therapy. Many identified mutations are target in transcriptional and epigenetic regulation as a mechanism of resistance in ALL. It is worth outlining that the high incidence of *CREBBP* mutations found in relapse-prone HD ALL cases discloses the possibility of a targeted customized treatment in this genetic subgroup [73].

In our laboratory we have investigated the role of PI3K/Akt pathway and CREB family members in a number of lymphoid and erythroleukaemia cell lines treated with chemical and physical agents inducing cell death by apoptosis or necrosis [20, 21, 47, 77-80]. We first detected with Western Blotting a high constitutive level of CREB phosphorylation at Ser133 in Jurkat T cells under normal serum culture conditions [20]. Under low serum culture conditions, an early (within 1 h) and transient increase in CREB phosphorylation was observed in response to TRAIL treatment and reduced upon pre-treatment with LY294002 or SB253580, demonstrating the PI3K/Akt- and p38 MAPK-dependency of this effect. Interestingly, both phospho-CREB and phospho-ATF-1 were down-regulated in response to TRAIL treatment of normal primary cells derived from haematopoietic precursors (HUVEC, HEMA), whereas both of them were up-regulated in the neoplastic counterparts (K562 cell line) [20, 21]. The PI3K/Akt pathway dependency of CREB/ATF-1 phosphorylation induced by TRAIL treatment was demonstrated both in primary cells and in leukaemia cell lines of different origin and TRAIL sensitivity, showing that the observed phenomenon is a general feature of TRAIL action in leukaemia [77, 80]. In addition, the observation of CREB cleavage products upon TRAIL/LY294002 combined treatment of sensitive leukaemia cells was consistent with previous reports on other neoplastic cell lines [81] and compatible with the TRAIL-mediated activation of the caspase cascade and cleavage of anti-apoptotic molecules. The parallel analysis with immune fluorescence demonstrated the nuclear translocation of the phosphorylated form of CREB upon treatment with 100 ng/mL TRAIL, whereas the immune labelling was mainly detectable in the cytoplasm compartment upon the higher more cytotoxic dose (1000 ng/mL) as shown in Fig. 2. A further enhancement of apoptotic cell death was obtained with the use of CREB1 siRNA technology leading us to hypothesize that CREB activation can have an important role in the complex crosstalk among pro- and anti-apoptotic pathways in Jurkat T cells [20, 80].

5.3. Chronic myelogenous leukaemia

Chronic myelogenous leukaemia (CML) is characterized in the 85-90% of the cases by the presence of the Philadelphia (Ph) chromosome and the *BCR-ABL* fusion gene. A further 5-10% of the cases display other translocations, most commonly complex variants, that involve one or more chromosomal regions in addition to bands 9q34 and 22q11, but also simple variants that typically involve 22q11 and a chromosome other than 9q34. However, genes that cooperate with *BCR-ABL* leading to acute leukaemia are not well understood neither the role played by CREB in CML has been clarified. Preliminary observations of the group of Kathleen Sakamoto indicate that CREB is highly expressed in blood and bone marrow cells from patients with CML in chronic phase, but not in normal bone marrow cells

[82]. The same authors previously showed that inhibition of CREB by using RNA interference (RNAi) technology resulted in decreased proliferation and survival of bcr-abl-expressing K562 cells [45, 83], whereas other authors reported that CREB antisense oligonucleotides were able to induce death of human leukaemia cells and bone marrow cells from patients affected with both AML and CML [84]. A critical factor for the genesis of acute leukaemia or acute transformation of CML appears to be the formation of fusion genes between *NUP98* and members of the *HOX* gene family [85]. Interestingly, all the NUP98-HOX-involved fusion products exhibit dual binding ability to both CREB binding protein, a co-activator, and histone deacetylase 1, a co-repressor, acting as both trans-activators and trans-repressors and contributing to the genesis of acute leukaemia or acute transformation of CML [86].

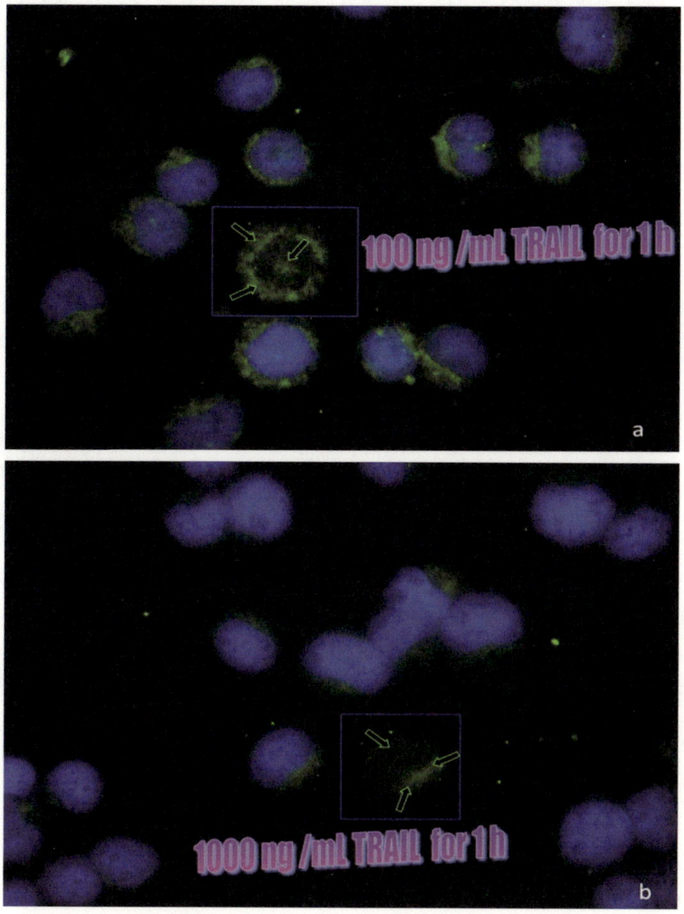

Figure 2. a, b: Phospho-CREB localization in Jurkat T cells upon TRAIL treatment. An evident nuclear translocation of phospho-CREB (green fluorescence) was detected upon 1 h treatment only with the lower dose of TRAIL (panel a), whereas the labelling was located at cytoplasm level upon the higher more cytotoxic dose (panel b). Nuclei were counterstained with 6-diamino-2-phenylindole (DAPI) (blue fluorescence). Green and blue fluorescence single emissions are overlapped in the merge panels. The insets show green fluorescence single emission. Original magnification: 40X. The figure has been adapted from [20].

5.4. Chronic lymphocytic leukaemia

Chronic lymphocytic leukaemia (CLL) originates from the abnormal accumulation of antigen-stimulated B cells that escape normal cell death mechanisms and/or undergo increased proliferation [87]. CLL is the most prevalent adult leukaemia in the Western world, yet no curative treatment exists. Many studies have explored the use of family-specific cyclic nucleotide phosphodiesterase (PDE) inhibitors in light of the potent effects of cAMP signalling on immune system function [88, 89]. Among the 11 currently known families of cyclic nucleotide PDEs, all but three are capable of catabolizing cAMP and at least 5 PDE families (PDE1-4, PDE7 and PDE8) are expressed in lymphoid cells and regulated by either mitogens or agents that induce cAMP-mediated signalling. Previous work has established that inhibition of PDE4 is sufficient to selectively induce apoptosis in CLL cells by increasing the concentration of cAMP [88]. In a recent paper Meyers et al. [89] examined how CLL cells differ from normal haematopoietic cells with regard to their sensitivity to PDE4 inhibitor-mediated cAMP accumulation, CREB phosphorylation and gene expression. Interestingly, it was discovered that upon exposure to rolipram, a prototypical PDE4 inhibitor, cAMP intracellular levels rapidly rose in both CLL and normal B cells, whereas no such increase was detected in T cells. Likewise, ATF-1/CREB Ser63/133 phosphorylation was induced by rolipram in nearly all CLL and B cells, whereas normal T cells displayed a lower response. Based on these findings and on previous observations of a reduced basal cAMP signalling in CLL cells, the authors suggested the involvement of specific PDE or splice isoforms in the reduced basal apoptotic index of CLL cells [89]. Looking for etiological agents, other authors have identified a stromal cell–derived factor-1 (SDF-1)-dependent mechanism as a microenvironmental regulatory mechanism of CLL cell survival [90]. It is known that SDF-1 is a chemokine that plays an important role in B-cell development. In fact, high levels of SDF-1 are produced by stromal cells within the marrow to retain B-cell precursors in close contact with them, within the supportive haematopoietic microenvironment [91], and to prevent their premature release into the circulation. Upon *in vitro* treatment of CLL cells with synthetic SDF-1α, a rapid and transient activation of p44/42 MAPK (ERK1/2) signalling pathway was observed and related to CLL cell survival. Downward MAPK activation transcription-dependent and -independent mechanisms were involved. In fact, MAPK was able to promote cell survival directly by inactivating the pro-apoptotic BAD protein and indirectly by activating CREB, which, in turn, is important for the transcriptional up-regulation of the anti-apoptotic *BCL-2* gene [92]. Thus, SDF-1 engages B lineage CLL cells through the stromal cell receptor CXCR4 and affects components of the cell death machinery, leading to the noted resistance of CLL cells to apoptosis.

5.5. Human T Lymphotropic Virus 1 (HTLV-1) related T cell leukaemia

Human T-cell leukaemia virus type-I (HTLV-1) is the first discovered human retrovirus [93]. It has been recognized as the etiological agent of an aggressive malignancy known as adult T-cell leukaemia (ATL) as well as of the neurological syndrome TSP/HAM and of other clinical disorders. *In vitro* HTLV-1 is able to infect a number of different cell types, whereas in natural human infections it generally targets mature CD4+ helper T cells or, less frequently, CD8+ T cells. Although the mechanism of HTLV-1 pathogenicity is not fully understood yet, it is widely believed that a virally encoded trans-activator protein, called Tax, is centrally involved in this mechanism. In a recent review Azran et al. [94] provide valuable insights into the molecular mechanisms of HTLV-1 leukemogenesis. In particular, the authors detail the signalling pathways recruited by Tax to set infected T cells into continuous uncontrolled replication and to destabilize their genome, enabling, thereby, accumulation of mutations that can contribute to the leukemogenic process. Tax is able to modulate the expression of many viral genes via the viral long terminal repeat (LTR) and cellular genes through the CREB/ATF-, AP-1-, serum responsive factor (SRF)- and NF-κB-associated pathways, employing the CBP/p300 and p/CAF (p300/CBP-associated factor) co-activators for achieving the full transcriptional activation competence of each of these pathways. It is worth noting that Tax responsive elements (TxRE) contain a centered sequence TGACG(T/A)(C/G)(T/A) that is imperfectly homologous to the consensus cAMP responsive element (CRE; TGACGTCA). Thus, the presence of Tax is necessary for CREB to form a stable complex with the viral CRE. In fact, by interacting with the bZIP region of CREB, Tax enhances CREB dimerization and increases, thereby, its affinity to CRE. In particular, it has been recently shown that CREB is the most prominent factor that cooperates with Tax in activating HTLV-1 LTR region expression [95]. Moreover, it has been demonstrated that while, in the absence of Tax, CREB can activate HTLV-1 LTR expression only if phosphorylated by PKA, another member of the family, namely CREB2, can markedly activate the viral LTR without phosphorylation and can mediate a much stronger activation of the viral LTR by Tax than CREB does [94, 96]. Interestingly, mutant models disrupting Tax activation of the CREB protein resulted in the preferential immortalization of CD8+ lymphocytes, rather than CD4+ lymphocytes, whereas the disruption of Tax interaction with CBP did not affect lymphocyte immortalization [97].

5.6. Lymphoma

Lymphomas are haematological malignancies of the lymphoid system. Deregulated gene expression is a hallmark of cancer and is well documented in B-cell lymphomas [98]. B cells are particularly susceptible to malignant transformation since the mechanisms involved in antibody diversification can cause chromosomal translocations and oncogenic mutations. B-cell lymphomas include Hodgkin lymphoma (HL) and non-Hodgkin lymphoma (B-NHL). B-NHL consists of a heterogeneous group of diseases whose pathogenesis is associated with multiple genetic lesions affecting oncogenes and tumour-suppressor genes and whose treatment is related to the different grade of malignancy. The most common type of B-NHL is represented by the diffuse large B-cell lymphoma (DLBCL), which generally arises as a clinical evolution of the follicular lymphoma (FL). A number of papers have demonstrated the involvement of CREB family members in the pathogenesis of lymphoma. It has been previously found that CREB acts as a positive regulator of the translocated *BCL-2* allele in FLs with the t(14;18) translocation [60] and that the high constitutive expression of *ATF-3* is linked to the viability of Hodgkin/Reed-Sternberg cells and, thus, considered as a molecular hallmark of classical HL [99]. More recently, a number of studies have disclosed the implication of the HAT proteins CBP and p300 as tumour suppressors in B-cell neoplasms [100-102]. Nevertheless, the various mechanisms through which each of these cofactors specifically contributes to lymphomagenesis are still to be elucidated. As before mentioned, CBP and p300 function as co-activators of transcription factors and acetylate proteins relevant to lymphomagenesis such as p53, NF-κB, Bcl-6 and Hsp90 [100, 103, 104]. In particular, p300 acts as a co-activator of NF-κB, activates p53 but attenuates Hsp90 chaperone functions and, moreover, transcriptional repressor *BCL-6* is frequently translocated and hyper-mutated in DLBCL where it results inversely correlated with p300 [100]. Importantly, de-acetylated Hsp90 represses p53 but maintains *BCL-6* expression, which suppresses p300 and its essential cofactor BAT3, which is necessary for p53 acetylation and activation. Somatic heterozygous mutations or deletions of the *CREBBP* locus occur in more than the 50% of DLBCL and the 32% of FL cases, whereas *EP300* mutations occur in the 10% of DLBCLs. All cases seem to have in common the disruption of the HAT catalytic domain, and the resulting truncated or mutant proteins may have dominant negative or gain of function properties, or may simply result in a reduced dosage of histone acetyltransferases. Structural alterations inactivating *CREBBP* and, less often, *EP300* have been recently documented and linked to the pathogenesis of both most common types of B-NHL [102]. According to Pasqualucci et al. [102] point mutations at the HAT coding domain of *CREBBP* and *EP300* result in specific defects in acetylation-mediated inactivation of the Bcl-6 oncoprotein and activation of the p53 tumour-suppressor, representing major pathogenetic mechanisms shared by the most common forms of B-NHL. Suppression of p300 either through Bcl-6 or inactivating mutations plays a key role in DLBCL. In fact, treatment of DLBCL cells with Bcl-6 inhibitors leads to p300 protein expression and acetyltransferase activity with subsequent acetylation of p53 (which induces p53 transcriptional functions) and Hsp90 (which suppresses Hsp90 chaperone activity) [100]. Moreover, the combination of Bcl-6 and histone deacetylase inhibitors (HDACI) leads to even higher p300 activity and synergistic killing of lymphoma cells *in vitro* and *in vivo* [100]. Interestingly, the direct effect of HDACI on non-histone proteins as DNA binding transcriptional factors (NF-κB, p53, CREB, GATA, c-myc, Bcl-6, E2F, IRF) can also affect cell growth and differentiation [101]. Furthermore, in light of HDACI effects on cell cycle regulatory molecules (Cyclin D1, p21 and p27) there is enough evidence that indicates these novel pleiotropic drugs as promising compounds for the treatment of B- and even T-cell malignancies in addition to conventional chemotherapy [105].

5.7. Multiple myeloma

Multiple myeloma (MM), also known as plasma cell myeloma or Kahler's disease, is a B-cell malignancy characterized by the accumulation in the bone marrow of plasma cells with a low proliferation index and an extended life span. Most cases of myeloma also feature the production of a paraprotein, an abnormal antibody that can cause kidney problems. MM cell lines as well as *de novo* MM cells express multiple anti-apoptotic proteins, often do not encode functional p53 and frequently contain a dysregulated Akt pathway [104-107]. A number of factors related to MM cell growth and survival and linked to CREB family members have been identified [108]. Among these factors, the myeloid cell leukaemia-1 (Mcl-1) protein, an anti-apoptotic member of the Bcl-2 family, has been considered as a critical regulator of MM cell survival and proposed as an attractive therapeutic target [108]. *Mcl-1* is an immediate early gene activated in response to GM-CSF and IL-3. It has been previously reported that *Mcl-1* activation can occur in dependence of the PI3K/Akt pathway through a transcription factor complex containing CREB [109]. Recent reports have demonstrated that Mcl-1 specific down-regulation or repression is able to initiate apoptosis in MM [110]. To this end, proteasome inhibitors like bortezomib have been used though with contrasting results. In fact, it has been shown that accumulated and cleaved Mcl-1 products by proteasome inhibition have either a pro- or an anti-apoptotic function. In particular, Hu et al. [111] have investigated the role of endoplasmic reticulum unfolded protein response (UPR) in order to unravel the mechanisms underlying Mcl-1 accumulation following treatment with proteasome inhibitors, discovering the enhanced translation of ATF-4, an important effector of UPR, upon proteasome inhibition, and indicating ATF-4 as responsible for bortezomib resistance of MM [111]. Besides Mcl-1, novel factors are being identified as important players in the pathogenesis of MM. Recent studies have suggested that X-box–binding protein 1 (XBP1), a bZIP transcription factor of the CREB/ATF family, has an important role in the survival of MM cells [112]. XBP1 is required for B lymphocyte terminal differentiation to plasma cells and is essential for immunoglobulin secretion. Abundant or deregulated expression of *XBP1* has been detected in MM cells [113, 114] and in hepatocellular carcinomas [115]. Due to the production of abundant immunoglobulins and cytokines, MM cells must be able to survive under conditions of chronic ER stress involving UPR and including constitutive activation of the ER-located transmembrane kinase/endoribonuclease (RNase) protein IRE1α-XBP1 pathway. This pathway, implicated in the proliferation and survival of MM cells, has been considered as a prognostic factor [116] and, moreover, as a possible target of chemo/immunotherapy [114, 117]. A growing body of evidence attributes a pathogenetic role to several microRNAs (miRNA) resulting up-regulated in MM and targeting p/CAF, a positive regulator of p53 [118]. Other authors have indicated a possible role of CREB family members in IL-6-mediated effects on myeloma cell growth and survival [119].

6. Concluding remarks

CREB/ATF family is a growing family of transcription factors involved in a number of physiological and pathological processes. Day by day, new family members are being identified for their primary role in normal or aberrant haematopoiesis and proposed as therapeutic targets of anticancer drugs [112]. In fact, by regulating gene expression, transcription factors are often the final mediators of such central processes as proliferation, survival, self-renewal and invasion. Based on these effects, it is conceivable that inhibition of transcription factors can revert the malignant behaviour of many tumour types and can potentially achieve a very high therapeutic index [86]. Actually, in light of its important role in the pathogenesis of leukaemia, CREB has been indicated as a potential prognostic marker of disease progression in AML and a molecular target for future treatment of leukaemia. In addition, CREB has also been implicated in many solid tumours including hepatocellular carcinoma, osteosarcoma, lung adenocarcinoma, melanoma and lymphoma [46]. Indeed, since *CREB* overexpression results in a poor prognosis for the patient, the regulation of CREB activity might represent a useful strategy to treat solid tumours like prostate, breast and lung cancer, as well as haematological malignancies like AML and lymphoma. However, a key question concerns whether the activation of CREB (or other transcription factors) seen in cancer cells is directly driving the cell malignant phenotype, or whether it is merely a by-product of activation of one of the upstream pathways or only a partner in a more complex scenario. This is a crucial point, since CREB would represent a good molecular target only if it were a main player in the specific tumour biology. Unfortunately, clinical and experimental evidences suggest that several functionally cooperating genetic alterations, including chromosomal translocations, lead to the expression of fusion proteins that play a key role in the pathogenesis of the leukaemia phenotype. CREB itself can promote cellular transformation as a fusion protein or by cooperating with other oncogenes or transcription factors. Furthermore, due to the recruitment of chromatin modulating mechanisms in the transforming activity of leukemogenic factors, transcriptional therapies aimed at inhibiting DNA methyltransferases, histone deacetylases or acetyltransferases, like CBP and p300, are emerging as new frontiers for cancer treatment. Unlike HDACI, which have been used in several phase I/II clinical trials, HAT inhibitors have been less extensively investigated for their potential use in cancer therapy. Indeed, interesting results obtained with clinical treatment of solid tumours [120] suggest that p300 inhibition may be a promising anticancer approach. To overcome the numerous side effects and the mostly transient clinical responses exerted by epigenetic compounds used as a single treatment [121], combinatorial therapy involving epigenetic agents together with conventional or targeted agents is increasingly seen as a more attractive opportunity. Therefore, further preclinical investigations aimed at better dissecting epigenetic mechanisms driving induction, maintenance and potential reversibility of the leukaemia state are welcome and functional to select the most potent drugs and combinations and to develop more efficient and long-lasting targeted therapeutic strategies. We hope to have contributed with this chapter to make the state of the art on the role of CREB in leukaemia and lymphoma neoplasms in order to allow further steps moving ahead from bench to bedside.

Acknowledgements

This book chapter was supported by funds of the Italian Ministry of University and Research (MIUR) granted in 2011 to Prof. Roberta Di Pietro.

Author details

Francesca D'Auria[1] and Roberta Di Pietro[2*]

*Address all correspondence to: r.dipietro@unich.it

1 Department of Cardiac and Vascular Surgery, Campus Bio-Medico University of Rome, Italy

2 Department of Medicine and Ageing Sciences, G. d'Annunzio University of Chieti-Pescara, Italy

References

[1] Sassone-Corsi P. Transcription factors responsive to cAMP. Annu Rev Cell Dev Biol. 1995;11: 355-77.

[2] Alberini CM. Transcription factors in long-term memory and synaptic plasticity. Physiol Rev. 2009;89(1): 121-45.

[3] Montminy M. Transcriptional regulation by cyclic AMP. Annu Rev Biochem.1997;66: 807–22.

[4] Persengiev SP, Green MR. The role of CREB/ATF family members in cell growth, survival and apoptosis. Apoptosis. 2003;8(3): 225-28.

[5] Lu D, Wolfgang CD, Hai T. Activating transcription factor 3, a stress-inducible gene, suppresses Ras-stimulated tumorigenesis. J Biol Chem. 2006;281(15): 10473-81.

[6] Don J, Stelzer G. The expanding family of CREB/CREM transcription factors that are involved with spermatogenesis. Mol Cell Endocrinol. 2002;187(1-2): 115-24.

[7] Mayr B, Montminy M. Transcriptional regulation by the phosphorylation-dependent factor CREB. Nat Rev Mol Cell Biol. 2001;2: 599-609.

[8] Salameh A, Galvagni F, Anselmi F, De Clemente C, Orlandini M, Oliviero S. Growth factor stimulation induces cell survival by c-Jun. ATF2-dependent activation of Bcl-XL. J Biol Chem. 2010;285(30): 23096-104.

[9] Hai T, Curran T. Cross-family dimerization of transcription factors Fos/Jun and ATF/CREB alters DNA binding specificity. Proc Natl Acad Sci U S A. 1991;88(9): 3720-24.

[10] De Cesare D, Vallone D, Caracciolo A, Sassone-Corsi P, Nerlov C, Verde P. Heterodimerization of c-Jun with ATF-2 and c-Fos is required for positive and negative regulation of the human urokinase enhancer. Oncogene. 1995;11(2): 365-76.

[11] Benbrook DM, Jones NC. Different binding specificities and transactivation of variant CRE's by CREB complexes. Nucleic Acids Res. 1994;22(8): 1463-69.

[12] Hayes, JD, McMahon M. Molecular basis for the contribution of the antioxidant response element to cancer chemoprevention. Cancer Letters. 2001;174(2): 103-13.

[13] Hai T, Wolfgang CD, Marsee DK, Allen AE, Sivaprasad U. ATF3 and stress responses. Gene Expr. 1999;7(4-6): 321-35.

[14] Wek RC, Anthony TG. EXtENDINg beta cell survival by UPRegulating ATF4 translation. Cell Metab. 2006;4(5): 333-34.

[15] Hai T, Wolford CC, Chang YS. ATF3, a hub of the cellular adaptive-response network, in the pathogenesis of diseases: is modulation of inflammation a unifying component? Gene Expr. 2010;15(1): 1-11.

[16] Han SI, Yasuda K, Kataoka K. ATF2 interacts with beta-cell-enriched transcription factors, MafA, Pdx1, and beta2, and activates insulin gene transcription. J Biol Chem. 2011;286(12): 10449-56.

[17] Conkright MD, Canettieri G, Screaton R, Guzman E, Miraglia L, et al. TORCs: transducers of regulated CREB activity. Mol Cell. 2003;12: 413-23.

[18] Drozdov I, Svejda B, Gustafsson BI, Mane S, Pfragner R, Kidd M, Modlin IM. Gene network inference and biochemical assessment delineates GPCR pathways and CREB targets in small intestinal neuroendocrine neoplasia. PLoS One. 2011;6(8): e22457.

[19] Wu X, Jin W, Liu X, Fu H, Gong P, et al. Cyclic AMP response element modulator-1 (CREM-1) involves in neuronal apoptosis after traumatic brain injury. J Mol Neurosci. 2012;47(2): 357-67.

[20] Caravatta L, Sancilio S, di Giacomo V, Rana R, Cataldi A, Di Pietro R. PI3-K/Akt-dependent activation of cAMP-response element-binding (CREB) protein in Jurkat T leukemia cells treated with TRAIL. J Cell Physiol. 2008;214(1): 192-200.

[21] Di Pietro R, di Giacomo V, Caravatta L, Sancilio S, Rana RA, Cataldi A. Cyclic nucleotide response element binding (CREB) protein activation is involved in K562 erythroleukemia cells differentiation. J Cell Biochem. 2007;100(4): 1070-79.

[22] Migliaccio G, Di Pietro R, di Giacomo V, Di Baldassarre A, Migliaccio AR, et al. In vitro mass production of human erythroid cells from the blood of normal donors and of thalassemic patients. Blood Cells Mol Dis. 2002;28(2): 169-80.

[23] Lau E, Ronai ZA. ATF2 - at the crossroad of nuclear and cytosolic functions. J Cell Sci. 2012;125(Pt 12): 2815-24.

[24] Hai T, Hartman MG. The molecular biology and nomenclature of the activating transcription factor/cAMP responsive element binding family of transcription factors: activating transcription factor proteins and homeostasis. Gene. 2001;273: 1–11.

[25] Llarena M, Bailey D, Curtis H, O'Hare P. Different mechanisms of recognition and ER retention by transmembrane transcription factors CREB-H and ATF6. Traffic. 2010;11(1): 48-69.

[26] Chan HM, La Thangue NB. p300/CBP proteins: HATs for transcriptional bridges and scaffolds. J Cell Sci. 2001;114(Pt 13): 2363-73.

[27] Janknecht R. The versatile functions of the transcriptional coactivators p300 and CBP and their roles in disease. Histol Histopathol. 2002;17(2): 657-68.

[28] Chrivia JC, Kwok RP, Lamb N, Hagiwara M, Montminy MR, Goodman RH. Phosphorylated CREB binds specifically to the nuclear protein CBP. Nature. 1993;365(6449): 855-59.

[29] Arany Z, Sellers WR, Livingston DM, Eckner R. E1A-associated p300 and CREB-associated CBP belong to a conserved family of coactivators. Cell. 1994;77(6): 799-800.

[30] Yuan W, Condorelli G, Caruso M, Felsani A, Giordano A. Human p300 protein is a coactivator for the transcription factor MyoD. J Biol Chem. 1996;271: 9009-13.

[31] Kwok RP, Lundblad JR, Chrivia JC, Richards JP, Bächinger HP, et al. Nuclear protein CBP is a coactivator for the transcription factor CREB. Nature. 1994;370(6486): 223-26.

[32] Nakajima T, Uchida C, Anderson SF, Parvin JD, Montminy M. Analysis of a cAMP-responsive activator reveals a two-component mechanism for transcriptional induction via signal-dependent factors. Genes Dev. 1997;11(6): 738-47.

[33] Ogryzko VV, Schiltz RL, Russanova V, Howard BH, Nakatani Y. The transcriptional coactivators p300 and CBP are histone acetyltransferases. Cell. 1996;87(5): 953-59.

[34] Kalkhoven E. CBP and p300: HATs for different occasions. Biochem Pharmacol. 2004;68: 1145-55.

[35] Fu M, Wang C, Zhang X, Pestell RG. Acetylation of nuclear receptors in cellular growth and apoptosis. Biochem Pharmacol. 2004;68: 1199-208.

[36] Petrij F, Dorsman JC, Dauwerse HG, Giles RH, Peeters T, et al. Rubinstein-Taybi syndrome caused by a de novo reciprocal translocation t(2;16)(q36.3; p13.3). Am J Med Genet. 2000;92: 47-52.

[37] Shima Y, Kitabayashi I. Deregulated transcription factors in leukemia. Int J Hematol. 2011; 94(2): 134-41.

[38] Blobel GA. CREB-binding protein and p300: molecular integrators of hematopoietic transcription. Blood. 2000; 95(3): 745-55.

[39] Kasper LH, Boussouar F, Ney PA, Jackson CW, Rehg J, et al. A transcription-factor-binding surface of coactivator p300 is required for haematopoiesis. Nature. 2002; 419(6908): 738-43.

[40] Blobel GA. CBP and p300: versatile coregulators with important roles in hematopoietic gene expression. J Leukoc Biol. 2002; 71(4): 545-56.

[41] Zimmer SN, Zhou Q, Zhou T, Cheng Z, Abboud-Werner SL, et al. Crebbp haploinsufficiency in mice alters the bone marrow microenvironment, leading to loss of stem cells and excessive myelopoiesis. Blood. 2011;118(1): 69-79.

[42] Rebel VI, Kung AL, Tanner EA, Yang H, Bronson RT, Livingston DM. Distinct roles for CREB-binding protein and p300 in hematopoietic stem cell self-renewal. Proc Natl Acad Sci U S A. 2002;99(23): 14789-94.

[43] Heissig B, Hattori K, Dias S, Friedrich M, Ferris B, et al. Recruitment of stem and progenitor cells from the bone marrow niche requires MMP-9 mediated release of kit ligand. Cell. 2002;109(5): 625-37.

[44] Kwon EM, Raines MA, Blenis J, Sakamoto KM. Granulocyte-macrophage colony-stimulating factor stimulation results in phosphorylation of cAMP response element-binding protein through activation of pp90RSK. Blood. 2000;95: 2552-58.

[45] Cheng JC, Kinjo K, Judelson DR, Chang J, Wu WS, et al. CREB is a critical regulator of normal hematopoiesis and leukemogenesis. Blood. 2008;111(3): 1182–92.

[46] Sandoval S, Pigazzi M, Sakamoto KM. CREB: A Key Regulator of Normal and Neoplastic Hematopoiesis. Adv Hematol. 2009; 2009: 634292-300.

[47] di Giacomo V, Sancilio S, Caravatta L, Rana RA, Di Pietro R, Cataldi A. Regulation of CREB activation by p38 MAPKinase during human primary erythroblasts differentiation. Int J Immunopathol Pharmacol, 2009;22(3): 679-88.

[48] Zauli G, Gibellini D, Vitale M, Secchiero P, Celeghini C, et al. The induction of megakaryocyte differentiation is accompanied by selective Ser133 phosphorylation of the transcription factor CREB in both HEL cell line and primary CD34 cells. Blood. 1998;92: 472–80.

[49] Wen AY, Sakamoto KM, Miller LS. The role of the transcription factor CREB in immune function. J Immunol. 2010;185(11): 6413-19.

[50] Mantamadiotis T, Papalexis N, Dworkin S. CREB signalling in neural stem/progenitor cells: recent developments and the implications for brain tumour biology. Bioessays. 2012;34(4): 293-300.

[51] Hawk JD, Abel T. The role of NR4A transcription factors in memory formation. Brain Res Bull. 2011;85(1-2): 21-29.

[52] Montminy MR, Gonzalez GA, Yamamoto KK. Characteristics of the cAMP response unit. Metabolism. 1990;39(9 Suppl 2): 6-12.

[53] Shaywitz AJ, Greenberg ME. CREB: A Stimulus-Induced Transcription Factor Activated by A Diverse Array of Extracellular Signals. Annual Rev Biochem. 1999;68: 821-61.

[54] Wang Z, Iwasaki M, Ficara F, Lin C, Matheny C et al. GSK-3 promotes conditional association of CREB and its co-activators with MEIS1 to facilitate HOX-mediated transcription and oncogenesis. Cancer Cell. 2010;17(6): 597–608.

[55] Xing J, Kornhauser JM, Xia Z, Thiele EA, Greenberg ME. Nerve growth factor activates extracellular signal-regulated kinase and p38 mitogen-activated protein kinase pathways to stimulate CREB serine 133 phosphorylation. Mol Cell Biol. 1998;18(4): 1946-55.

[56] Brunet A, Bonni A, Zigmond MJ, Lin MZ, Juo P, et al. Akt promotes cell survival by phosphorylating and inhibiting a Forkhead transcription factor. Cell. 1999;19;96(6): 857-68.

[57] Screaton RA, Conkright MD, Katoh Y, Best JL, Canettieri G, et al. The CREB coactivator TORC2 functions as a calcium- and cAMP-sensitive coincidence detector. Cell. 2004;119(1): 61-74.

[58] Wang L, Gural A, Sun XJ, Zhao X, Perna F, et al. The Leukemogenicity of AML1-ETO Is Dependent on Site-Specific Lysine Acetylation. Science. 2011;333(6043): 765–69.

[59] Chevalier SA, Durand S, Dasqupta A, Radonovic M, Cimarelli A, et al. The Transcription Profile of Tax-3 Is More Similar to Tax-1 than Tax-2: Insights into HTLV-3 Potential Leukemogenic Properties. PLoS One. 2012;7(7): e41003.

[60] Shankar DB, Cheng JC, Kinjo K, Federman N, Moore TB, et al. The role of CREB as a proto-oncogene in hematopoiesis and in acute myeloid leukemia. Cancer Cell. 2005;7(4): 351-62.

[61] Cho EC, Mitton B, Sakamoto KM. CREB and Leukemogenesis. Crit Rev Oncog. 2011;16(1-2): 37–46.

[62] Sobulo OM, Borrow J, Tomek R, Reshmi S, Harden A, et al. MLL is fused to CBP, a histone acetyltransferase, in therapy-related acute myeloid leukemia with at(11;16)(q23;p13.3). Proc Natl Acad Sci U S A. 1997;94(16): 8732–37.

[63] Kinjo K, Sandoval S, Sakamoto KM, Shankar DB. The role of CREB as a proto-oncogene in hematopoiesis. Cell Cycle. 2005;4(9): 1134-35.

[64] Sandoval S, Kraus C, Cho EC, Cho M, Bies J, et al. Sox4 cooperates with CREB in myeloid transformation. Blood. 2012;120(1): 155-65.

[65] Peters AH, Schwaller J. Epigenetic mechanisms in acute myeloid leukemia. Prog Drug Res. 2011;67: 197-219.

[66] Rowley JD, Reshmi S, Sobulo O, Musvee T, Anastasi J, et al. All patients with the T(11;16)(q23;p13.3) that involves MLL and CBP have treatment-related hematologic disorders. Blood. 1997;90(2): 535-41.

[67] Ernst P, Mabon M, Davidson AJ, Zon LI, Korsmeyer SJ. An Mll-dependent Hox program drives hematopoietic progenitor expansion. Current Biology. 2004;14(22): 2063-69.

[68] Ma X. Epidemiology of myelodysplastic syndromes. Am J Med. 2012;125(7 Suppl): S2-5.

[69] Zimmer SN, Lemieux ME, Karia BP, Day C, Zhou T, et al. Mice heterozygous for CREB binding protein are hypersensitive to γ-radiation and invariably develop myelodysplastic/myeloproliferative neoplasm. Exp Hematol. 2012;40(4): 295-306.

[70] Pigazzi M, Manara E, Baron E, Basso G. ICER expression inhibits leukemia phenotype and controls tumor progression. Leukemia. 2008;22(12): 2217–25.

[71] Pigazzi M, Manara E, Baron E, Basso G. miR-34b targets cyclic AMP-responsive element binding protein in acute myeloid leukemia. Cancer Res. 2009;69(6): 2471-78.

[72] Pui CH, Mullighan CG, Evans WE, Relling MV. Pediatric acute lymphoblastic leukemia: where are we going and how do we get there? Blood. 2012;120(6): 1165-74.

[73] Inthal A, Zeitlhofer P, Zeginigg M, Morak M, Grausenburger R, et al. CREBBP HAT domain mutations prevail in relapse cases of high hyperdiploid childhood acute lymphoblastic leukemia. Leukemia. 2012;26(8): 1797-803.

[74] Mullighan CG, Zhang J, Kasper LH, Lerach S, Payne-Turner D, et al. CREBBP mutations in relapsed acute lymphoblastic leukaemia. Nature. 2011;471(7337): 235-39.

[75] Kung AL, Rebel VI, Bronson RT, Ch'ng LE, Sieff CA, et al. Gene dose-dependent control of hematopoiesis and hematologic tumor suppression by CBP. Genes Dev. 2000;14(3): 272-77.

[76] Shigeno K, Yoshida H, Pan L, Luo J.M, Fujisawa S, et al. Disease-related potential of mutations in transcriptional cofactors CREB-binding protein and p300 in leukemias. Cancer Lett. 2004;213(1): 11-20.

[77] Di Pietro R, Zauli G. Emerging non-apoptotic functions of Tumor necrosis factor-Related Apoptosis Inducing Ligand (TRAIL)/Apo2L. J Cell Physiol. 2004;201(3): 331-40.

[78] Sabatini N, Di Pietro R, Rapino M, Sancilio S, Comani S, Cataldi A. PI-3-kinase/NF-κB mediated response of Jurkat T leukemic cells to two different chemotherapeutic drugs, Etoposide and TRAIL. J Cell Biochem. 2004;93(2): 301-11.

[79] Zauli G, Sancilio S, Cataldi A, Sabatini N, Bosco D, Di Pietro R. PI-3K/Akt and NF-κB/IκBα pathways are activated in Jurkat T cells in response to TRAIL treatment. J Cell Physiol. 2005;202(3): 900-11.

[80] R. Di Pietro. Signalling pathways leading to TRAIL resistance. In Advances in Cancer Therapy, Book 3, ISBN 979-953-307-209-7, Eds. Hala Gali-Muhtasib, 2011; 201-26.

[81] Milani D, Zauli G, Rimondi E, Celeghini C, Marmiroli S, et al. Tumour necrosis factor–related apoptosis-inducing ligand (TRAIL) sequentially activates pro-survival and pro-apoptotic pathways in SK-N-MC neuronal cells. J Neurochem. 2003;86: 126–35.

[82] Cheng HC, Sakamoto KM. Report on the workshop "New Technologies in Stem Cell Research" Society for Pediatric Research, San Francisco, California. Stem Cells. 2007;25: 1070-88.

[83] Pellegrini M, Cheng JC, Voutila J, Judelson D, Taylor J, et al. Expression profile of CREB knockdown in myeloid leukemia cells. BMC Cancer. 2008;8: 264-76.

[84] Saeki K, Yuo A, Koizumi M, Fujiwara K, Kaneko M, et al. CREB antisense oligonucleotides induce non-apoptotic cell death in proliferating leukemia cells, but not nor-

mal hematopoietic cells, by a bizarre non-antisense mechanism. Leukemia. 2001;15: 238-45.

[85] Bai XT, Gu BW, Yin T, Niu C, Xi XD, et al. Trans-repressive effect of NUP98-PMX1 on PMX1-regulated c-FOS gene through recruitment of histone deacetylase 1 by FG repeats. Cancer Res. 2006;66(9): 4584-90.

[86] Sakamoto KM, Frank DA. CREB in the Pathophysiology of Cancer: Implications for Targeting Transcription Factors for Cancer Therapy. Clin Cancer Res. 2009;15: 2583-87.

[87] Chiorazzi N, Hatzi K, Albesiano E. B-cell chronic lymphocytic leukemia, a clonal disease of B lymphocytes with receptors that vary in specificity for (auto)antigens. Ann N Y Acad Sci. 2005;1062: 1-12.

[88] Lerner A, Epstein PM. Cyclic nucleotide phosphodiesterases as targets for treatment of haematological malignancies. Biochem J. 2006;393(Pt 1): 21-41.

[89] Meyers JA, Su DW, Lerner A. Chronic lymphocytic leukemia and B and T cells differ in their response to cyclic nucleotide phosphodiesterase inhibitors. J Immunol. 2009;182(9): 5400-11.

[90] Burger JA, Tsukada N, Burger M, Zvaifler NJ, Dell'Aquila M, Kipps TJ. Blood-derived nurse-like cells protect chronic lymphocytic leukemia B cells from spontaneous apoptosis through stromal cell-derived factor-1. Blood. 2000;96(8): 2655-63.

[91] Ma Q, Jones D, Springer TA. The chemokine receptor CXCR4 is required for the retention of B lineage and granulocytic precursors within the bone marrow microenvironment. Immunity. 1999;10: 463-71.

[92] Bonni A, Brunet A, West AE, Datta SR, Takasu MA, Greenberg ME. Cell survival promoted by the Ras-MAPK signaling pathway by transcription-dependent and -independent mechanisms. Science. 1999;286(5443): 1358-62.

[93] Poiesz BJ, Ruscetti FW, Gazdar AF, Bunn PA, Minna JD, Gallo RC. Detection and isolation of type C retrovirus particles from fresh and cultured lymphocytes of a patient with cutaneous T-cell lymphoma. Proc Natl Acad Sci USA. 1980;77: 7415–19.

[94] Azran I, Schavinsky-Khrapunsky Y, Aboud M. Role of Tax protein in human T-cell leukemia virus type-I leukemogenicity. Retrovirology. 2004;1: 20-44.

[95] Ching YP, Chun ACS, Chin KT, Jeang KT, Jin DY. Specific TATAA and bZIP requirements reveal that HTLV-I Tax has transcriptional activity subsequent to the assembly of an initiation complex. Retrovirology. 2004;1: 18-30.

[96] Gachon F, Thebault S, Peleraux A, Devaux C, Mesnard JM. Molecular interactions involved in the transactivation of the human T-cell leukemia virus type 1 promoter mediated by Tax and CREB-2 (ATF-4). Mol Cell Biol. 2000;20: 3470-81.

[97] Robek MD, Ratner L. Immortalization of T Lymphocytes by Human T-Cell Leukemia Virus Type 1 Is Independent of the Tax-CBP/p300 Interaction. J Virol. 2000;74(24): 11988-92.

[98] Shaknovich R, Melnick A. Epigenetics and B-cell lymphoma. Curr Opin Hematol. 2011;18(4): 293-99.

[99] Janz M, Hummel M, Truss M, Wollert-Wulf B, Mathas S, et al. Classical Hodgkin lymphoma is characterized by high constitutive expression of activating transcription factor 3 (ATF3), which promotes viability of Hodgkin/Reed-Sternberg cells. Blood. 2006;107(6): 2536-39.

[100] [100] Cerchietti LC, Hatzi K, Caldas-Lopes E, Yang SN, Figueroa ME, et al. BCL6 repression of EP300 in human diffuse large B cell lymphoma cells provides a basis for rational combinatorial therapy. J Clin Invest. 2010;120(12): 4569–82.

[101] Zain J, O'Connor OA. Targeting histone deacetyalses in the treatment of B- and T-cell malignancies. Invest New Drugs. 2010;Suppl 1: S58-78.

[102] Pasqualucci L, Trifonov V, Fabbri G, Ma J, Rossi D, et al. Analysis of the coding genome of diffuse large B-cell lymphoma. Nat Genet. 2011;43(9): 830-37.

[103] Gu W, Roeder RG. Activation of p53 sequence-specific DNA binding by acetylation of the p53 c-terminal domain. Cell. 1997;90(4): 595–606.

[104] Rothgiesser KM, Fey M, Hottiger MO. Acetylation of p65 at lysine 314 is important for late NF-κB-dependent gene expression. BMC Genomics. 2010;11: 22-33.

[105] Zain J. Role of histone deacetylase inhibitors in the treatment of lymphomas and multiple myeloma. Hematol Oncol Clin North Am. 2012;26(3): 671-704, ix.

[106] Portier M, Moles JP, Mazars GR, Jeanteur P, Bataille R, et al. p53 and RAS gene mutations in multiple myeloma. Oncogene. 1992;7: 2539-43.

[107] Hyun T, Yam A, Pece S, Xie X, Zhang J, et al. Loss of PTEN expression leading to high Akt activation in human multiple myelomas. Blood. 2000;96: 3560-68.

[108] Zhang B, Fenton RG. Proliferation of IL-6-independent multiple myeloma does not require the activity of extracellular signal-regulated kinases (ERK1/2). J Cell Physiol. 2002;193(1): 42-54.

[109] Wang JM, Chao JR, Chen W, Kuo ML, Yen JJ, Yang-Yen HF. The antiapoptotic gene mcl-1 is up-regulated by the phosphatidylinositol 3-kinase/Akt signaling pathway through a transcription factor complex containing CREB. Mol Cell Biol. 1999;19: 6195-206.

[110] Gomez-Bougie P, Wuillème-Toumi S, Ménoret E, Trichet V, Robillard N, et al. Noxa up-regulation and Mcl-1 cleavage are associated to apoptosis induction by bortezomib in multiple myeloma. Cancer Res. 2007;67(11): 5418-24.

[111] Hu J, Dang N, Menu E, De Bryune E, Xu D, et al. Activation of ATF4 mediates unwanted Mcl-1 accumulation by proteasome inhibition. Blood. 2012;119(3): 826-37.

[112] Ri M, Tashiro E, Oikawa D, Shinjo S, Tokuda M, Yokouchi Y, et al. Identification of Toyocamycin, an agent cytotoxic for multiple myeloma cells, as a potent inhibitor of ER stress-induced XBP1 mRNA splicing. Blood Cancer J. 2012;2(7): e79.

[113] Carrasco DR, Sukhdeo K, Protopopova M, Sinha R, Enos M, et al. The differentiation and stress response factor XBP-1 drives multiple myeloma pathogenesis. Cancer Cell. 2007;11(4): 349-60.

[114] Bae J, Carrasco R, Lee AH, Prabhala R, Tai YT, et al. Identification of novel myeloma-specific XBP1 peptides able to generate cytotoxic T lymphocytes: a potential therapeutic application in multiple myeloma. Leukemia. 2011;25: 1610-19.

[115] Shuda M, Kondoh N, Imazeki N, Tanaka K, Okada T, et al. Activation of the ATF6, XBP1 and grp78 genes in human hepatocellular carcinoma: a possible involvement of the ER stress pathway in hepatocarcinogenesis. J Hepatol. 2003;38(5): 605-14.

[116] Bagratuni T, Wu P, Gonzalez de Castro D, Davenport EL, Dickens NJ, et al. XBP1s levels are implicated in the biology and outcome of myeloma mediating different clinical outcomes to thalidomide-based treatments. Blood. 2010;116: 250–53.

[117] Papandreou I, Denko NC, Olson M, Van Melckebeke H, Lust S, et al. Identification of an Ire1alpha endonuclease specific inhibitor with cytotoxic activity against human multiple myeloma. Blood 2011;117: 1311–14.

[118] Pichiorri F, Suh SS, Ladetto M, Kuehl M, Palumbo T, et al. MicroRNAs regulate critical genes associated with multiple myeloma pathogenesis. Proc Natl Acad Sci U S A. 2008;105(35): 12885-90.

[119] Xiao W, Hodge DR, Wang L, Yang X, Zhang X, Farrar WL. NF-kappaB activates IL-6 expression through cooperation with c-Jun and IL6-AP1 site, but is independent of its IL6-NFkappaB regulatory site in autocrine human multiple myeloma cells. Cancer Biol Ther. 2004;3(10): 1007-17.

[120] Santer FR, Höschele PP, Oh SJ, Erb HH, Bouchal J, et al. Inhibition of the acetyltransferases p300 and CBP reveals a targetable function for p300 in the survival and invasion pathways of prostate cancer cell lines. Mol Cancer Ther. 2011;10(9): 1644-55.

[121] Boumber Y, Issa JP. Epigenetics in cancer: what's the future? Oncology (Williston Park). 2011;25(3): 220-6, 228.

Chapter 24

Life-Cycling of Cancer: New Concept

Marina Shaduri and Marc Bouchoucha

Additional information is available at the end of the chapter

http://dx.doi.org/10.5772/55385

1. Introduction

The best way to deal with a tricky and unpredictable disease is to understand its essence, causes and triggers.

- Why and how become some normal cells "rebellious" and aggressive? Are there any common processes and rules that govern the transformation of normal cells into malignant neoplasm?
- What is the main cause of cancer diversity and individualism?
- Why do some cancers give metastasis and some do not?
- There are overlaps between benign and malignant lesions. Can we define cancer accurately? Is there a clear margin or a criterion that differentiates benign and slowly progressing malignant neoplasm?

The basic questions about cancer must be answered to demystify this scary disease and solve the "Oncogenic Paradox" described by the Nobel Prize laureate Albert Szent-Gyorgyi [1]: "The malignant transformation of tissues … is a very specific process which must involve very specific changes in a very specific chemical machinery. Accordingly, one would expect that such transformation can be brought about only by a very specific process, as locks can be opened only by their own keys. Contrary to this, a malignant transformation can be brought about by an infinite number of unspecific influences, such as pieces of asbestos, high-energy radiation, irritation, chemicals, viruses, etc. It is getting more and more difficult to find something that is not carcinogenic".

A new promising way of understanding malignant neoplasia and its paradoxes rests upon integrating biomedical and physical knowledge. Several years ago the US National Cancer Institute funded a major research program to bring insights into the cancer problem from the standpoint of physical science; the hope was that physicists could introduce some radical new ideas to the table. In the manuscript we focus mainly on the physical aspects of cancer origin pushing aside biochemical, immunological and gene-associated findings that do not presently add much to the conceptual framework for cancer theory. Our model of carcinogenesis incorporates certain recently discovered physical phenomena [2-4] that elucidate many peculiarities of malignant processes.

New concept of cancer origin is a particular example of the more general model of system-genesis published last year [5]. According to this hypothesis, a malignant neoplasm originates within a small isolated area of a larger organism as a new functional unit with its individual mechanisms of self-control and self-regulation; the cells that are deprived of nutrients and oxygen do pass through several stages of dramatic transformations that lead to the formation of toti- or pluripotent cells with altered genetic makeup. The future fate of this "potential neoplasm" depends on a combination of some physical factors and on the proper timing of successive events that include the unification of enclosed cells and their preparation for aggressive expansion through the physical effect of "Random Lasing" [2]. Hence, contrary to a widely spread opinion of cancer being a chaotic and poorly controlled pull of rebellious cells that are "driven mad" by some mutations, we consider malignant neoplasm to be a strictly controlled and adaptive system of cooperatively acting primitive cells. Some researchers share this point of view regarding cancer as a self-organizing adaptive system or a parasite-like organism [6, 7].

Our model of carcinogenesis is the result of 12-year-long experimental and clinical work in the emerging scientific field of Biological Holography. All illustrations presented in the manuscript are obtained with the computer-assessed device (CID-system) developed specially for cancer detection and visualization [5]. This hardware-software system is the ever first cancer-detecting and monitoring tool convenient for mass-screening purposes; it is capable of detecting and monitoring of any malignant process disregarding its type and location in the body. The non-invasive and automatable method of any cancer detection through a single and short-term procedure is already implemented in diagnostic practice: the patients with and without malignancies are distinguished by spectral information emitted from their body surfaces.

2. Cancer origin theories: State-of-the-art

Malignant neoplasia of normal cells remains a source of misunderstanding and controversy. There is a vast literature on cancer theories. In this section we briefly describe only some of the most acknowledged and interesting ideas. Although none of the debatable hypothesis of carcinogenesis elucidates the general scenario applicable to all cases of cancer, they are nevertheless helpful in generalization of the state-of-the-art knowledge.

A central feature of today's view of cancer is that it does not develop all at once but evolves as a result of complex succession of events over time. According to Hanahan and Weinberg [8] there are several essential alterations in cell physiology typical for malignant cell growth. These hallmarks of cancers include: 1) Self sufficiency in growth signals, 2) Insensitivity to anti-growth signals, 3) Evading apoptosis, 4) Limitless replicative potential 5) Sustained angiogenesis, 6) Tissue invasion and metastasis, and 7) Genome instability. It is also widely accepted that cancers express aerobic glycolysis regardless of their tissue or cellular origin [9]. Abnormal segregation of chromosomes during mitosis (aneuploidy) and genome instability are found almost in all cancers [10], though the reason(s) of these abnormalities are not clarified.

The somatic mutation theory of carcinogenesis has been dominant since the beginning of the 20th century. It is known that cancer cell genomes carry somatic mutations in DNA that may include base substitutions, small insertions and deletions, rearrangements, and copy number alterations. As the tumor progresses, mutations accumulate and the cell eventually becomes cancerous. Apart of successive alterations in genetic material (somatic events), some germ-line mutations can also predispose a person to heritable or familial cancer. Certain defects in DNA are known to be responsible for a variety of hereditary cancer predisposition syndromes including non-polyposis colorectal carcinoma, Bloom syndrome, ataxia-telangiectasia, Fanconi anaemia, etc. [11,12]. Molecular genetics has identified some oncogenes that, along with tumor suppressor genes, can reproduce many aspects of cancer progression. In fact, each tumor is unique in its genetic makeup [13] and, correspondingly, has a unique phenotype akin to an individual organism. Many researchers consider the above theory unsatisfactory because no strict correlation exists between gene mutations and malignancy; besides, it is unclear which factors trigger the gen-associated events that lead to neoplasia. Evidently, the genomic instability per se is not sufficient to initiate a malignant tumor. The somatic mutation theory can explain neither genetic variability within individual tumors, nor many other observable phenomena in cancer biology.

The **cancer-stem-cell (CSC) concept** is becoming increasingly popular, since non-differentiated, relatively primitive and pluri- or totipotent cells have the ability to self-renew and to give rise to distinct types of malignant cells. It is now generally accepted that the CSC sub-population of cancer cells plays significant role in initiation, progression and recurrence of cancer. The CSC concept was first demonstrated in the study of leukemia, which was found to be associated with the "stem-cells" having specific surface antigen profiles [14, 15]. Italian researchers who spotted CSCs in human primary bone sarcomas highlighted CD133 as a pivotal marker for their identification [16]. In recent years similar cells were found in human cancers of brain, breast, colon, pancreas and other tissues [17]. Kornelia Polyak from Dana-Farber Cancer Institute (Boston, US) demonstrated that the frequency of tumor cells positive for stem cell–like and more differentiated cell markers varies according to tumor subtype and histological stage [18]; the question whether malignancy arises from normal stem cells due to maturation arrest or due to transformation of mature cells into CSC is still open.

The Viral/Microbial Theory of Cancer that regards viruses/microbes as potential triggers of a neoplastic process has long history. First finding concerned the avian leucosis virus as a cause of leukemia in chickens [19]; Two years later after this discovery P. Rous presented his theory about ultramicroscopic organisms capable to induce cancer in humans and animals [20]. Since then many viral infections have been linked to malignant processes. Recent studies have provided cogent evidence that some "oncoviruses", e.g., human papillomavirus, hepatitis B and hepatitis C virus, Epstein-Barr virus, etc. are indeed associated with increased incidence of human cancers [21, 22]. Over the years, scientists have proposed a number of mechanisms to explain this link. However, numerous cases of cancer can originate and develop independently of any viruses, fungi or bacteria.

A major cohort of scientists supports the **embryonal theory of cancer.** A type of similarity between embryogenesis and carcinogenesis was first mentioned by John Beard, who put forward The Unitarian Trophoblastic Theory of cancer [23]. The main idea behind his theory is that certain fetal cells or atavistic genes give rise to a neoplasm. Prominent physicist Paul Davis argues that ancient genetic toolkit active in the earliest stages of embryogenesis gets switched back on, re-activating the Proterozoic developmental plan for building cell colonies [7]. Rippert [24] suggested that cells expressing embryonic potential arise due to the process of dedifferentiation. According to the proponents of the embryonal theory, some immature cells such as the remnants of fetal tissues, become eventually malignant due to altered blood supply, e.g., after tissue traumas or mechanical isolation of a small area from nutrients and oxygen. Remarkably, the development of the zygote up to the blastula stage is more or less the same in all mammals, so one can assume that the early phases of cancer "prenatal life" would be of the same nature. Whether we should blame the atavistic genes or there are some other factors that eventually "fertilize" the host-cells producing neoplasm remains an open question.

The embryonal theory is closely related to the hypothesis dubbed **the "speciation theory"** that regards cancers as new species. Duesberg and his UC Berkeley colleagues, who studied aneuploid nature of a cell karyotype across numerous cell cultures, came to a conclusion that some cell-destructive events cause chromosomal mutations and result in cells with totally new phenotypes [25]. The authors argue that carcinogenesis is initiated by a disruption of chromosomes that alters the balance of tens of thousands of genes. The result of these processes is a cell with new traits – that is, a new phenotype or a new organism. According to these researchers, "cancer is comparable to a bacterial level of complexity, but still autonomous; ... it doesn't follow orders like other cells in the body, and it can grow where, when and how it likes" [ibid]. M. Vincent [26] also considers cancer as a programmed and evolutionarily conserved formation rather than just a random series of disease-causing mutations.

Malignant neoplasm develops within host tissues, so the state of entire body and traits of **the micro-environment** of a "cancer-nursery" must be taken in account while searching cancer initiation factors. Gene mutations are only part of the process that leads to cancer, which involves an interaction between neoplasm and surrounding tissue. The importance of changes in the micro-environment during tumor progression has been recognized thanks to pertinent enthusiastic scientists, who were moving against the mainstream science to prove their hypothesis [27-29]. The existence of histologically abnormal tissue beyond a neoplastic area that predisposes to tumor formation is a characteristic feature of many cancers. Interesting data were published by a team of American researchers who established that in the course of tumor development the normal cells in tumor stroma may lose more regions of DNA than do the cancer cells [30]. Another team of American scientists demonstrated that stromal cells actively participate in carcinogenesis [31]. Sonnenschein and Soto from Tufts University in Boston [32] put forward the tissue organization field theory arguing that dynamic breakdown of cellular communication and signal transduction prompts disoriented cells to mistakenly revert to pro-growth patterns of behavior.

The theoretical considerations listed above are substantiated by empiric evidence, but they deal with particular events and manifestations of carcinogenesis. These hypotheses are essentially complementary to each other rather than contradictory; they describe various contributing factors and peculiarities of a neoplasm but no data are available concerning the general scenario and common physical processes that take place at early stages of any cancer genesis. No doubt that there is an urgent need for such a theory capable to reconcile existing hypotheses and empiric findings by establishing the reasons and physical laws that drive normal cells towards malignant neoplasia.

3. Malignant neoplasm as a new organism

Our model of cancer origin has much in common with the embryonal and speciation hypotheses mentioned above; however, it brings new insights into physical mechanisms of cancer emergence and elucidates some details of its "prenatal" life. In this section we will discuss the general peculiarities of complex adaptive systems and show that malignant neoplasm being a system of cooperatively acting cells, behaves as an autonomous organism with its own mechanisms of self-control and self-regulation. Evidently, the whole spectrum of distinct cells, tissues and organs in human body comes out from a bunch of initially identical cells produced by a single zygote - the same processes would be expected in cancers. Lloyd J. Old has found common genetic programs at work in tumor cells and gametes that led him to describe cancer as a "somatic cell pregnancy" [33]. In sections 6 and 7 of the manuscript we will search an answer to the question: how a normal and well-differentiated (somatic) cell becomes "pregnant" in the absence of fertilizing agents?

One can suggest that a cluster of young cancer-cells would not survive in the heavily populated competitive environment unless their development is driven by powerful autonomous mechanisms of self-regulation and adaptation. Such self-organizing entities belong to the class of complex adaptive systems (CAS) which are capable to learn from their experience while functioning in variable ambience. Adaptive evolution (evolvability) and the emergence phenomenon are their yet unexplained characteristics. Emergence implies appearance of certain unpredictable and qualitatively new functions that pop up out of the multiplicity of relatively simple interactions.

It is widely accepted, that all CASs share the following common characteristics: 1) robustness – the ability to maintain a basic level of dynamic equilibrium; 2) resilience – all CASs are capable to restore the quasi-equilibrium state after various perturbations; 3) multi-level organization in terms of complex structural and functional hierarchy; 4) self-organization that implies creation of more complex internal structures without external resources or information and, of course, 5) adaptability in the sense that any CAS can vary its strategy and tactics according to a new or previously experienced situation. The listed hallmarks of autonomously functioning systems are unimaginable without synergy, which implies an orchestrated, synchronized and interdependent behavior of all system-components.

We argue that cancer has all the traits typical for any CAS: cancer cells are hard to destroy even by chemical toxins and radiation, since they coordinate their action in order to survive as an entity. Only united and self-organizing system of cooperating cells would be able to start the vital struggle against the powerful host-organism. The cancer-system shares the phase-space with the host-CAS which is its rival and breadwinner at the same time. New organism should either defeat its host, or, alternatively, obey its rules and commands adapting to the variable ambience.

3.1. Adaptive behavior and diversity of cancers

There are about 200 types of cancers each type comprising multiple "families" and sub-types of cells. The scientists from the Wellcome Trust Sanger Institute in Hinxton, England, recently announced 73 different combinations of disease-causing mutations in the breast tumors each involving up to six different genes from a set of 40 driver genes [34]. Canadian researchers have shown that the cells taken from patients with acute lymphoblastic leukemia are actually composed of multiple families of genetically distinct leukemia cells [35]. No doubt, that the treatment of such a diverse pathology would not be efficient without understanding of the most general regulatory mechanisms common for all cancers.

What is the reason of cancer diversity? Are its cells the clones of distinct "cancer-stems" that originate simultaneously, or they emerge as new cells due to clashes with surrounding cells that produce odds and ends of damaged cellular components?

We assume that an interaction of poorly differentiated cells with the bystander elements of stroma can yield various karyo- and phenotypes through the same mechanisms that take place in the first "nursery" of emerging cancer. The tumor micro-environment is a complex system of many cell types, including endothelial cells and their precursors, smooth-muscle cells, fibroblasts, granulocytes, lymphocytes, macrophages, etc. Taking into consideration the features of CAS, one can suggest that adaptation of young, meta-stable and extremely motile cancer cells to variable and heterogeneous micro-environment plays crucial role in the process of cell diversification; however, there is another possibility to provide diverse "stems" and their clones. This "fresh" idea about recurrent (iterative) cycles of carcinogenesis that imply successive production of less complex generations of malignant cells is described in section 7.

Many cancers adapt to chemo- and radiation therapy: according to some researchers, the clonal selection leads to the resistance of recurrent tumors [36]. If "cancer-embryos" are nurtured in various conditions before they proceed to active life-cycling, they might give birth to distinct "clones". This process cannot be considered as selection, but as the emergence of new organisms by the same scenario as in the first act of carcinogenesis.

It should be noted that the adaptation itself is not a well understood phenomenon. Elusive non-molecular processes of information exchange between the cells/tissues are difficult to study. As a result, we often ignore an obvious fact that no process of learning (gaining experience) is possible without data storage. No doubt that some mechanisms of data memorizing should exist in all, even in simplest entities capable to adapt and develop: ambient information has to be perceived, processed and stored in a readily accessible (usable) form. We argue that a kind of associative memory must be an embedded feature of all adaptive systems, among them, of cancers, since autonomous functioning, adaptation and development are unimaginable without the available information on previously experienced states [5]. The physical basis of a system memory is closely related to real-time holographic mechanisms that are basic for any CAS. These poorly understood mechanisms that imply the wave-wave and wave-matter interactions ensure the unification and integration of many separate elements into an autonomously functioning system of interdependent agents (see below).

3.2. Collective behavior of malignant cells

Cells and other elements of complex biological systems are functionally interdependent – they exhibit evident signs of collective behavior being organized as a hierarchy [37-39]. If cancers are integral and adaptive organisms, the action of malignant cells should be strictly coordinated. Indeed, nontrivial spatial correlations between malignant cells have been found by various researchers. The cooperative behavior, namely, collective migration of malignant cells during their invasion into healthy tissues seems to follow essentially the same pathways as healthy cells that participate in embryological development and damaged tissue reparation [40]. Cells performing collective migration share many biological characteristics with independently migrating cells but, by affecting one another mechanically and via signaling, these cell groups are subject to additional regulation and constraints [41, 42].

Experimental and clinical observations support the suggestion that cancer cells form a complex and integrated system. G. Lambert studied the collective response of breast cancer tissues to drug-induced stress and found a similarity between the rapid evolution of drug resistance in cancers and the behavior of bacterial colonies under starvation conditions [43]. Professor P. Davies, principal investigator of a major research program funded by the National Cancer Institute, argues that cancer is not a random bunch of selfish rogue cells behaving badly, but a highly-efficient pre-programmed response to stress, honed by a long period of evolution. [7, 44].

Hence, one can regard cancer as a life-tenacious organism created by and incorporated into relatively mature tissues of the host-body. This complex adaptive system, which is doomed to conduct a life-long battle with its superior ancestor - parental body, has its own powerful self-regulation mechanisms, a flexible primitive structure and enough power to hunt the preys – host cells.

4. New approach to the cancer non-invasive study

Cancer remains an elusive, unpredictable and scary disease mostly because the malignant processes are difficult to detect and monitor. The most efficient methods of cancer conventional diagnostics are either harmful or too costly to be used in vivo as often as necessary. Oncologists lack a non-invasive, reliable, user-friendly, automatable and non-expensive test for tracking the malignant processes on the organism-level. We were lucky to find the solution to this problem thanks to an unexpected discovery of a previously unknown physical effect - "the holographic diffraction" which turned out to be characteristic of all biological objects [4-5, 45]. Detailed description of the innovative technology developed and tested by the authors was published earlier [46, 47]; in this manuscript we present concise information about this principally new approach to the detection and monitoring of malignant processes for a better understanding of our empiric data.

The computer-assessed diagnostic system "CID" provides reliable and comprehensive spectral information valuable for non-invasive detection and monitoring of malignant processes of any location and type [5]. The CID-system belongs to the class of the imaging technology dubbed BHT (Bio-holographic tomography) which is both – a diagnostic and research tool. The device is not cumbersome or difficult to operate: examinations can be conducted right at a patient's bed and the interface is so simple that even novice users can collect data in the form of BHT-grams. The whole procedure of the BHT-examination lasts several minutes: distal body-parts (usually 10 fingertips) are exposed to the pulsed electric fields that are strong enough to initiate the discharge of air; the relaxation of excited atoms and molecules in ionized gas produces optical radiation, which is captured for further processing and analysis; cancer-specific optical signatures are determined by analyzing effects of electric impulses on the body distal "terminals". A computer operates the device and performs analyses of recordings (fig. 1).

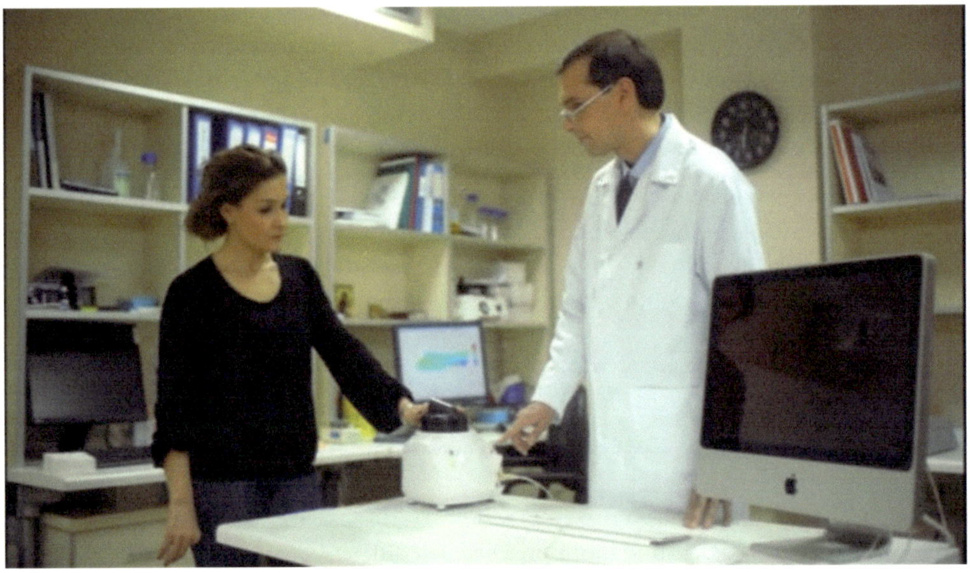

Figure 1. BHT-examination implies the recording of ten fingertips' emission that takes only 2-3 minutes.

In observational research, results can be changed or biased by the act of measurement itself. The distal areas of human body are used as a source of information because they provide less distorted spectral information about entire body-state avoiding "an observer/measurement effect". A set of images-tomograms of 10 fingertips (each showing a 2D momentary "slice" of the 3D system) is recorded for the detection and monitoring of malignant processes in human body. The fingertips are exposed to electric impulses of distinct frequencies, so that one gets comparable information on the character of resonant responses to electric impulses of particular frequencies in 10 distant areas of human body (necessary for mapping of pathological process). The harmless and short-term procedure of a person examination can be conducted as often as necessary.

In clinical practice various modalities are used for imaging of body parts, including radiography, computed tomography, magnetic resonance imaging (MRI), and positron emission tomography-computed tomography (PET-CT). All these modalities focus on particular areas of human body in order to get the images of organs/tissues that physicians need to examine. In BHT there is no necessity to screen entire body part by part, since the holography-based mechanisms spread the scaled information about the deviations from normal functioning of cells and tissues throughout the whole body acting akin to a wireless system of bio-communication. Experimental and clinical study of various patients (with and without diseases) enabled us to reveal some cancer-specific spectral signatures in fingertip BHT-grams [5, 48] that prompted subsequent research in oncology. The CID is a portable, easy-to-use and non-costly tool of the whole body examination; it allows the determination of the spatiotemporal distribution of malignant processes throughout an intact organism. The CID-system is already implemented in routine diagnostic practice.

Pre-existing devices of the same class [49, 50] failed to provide reliable and reproducible information on cancer-specific emission and on the dynamics of systems. In order to stabilize the air discharge plasma and obtain the informative optical data it became indispensable to modify the device and alter the examination procedure. We have filtered out the most variable and non-informative spectral components thus getting reproducible and comparable recordings of fingertip emission. Stabilization of the discharge plasma and improvement of data quality have been achieved through the limitation of the gas transit-time across the discharge zone, the restriction of particle upward scattering/dissipation, etc.

It became necessary to conduct a plethora of probes on hundreds of patients with distinct types and stages of cancer before we understood the principles of the holographic imaging and developed the system of data interpretation. Close collaboration with clinicians made it possible to define the matrix of correlations between clinical diagnoses and spectral information obtained in various conditions of data acquisition. Experimental and clinical work conducted during several years led us to the conclusion that interference patterns emitted from body surfaces in response to high frequency electric impulses carry encoded information on the shapes, densities, complexity and dynamic features of the most problematic areas/processes disregarding their type, size and location in human body (fig. 2).

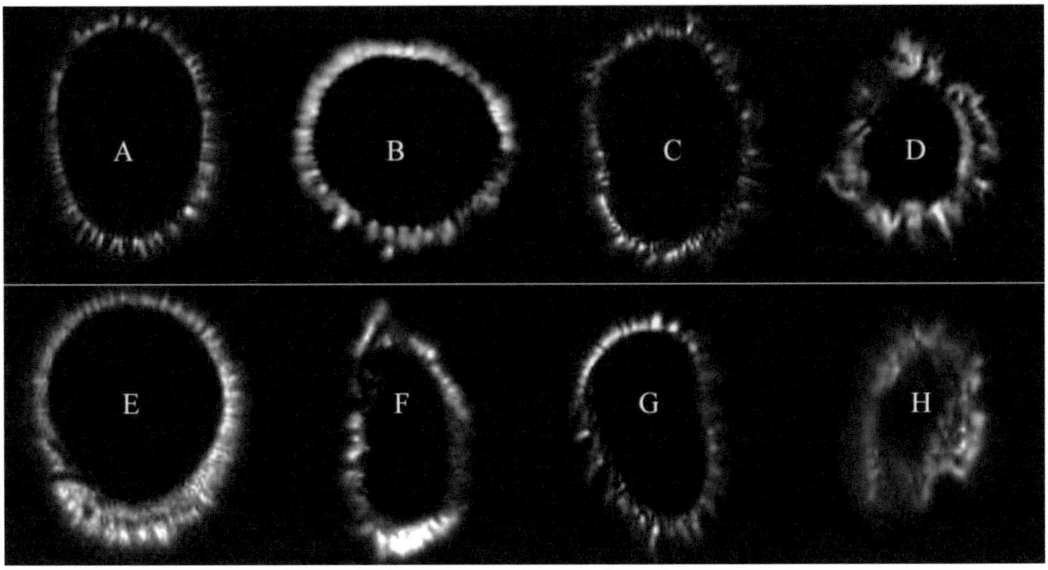

Figure 2. The geometry and texture of fingertip BHT-grams is altered according to certain characteristics of the most affected tissues and organs: A - a healthy person's uniform emission; B – a case of prostate cancer (a chestnut–like flattened shape); C – cancer of the left kidney (the shape of a bean); D – the lactation state; E – gastrointestinal cancer; F – the shoulder malfunctioning (complex elongated shape); G – lung cancer, advanced stage; H – colorectal cancer (terminal stage).

A system in a quasi-balanced state radiates evenly thanks to intrinsic processes of the destructive interference (similar waves propagating in opposite directions cancel one other and do not affect neighboring waves), whereas any perturbation caused by pathological processes results in constructive interference and phase-shifts that upsets the whole system of interdependent waves. Actually, all non-uniformities on fingertip BHT-grams represent the interference patterns, namely the replicas-holograms of the most malfunctioning tissues and cells – the source of wave-imbalance.

This extraordinary capability of system-waves to scale the information on any abnormal process and to deliver it to all body-elements enables the BHT-analysts to observe many structural nuances of pathological areas like in a microscope (fig.3).

The discovery of the astonishing peculiarity of biological systems that act like "bio-microscopes" became a great stimulus for subsequent theoretical and experimental research. This natural phenomenon enabled us to get and analyze the interference patterns/holograms of real anatomic structures using human fingertips as a source of the otherwise invisible and non-measurable information. New approach to the evaluation of the body problematic areas can be referred to as the "Holographic Imaging". Owing to non-locality of holographic information and because of spectral differences between immature cancer-cells and differentiated host-cells, it has become possible to detect malignant pathology with high accuracy [45]. It should be noted that contrary to the spectral analysis of BHT-grams, the visual interpretation of the holographic replicas is not an automatable task.

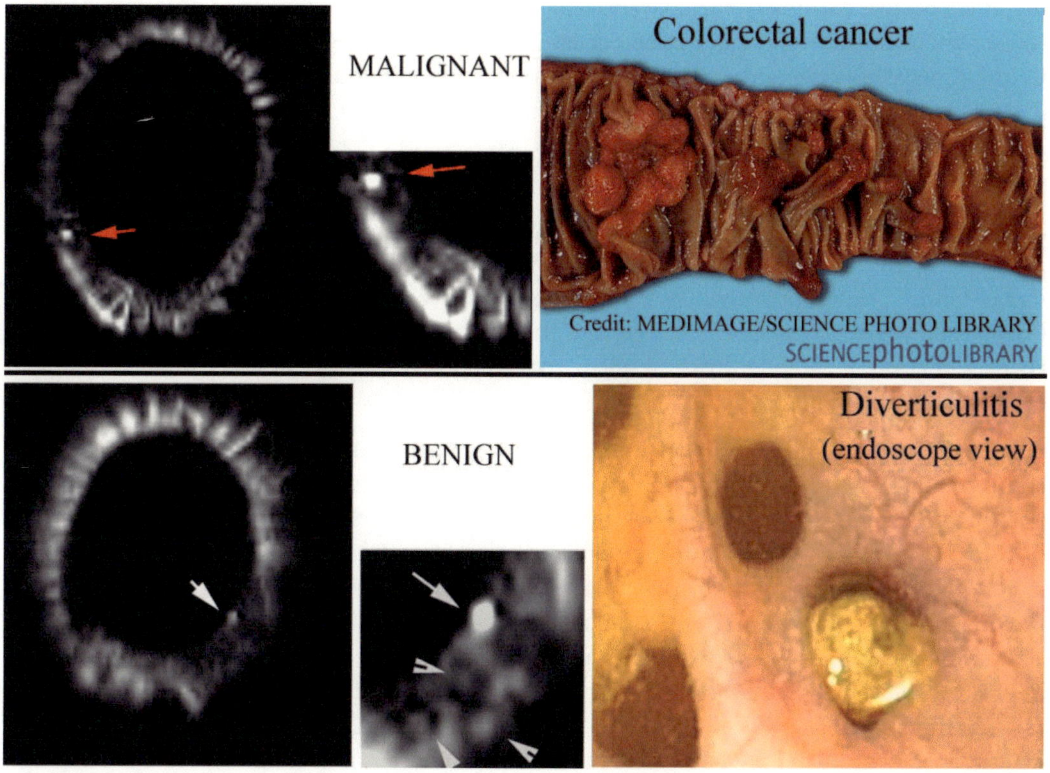

Figure 3. Holograms of the small body-structures are displayed on BHT-grams like in a microscope (see section 5 for explanations of the scaling effects). Two fingertip "coronas" and their enlarged parts are shown next to photographs of similar pathologies. Red arrows (upper images) point to a very bright inclusion embedded into a dark zone. Such a contrast between bright "spot" and dark background is typical for invasive cancer: the degrading host-cells around invasive tumors emit weakly. In the case of benign diverticula (bottom image, white arrows) no signs of degradation are present next to rounded inclusions and the center of relatively intensive emission.

5. Spectral information is distinct in benign and malignant cases of pathology

Waves play enormous role in integration and self-organization of complex adaptive systems, though their contribution to the functioning of human body is still grossly underestimated. Some oscillatory and cyclic bio-activities are studied in the process of functional diagnostics in conventional medicine (e.g., ECG, EEG, etc.); however, organization of nonlinear waves within intact body (especially on micro- and nano-scales) was never explored experimentally.

All physical objects radiate in response to incident electromagnetic waves that are always present in the environment. The spectrum emitted by simple objects such as particles, atoms, molecules and chemical substances, can be recorded and studied much easier than that of complex dynamical systems where internal waves interact with each other. Natural radiation of human body is extremely variable and weak; besides, any perturbation of observable waves causes their instant change, so direct measurements cannot provide reliable spectral information. Only resonant enhancement of body emission and its distant probing can bring the relevant data on the dynamics and character of intrinsic processes. In our model of carcinogenesis we focus mainly on dynamic processes and interactions rather than on various participants (the solid components) in biological processes.

The hardware-software system "CID" records a resonant response of a body to applied electric impulses of high frequencies. This spectral information is valuable for investigation and understanding of yet unknown functional mechanisms in human organism. An elusive and extremely fragile system of organized and interdependent physical waves of various types ensures not only the self-control and self-regulation of the system, but also its interaction with ambient waves and fields [5].

Waves are carriers of energy and information, so their internal "life" and exchange with environment is worth to study. One can ask whether various non-molecular signals, waves and their interference patterns emitted by nontransparent and dynamic organisms carry non-distorted (and interpretable) information on the state of various tissues, cells, intercellular communications and other peculiarities of internal processes. Experimental findings of many researchers prove that the answer to the posed question is positive: G. Hyland has shown that some biological objects emit highly focused coherent electromagnetic waves of ultra-low intensity. The author assumes that such an emission is an outward sign of an orderly functioning metabolism [51]. Japanese researchers caught sound waves generated by bacteria and showed that bacterial cells can enhance the proliferation of neighboring cells through acoustic waves. It is suggested that sounds can function as growth-regulatory signals for entire colony of cells [52]. The alteration of bacterial growth and the synchronization of light emission of adjacent cultures were observed by M. Trushin [53]. An ability of placental mammalian cells to generate pulsating light signals in response to near-ultraviolet light irradiation was discovered by G. Albrecht-Buehler [54]. Such a reversible enhancement of autofluorescence can be used by cells for the "quorum sensing" and coordinated action. And finally, our own experimental and clinical data provide arguments on behalf of the well organized system of interacting waves whose rules and mechanisms are already disclosed (at least partially). The coordinated vibrations and waves of a system medium turned out to be crucial for system integrity and self-regulation via real-time holographic mechanisms (see below).

Although the study of weak radiation of complex biological objects is still in its infancy, spectral analysis of cells, tissues and entire organisms offers great potential being a source of readily automatable biomedical information. The development of spectral methods for Biomedicine was prompted by recent advances in computer sciences, since enormous amount of spectral data requires specific tools and appropriate concepts for data interpretation. There are many approaches to spectroscopic studies of biological samples. Here are some examples that demonstrate the usefulness of spectra for medical studies:

- American researchers developed a novel microscopy technique, called nonlinear interferometric vibrational imaging (NIVI) intended for quantitative analysis of tissue specimens [55]. The NIVI can differentiate cancer versus normal tissue sections with greater than 99% confidence interval in a preclinical rat breast cancer model and define cancer boundaries in fresh unstained tissues.

- Extremely detailed study of cells in their natural state without the need of fixatives has been performed through Raman spectroscopic analysis [56].
- Surface-enhanced Raman spectroscopy in conjunction with imaging was found to be informative in the studies of the chemical composition of the live cells [57].
- Fluorescence emission spectrum of blood components was found to be efficient in distinguishing normal from early-stage and advanced-stage breast cancer. The sensitivity and specificity of the method are 80.4% and 100%, respectively, in distinguishing subjects with breast cancer from normal controls [58].
- Fourier Transform Infrared (FTIR) spectroscopic studies and Fluorescence Emission Spectroscopy (FES) have been effectively employed in the qualitative and quantitative analyses of rat tissues. The study showed that the spectral profiles are different when the tissue of a particular organ is affected with tumor [59].
- Near-infrared light (NIR) is used to differentiate oxygenated vs. deoxygenated forms of hemoglobin and myoglobin. Illumination of intact tissue with NIR allows qualitative assessment of changes in the tissue concentration of these molecules [60].
- Over the last few years infrared microspectroscopy has been used to study cells and tissues. Research work is now aimed at characterizing spectral biomarkers for cancer diagnosis [61]. Dynamic IR imaging with image-processing-guided frequency analysis is a promising modality for breast cancer detection and may not have the tissue-dependent limitations of mammography. The IR imaging process recognizes the cancer area independently of tissue density, cancer size, and cancer appearance on mammography [62].
- Photoacoustic tomography (PAT) is an automatable emerging technique for spectroscopic analysis and imaging live tissue at depths up to 10 cm for detecting tumors and cancer research. The method enables in vivo study of melanomas with both exquisite sensitivity and high specificity [63, 64]. Besides, it can provide anatomical, functional, metabolic, molecular, and genetic contrasts of vasculature, hemodynamics, oxygen metabolism, biomarkers, and gene expression.
- Angle-resolved low coherence interferometry (a/LCI) during endoscopic examination has been found to be convenient for esophageal cancer diagnosis [65]. Physicians shine short bursts of light at locations of suspected disease and sensors capture and analyze the light as it is reflected back.

It is evident that spectral characteristics of actively developing immature cells differ from the emission of normal cells due to increased metabolic rate and proliferative activity of cancer-cells. Much more difficult is to explain how a small cluster of malignant cells alters the emission of distant body-parts, e.g., human fingertips.

The "Holographic Imaging" of abnormally functioning internal structures through non-transparent body is, in fact, a mind-boggling effect. Nobody could ever imagine that it was possible to observe the structural and functional nuances of internal cells, tissues and microscopic areas via assessment of fingertip emission; neither could it be suspected that our organism is able to scale the holograms of real anatomic structures and to expose on a huge scale only those cells and tissues that do not obey the general rules of entire system. This "holographic imaging" is a physical phenomenon and it has been explained as a manifestation of background activity of the system nonlinear medium (phase-space) that acts akin to an organizing holographic grating of a body [5].

In complex adaptive systems (CAS), where all components are well-controlled and there exists a strong subordination between the levels of a system hierarchy, a permanent interaction of "each" and "all" (non-locality) is of utmost importance. In order to achieve interdependence of all agents of a CAS, the periodic grating and synchronicity of vibrations within whole medium must be set from the very first moments of a new system emergence. In the next section we will discuss the role of focused coherent waves in the processes of a system-unification that makes it possible to create an integral system of cooperatively acting agents out of separate elements.

Can the waves generated within human body affect the motion of small neutral particles, molecules and cells? Physicists know that certain waves (e.g., light) can serve to bind neutral matter in new organized forms. It has been established that high frequency oscillations of intense fields interact with micron-size dielectric objects trapping and bounding small particles. The artificial holographic/diffractive setups allow the simultaneous production of very high numbers of such traps generated by superimposing coherent beams either through the wave-interference or through the interaction of several beams previously fanned-out by diffractive optical elements [66]. Hence, a kind of feedback interactions really exists between the waves and solid particles of a CAS. If the suggestion about interdependent action of all system-waves and solid "particles" is correct, the medium waves of a biological system would mirror the state of corresponding solid elements (atoms, molecules, cells, etc.) as all these "agents" are enclosed in the partially bounded space. Any alteration in one of these two complementary realms would affect another - either directly or via some intermediate mechanisms; so, one can evaluate the system-wave behavior/patterns (interference) in order to get information on both - the features of background waves and the state of their complementary (solid) structures.

The permanent wave-wave and wave-matter interactions within a bounded space can explain the effect of the "holographic imaging" discovered by our team 12 years ago; it was an exciting day when we were all huddled round the computer puzzled by the similarity between some BHT-grams and real anatomic structures (see section 8).

As mentioned earlier, an integral system of interfering waves is too sensitive to be studied directly: the wave functions collapse as soon as an observer tries to probe this fragile "structure". That is why we take only the most distant minor areas of human body for BHT-examination – the minor "terminals" of a system provide us with less perturbed system-information.

The background order within the medium/space of a system can explain many peculiarities of CASs. This unifying and organizing realm of a system must be preserved during the whole life-cycle; obviously, the ordered motion of a system-medium and the wave interactions set at initial stage of the system-genesis become more and more complex in parallel with its growth and development. The invisible activity of waves in the phase-space occupied by a CAS can be considered as a "wireless" system of communication between all system-components.

Information propagates in the form of a signal or a message that cannot alter behavior of the solid matter directly but can instead be sent simultaneously to all system-waves. Obviously, diverse "recipients" of information would not react to one and the same message in a similar way; however, weak interactions ensure delivering of a message to a large "audience", actually to the whole system, so that the instructions and commands would not miss their targets.

The question arises whether there are any specific mechanisms that a biological system utilizes for the reinforcement/amplification of the most urgent and/or essential information; it is also very important to understand how a system controls its "misbehaving agents" and which mechanisms are able to transform weak signals into an effective force? We have reasoned that the system-mechanisms of self-control and self-organization require the interaction between weak (information-associated) and strong (energy-associated) waves; powerful or focused waves can play the role of mediators between the information-associated processes and the processes that affect distinct particles, molecules and cells. The reinforcement of information without actual participation of the solid matter in the process of signal amplification is possible via the holography-based mechanisms.

The holographic principle and real-time holography are the only concepts that can explain the imaging of scaled internal structures on the surfaces of autonomous systems. A characteristic feature of any static and dynamic hologram is that any part of a holographic record can be used for the reconstruction of the whole recorded scene. In physics the principle of holography implies that information about a 3D space-volume is encoded in 2D form on its boundary [67-69]. We argue that permanent encoding and decoding of information is a natural phenomenon specific for all autonomously functioning systems; it should not be confused with the conventional process of technical holography.

The real-time holography enables a rapid successive recording and read-out of the information (interference patterns); in the case of a CAS the amount of the processed information can be very high (terabits/s), since the operation is performed in parallel within the entire volume. When creating a hologram, the ordered reference waves (aka the ordered medium-waves of the body) interfere with disordered waves generated by perturbed waves/particles. This information can be reconstructed if the reference waves are subtracted, e.g., by conjugated waves that propagate in the opposite direction. The original object's field/image is reconstructed when the waves deflect in the hologram structure. The refresh rate (update) of information correlates with the periods of phase-conjugated waves, so the reaction of the entire system to any disorder in a high frequency range would be much more "acute" than in the case of a mismatch in slower processes.

We argue that the holographic mechanisms play crucial role in the self-organization of any CAS. These mechanisms imply existence of a hidden order in the background medium where all waves comprise a harmonious structure of vibrations and standing waves; the same mechanisms are critical for the adaptation (decentralized memory) and the resilience of biological systems. Any perturbation, disregarding its actual cause and culprit, would result in constructive interference and phase-shifts of corresponding waves thus altering the entire (scale-invariant) system of background harmonics. Besides, the principle of holography makes it possible to observe the most disordered tissues and organs via assessment of their holographic replicas on distant surfaces of a system (e.g., fingertip BHT-grams), since the "whole" and its "part" can equally reconstruct the entire "holo-image".

The scaling of information in a system of natural origin depends greatly on the frequency/wavelengths of the most perturbed intrinsic waves. Thanks to the fractal nature of body wave-structure, its self-similarity and scale-invariance, the high frequency signals from excited cells (short waves correspond to small structures) can reach the body surface only after their scaling through the waves of lower frequency (longer waves correspond to larger structures of a system): the fingertips BHT-grams display the interference patterns with the resolution that is proportional to the frequency of constructively interfering waves.

On the way towards the body surface, the upward propagating waves of high frequency (complementary to cells and other microscopic structures) are scaled through the doubling of their amplitudes and periods at each successive level of the hierarchy; that is why the interference patterns/holograms of cells and their constellations are emitted with higher resolution compared to holograms of larger parts of the body. This peculiarity of the multilevel and self-similar structure of interacting waves enables us to observe and analyze the most active processes and also malignant cells/tissues via assessment of fingertip BHT-grams (see section 8 for examples of the cell-holograms).

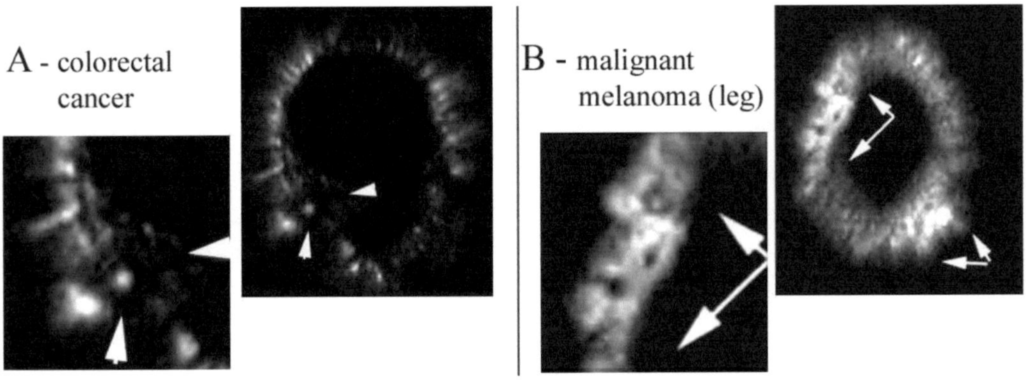

Figure 4. Examples of cancer-signatures on fingertip BHT-grams. In the case of colorectal cancer (A) a part of growing neoplasm paves its way through degrading surrounding tissues (dark zone around to bright inclusion). In the case of malignant melanoma (B) the rapidly proliferating cancer-cells produce an effect of diffuse illumination. The multidirectional radiation that illuminates major parts of BHT-grams is a hallmark of the high frequency coherent emission generated by large conglomerates of poorly differentiated cells (see section 6 for more explanations).

In the cases of cancer, two autonomously functioning entities occupy a shared phase-space and compete for available resources. The conflicting organisms that are "trapped" within a shared body are not able to synchronize their individual rhythms and achieve a state of a quasi-balance. Hence, the BHT-grams of the patients with cancer would display the replicas (interference patterns) of aggressive neoplasm with huge resolution. In certain cases of malignant pathology the fingertip "coronas" demonstrate dark areas around brighter inclusions that present the "remnants" of cells destroyed by cancer-cells (fig.3 and fig. 4,a); The effect of illumination by diffuse light is a BHT-characteristic of actively proliferating non-differentiated cells (fig. 4,b).

6. Emergence of cancer via random lasing

Waves – the carriers of energy and information - are the sole candidates to perform the task of information reinforcement in living systems. In a bounded system of interdependent mechanical and electromagnetic waves of various intensities, wavelengths and frequencies, any perturbation propagates throughout the entire system. The higher coherence and intensity of waves the greater their influence on the solid matter. The interaction of the information- and energy-associated events ensures synergy and coordination of all system-components.

The recently discovered physical effect of "Random Lasing" [2, 3] which implies the focusing and amplification of light in a non-uniform and disordered medium, e.g., in biological tissues, casts new light on the interaction between information and energy-related biological mechanisms. The reinforcement of information through the real-time holographic mechanisms differs from the principles that focus and amplify waves in random lasing; the random lasing implies a complex process of wave-trapping and releasing by disordered excitable material. Emitted waves become much more focused and coherent than those that have been initially "arrested", which explains the term "lasing" (light amplification by lasers).

Conventional lasers that amplify light through the stimulation of photonic emission, require an excitable medium (gain medium) and some feedback mechanisms that temporarily trap the light before emitting a narrower spectrum beams. Usually the gain medium in lasers is excited by pumped energy supplied as an electrical current, or as light of different wavelength, while the photons are confined between mirrors in optical resonator.

Back in 2000, several teams of researchers announced the creation of microlasers exploiting a disordered dielectric material as gain medium [70, 71]. A disordered material that comprises the scattering elements in random positions was found capable to exhibit a laser-like behavior [72]. Electromagnetic waves bounce from one scattering center/cavity to another and such a recurrent scattering on a microscopic length scale temporarily traps light. Hence, the random lasers do not possess large cavity or mirrors typical for conventional lasers; they contain only multiple non-uniformities that scatter light (or other waves). Small irregularities in the material act just like artificial mirrors in laser resonators preventing the light from escaping too quickly. These non-uniformities can be presented by particles, bubbles, droplets of dye, density fluctuations in fluids, surface roughness, cells in organisms, textile fibers in clothing, etc. In polymer films and biological tissues the lasing effects take place because of naturally formed cavities and non-uniformities that temporarily trap energy of waves through internal resonances.

Coherent amplified emission and dramatic spectral narrowing take place only if excitable medium gains energy above the threshold of its excitation [73, 74]. The random micro-laser characteristics can be tuned by varying the geometry of the scatterers' clusters, since each cluster operates at its own specific wavelength, depending on its shape and size.

In some cases constructive interference of backscattered waves brings transport of light to a complete halt (Anderson localization). Philip Anderson was awarded the Nobel Prize in physics for the theory of light localization in disordered medium [75]. In principle, not only electrons and photons, but actually any wave can be localized in a similar way: successful experiments aimed at the sound-wave localization in the strongly disordered 3D samples (composed of aluminum beads) have been described in 2008 [76].

The effects of light amplification and lasing have been found in various vegetable and animal tissues as well as in human tissues from various organs [77]. Even individual cells are capable to produce narrowband laser emission remaining alive after prolonged lasing action: these data were published by researchers from Harvard Medical School, who created biological cell "lasers" based on green fluorescent protein [78]. The team engineered human embryonic kidney cells to produce this protein; when they placed such a cell in the optical micro-resonator and exposed it to pulsed blue light, the cell started to emit a directional laser beam visible with the naked eye.

We have described the random lasing effect and wave interactions in detail because these findings elucidate the energy-mediated mechanism by which information in the form of weak waves affects inert material and creates an "order out of chaos" within the whole system (essential for the system-resilience); besides, the random lasing can account for the appearance of anaplastic cells – the process referred to as the "dedifferentiation" [79]. The spectra narrowing and light amplification are equally important for the understanding of cancer aggressive behavior as the focused light can readily destroy surrounding tissues and facilitate the neoplasm progression.

Indeed, intensity and character of lasing in malignant neoplasm were found to be distinct from benign tissues of the same origin. The Utah University researchers have demonstrated that the malignant colon tissues, when soaked in the laser dye Rhodamine 6G and excited by laser light, emit many more coherent lines than benign tissues in the same colon [2]. The disorder in cancerous tissue was much more chaotic than that in a benign tissue due to a mixture of distinct cells and processes of degradation; however, the increased intensity of coherent radiation in cancerous tissues is indicative of the aggressive behavior and active signaling between elements of neoplasm. The Utah University scientists have experimented with various healthy and cancerous colon tissues taken from different patients, as well as from other parts of the human body such as kidney, with very similar results.

It is acknowledged that the radiation pressure from the focused laser beams is able to trap and physically move small dielectric particles acting like a kind of tweezers. S. Kawata and T.

Sugiura were the first to demonstrate that the field can be coupled to the particles in proximity on the order of 100 nanometers [80]. Optical interaction forces are able to organize microscopic objects with sub wavelength accuracy; they can be very long range and oscillate in sign at the optical wavelength [66, 81]. Continuous evanescent field that originates in conditions of multiple internal reflections within a small bounded area can guide a large number of particles into a preferred direction.

The field-wave-matter interactions discussed above can be considered the key mechanisms of the self-organization in live cells, since a complex system of organized waves is able to direct and unify diverse elements into an indivisible "whole".

Random lasing creates a perfect order out of extreme disorder. This effect takes place in a chaotic excited medium and it might facilitate creation of a new ordered system out of "ashes" of the host-body degrading cells. Such "Phoenix Paradigm" was proposed by researchers of the Pittsburgh Cancer Institute: their experiments with the Kaposi Sarcoma-associated Herpesvirus resulted in the conclusion that excessive cell death, rather than its absence, may be a defining force that drives the cancer emergence [82]. In a stressful situation, e.g., when deprived of energy and oxygen, living cells can act as a gain medium for wave reinforcement. The increase in internal pool of energy that results in excitement of cellular matrix can be caused by many "cancer-promoting" factors: the degradation of intracellular substances, intrusion of some toxic substances or viruses/microbes into cells, increased temperature during inflammatory reactions, etc. can contribute to random lasing within a small bounded area; however, all these factors should be evaluated from the standpoint of their energy-associated effects upon an emerging system.

Coherent radiation of any cellular constellation can reach the body surface if cellular emission is strong and distinct from less intensive radiation of surrounding tissues. The signatures of random lasing are especially prominent on BHT-grams of the patients with aggressive malignant processes (fig. 5).

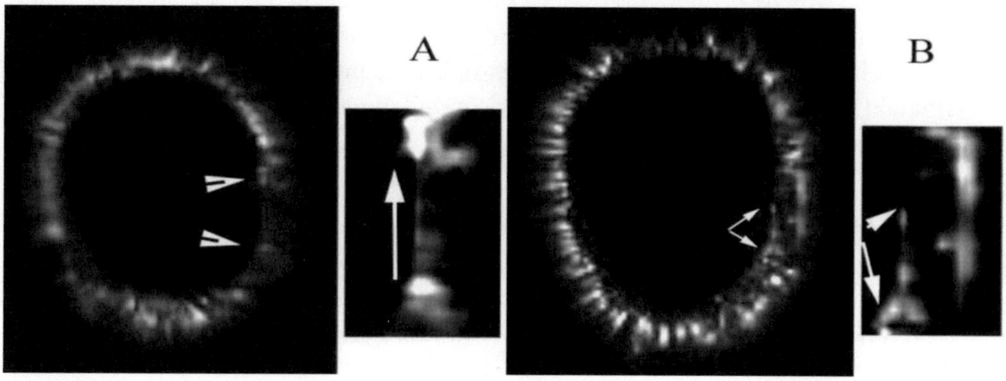

Figure 5. Examples of coherent beams produced by cancer cells. Enlarged and slightly contrasted parts of fingertip coronas are shown next to the raw BHT-grams. A – gastrointestinal cancer, ongoing radiation therapy; B – non-treated renal cancer with spreading metastasis. White arrows point to the scaled holograms of straight tiny lines (focused light).

7. New concept of cancer origin: Dramatic events within a "cancer-nursery"

Cancer, as a new system with altered karyo- and phenotype, originates within a larger and more mature host-system only if a cluster of genetically altered cells builds up its real-time holographic mechanisms of control and regulation. The physical processes within a bounded area of the host-organism play critical role in the cancer-emergence.

We argue that the early carcinogenesis is a multistep process and it starts in a small "nursery", isolated from the matter, energy and information. Such a segregated "nursery" is deprived of oxygen and nutrients having no access to blood supply for this or that reason (a trauma, fibrosis, etc.). A number of starving ischemic cells undergo a chain of metabolic and structural alterations that include the shift of metabolism from aerobic to anaerobic glycolysis, significant increase of Hypoxia-Inducible Factors [83], activation of cell-death programs, disruption of cellular membranes, release of energy from complex substances through their degradation, and other dramatic events typical for metabolic and hypoxic stress in "cut out tissues".

A growing body of evidence supports the view that hypoxia can contribute to the development of cancer. Some researchers established that hypoxia drives cancer progression by promoting genomic instability and that inactivation of apoptosis is essential for tumor-cell survival during this process [84, 85]. Chinese researchers demonstrated that hypoxia inhibits serum withdrawal-induced apoptosis in endothelial progenitor cells [86], while Australian scientists determined that certain monocyte/macrophage populations survive better under conditions of low oxygen [87].

Low oxygen levels characterize the micro-environment of both stem cells and rapidly growing tumors. Moreover, hypoxia is associated with the maintenance of stem-cell–like phenotypes and increased invasion, angiogenesis and metastasis in cancer patients [88]. Recent observations demonstrate the parallelism existing in hypoxia responses of embryonic, adult and cancer stem cells: the mechanisms involved in hypoxia-dependent processes related to stem cell features and tumor progression include the maintenance of the undifferentiated state, cell proliferation, tumor neovascularization, extra-cellular matrix degradation and motility factor up-regulation [89]. Hypoxia often leads to increased aggressiveness and tumor resistance to chemotherapy and radiation [90]. All the findings about the effects of hypoxia and starvation on the state of bounded cellular constellations were taken into account while working on the new concept of cancer emergence.

According to our hypothesis, not only hypoxia, but also isolation from other environmental processes should be considered as the key factors that initiate carcinogenesis. The degradation of starving cells should be tightly regulated in order to rescue at least some of confined cells. It is well known that autophagy is a highly conserved self-digestion process to promote cell survival in response to nutrient starvation and other metabolic stresses [91-92]; however, the role of autophagy that may lead either to cell survival or to cell death is poorly understood in the context of early carcinogenesis.

The autophagy is the chief machinery for bulk elimination and reutilization of aberrant cell components - constituents of cytoplasm and organelles. In the cases of cancer this "self-digesting" mechanism plays an essential role at all stages of the disease, since it helps to prevent tumor cell necrosis by mitigating metabolic stress while acting in concert with apoptosis [93]; the autophagy provides an alternate energy source by degrading damaged proteins and organelles that allow some tumor cells to survive during extended periods of starvation [94]. In the absence of phagocytes, apoptosis would be less efficient as the debris cannot be eliminated from the isolated "nursery" (the disposal of debris is necessary in apoptosis). So, the autophagy seems to dominate over apoptosis in early carcinogenesis though cooperation or alternated action of both mechanisms is not excluded especially just after cessation of the blood supply. Increasing evidence points to the selectivity of autophagy: it helps to "sort" vacuolar enzymes, to remove the aggregate-prone proteins and to destruct only excessive organelles [95].

There is a kind of similarity between neoplasm and budding primitive organisms (see fig.11 in section 8 – holograms of proliferating cells). A key role of recycling of cellular organelles via autophagy and *de novo* purine biosynthesis was found while studying caloric restriction effects on the longevity of budding yeast (Saccharomyces cerevisiae). This yeast is an effective model for the analysis of genes and cellular pathways. Researchers have shown that additional genes appear to contribute to the restriction of either amino acids or sugar, and that defects in autophagy prevent lifespan extension induced by limitation of nutrients in the growth media [96]. An international team of researchers found that the autophagy helps some starving cells to recover, whereas the cells with a disrupted mitochondrial transmembrane potential inexorably die even under optimal culture conditions [97].

Taking all the above findings into account, one can speculate that a complex action of death-programs maintains viability of some cells at the expense of others and that debris of sacrificed cells serve as the sources of energy and nutrients for a cluster of rescued cells. The most viable cells with primitive organization, increased pool of free energy, altered genetic material and the capability to proliferate without additional resources, start to colonize the "nursery" and prepare themselves for the cooperative functioning.

New genetic makeup of surviving cells might have many reasons, such as partial degradation of cellular DNA, abnormal mitosis due to metabolic stress [98], fusion of cells or their "remnants", functional impairment of DNA repair pathways, the shattering and rebuilding of chromosomes named chromothripsis [99, 100], etc. In chromothripsis the chromosomes exhibit a Humpty Dumpty-like behavior: multiple fragments of chromosomes stuck back together after almost complete "pulverization". Such a massive genomic rearrangement acquired in a single catastrophic event can lead stressed cells towards neoplasia [ibid]; however, the effect of coherent waves on the genetic material of cells should not be ignored, since extreme disorder in overexcited biological tissues would initiate the random lasing processes and the laser-like coherent beams would be able to cut/weld distinct macromolecules and other cellular structures.

Thus, dramatic events within a bounded area are accompanied by the release of free energy that excites the trapped mass of degrading cells. Random lasing takes place in the extremely disordered overexcited medium full of debris where the clusters of nanoparticles, macromolecules and the remnants of cells have their own unique sets of lasing frequencies

[73,74]. Intensive motion of the enclosed mass becomes ordered thanks to the organizing effects of powerful waves in the medium [66, 80, 81].

The wave interactions and the motion of solid matter within an isolated area inevitably reach a state when all dynamic processes become synchronous and coordinated. Increasing laser-like radiation of excited cells can help them to break through the isolation and invade host-tissues. "Cancer embryos" do not and cannot manage their logistic problems at the stages of division, compaction and unification that take place in isolation (prenatal phase); such a neoplasm needs to gain power and become "armed" with laser-weapons before it proceeds to the stages of expansion and growth. At the stage of unification via ordered vibrations and organized motion, the entire cluster of new cells acquires its individual rhythm of functioning and becomes a self-organizing entity ready to grow and struggle for resources.

Duration and timing of all "prenatal" stages are the factors of great importance in any system-genesis. For example, one can deduce that if a "cancer-embryo" is ready for independent functioning but the barrier around its nursery cannot be breached yet, the cells would continue to "chop" internal structures and eventually die. Without supply of nutrients, oxygen and some "building blocks" from surroundings, the trapped energy would be spent on the self-destructive work yielding a cyst filled with fluids/semi-solid material; if, on the contrary, the passage of nutrients through the isolating barrier is open earlier than enclosed cells become integrated and "armed", the neoplasm would grow and develop like a benign tumor.

In the manuscript we do not discuss the "postnatal" behavior of the neoplasm in detail; however, once adaptive malignant organism left its nursery and started the life-long battle with its host-rival, it would repeat the same (formerly experienced) scenario whenever possible by blocking blood supply to minor areas and creating the nurseries for new "generations" within the host or its own tissues (the latter is a source of metastasis). Cancer easily adapts to variable situation thanks to the holographic mechanisms of data storage [5] and its first "experience" determines the behavior of its clones. This proclivity of the neoplasm to execute the learned schema of action multiple times in the same or in a slightly changed form can explain the exponential progression, diversity, resistance to the stress posed by "aggressive treatment" and other yet unsolved peculiarities of cancer. The arrangement of new nurseries in various host tissues can be regarded as a kind of adaptive de-evolution: malignant cells produce new generations of "stems" whose structure becomes more and more primitive in each successive cycle.

The schema presented on figure 6 describes the main stages of such an iterative carcinogenesis.

It is established that non-differentiated stem-cell-like sub-populations of cancer (CSCs) are resistant to chemo- and radiation therapy [101]. Since a "cancer-stem" that yields CSCs originates from the remnants of partially degraded progenitor cells, a kind of genetic kinship exists between the host and malignant tissues. The same can be said about a relatively mature neoplasm and its metastasis: the features of metastasis though distinct from primary cancer cells are usually distinguishable from the metastasis of other types of cancer.

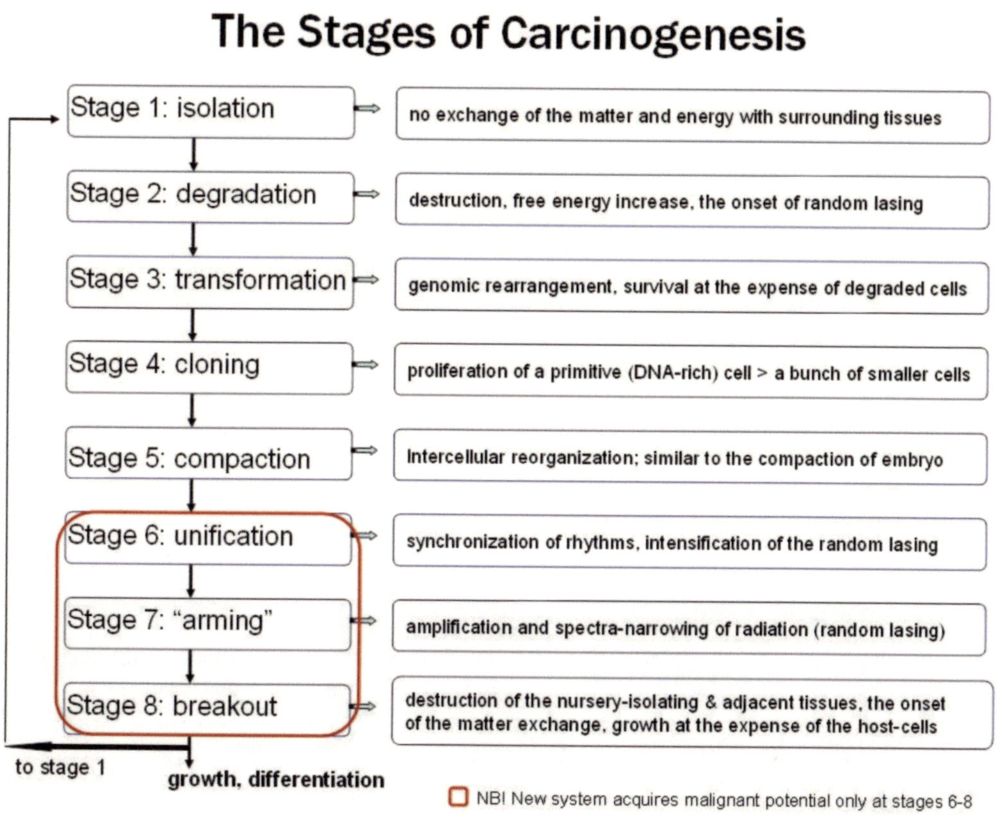

Figure 6. The host-cells should pass through "prenatal" stages before the malignant system leaves its "nursery". Note, that some malignant tissues can start the whole process anew. Each successive cycle would generate less differentiated cells.

To summarize, we argue that malignant neoplasia presents an iterative process of the recurrent system-genesis: one and the same scenario is repeated multiple times within various tissues, in various conditions and with accelerated "prenatal" periods. Such course of the disease can explain the capability of many types of neoplasm to give metastasis through successive rejuvenation of its "daughter-spores". Multiple execution of described tactics of the self-reproduction and the creation of new (younger and less differentiated) generations enables the primary clone of malignant neoplasm to progress exponentially, conquer more and more space at the expense of diverse tissues, resist new stresses and ultimately destroy its breadwinner host. From this point of view, certain stresses posed by standard chemo- and radiation therapy should be considered as the factors that in some cases facilitate the genesis of extremely aggressive and resistant clones of new primitive "organisms".

An unpredictable nature of cancer and dubious efficiency of the methods of its treatment often raise the question whether intervention into the disease course is better than the watchful waiting. For instance, the breast ductal carcinoma in situ, which is a low grade (well differentiated) malignant tumor, can become invasive after more than 30 years since its first manifestation [102]; many patients with low-risk prostate cancer lead a normal life for about 10 years without any treatment: "some prostate cancers might never have developed into serious disease… surgery or radiation therapy may not outweigh the substantial side effects of these treatments" [103].

No doubt, it is urgent and critical to understand the most common rules and principles of malignant neoplasia. We hope that an interdisciplinary approach to the problem and fresh ideas would help everyone involved in healthcare and medical decision-making to plot a clear course through the cancer-paradoxes.

8. Holo-imaging: Some examples

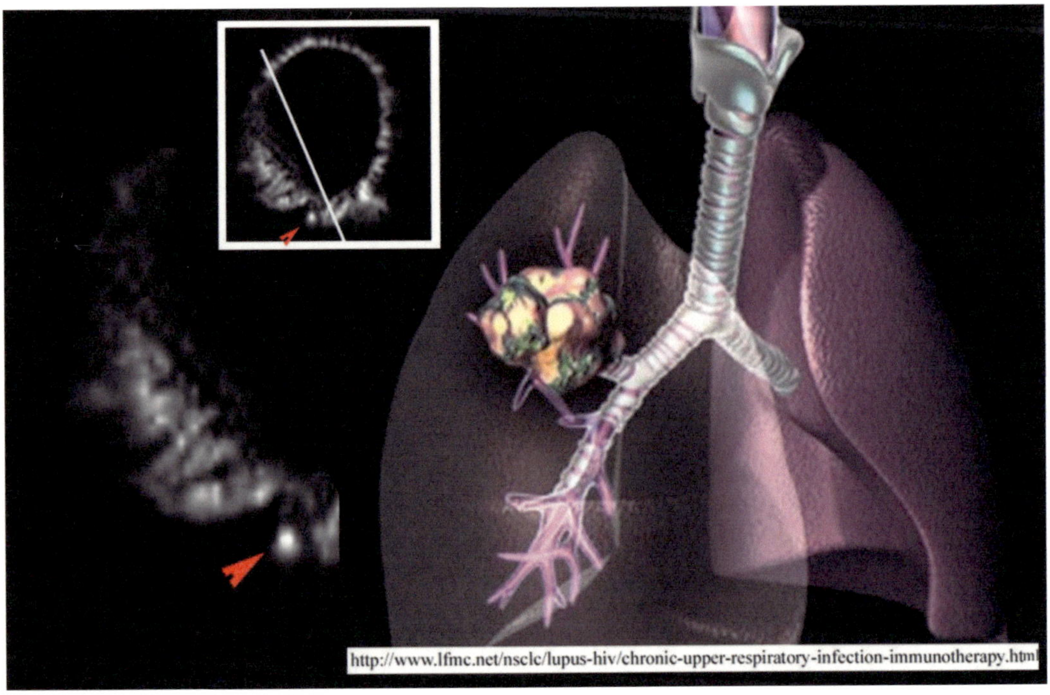

Figure 7. BHT-gram of the patient with treated lung carcinoma. Prominent functional and/or structural disorder in large areas of the body alters major parts of coronas displaying characteristic features of affected tissues in a slightly distorted form. The holographic replica of the most affected lobe of the lung occupies 2/3 of the index finger BHT-gram. Red arrow points to the replica of a growing metastasis.

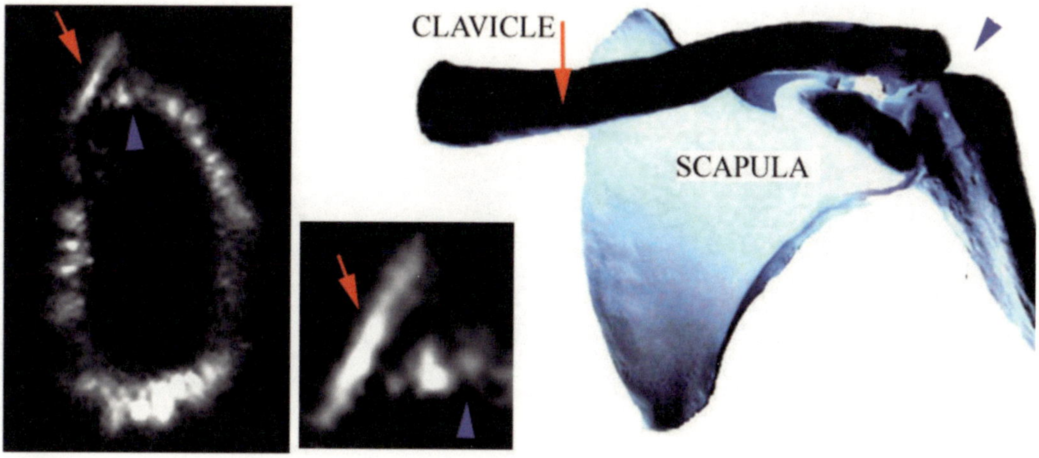

Figure 8. Shapes of presented corona's parts are distorted resembling a shoulder joint (blue arrows); a replica of the most affected bone – clavicle - is displayed with higher quality (red arrows). This is a case of the shoulder malfunctioning (former trauma).

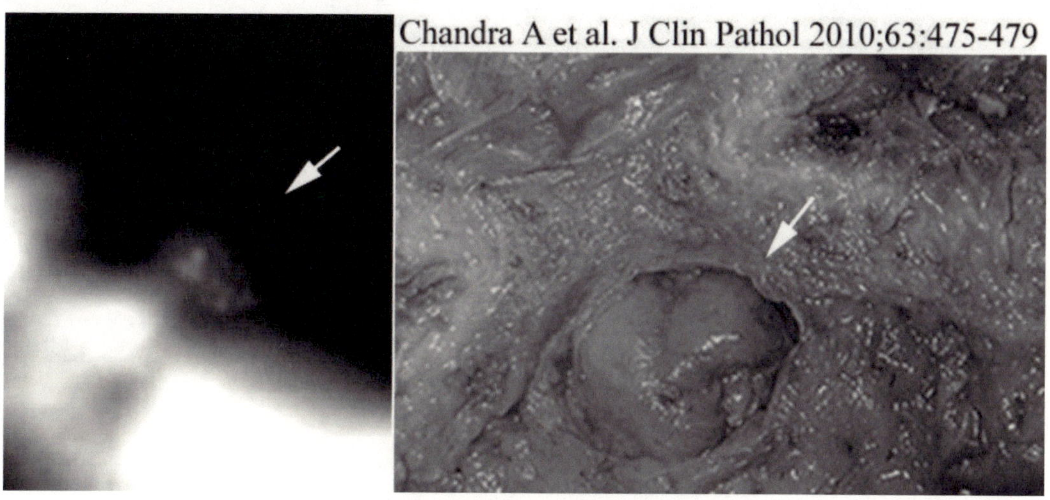

Figure 9. Small areas provide their holographic replicas with higher resolution than the large ones. A case of malignant polyp in the urinary bladder (left) is shown next to the photograph of the bladder cancer.

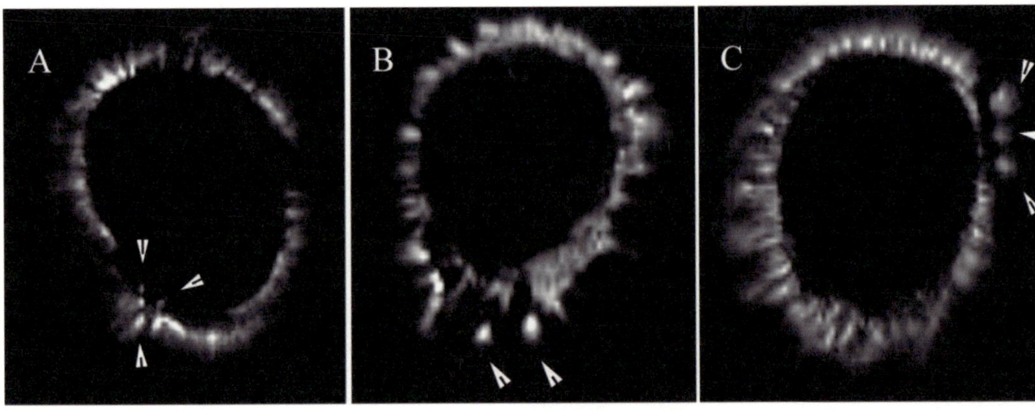

Figure 10. Spreading metastases are displayed on BHT-grams as bright balls on a dark background (indicated): A – Colorectal carcinoma with liver metastasis; B – Colorectal carcinoma with regional metastasis; C – Renal carcinoma with metastasis in regional lymph-nodes.

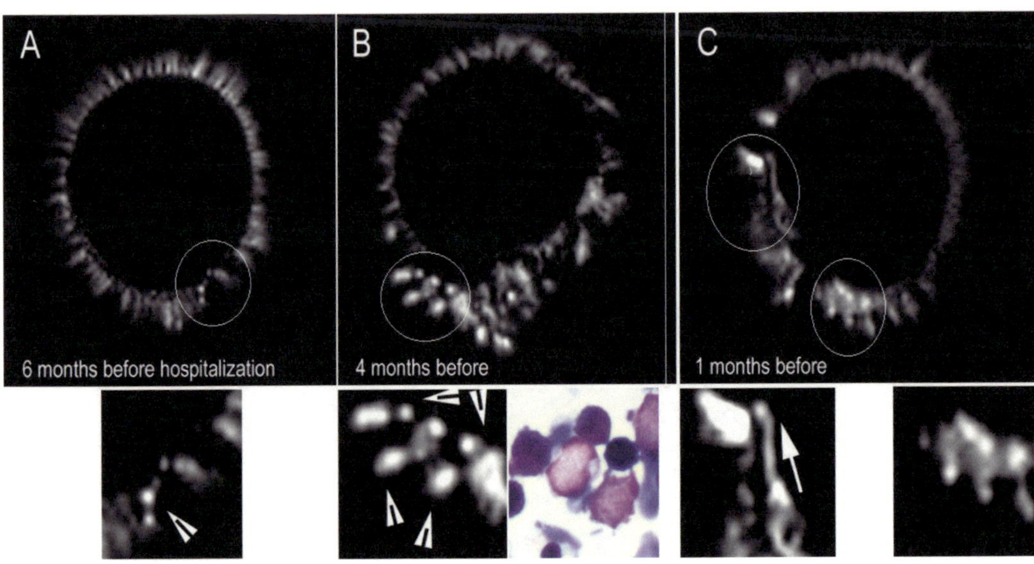

Figure 11. A case of refractory dysmyelopoietic anemia transformed to acute leukemia and liver metastasis. BHT-signs of the disease aggravation have been revealed 4 months before the clinical manifestation of acute leukemia (B). Lab-analyses were not informative a month prior to urgent hospitalization of the patient (C). Abnormally proliferating cells are displayed with huge resolution (B, enlarged part). Compare these holograms of "budding" cancer-cells to the bone marrow smear of a patient with acute leukemia (color-image from http://www.washington.edu/news/2011/09/06/gene-defect-that-predisposes-people-to-leukemia-discovered/).

http://dx.doi.org/10.5772/55385

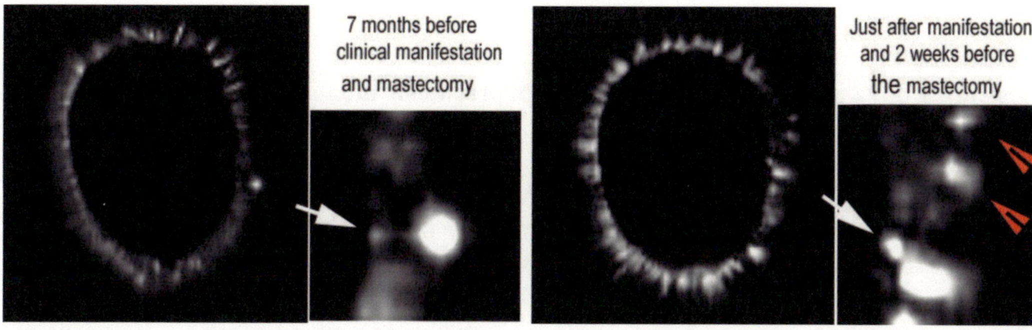

Figure 12. The case of the breast cancer (relapse). BHT revealed the tumor 7 months prior to its detection by conventional imaging methods. Pay attention to powerful diffuse light that consists of multidirectional coherent beams. Such a "fireball" is typical for the neoplasm that just came out of its "nursery" (dark surroundings). Several months later the neoplasm became less uniform and poorly outlined; it grows, multiplies and creates the nurseries for new generations (red arrowheads).

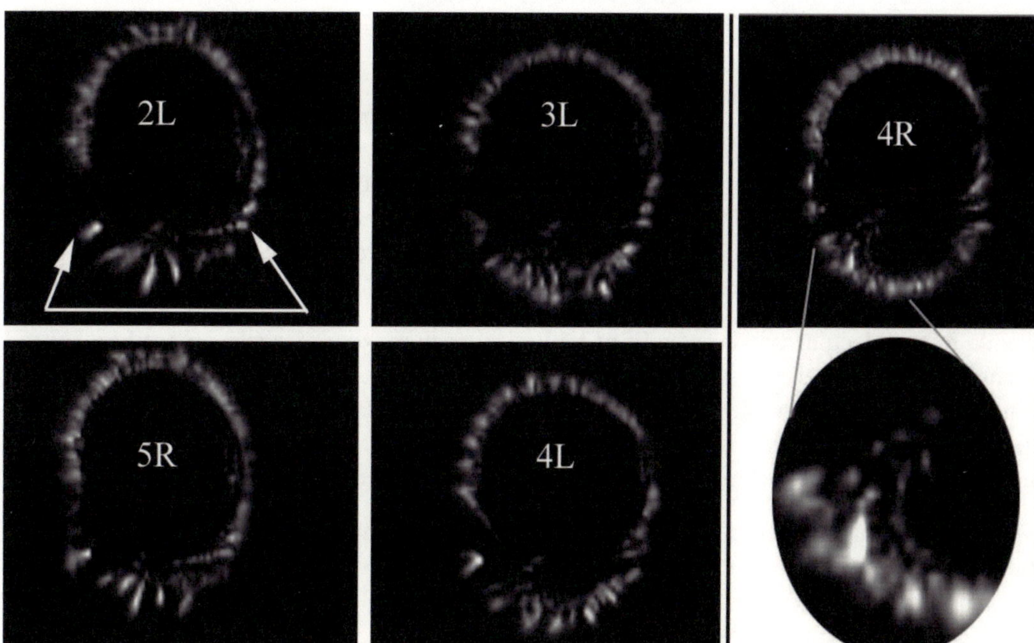

Figure 13. A case of the breast cancer (treated). Almost all BHT-grams display similar replicas of unusually shaped structures. Such a similarity of disordered coronas is typical for an aggravating (sub-acute, transitory) state. A chain of enlarged lymph-nodes in the upper thorax-neck was found to be responsible for the similarity of interference patterns.

9. Conclusion

Presented work was inspired by the discovery of previously unknown physical effects specific to complex adaptive systems of natural origin [5]. The model of carcinogenesis discussed above is a particular example of the more general scenario of system-genesis [5]. According to our data, the "prenatal" life of malignant cells starts in isolation from normally functioning host-tissues. This segregated "nursery" of cancer cells can be compared to a closed box with the famous "Schrödinger's cat" whose fate is totally unpredictable: no direct observation is possible unless the box is transparent to the observer's eye. Conventional biomedical approaches to *in vivo* diagnostics and monitoring are not efficient in such cases. However, we managed to look into the "cancer-nursery" with the help of the waves that in autonomously functioning systems of natural origin act as "wireless" means of the communication between all system-components; back in 2000 we found that cancer provides specific spectral signatures and that aggressive behavior of its cells can be detected via non-invasive analysis of the body-surface radiation. Thanks to complex nonlinear mechanisms of information scaling and transfer across the system, it became possible to conduct a non-perturbing observation of some physical processes that take place in early carcinogenesis. Presented hypothesis focuses on very early stages of cancer emergence; however, we suggest that the described scenario of the system-genesis within more mature organism is equally responsible for the generation of distinct clones and metastasis.

The general model of iterative carcinogenesis reconciles many existing hypotheses and also significantly reduces the number of possible causes and triggers of malignant neoplasia; besides, it opens wide horizons for new experiments and theoretical considerations that can result in the development of more targeted methods of cancer treatment. Apart of the widely known facts about biochemical and genetic features of cancer cells, our model takes into account some physical aspects of malignant neoplasia.

Fragile non-molecular processes within biological systems were largely ignored by official science due to their elusive and non-measurable nature. The findings of the physicists who demonstrated the ability of live cells to manipulate and focus intra- and intercellular waves (e.g., light) should be acknowledged as a giant leap forward, towards the official recognition of the critical role that background nonlinear processes play in the system life-cycling.

We hope that empiric generalization of the biomedical and physical information together with the new possibility to study the "secret" life of the neoplasm would cast light on many puzzles and paradoxes of malignant processes and also help to build foundation for more efficient diagnostic and cancer-treatment strategies.

Acknowledgements

This research would not have been possible without the support of many enthusiastic and open-minded people. Medical professionals, engineers, software developers, biologists, physicists and friends contributed to this work. We would like to extend our sincere thanks to all of them. We express our gratitude to Dr. Raymond Samak – the oncologist from Nice, France and to Dr. Marina Abuladze from the Institute of Physics (Tbilisi, Georgia), who kindly assisted us in the course of the manuscript preparation. We are also much indebted to Professor Andrea Peracino and Dr. Emanuela Folco from the Lorenzini Foundation (Milan, Italy) for their help, valuable advices and encouragement. Deepest gratitude is due to the staff of many collaborating hospitals, clinics and private medical cabinets in France and Italy; without their assistance our work would not have been successful.

Author details

Marina Shaduri[1,2] and Marc Bouchoucha[1]

1 Center of Bioholography, Tbilisi, Georgia

2 Advanced BioResearch & Technology, Luxemburg

References

[1] Szent-Gyorgyi A. The Living State and Cancer. Proc. Natl. Acad. Sci. Biophysics 1977; 74(7) 2844-2847.

[2] Polson R, Vardeny Z. Random lasing in human tissues. Appl. Phys. Lett 2004; 85: 1289-1292

[3] Martorell J, Lawandy N. Observation of inhibited spontaneous emission in a periodic dielectric structure. Phys. Rev. Lett 1990; 65, 1877–1880.

[4] Shaduri M. The Holographic Principle and Emergence Phenomenon. In: Rosen J. (ed.) Holography, Research and Technologies. Rijeka: InTech; 2012. p27-54. Available from: http://www.intechopen.com/books/holography-research-and-technologies/the-holographic-principle-and-emergence-phenomenon

[5] Shaduri M. Secondary holodiffractional radiation of biological systems. Kybernetes – The International Journal of Systems & Cybernetics 2005; 34 (5) 666-680.

[6] Deisboeck T, Berens M, Kansal A. et al. Pattern of Self-Organization in Tumour Systems: Complex Growth Dynamics in a Novel Brain Tumour Spheroid Model, Cell Prolif 2001; 34 115-134

[7] Davies P, Lineweaver C. Cancer Tumors as Metazoa 1.0: Tapping Genes of Ancient Ancestors, Phys. Biol 2011; 8 015001, p. 7

[8] Hanahan D, Weinberg R. The Hallmarks of Cancer. Cell 2000; 100 57-70

[9] Seyfried T, Shelton L. Cancer as a Metabolic Disease (review). Nutrition & Metabolism 2010; 7: 7. Available from http://healthycuriousity.blogspot.com/2012/01/cancer-as-metabolic-disease.html

[10] Nikholson J, Duesberg P. On the Karyotypic Origin and Evolution of Cancer Cells. Cancer Genet Cytogenet 2009;194(2):96-110.

[11] Croce C. Oncogenes and Cancer, N Engl J Med 2008; 358: 502-511

[12] Charames G, Bapat B. Genomic Instability and Cancer, Curr Mol Med 2003; 7: 589-596.

[13] Hameroff S. A New Theory of the Origin of Cancer: Quantum Coherent Entanglement, Centrioles, Mitosis, and Differentiation. BioSystems 2004;77:119–136

[14] Lapidot T. A Cell Initiating Human Acute Myeloid Leukaemia After Transplantation into SCID Mice. Nature 1994; 367: 645–648

[15] Dick J, Lapidot T. Biology of Normal and Acute Myeloid Leukemia Stem Cells. Int J Hematol 2005: 82(5) 389-396

[16] Tirino V, Desiderio, Paino F, et al. Human Primary Bone Sarcomas Contain CD133+ Cancer Stem Cells Displaying High Tumorigenicity In Vivo. FASEB J 2011 Jun;25(6): 2022-30

[17] Avall Lundqvist E, Sjövall K, Eneroth P. Initial Experiences with Serum Alkaline DNase Activity in Monitoring the Effects of Therapy for Carcinoma of the Uterine Cervix. Eur J Cancer 1991;27(10): 1313-1315.

[18] Polyak K. Heterogeneity for Stem Cell–Related Markers According to Tumor Subtype and Histologic Stage in Breast Cancer. Clin Cancer Res 2010; 16(3): 876–887

[19] Ellerman V, Bang O. Experimentelle Leukaemia bei Hühnern, Zentralbl. Bakt 1908; 46:595:7

[20] Rous P. A Sarcoma of the Fowl Transmissible by an Agent Separable from the Tumor Cells (1911) Downloaded from jem.rupress.org on August 3, 2012.

[21] Thompson M, Kurzrock R. Epstein-Barr Virus and Cancer. Clin Cancer Res 2004;10:.803OF

[22] Yu Y, Clippinger A, Alwin J. Viral Metabolism: Changes in Glucose and Glutamine Utilization During Human Cytomegalovirus Infection. Trends in Microbiology 2011; 19(7): 360-367

[23] Beard J. The Enzyme Treatment of Cancer and its Scientific Basis, 1911; Available from http://vitamincfoundation.org/beard/ (accessed 06 August 2012).

[24] Rippert H. Das Carcinom des Menschen. Geschwulstlehre. 2011; Cohen(ed), Bonn.

[25] Duesberg P, Mandrioli D, McCormack A, Nicholson JM. Is Carcinogenesis a Form of Speciation? Cell Cycle 2011; 10(13):2 100-114.

[26] Vincent M. Cancer: A De-repression of a Default Survival Program Common to All Cells? BioEssays 2012; 34(1): 72–82

[27] Hu M, Yao J, Carroll D. et al. Regulation of in situ to Invasive Breast Carcinoma Transition. Cancer Cell 2008; 13(5): 394-406.

[28] Rønnov-Jessen L, Bissell M. Breast Cancer by Proxy: Can the Microenvironment be Both the Cause and Consequence? Trends Mol Med 2009; 5: 5–13

[29] Kenny P, Lee G, Bissell M. Targeting the Tumor Microenvironment. Frontiers in Bioscience.2007; 12: 3468-3474.

[30] Fukino K, Shen L, Matsumoto S. et al. Combined Total Genome Loss-of-heterozygosity Scan of Breast Cancer Stroma and Epithelium Reveals Multiplicity of Stromal Targets, Cancer Res 2004; 64: 7231-7236.

[31] Tlsty T, Coussens L. Tumor Stroma and Regulation of Cancer Development. Annual Review of Pathology 2005; 1: 119-150.

[32] Sonnenschein C, Soto A. Theories of Carcinogenesis: An Emerging Perspective. Semin Cancer Biol 2008; 18(5): 372–377.

[33] Old LJ. Cancer is a Somatic Cell Pregnancy. Cancer Immun 2007; 7: 19-21

[34] Stratton M, Campbell P, Futreal P. The Cancer Genome. Nature 2009; 458: 719-724.

[35] Wang J, Dick J. Cancer Stem Cells: lessons from leukemia. Trends in Cell Biology 2005; 15(9) 494-501.

[36] Radosevich J, Elseth K, Vesper B. et al. Long-Term Adaptation of Lung Tumor Cell Lines with Increasing Concentrations of Nitric Oxide Donor. The Open Lung Cancer Journal 2009; 2: 35-44

[37] Deisboeck T, Berens M, Kansal A. et al. Pattern of Self-Organization in Tumour Systems: Complex Growth Dynamics in a Novel Brain Tumour Spheroid Model. Cell Prolif 2001; 34(2): 115–134.

[38] Kenny P, Nelson C, Bissell, M. The Ecology of Tumors. The Scientist 2006; 20(4): 31–35.

[39] Bonnet D, Dick J. Human Acute Myeloid Leukemia is Organized as a Hierarchy that Originates from a Primitive Hematopoietic Cell. Nature Medicine 1997; 3: 730 – 737.

[40] Friedl P, Hegerfeldt Y, Tusch M. Collective cell migration in morphogenesis and cancer. Int. J. Dev. Biol 2004; 48: 441-449.

[41] Rørth P. Collective Cell Migration. Annual Review of Cell and Developmental Biology 2009;25: 407-429.

[42] Subra Suresh S. Biomechanics and Biophysics of Cancer Cells. Acta Biomater 2007; 3(4): 413–438.

[43] Lambert G. Emergent Collective Behavior of Microorganisms. PhD thesis. Princeton University; 2011.

[44] Davies P, Demetrius L, Tuszynski J. Cancer as a Dynamical Phase Transition, Theoretical Biology and Medical Modelling 2011; 8:3. doi:10.1186/1742-4682-8-30.

[45] Shaduri M, Benford M, Bouchoucha M, Sukhin D, Lebedev V. Holo-imaging - the principle of holography and its practical application: proceedings of the Int. conf. Actual problems of modern physics, 15 June 2008, Krasnodar, Russia. Kuban State University; 2009.

[46] Shaduri M, Tshitshinadze G, Davitashvili T. Investigation of biological systems' holographic properties. Bulletin of the Georgian Academy of Sciences 2002; 2: 264-267.

[47] Shaduri M. A Device to Detect Malignant Processes in Living Organisms - patent. International Application No.: PCT/GE2008/000003.

[48] Shaduri M. Principle of holography in complex adaptive systems. Kybernetes – The International Journal of Systems & Cybernetics 2008; 37(6): 732-738.

[49] Korotkov K. Human Energy Field: study with GDV Bioelectrography. NewYork, USA: Backbone Publishing Co; 2002.

[50] Canetos J, Herbepin P, Reynes J. Method and Installation for Determining the Physical Properties of an Object. US Patent Application, Publication No AU2001031853, May 22, 2003.

[51] Hyland G. Physics and biology of mobile telephony. The Lancet 2000; 356 (9244) 1833 – 1836.

[52] Matsuhashi M, Shindo A, Ohshima H, et al. Cellular Signals Regulating Antibiotic Sensitivities of Bacteria. Microb Drug Resist 1996; 2(1):91-3.

[53] Trushin M. Studies on Distant Regulation of Bacterial Growth and Light Emission. Microbiology 2003; 149: 363–368

[54] Albrecht-Buehler G. Reversible Excitation Light-Induced Enhancement of Fuorescence of Live Mammalian Mitochondria. FASEBJ. 2000; 14: 1864-1866.

[55] Chowdary P, Jiang Z, Chaney E, et al. Molecular Histopathology by Spectrally Reconstructed Nonlinear Interferometric Vibrational Imaging. Cancer Res 2010; 70(23): 9562-9.

[56] Salzer R, Steiner G, Mantsch H. et al. Infrared and Raman Imaging of Biological and Biomimetic Samples. Fresenius' J Anal Chem 2000; 366:712-716.

[57] Kneipp K, Haka AS, Kneipp H, et al. Surface-enhanced Raman Spectroscopy in Single Living Cells Using Gold Nanoparticles. Appl Spec 2002; 56:150–154.

[58] Kalaivani R, Masilamani V, Sivaji K, et al. Fluorescence Spectra of Blood Components for Breast Cancer Diagnosis. Photomed Laser Surg. 2008; Jun;26(3):251-6.

[59] Sankari G, Aishwarya T, Gunasekaran S. Fourier Transform Infrared Spectroscopy and Fluorescence Emission Spectroscopic Investigations on Rat Tissue. Recent Research in Science and Technology 2010; 2(11): 20-31.

[60] Gussakovsky E, Jilkina O, Yang Y. et al. Non-invasive Measurements of Hemoglobin + Myoglobin, their Oxygenation and NIR Light Pathlength in Heart in vivo by Diffuse Reflectance Spectroscopy. Proc. of SPIE 2009; 7161 71612L. doi: 10.1117/12.807715.

[61] Sulé-Suso J, Cinque G. Infrared Microspectroscopy in Cancer Diagnosis. Do We Need Synchrotron Light? Microscopy and Analysis 2010; 140: 25-28.

[62] Lääperi J, Järvenpää D, Kuukasjärvi R. et al. A Dynamic Infrared Imaging-Based Diagnostic Process for Breast Cancer. Acta Radiol. 2009; 50(8):860-9.

[63] Chulhong Kim, Eun Chul Cho, Jingyi Chen et al. In Vivo Molecular Photoacoustic Tomography of Melanomas Targeted by Bioconjugated Cold Nanocages. ACS Nano 2010; 4(8) 4559–4564.

[64] Geng Ku, Bruno D, Fornage M. Et al. Thermoacoustic and Photoacoustic Tomography of Thick Biological Tissues Toward Breast Imaging. Technology in Cancer Research & Treatment 2005; 4(5): 559-565.

[65] Terry N, Zhu Z, Rinehart M. et al. Detection of Dysplasia in Barrett's Esophagus With In Vivo Depth-Resolved Nuclear Morphology MeasurementsGastroenterology 2011; 140(1): 42-50.

[66] Fournier J, Burns M, Golovchenko J. Writing Diffractive Structures by Optical Trapping. Proc. SPIE 1995; 2406: 101-111.

[67] Bousso R. The holographic principle. Reviews of Modern Physics 2002; 74: 825-870.

[68] Bekenstein, J. Universal Upper Bound on the Entropy-to-Energy Ratio for Bounded Systems. Physical Review D 1981; 23(2) 287-298.

[69] Shaduri M, Davitashvili T. Holo-diffraction in Biological Systems. Bulletin of the Georgian Academy of Sciences 2004; 3: 477-481.

[70] Van Soest G, Poelwijk F, Sprik R, Lagendijk A. Dynamics of a Random Laser above Threshold. Phys. Rev. Lett 2001; 86: 1522–1525.

[71] Polson R, Chipouline A, Vardeny Z. Random Lasing in π-Conjugated Films and Infiltrated Opals. Advanced Materials 2001; 13(10): 760–764.

[72] Lawandy Nabil M. Disordered Media: Coherent Random Lasing. Nature Physics 2010. 6: 246 – 248.

[73] Apalkov V., Raikh M and Shapiro B. Random Resonators and Prelocalized Modes in Disordered Dielectric Films. Phys. Rev. Lett. 2002; 89(1), 016802: 4

[74] Cao H. Waves in Random Media. Institute of Physics Publishing; 2003;13 R1PII: S0959-7174(03)39997-5.

[75] Folli V, Conti C. Anderson Localization in Nonlocal Nonlinear Media. Optics Letters 2012; 37(3) 332-334.

[76] Hefei H, Strybulevych A, Page J. et al. Localization of Ultrasound in a Three-Dimensional Elastic Network. Nature Physics 2008; 4: 945 – 948.

[77] Song Qinghai, Xiao, Shumin, Xu, Zhengbin et al. Random Lasing in Bone Tissue. Optics Letters 2010; 35(9) 1425-1427.

[78] Malte C, Gather M, Seok Hyun Yun. Single-Cell Biological Lasers. Nature Photonics 2011; 5: 406–410.

[79] Jopling C, Boue S, Belmonte J. Dedifferentiation, Transdifferentiation and Reprogramming: Three Routes to Regeneration. Nature Reviews Molecular Cell Biology 2011; 12: 79-89.

[80] Kawata S, Sugiura T. Movement of Micrometer-Sized Particles in the Evanescent Field of a Laser Beam". Optics letters 1992; 17 (11): 772.

[81] Mohanty S, Andrews J, Gupta P. Optical Binding Between Dielectric Particles. Optics Express 2004; 12(12) 2746-2753.

[82] Zhao J, Punj V, Matta H, Mazzacurati L, Schamus S, et al. K13 Blocks KSHV Lytic Replication and Deregulates vIL6 and hIL6 Expression: A Model of Lytic Replication Induced Clonal Selection in Viral Oncogenesis. PLoS ONE 2007: 2(10): e1067.

[83] Ke Q, Costa M. Hypoxia-Inducible Factor-1 (HIF-1). Mol Pharmacol 2006;70:1469–80.

[84] Nelson D., Tan T, Rabson B, et al. Hypoxia and Defective Apoptosis Drive Genomic Instability and Tumorigenesis, Genes Dev. 2004; 18: 2095–2107.

[85] Harris A. Hypoxia — a key regulatory factor in tumour growth. Nature Rev. Cancer 2001; 2: 38–47.

[86] Dai T, Zheng H, Fu GS. Hypoxia Confers Protection Against Apoptosis via the PI3K/Akt Pathway in Endothelial Progenitor Cells. Acta Pharmacol Sin 2008; 29: 1425–1431.

[87] Roiniotis J, Hang Dinh, Masendycz P, et al. Hypoxia Prolongs Monocyte/Macrophage Survival and Enhanced Glycolysis Is Associated with Their Maturation under Aerobic Conditions. The Journal of Immunology 2009; 182(12) 7974-7981.

[88] Quail D, Taylor M, Walsh L, et al. Low Oxygen Levels Induce the Expression of the Embryonic Morphogen Nodal. Mol Biol Cell 2011;22(24):4809-21.

[89] Silván U, Díez-Torre A, Arluzea J, Andrade R, Silió M, Aréchaga J. Hypoxia and Pluripotency in Embryonic and Embryonal Carcinoma Stem Cell Biology. Differentiation 2009;78:159–168.

[90] Amberger-Murphy V. Hypoxia Helps Glioma to Fight Therapy. Curr. Cancer Drug Targets 2009; 9:381–390.

[91] Chan Gao, Weipeng Cao, Lan Bao, et al. Autophagy Negatively Regulates Wnt Signalling by Promoting Dishevelled Degradation. Nature Cell Biology 2010; 12, 781.

[92] Kanamori H, Takemura G, Maruyama R, et al. Functional Significance and Morphological Characterization of Starvation-Induced Autophagy in the Adult Heart. Am J Pathol. 2009; 174(5):1705-14.

[93] Degenhardt K, Mathew R, Beaudoin B, et al. Autophagy Promotes Tumor Cell Survival and Restricts Necrosis, Inflammation, and Tumorigenesis. Cancer Cell 2006; 10(1) 51–64.

[94] White E. Role of Metabolic Stress Responses of Apoptosis and Autophagy in Tumor Suppression. Ernst Schering Found Symp Proc. 2007; (4): 23–34.

[95] Komatsu M, Ichimura Y. Selective Autophagy Regulates Various Cellular Functions. Genes Cells. 2010;15(9):923-33.

[96] Matecic M, Smith DL Jr, Pan X, Maqani N, et al. A Microarray-Based Genetic Screen for Yeast Chronological Aging Factors. PLoS Genet 2010; 6(4): e1000921. doi:10.1371/journal.pgen.1000921.

[97] Boya P, González-Polo R, Casares N, et al. Inhibition of Macroautophagy Triggers Apoptosis. Mol Cell Biol. 2005; 25(3): 1025-1040.

[98] Huang L, Bindra R, Glazer P, Harris A. Hypoxia-Induced Genetic Instability—a Calculated Mechanism Underlying Tumor Progression. Journal of Molecular Medicine 2007; 85(2) 139-148.

[99] Stephens P, Greenman C, Fu B, et al. Massive Genomic Rearrangement Acquired in a Single Catastrophic Event during Cancer Development. Cell, 2011; 144(1) 27-40.

[100] Kloosterman V, Tavakoli-Yaraki M, Roosmalen M. et al. Constitutional Chromothripsis Rearrangements Involve Clustered Double-Stranded DNA Breaks and Nonhomologous Repair Mechanisms. Cell Reports 2012; 1(6) 648-655.

[101] Rich J. Cancer Stem Cells in Radiation Resistance. Cancer Res 2007; 67: 8980-8984

[102] Evans A. Ductal Carcinoma in situ (DCIS): Are We Overdetecting it? Breast Cancer Research 2004; 6: 23.

[103] Stattin P, Holmberg E, Johansson J. et al. Outcomes in Localized Prostate Cancer: National Prostate Cancer Register of Sweden Follow-up Study, JNCI J. Natl. Cancer Inst. 2010; 102(13) 950-958.